OTHER TITLES OF INTEREST

⟁ **W9-BTF-319**

CODING AND REIMBURSEMENT
Codelink® CPT & ICD-9-CM Code Linkage Series
Collections Made Easy!
CPT & HCPCS Coding Made Easy!
E/M Coding Made Easy!
4-in-1 Master Coder Series
HCPCS Coders Choice®, Color Coded, Thumb Indexed
Health Insurance Carrier Directory
ICD-9-CM, Coders Choice®, Thumb Indexed
ICD-9-CM, TimeSaver®, Ring Binder, Tab Indexed
ICD-9-CM Coding For Physicians' Offices
ICD-9-CM Coding Made Easy!
Medicare Rules and Regulations
Physicians Fees
Reimbursement Manual for the Medical Office
Working with Insurance and Managed Care Plans

PRACTICE MANAGEMENT
365 Ways to Manage the Business Private Practice
Capitation: Tools, Trends, Traps & Techniques
Computerizing Your Medical Office
Designing and Building Your Professional Office
Doctor Business
Encyclopedia of Practice and Financial Management
Getting Paid for What You Do
Health Information Management
The Managed Care Handbook
Managing Medical Office Personnel
Marketing Strategies for Physicians
McGraw-Hill Pocket Guide to Managed Care
Medical Marketing Handbook
Medical Office Policy Manual
Medical Practice Forms
Medical Practice Handbook
Medical Staff Privileges
Negotiating Managed Care Contracts
Patient Satisfaction
Patients Build Your Practice
Physician's Office Laboratory
Professional and Practice Development
Promoting Your Medical Practice
Surviving a Competitive Health Care Market

AVAILABLE FROM YOUR LOCAL MEDICAL BOOK STORE OR CALL 1-800-MED-SHOP

OTHER TITLES OF INTEREST

FINANCIAL MANAGEMENT
Accounts Receivable Management for the Medical Practice
Achieving Profitability with a Medical Office System
Business Ventures for Physicians
Financial Planning Workbook for Physicians
Financial Valuation of Your Practice
Pension Plan Strategies
Physician Financial Planning in a Changing Environment
Securing Your Assets
Selling or Buying a Medical Practice

RISK MANAGEMENT
Behavioral Types and the Art of Patient Management
Belli: For Your Malpractice Defense
Law, Liability and Ethics for Medical Office Personnel
Malpractice Depositions
Medical Malpractice: A Physician's Guide
Testifying in Court

DICTIONARIES AND OTHER REFERENCE
Health & Medicine on the Internet
Isler's Patient Guide to Medical Terminology
Medical Acronyms, Eponyms and Abbreviations
Medical Phrase Index
Medical Word Building
Medico Mnemonica
Medico-Legal Glossary
Spanish/English Handbook for Medical Professionals

MEDICAL REFERENCE AND CLINICAL
Drugs of Abuse
Gastroenterology: Problems in Primary Care
Hematology: Diagnosis and Treatment of Blood Disorders
Medical Procedures for Referral
Neurology: Problems in Primary Care
Orthopaedics: Problems in Primary Care
Patient Care Emergency Handbook
Patient Care Flowchart Manual
Patient Care Procedures for Your Practice
Pulmonary Medicine: Problems in Primary Care
Urology: Problems in Primary Care

**AVAILABLE FROM YOUR LOCAL MEDICAL
BOOK STORE OR CALL 1-800-MED-SHOP**

H·C·P·C·S

Health Care
Procedure Coding System

National Level II
Medicare Codes

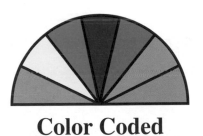

Color Coded

2006

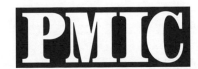

ISBN 1-57066-369-6 (Coder's Choice)
ISBN 1-57066-371-8 (Timesaver Binder)
ISBN 1-57066-392-0 (Codes on Disk)

Practice Management Information Corporation (PMIC)
4727 Wilshire Boulevard, Suite 300
Los Angeles, California 90010
1-800-MED-SHOP

http://pmiconline.com

Printed in China

Copyright© 2005 by Practice Management Information Corporation, Los Angeles, California 90010. All rights reserved. None of the content of this publication may be reproduced, stored in a retrieval system, or transmitted in any form or by any means (electronic, mechanical, photocopying, recording or otherwise) without the prior written permission of the publisher.

Additional copies of this book may be purchased from any medical book store, from PMIC by mail to the above address, by visiting our web site at http://pmiconline.com or by calling 1-800-MED-SHOP.

FOREWORD

The Health Care Procedure Coding System (HCPCS), National Level II, is a listing of codes and descriptive terminology used for reporting the provision of supplies, materials, injections and certain services and procedures to Medicare. HCPCS 2006 is the most recent revision of the HCPCS National Level II codes. The changes that appear in this revision have been prepared by our editorial staff using the HCPCS revisions released by the Center for Medicare and Medicaid Services (CMS), which is overseen by the Department of Health and Human Services (DHHS). HCPCS National Level II codes are now effective January 1st of each year.

Even though HCPCS National Level II codes have been in use since 1983, there is still some confusion among health care professionals regarding when and how to use these codes instead of the more familiar CPT codes. In addition, due to what is known as "carrier discretion," the use, interpretation, and reimbursement policies for HCPCS National Level II codes, which should be uniform nationwide, vary from carrier to carrier.

One of our goals as a publisher is to educate our customers about the business of medicine. One of our most successful methods of accomplishing this goal is to create publications about new or unfamiliar concepts, such as HCPCS, that are similar in format and content to related publications, such as CPT. This provides our customers with an opportunity to learn and implement new concepts of vital importance to their medical practice using formats, conventions and terminology that they already use and understand.

James B. Davis, President

DISCLAIMER

This publication is designed to offer basic information regarding coding and billing of medical services, supplies and procedures using the HCPCS coding system. The information presented is based upon material obtained from the Center for Medicare and Medicaid Services (CMS), and the experience and interpretations of the editors and publisher. Though all of the information has been carefully researched and checked for accuracy and completeness, the publisher accepts no responsibility or liability with regard to errors, omissions, misuse or misinterpretation.

CONTENTS

INTRODUCTION 1

    Structure of HCPCS 1

    Sections 2

    Instructions for Use of HCPCS National Level II Codes 3

    Format of the Terminology 3

    Guidelines 4

    HCPCS Modifiers 4

    Unlisted Procedure or Service 5

    Special Report 5

    HCPCS Code Changes 6

    Special Coverage Symbols 7

    Durable Medical Equipment Regional Carriers (DMERCs) 8

    Appendices 10

    HCPCS 2006 on CD-ROM 10

TRANSPORTATION SERVICES 11

MEDICAL AND SURGICAL SUPPLIES 17

ADMINISTRATIVE, MISCELLANEOUS AND
INVESTIGATIONAL 57

ENTERAL AND PARENTERAL THERAPY 63

HOSPITAL OUTPATIENT PPS CODES 69

DENTAL PROCEDURES 81

DURABLE MEDICAL EQUIPMENT 117

PROCEDURES AND PROFESSIONAL SERVICES 161

REHABILITATIVE SERVICES 181

DRUGS ADMINISTERED OTHER THAN ORAL METHOD 187

CHEMOTHERAPY DRUGS...219

K CODES: FOR DMERCS' USE ONLY 227

ORTHOTIC PROCEDURES..235

PROSTHETIC PROCEDURES...277

MEDICAL SERVICES...313

PATHOLOGY AND LABORATORY 317

TEMPORARY CODES 323

DIAGNOSTIC RADIOLOGY SERVICES..339

PRIVATE PAYER CODES...341

STATE MEDICAID AGENCY CODES...379

VISION SERVICES...387

HEARING SERVICES 397

APPENDIX A: MODIFIERS...403

APPENDIX B: SUMMARY OF CHANGES 421

APPENDIX C: TABLE OF DRUGS..485

APPENDIX D: MEDICARE REFERENCES 547

INDEX..701

INTRODUCTION

HCPCS is an acronym for Health Care Procedure Coding System. This coding system was developed in 1983 by the Health Care Financing Administration (HCFA) for the purpose of standardizing the coding systems used to process Medicare claims. In 2001, HCFA changed its name to the Center for Medicare and Medicaid Services (CMS) to reflect its increased emphasis on improving Medicare and Medicaid beneficiary services and information.

The HCPCS coding system is primarily used to bill Medicare for supplies, materials and injections. It is also used to bill for certain services and procedures which are not defined in CPT. HCPCS codes must be used when billing Medicare carriers, and in some states, Medicaid carriers. Some private insurance carriers also allow or mandate the use of HCPCS codes, mostly those that are processing Medicare claims.

STRUCTURE OF HCPCS

HCPCS is a systematic method for coding supplies, materials, injections and services performed by health care professionals. Each supply, material, injection or service is identified with a five digit alphanumeric code. With the HCPCS coding system, the supplies, materials and injections can be accurately identified and properly reimbursed. There are three levels of codes within the HCPCS coding system.

LEVEL I CPT CODES

The major portion of the HCPCS coding system, referred to as Level I, is CPT. Most of the procedures and services you perform, even for Medicare patients, are billed using CPT codes. However, one of the major deficiencies of CPT is that it has limited code selections to describe supplies, materials and injections.

LEVEL II NATIONAL CODES

HCPCS National Level II codes are alphanumeric codes which start with a letter followed by four numbers. The range of HCPCS National Level II codes is from A0000 through V0000. There are also HCPCS National Level II modifiers. HCPCS National Level II codes are uniform in description throughout the United States. However, due to what is known as "carrier discretion" the processing and reimbursement of HCPCS National Level II codes is not necessarily uniform.

There are over 2,400 HCPCS National Level II codes covering supplies, materials, injections and services. A fundamental understanding of when and how to use HCPCS National Level II or Local Level III codes can have a significant impact on your Medicare reimbursement. The majority of health care professionals use codes from the Medical and Surgical Supplies section and Drugs Administered by Other Than Oral Method, commonly referred to as "A" codes and "J" codes.

HCPCS CODE OVERLAP

As may be expected, there is some overlap among the three HCPCS code levels. On occasion you may have a coding situation where a specific code exists at all three levels for the same service or material. When faced with this situation, the general rule is that Local Level II codes have the highest priority, followed by CPT codes. You should consult your local Medicare carrier if you have any questions regarding HCPCS code overlap.

SECTIONS

The main body of HCPCS National Level II codes is divided into 22 sections. The supplies, materials, injections and services are presented in alphanumeric order within each section. The sections of HCPCS National Level II are:

Transportation Services	A0000-A0999
Medical And Surgical Supplies	A4000-A7509
Miscellaneous And Experimental	A9000-A9999
Enteral And Parenteral Therapy	B0000-B9999
Temporary Hospital Outpatient PPS	C0000-C9999
Dental Procedures	D0000-D9999
Durable Medical Equipment (DME)	E0000-E9999
Temporary Procedures & Professional Services	G0000-G9999
Rehabilitative Services	H0000-H9999
Drugs Administered Other Than Oral Method	J0000-J8999
Chemotherapy Drugs	J9000-J9999
Temporary Codes For DMERCS	K0000-K9999
Orthotic Procedures	L0000-L4999
Prosthetic Procedures	L5000-L9999
Medical Services	M0000-M9999
Pathology And Laboratory	P0000-P9999
Temporary Codes	Q0000-Q9999
Diagnostic Radiology Services	R0000-R9999

Private Payer Codes	S0000-S9999
State Medicaid Agency Codes	T0000-T9999
Vision Services	V0000-V2999
Hearing Services	V5000-V5999

INSTRUCTIONS FOR USE OF HCPCS NATIONAL LEVEL II CODES

A health care professional using the HCPCS National Level II codes selects the name of the material, supply, injection, service or procedure that most accurately identifies the service performed or supply delivered. Most often, HCPCS National Level II codes will be used instead of, or in addition to, CPT codes for visits, evaluation and management services, or other procedures performed at the same time or during the same visit. All services, procedures, supplies, materials and injections should be properly documented in the medical record.

The listing of a supply, material, injection or service and its code number in a specific section of HCPCS does not usually restrict its use to a specific profession or specialty group. However, there are some HCPCS National Level II codes that are by definition, profession or specialty specific.

FORMAT OF THE TERMINOLOGY

HCPCS National Level II terminology has been developed as stand-alone descriptions of supplies, materials, injections, services and procedures. However, some of the procedures in HCPCS National Level II are not printed in their entirety but refer back to a common portion of the procedure listed in a preceding entry. This is evident when an entry is followed by one or more indentations. For example:

L1610 Hip orthosis (HO), abduction control of hip joints; flexible, (Frejka cover only), prefabricated, includes fitting and adjustment

L1640 static, pelvic band or spreader bar, thigh cuffs, custom fabricated

Note that the common part of code L1610 (the part before the semicolon) should be considered part of code L1640. Therefore the full procedure description represented by code L1640 would read:

L1640   Hip orthosis (HO), abduction control of hip joints; static, pelvic band or spreader bar, thight cuffs, custom fabricated

GUIDELINES

Specific GUIDELINES are presented at the beginning of most of the sections. These GUIDELINES define items that are necessary to appropriately interpret and report the supplies, materials, injections, services and procedures listed in that section.

HCPCS MODIFIERS

A modifier provides the means by which the health care professional can indicate that a service or procedure that has been performed has been altered by some specific circumstance but not changed in its definition or code. HCPCS modifiers may be used to indicate the following:

- A service was supervised by an anesthesiologist

- A service was performed by a specific health care professional, for example, a clinical psychologist, clinical social worker, nurse practitioner, or physician assistant.

- A service was provided as part of a specific government program

- A service was provided to a specific side of the body

- Equipment was purchased or rented

- Single or multiple patients were seen during nursing home visits

It is important to note that HCPCS National Level II modifiers can be combined with CPT codes when reporting services to Medicare.

An example of the use of HCPCS National Level II modifiers is:

E1280-NR   Heavy duty wheelchair; detachable arms (desk or full length) elevating leg rests - new when rented

A listing of modifiers pertinent to each section of HCPCS National Level II are located in the GUIDELINES of each section. A complete listing of HCPCS National Level II modifiers is found in APPENDIX A.

UNLISTED PROCEDURE OR SERVICE

A service or procedure may be provided that is not listed in this edition of HCPCS National Level II. When reporting such a service, the appropriate "unlisted procedure" code may be used to indicate the service, identifying it by "special report" as defined below. HCPCS National Level II terminology is inconsistent in defining unlisted procedures. The procedure definition may include the term(s) "unlisted," "not otherwise classified," "unspecified," "unclassified," "other" and "miscellaneous." Prior to using these codes, try to determine if a Local Level III or CPT code is available. When an unlisted procedure code is used, the supply, material, injection, service or procedure must be described. Each of these unlisted procedure codes relates to a specific section of HCPCS National Level II and is presented in the GUIDELINES of that section.

SPECIAL REPORT

A supply, material, injection, service or procedure that is rarely provided, unusual, variable or new may require a special report for reimbursement purposes. Pertinent information should include an adequate definition or description of the nature, extent, and need for the supply, material, injection, service or procedure.

HCPCS CODE CHANGES

Each year numerous codes are added, changed or deleted. A summary of revisions to HCPCS 2006 is found in APPENDIX B. The following symbols, identical to those used in CPT, are used to indicate additions, changes and deletions in HCPCS National Level II.

ADDITIONS TO HCPCS

New HCPCS National Level II codes are identified with a small black circle placed to the left of the code number. An example of a new code in HCPCS 2006 is:

● **G0375**   Smoking and tobacco use cessation counseling visit; intermediate, greater than 3 minutes up to 10 minutes

CHANGES TO HCPCS

Changes in HCPCS National Level II code definitions are identified with a small black triangle placed to the left of the code number. An example of a changed code in HCPCS 2006 is:

▲ **A9530**   Iodine I-131 sodium iodide solution, therapeutic, per millicurie

DELETIONS FROM HCPCS

Deleted HCPCS National Level II codes are enclosed within parentheses, along with an italicized reference to replacement codes when available. An example of a code deleted from HCPCS 2006 is:

(C9400) Code deleted December 31, 2005; use A9505

SPECIAL COVERAGE SYMBOLS

NOT VALID FOR MEDICARE

There are codes listed in HCPCS which are not valid for Medicare. These codes are identified by a red bar over the HCPCS code. These codes should not be used to report services to Medicare.

NON-COVERED BY MEDICARE

There are numerous supplies, materials, injections, services and procedures which are not covered by Medicare, either by program definition or by legislative statute. Examples of non-covered services include routine services and appliances, foot care and supportive devices for feet, custodial care, personal comfort items, and cosmetic surgery. These codes are identified by an orange bar over the HCPCS code. These codes should not be used to report services to Medicare; however, in most cases, you may bill the patient directly for non-covered services.

SPECIAL COVERAGE INSTRUCTIONS

Your local Medicare carrier has specific coverage instructions for processing certain HCPCS codes. These codes are identified by a yellow bar over the HCPCS code. While these codes are covered by the Medicare program, the use of these codes does not guarantee payment. If you have a question about a specific code in this category, review your Medicare provider manual or consult with your local Medicare carrier.

CARRIER DISCRETION

Processing and payment for these codes is done at the discretion of each insurance carrier. These codes are identified by a blue bar over the HCPCS code. For codes in this category, you should check with your Medicare carrier for proper billing instructions prior to filing an insurance claim.

DURABLE MEDICAL EQUIPMENT REGIONAL CARRIERS (DMERCs)

All Medicare claims for durable medical equipment (DME), prosthetics, orthotics and supplies go to one of four durable medical equipment regional carriers, or DMERCs.

MEDICARE SUPPLIER NUMBER

Before submitting claims to DMERCs, you must apply for a supplier number. You must use this number when submitting claims to all four carriers. To find out more information, go to the Medicare website at http://www.cms.gov.

REGIONALIZATION OF CLAIM PROCESSING

In accordance with Section 1834(a) of Title XVIII of the Social Security Act, the Center for Medicare and Medicaid Services has contracted with four carriers to process Part B Medicare claims for durable medical equipment, prosthetics, orthotics, and supplies. Listed below are the contracted carriers and the states that they serve. The residence of the beneficiary is what determines which regional carrier processes the claim.

Region A: CT, DE, MA, ME, NH, NJ, NY, PA, RI, VT

HealthNow New York Inc.
DMERC A
P.O. Box 6800
Wilkes-Barre, PA 18773-6800
(866) 419-9458
http://www.umd.nycpic.com/dmerc.html

Region B: DC, IL, IN, MD, MI, MN, OH, VA, WI, WV

Adminastar Federal, Inc.
DMERC B
8115 Knue Road, PO Box 240
Indianapolis, IN 46250
(866) 270-4909
http://www.adminastar.com

Region C: AL, AR, CO, FL, GA, KY, LA, MS, NC, NM, OK, PR, SC, TN, TX, VI

Palmetto Government Benefits Administrators (GBA)
DMERC C
P.O. Box 100141
Columbia, SC 29202-3141
(866) 270-4909

Region D: AK, AZ, CA, GU, HI, IA, ID, KS, MO, MT, ND, NE, NV, OR, SD, UT, WA, WY

CIGNA Medicare
DMERC D
P.O. Box 690
Nashville, TN 37202
(866) 243-7272
http://cignamedicare.com

CHANGE OF CLAIM JURISDICTION

Prior to October 1, 1993, Medicare carriers processed durable medical equipment (DME), prosthetics, and orthotics claims based on where the transaction for the sale or rental took place. This is called the point of sale. Beginning October 1, 1993 and according to the state by state transfer schedule, regional processing of supplier claims began using beneficiary residence to determine which regional carrier had claim jurisdiction.

ELECTRONIC CLAIM FILING

The Center for Medicare and Medicaid Services is strongly encouraging electronic claims submission to DMERCs. Suppliers submitting claims electronic must use the designated National Standard Format which meets all Medicare billing requirements and is accepted by other third-party insurance carriers. The regional carriers will assist you in converting to electronic claims submission. You can contact the Electronic Media Coordinator (EMC) at the DMERCs listed above.

APPENDICES

APPENDIX A: Modifiers: Lists all National Level II modifiers, ambulance service, and PET scan modifiers.

APPENDIX B: Summary of Changes: Includes a summary of official additions, changes, and deletions to the current edition of HCPCS.

APPENDIX C: Table of Drugs: Includes drug names, cross references along with selected dosage, administration route, and HCPCS codes from the official HCPCS Table of Drugs.

APPENDIX D: Medicare References: Includes the complete text from all Medicare Coverage Instruction Manual (CIM) and Medicare Carriers Manual (MCM) citations in the body of the HCPCS book.

HCPCS 2006 ON CD-ROM

HCPCS codes are available on CD-ROM. The HCPCS short description datafile includes all official HCPCS codes with descriptions of 35 characters or fewer. The datafile can be uploaded to your PC for inclusion in billing programs. For more information regarding HCPCS codes on CD-ROM, call PMIC at 1-800-MED-SHOP or visit http://pmiconline.com.

TRANSPORTATION SERVICES

Guidelines

In addition to the information presented in the INTRODUCTION, several other items unique to this section are defined or identified here:

1. VEHICLE AND CREW REQUIREMENTS: The ambulance must be designed and equipped for transporting the sick or injured and include patient care equipment, such as a stretcher, clean linens, first aid supplies, oxygen equipment and other safety and lifesaving equipment required by state or local authorities. The ambulance crew must have two members, one of which has medical training equivalent to the standard and advanced Red Cross training. The vehicle and personnel supplier must provide a statement that describes the first-aid, safety and other patient-care items in the vehicle, the extent of first-aid training of the personnel and the supplier's agreement to notify Medicare of any changes that could affect coverage.

2. AIR AMBULANCE SERVICE: Air ambulance services are covered when the point of pick-up is inaccessible by land vehicle; distances or other obstacles are involved in getting the patient to the nearest hospital with appropriate facilities; and, all other conditions of coverage are met.

3. AMBULANCE SERVICE CLAIMS: Reimbursement may be made for expenses incurred for ambulance services when specific conditions have been met and the appropriate medical documentation is provided.

4. MATERIALS SUPPLIED BY AMBULANCE SERVICE: Reusable devices, such as back boards, neck boards and inflatable leg and arm splints, are considered part of general ambulance services and included in the charge for the trip. A separate reasonable charge may be recognized for non-reusable items and disposable supplies, such as oxygen, gauze and dressings, that are required for patient care during the trip.

5. UNLISTED SERVICE OR PROCEDURE: A service or procedure may be provided that is not listed in this edition of HCPCS. When reporting such a service, the appropriate "unlisted procedure" code may be used to indicate the service, identifying it by "special report" as defined below. HCPCS terminology is inconsistent in defining

unlisted procedures. The procedure definition may include the term(s) "unlisted", "not otherwise classified", "unspecified", "unclassified", "other" and "miscellaneous". Prior to using these codes, try to determine if a Local Level III code or CPT code is available. The "unlisted procedures" and accompanying codes for TRANSPORTATION SERVICES are as follows:

A0999 Unlisted ambulance service

6. SPECIAL REPORT: A service, material or supply that is rarely provided, unusual, variable or new may require a special report in determining medical appropriateness for reimbursement purposes. Pertinent information should include an adequate definition or description of the nature, extent, and need for the service, material or supply.

7. MODIFIERS: Listed services may be modified under certain circumstances. When appropriate, the modifying circumstance is identified by adding a modifier to the basic procedure code. CPT and HCPCS National Level II modifiers may be used with CPT and HCPCS National Level II procedure codes. One digit codes are to be used in combination. The first digit should indicate the origin; the second digit should indicate the destination.

The Level II modifiers commonly used with TRANSPORTATION codes are as follows:

-GM   Multiple patients on one ambulance trip

-QM   Ambulance service provided under arrangement by a provider of services

-QN   Ambulance services furnished directly by a provider of services

AMBULANCE SERVICE MODIFIERS

For ambulance service, one-digit modifiers are combined to form a two-digit modifier that identifies the ambulance's place of origin with the first digit, and ambulance's destination with the second digit. They are used in items 12 and 13 on the CMS Form 1491.

One digit ambulance modifiers:

-D   Diagnostic or therapeutic site other than -P or -H when these are used as origin codes

-E   Residential, domiciliary, custodial facility (other than an 1819 facility)

-G   Hospital-based dialysis facility (hospital or hospital related)

-H   Hospital

-I   Site of transfer (for example, airport or helicopter pad) between types of ambulance

-J   Non-hospital-based dialysis facility

-N   Skilled nursing facility (SNF) (1819 facility)

-P   Physician's office (includes HMO non-hospital facility, clinic, etc.)

-R   Residence

-S   Scene of accident or acute event

-X   (Destination code only) Intermediate stop at physician's office on the way to the hospital (includes HMO non-hospital facility, clinic, etc.)

8. CPT CODE CROSS-REFERENCE: Unless specified otherwise, there is no equivalent CPT code for listings in this section.

Transportation Services Including Ambulance

A0021 Ambulance service; outside state per mile, transport (Medicaid only)

Ambulance Waiting Time Table

Units	Time (Hrs)	Units	Time (Hrs)
1	1/2 to 1	6	3 to 3 1/2
2	1 to 1 1/2	7	3 1/2 to 4
3	1 1/2 to 2	8	4 to 4 1/2
4	2 to 2 1/2	9	4 1/2 to 5
5	2 to 3	10	5 to 5 1/2

A0080 Non-emergency transportation, per mile—vehicle provided by volunteer (individual or organization), with no vested interest

A0090 Non-emergency transportation, per mile—vehicle provided by individual (family member, self, neighbor) with vested interest

A0100 Non-emergency transportation; taxi

A0110 Non-emergency transportation and bus, intra or inter state carrier

A0120 Non-emergency transportation: mini-bus, mountain area transports, or other transportation systems

A0130 Non-emergency transportation: wheel-chair van

A0140 Non-emergency transportation and air travel (private or commercial) intra or inter state

A0160 Non-emergency transportation: per mile—case worker or social worker

A0170 Transportation ancillary: parking fees, tolls, other

A0180 Non-emergency transportation; ancillary: lodging-recipient

A0190 ancillary: meals-recipient

● New code ▲ Revised code ( ) Deleted code

A0200   ancillary: lodging-escort

A0210   ancillary: meals-escort

A0225   Ambulance service; neonatal transport, base rate, emergency transport, one way

A0380   BLS mileage (per mile); Medicare use A0425

A0382   BLS routine disposable supplies

A0384   BLS specialized service disposable supplies, defibrillation (used by ALS ambulances and BLS ambulances in jurisdictions where defibrillation is permitted in BLS ambulances)

A0390   ALS mileage (per mile); Medicare use A0425

A0392   ALS specialized service disposable supplies; defibrillation (to be used only in jurisdictions where defibrillation cannot be performed in BLS ambulances)

A0394   ALS specialized service disposable supplies; IV drug therapy

A0396   ALS specialized service disposable supplies; esophageal intubation

A0398   ALS routine disposable supplies

A0420   Ambulance waiting time (ALS or BLS), one-half (1/2) hour increments

A0422   Ambulance (ALS or BLS) oxygen and oxygen supplies, life sustaining situation

A0424   Extra ambulance attendant, ground (ALS or BLS) or air (fixed or rotary winged); (requires medical review)

A0425   Ground mileage, per statue mile

A0426   Ambulance service, advanced life support, non-emergency transport, level 1 (ALS1)

A0427   Ambulance service, advanced life support, emergency transport, level 1 (ALS1-emergency)

Not valid
for Medicare   Non-covered
by Medicare   Special
coverage
instructions   Carrier
discretion   **15**

A0428   Ambulance service, basic life support, non-emergency transport (BLS)

A0429   Ambulance service, basic life support, emergency transport (BLS-emergency)

A0430   Ambulance service, conventional air services, transport, one way (fixed wing)

A0431   Ambulance service, conventional air services, transport, one way (rotary wing)

A0432   Paramedic intercept (PI), rural area, transport furnished by a volunteer ambulance company which is prohibited by state law from billing third party payers

A0433   Advanced life support, level 2 (ALS2)

A0434   Specialty care transport (SCT)

A0435   Fixed wing air mileage, per statute mile

A0436   Rotary wing air mileage, per statute mile

A0800   Ambulance transport provided between the hours of 7 p.m. and 7 a.m.

A0888   Noncovered ambulance mileage, per mile (e.g., for miles traveled beyond closest appropriate facility)
MCM: 2125

● **A0998**   Ambulance response and treatment, no transport

A0999   Unlisted ambulance service
MCM: 2120.1, 2125

MEDICAL AND SURGICAL SUPPLIES

Guidelines

In addition to the information presented in the INTRODUCTION, several other items unique to this section are defined or identified here:

1. SUBSECTION INFORMATION: Some of the listed subheadings or subsections have special needs or instructions unique to that section. Where these are indicated, special "notes" will be presented preceding or following the listings. Those subsections within the MEDICAL AND SURGICAL SUPPLIES section that have "notes" are as follows:

Subsection	Code Numbers
External urinary supplies	A4356-A4359
Tracheostomy supplies	A4622-A4626
Supplies for ESRD	A4650-A4927

2. UNLISTED SERVICE OR PROCEDURE: A service or procedure may be provided that is not listed in this edition of HCPCS. When reporting such a service, the appropriate "unlisted procedure" code may be used to indicate the service, identifying it by "special report" as defined below. HCPCS terminology is inconsistent in defining unlisted procedures. The procedure definition may include the term(s) "unlisted", "not otherwise classified", "unspecified", "unclassified", "other" and "miscellaneous". Prior to using these codes, try to determine if a Local Level III code or CPT code is available. The "unlisted procedures" and accompanying codes for MEDICAL AND SURGICAL SUPPLIES are as follows:

A4335	Incontinence supply; miscellaneous
A4421	Ostomy supply; miscellaneous
A4649	Surgical supply; miscellaneous
A4913	Miscellaneous dialysis supplies, not otherwise specified
A6261	Wound filler, gel/paste, per fluid ounce, not elsewhere classified
A6262	Wound filler, dry foam, per gram, not elsewhere classified

3. SPECIAL REPORT: A service, material or supply that is rarely provided, unusual, variable or new may require a special report in determining medical appropriateness for reimbursement purposes.

Not valid for Medicare   Non-covered by Medicare   Special coverage instructions   Carrier discretion   **17**

Pertinent information should include an adequate definition or description of the nature, extent, and need for the service, material or supply.

4. MODIFIERS: Listed services may be modified under certain circumstances. When appropriate, the modifying circumstance is identified by adding a modifier to the basic procedure code. CPT and HCPCS National Level II modifiers may be used with CPT and HCPCS National Level II procedure codes. Modifiers commonly used with MEDICAL AND SURGICAL SUPPLIES are as follows:

-CC Procedure code change (use "CC" when the procedure code submitted was changed either for administrative reasons or because an incorrect code was filed)

-LT Left side (used to identify procedures performed on the left side of the body)

-RT Right side (used to identify procedures performed on the right side of the body)

5. CPT CODE CROSS-REFERENCE: Unless specified otherwise, the equivalent CPT code for all listings in this section is 99070.

6. DURABLE MEDICAL EQUIPMENT REGIONAL CARRIERS (DMERCS): Effective October 1, 1993 claims for supplies must be billed to one of four regional carriers depending upon the residence of the beneficiary. The transition dates for DMERC claims is from November 1, 1993 to March 1, 1994, also depending upon the state you practice in. See the Introduction for a complete discussion of DMERCs.

Medical and Surgical Supplies

A4206 Syringe with needle; sterile 1cc, each

A4207 sterile 2cc, each

A4208 sterile 3cc, each

A4209 sterile 5cc or greater, each

A4210 Needle-free injection device, each
CIM: 60-9

A4211 Supplies for self-administered injections
MCM: 2049

● New code   ▲   Revised code   ( )   Deleted code

A4212   Non-coring needle or stylet with or without catheter

A4213   Syringe, sterile, 20cc or greater, each

▲A4215   Needle, sterile, any size, each

▲A4216   Sterile water, saline and/or dextrose (diluent), 10 ml
MCM: 2049

A4217   Sterile water/saline, 500 ml
MCM: 2049

● A4218   Sterile saline or water, metercd dose dispenser, 10 ml

A4220   Refill kit for implantable infusion pump
CIM: 60-14

A4221   Supplies for maintenance of drug infusion catheter, per week (list drug separately)

A4222   Infusion supplies for external drug infusion pump, per cassette or bag (list drugs separately)

A4223   Infusion supplies not used with external infusion pump, per cassette or bag (list drugs separately)

A4230   Infusion set for external insulin pump, non needle cannula type
CIM: 60-14

A4231   Infusion set for external insulin pump, needle type
CIM: 60-14

A4232   Syringe with needle for external insulin pump, sterile, 3cc
CIM: 60-14

● A4233   Replacement battery, alkaline (other than j cell), for use with medically necessary home blood glucose monitor owned by patient, each

● A4234   Replacement battery, alkaline, j cell, for use with medically necessary home blood glucose monitor owned by patient, each

● A4235   Replacement battery, lithium, for use with medically necessary home blood glucose monitor owned by patient, each

---

Not valid   Non-covered   Special   Carrier   **19**
for Medicare   by Medicare   coverage   discretion
                                    instructions

● A4236   Replacement battery, silver oxide, for use with medically necessary home blood glucose monitor owned by patient, each

A4244   Alcohol or peroxide, per pint

A4245   Alcohol wipes, per box

A4246   Betadine or phisohex solution, per pint

A4247   Betadine or iodine swabs/wipes, per box

A4248   Chlorhexidine containing antiseptic, 1 ml

A4250   Urine test or reagent strips or tablets (100 tablets or strips)
MCM: 2100

A4253   Blood glucose test or reagent strips for home blood glucose monitor, per 50 strips
CIM: 60-11

(A4254   Code deleted December 31, 2005)

A4255   Platforms for home blood glucose monitor, 50 per box
CIM: 60-11

A4256   Normal, low and high calibrator solution/chips
CIM: 60-11

A4257   Replacement lens shield cartridge for use with laser skin piercing device, each

A4258   Spring-powered device for lancet, each
CIM: 60-11

A4259   Lancets, per box of 100
CIM: 60-11

(A4260   Code deleted December 31, 2005; use J7306)

A4261   Cervical cap for contraceptive use

A4262   Temporary, absorbable lacrimal duct implant, each

A4263   Permanent, long term, non-dissolvable lacrimal duct implant, each
MCM: 15030

A4265 Paraffin, per pound
CIM: 60-9

A4266 Diaphragm for contraceptive use

A4267 Contraceptive supply, condom, male, each

A4268 Contraceptive supply, condom, female, each

A4269 Contraceptive supply, spermicide (e.g., Foam, gel), each

A4270 Disposable endoscope sheath, each

A4280 Adhesive skin support attachment for use with external breast prosthesis, each

A4281 Tubing for breast pump, replacement

A4282 Adapter for breast pump, replacement

A4283 Cap for breast pump bottle, replacement

A4284 Breast shield and splash protector for use with breast pump, replacement

A4285 Polycarbonate bottle for use with breast pump, replacement

A4286 Locking ring for breast pump, replacement

A4290 Sacral nerve stimulation test lead, each

VASCULAR CATHETERS

A4300 Implantable access catheter, (eg, venous, arterial, epidural subarachnoid, or peritoneal, etc) External access
MCM: 2130

A4301 Implantable access total catheter, port/reservoir (eg, venous, arterial, epidural, subarachnoid, peritoneal, etc.)

INCONTINENCE APPLIANCES AND CARE SUPPLIES

A4305 Disposable drug delivery system, flow rate of 50 ml or greater per hour

---

| | Not valid for Medicare | | Non-covered by Medicare | | Special coverage instructions | | Carrier discretion | **21** |

A4306   Disposable drug delivery system, flow rate of 5 ml or less per hour

A4310   Insertion tray without drainage bag; and without catheter (accessories only)
MCM: 2130

A4311   Insertion tray without drainage bag; with indwelling catheter, foley type, two-way latex with coating (teflon, silicone, silicone elastomer or hydrophilic, etc.)
MCM: 2130

A4312   with indwelling catheter, foley type, two-way, all silicone
MCM: 2130

A4313   with indwelling catheter, foley type, three-way, for continuous irrigation
MCM: 2130

A4314   Insertion tray with drainage bag; with indwelling catheter, foley type, two-way latex with coating (teflon, silicone, silicone elastomer or hydrophilic, etc.)
MCM: 2130

A4315   with indwelling catheter, foley type, two-way, all silicone
MCM: 2130

A4316   with indwelling catheter, foley type, three-way, for continuous irrigation
MCM: 2130

A4320   Irrigation tray with bulb or piston syringe, any purpose
MCM: 2130

A4321   Therapeutic agent for urinary catheter irrigation
MCM: 2130

A4322   Irrigation syringe, bulb or piston, each
MCM: 2130

(A4324)   Code deleted December 31, 2004; use A4349

(A4325)   Code deleted December 31, 2004; use A4349

A4326   Male external catheter specialty type with integral collection chamber, each
MCM: 2130

   ●   New code   ▲   Revised code   ( )   Deleted code

A4327　Female external urinary collection device; meatal cup, each
MCM: 2130

A4328　　　pouch, each
MCM: 2130

A4330　Perianal fecal collection pouch with adhesive, each
MCM: 2130

A4331　Extension drainage tubing, any type, any length, with connector/adaptor, for use with urinary leg bag or urostomy pouch, each
MCM: 2130

A4332　Lubricant, individual sterile packet, each
MCM: 2130

URINARY CATHETERS

A4333　Urinary catheter anchoring device, adhesive skin attachment, each
MCM: 2130

A4334　Urinary catheter anchoring device, leg strap, each
MCM: 2130

A4335　Incontinence supply; miscellaneous
MCM: 2130

A4338　Indwelling catheter; foley type, two-way latex with coating (teflon, silicone, silicone elastomer, or hydrophilic, etc.), each
MCM: 2130

A4340　Indwelling catheter; specialty type, (e.g.; coude, mushroom, wing, etc.), each
MCM: 2130

A4344　Indwelling catheter, foley type; two-way all silicone, each
MCM: 2130

A4346　　　three-way for continuous irrigation, each
MCM: 2130

(A4347)　Code deleted December 31, 2004; use CPT

A4348　Male external catheter with integral collection compartment, extended wear, each, (e.g., 2 per month)
MCM: 2130

A4349   Male external catheter, with or without adhesive,
disposable, each
MCM: 2130

A4351   Intermittent urinary catheter; straight tip, with or without
coating (teflon, silicone, silicone elastomer, or
hydrophilic, etc), each
MCM: 2130

A4352   Intermittent urinary catheter; coude (curved) tip, with or
without coating (teflon, silicone, silicone elastomer, or
hydrophilic, etc), each
MCM: 2130

A4353   Intermittent urinary catheter, with insertion supplies
MCM: 2130

A4354   Insertion tray with drainage bag, but without catheter
MCM: 2130

A4355   Irrigation tubing set for continuous bladder irrigation
through a three-way indwelling foley catheter, each
MCM: 2130

EXTERNAL URINARY SUPPLIES

A4356   External urethral clamp or compression device (not to be
used for catheter clamp), each
MCM: 2130

A4357   Bedside drainage bag, day or night with or without
anti-reflux device, with or without tube, each
MCM: 2130

A4358   Urinary drainage bag, leg or abdomen, vinyl, with or
without tube, with straps, each
MCM: 2130

A4359   Urinary suspensory without leg bag, each
MCM: 2130

NOTE: See DME section for male or female urinals

OSTOMY SUPPLIES

A4361   Ostomy faceplate, each
MCM: 2130

A4362   Skin barrier; solid, 4 x 4 or equivalent; each
MCM: 2130

● **A4363** Ostomy clamp, any type, replacement only, each

A4364 Adhesive, liquid or equal, any type, per ounce
MCM: 2130

A4365 Adhesive remover wipes, any type, per 50
MCM: 2130

A4366 Ostomy vent, any type, each

A4367 Ostomy belt, each
MCM: 2130.A

A4368 Ostomy filter, any type, each

A4369 Ostomy skin barrier, liquid (spray, brush, etc.), per oz.
MCM: 2130

A4371 Ostomy skin barrier, powder, per oz.
MCM: 2130

▲ **A4372** Ostomy skin barrier, solid 4x4 or equivalent, standard wear, with built-in convexity, each
MCM: 2130

A4373 Ostomy skin barrier, with flange (solid, flexible or accordion), with built-in convexity, any size, each
MCM: 2130

A4375 Ostomy pouch, drainable, with faceplate attached, plastic, each
MCM: 2130

A4376 Ostomy pouch, drainable, with faceplate attached, rubber each
MCM: 2130

A4377 Ostomy pouch, drainable, for use on faceplate, plastic, each
MCM: 2130

A4378 Ostomy pouch, drainable, for use on faceplate, rubber, each
MCM: 2130

A4379 Ostomy pouch, urinary, with faceplate attached, plastic, each
MCM: 2130

A4380   Ostomy pouch, urinary, with faceplate attached, rubber, each
MCM: 2130

A4381   Ostomy pouch, urinary, for use on faceplate, plastic, each
MCM: 2130

A4382   Ostomy pouch, urinary, for use on faceplate, heavy plastic, each
MCM: 2130

A4383   Ostomy pouch, urinary, for use on faceplate, rubber, each
MCM: 2130

A4384   Ostomy faceplate equivalent, silicone ring, each
MCM: 2130

A4385   Ostomy skin barrier, solid 4x4 or equivalent, extended wear, without built-in convexity, each
MCM: 2130

A4387   Ostomy pouch, closed, with barrier attached, with built-in convexity (1 piece), each
MCM: 2130

A4388   Ostomy pouch, drainable, with extended wear barrier attached, (1 piece), each
MCM: 2130

A4389   Ostomy pouch, drainable, with barrier attached, with built-in convexity (1 piece), each
MCM: 2130

A4390   Ostomy pouch, drainable, with extended wear barrier attached, with built-in convexity (1 piece), each
MCM: 2130

A4391   Ostomy pouch, urinary, with extended wear barrier attached, (1 piece), each
MCM: 2130

A4392   Ostomy pouch, urinary, with standard wear barrier attached, with built-in convexity (1 piece), each
MCM: 2130

A4393   Ostomy pouch, urinary, with extended wear barrier attached, with built-in convexity (1 piece), each
MCM: 2130

A4394 Ostomy deodorant for use in ostomy pouch, liquid, per fluid ounce
MCM: 2130

A4395 Ostomy deodorant for use in ostomy pouch, solid, per tablet
MCM: 2130

A4396 Ostomy belt with peristomal hernia support
MCM: 2130

A4397 Irrigation supply; sleeve, each
MCM: 2130

A4398 Ostomy irrigation supply; bag, each
MCM: 2130

A4399 cone/catheter, including brush
MCM: 2130

A4400 Ostomy irrigation set
MCM: 2130

A4402 Lubricant, per ounce
MCM: 2130

A4404 Ostomy ring, each
MCM: 2130

A4405 Ostomy skin barrier, non-pectin based, paste, per ounce
MCM: 2130

A4406 Ostomy skin barrier, pectin-based, paste, per ounce
MCM: 2130

A4407 Ostomy skin barrier, with flange (solid, flexible, or accordion), extended wear, with built-in convexity, 4 x 4 inches or smaller, each
MCM: 2130

A4408 Ostomy skin barrier, with flange (solid, flexible or accordion), extended wear, with built-in convexity, larger than 4 x 4 inches, each
MCM: 2130

A4409 Ostomy skin barrier, with flange (solid, flexible or accordion), extended wear, without built-in convexity, 4 x 4 inches or smaller, each
MCM: 2130

A4410 Ostomy skin barrier, with flange (solid, flexible or accordion), extended wear, without built-in convexity, larger than 4 x 4 inches, each
MCM: 2130

● **A4411** Ostomy skin barrier, solid 4x4 or equivalent, extended wear, with built-in convexity, each

● **A4412** Ostomy pouch, drainable, high output, for use on a barrier with flange (2 piece system), without filter, each
MCM: 2130

A4413 Ostomy pouch, drainable, high output, for use on a barrier with flange (2 piece system), with filter, each
MCM: 2130

A4414 Ostomy skin barrier, with flange (solid, flexible or accordion), without built-in convexity, 4 x 4 inches or smaller, each
MCM: 2130

A4415 Ostomy skin barrier, with flange (solid, flexible or accordion), without built-in convexity, larger than 4x4 inches, each
MCM: 2130

A4416 Ostomy pouch, closed, with barrier attached, with filter (1 piece), each

A4417 Ostomy pouch, closed, with barrier attached, with built-in convexity, with filter (1 piece), each

A4418 Ostomy pouch, closed; without barrier attached, with filter (1 piece), each

A4419 Ostomy pouch, closed; for use on barrier with non-locking flange, with filter (2 piece), each

A4420 Ostomy pouch, closed; for use on barrier with locking flange (2 piece), each

A4421 Ostomy supply; miscellaneous
MCM: 2130

A4422 Ostomy absorbent material (sheet/pad/crystal packet) for use in ostomy pouch to thicken liquid stomal output, each
MCM: 2130

● New code ▲ Revised code ( ) Deleted code

A4423 Ostomy pouch, closed; for use on barrier with locking flange, with filter (2 piece), each

A4424 Ostomy pouch, drainable, with barrier attached, with filter (1 piece), each

A4425 Ostomy pouch, drainable; for use on barrier with non-locking flange, with filter (2 piece system), each

A4426 Ostomy pouch, drainable; for use on barrier with locking flange (2 piece system), each

A4427 Ostomy pouch, drainable; for use on barrier with locking flange, with filter (2 piece system), each

A4428 Ostomy pouch, urinary, with extended wear barrier attached, with faucet-type tap with valve (1 piece), each

A4429 Ostomy pouch, urinary, with barrier attached, with built-in convexity, with faucet-type tap with valve (1 piece), each

A4430 Ostomy pouch, urinary, with extended wear barrier attached, with built-in convexity, with faucet-type tap with valve (1 piece), each

A4431 Ostomy pouch, urinary; with barrier attached, with faucet-type tap with valve (1 piece), each

A4432 Ostomy pouch, urinary; for use on barrier with non-locking flange, with faucet-type tap with valve (2 piece), each

A4433 Ostomy pouch, urinary; for use on barrier with locking flange (2 piece), each

A4434 Ostomy pouch, urinary; for use on barrier with locking flange, with faucet-type tap with valve (2 piece), each

SUPPLIES

A4450 Tape, non-waterproof, per 18 square inches
MCM: 2130

A4452 Tape, waterproof, per 18 square inches
MCM: 2130

A4455 Adhesive remover or solvent (for tape, cement or other adhesive), per ounce
MCM: 2130

A4458 Enema bag with tubing, reusable

A4462 Abdominal dressing holder, each
MCM: 2079

A4465 Non-elastic binder for extremity

A4470 Gravlee jet washer
CIM: 50-4 MCM: 2320

A4480 Vabra aspirator
CIM: 50-10 MCM: 2320

A4481 Tracheostoma filter, any type, any size, each
MCM: 2130

A4483 Moisture exchanger, disposable, for use with invasive mechanical ventilation
MCM: 2130

A4490 Surgical stockings; above knee length, each
CIM: 60-9 MCM: 2079, 2100

A4495 thigh length, each
CIM: 60-9 MCM: 2079, 2100

A4500 below knee length, each
CIM: 60-9 MCM: 2079, 2100

A4510 full length, each
CIM: 60-9 MCM: 2079, 2100

A4520 Incontinence garment, any type (e.g. brief, diaper), each
CIM: 60-9

(A4521) Code deleted December 31, 2004; use CPT

(A4522) Code deleted December 31, 2004; use CPT

(A4523) Code deleted December 31, 2004; use CPT

(A4524) Code deleted December 31, 2004; use CPT

(A4525) Code deleted December 31, 2004; use CPT

(A4526) Code deleted December 31, 2004; use CPT

(A4527) Code deleted December 31, 2004; use CPT

(A4528) Code deleted December 31, 2004; use CPT

(A4529) Code deleted December 31, 2004; use CPT

(A4530) Code deleted December 31, 2004; use CPT

(A4531) Code deleted December 31, 2004; use CPT

(A4532) Code deleted December 31, 2004; use CPT

(A4533) Code deleted December 31, 2004; use CPT

(A4534) Code deleted December 31, 2004; use CPT

(A4535) Code deleted December 31, 2004; use CPT

(A4536) Code deleted December 31, 2004; use CPT

(A4537) Code deleted December 31, 2004; use CPT

(A4538) Code deleted December 31, 2004; use CPT

A4550　Surgical trays
MCM: 15030

A4554　Disposable underpads, all sizes, (e.g., chux's)
CIM: 60-9　MCM: 2130

A4556　Electrodes, (e.g., apnea monitor), per pair

A4557　Lead wires, (e.g., apnea monitor), per pair

A4558　Conductive paste or gel

A4561　Pessary, rubber, any type

A4562　Pessary, non rubber, any type

A4565　Slings

A4570　Splint
MCM: 2079

A4575　Topical hyperbaric oxygen chamber, disposable
CIM: 35-10

Not valid for Medicare　　Non-covered by Medicare　　Special coverage instructions　　Carrier discretion

A4580   Cast supplies (e.g., plaster)
MCM: 2079

A4590   Special casting materials (e.g., fiberglass)
MCM: 2079

A4595   Electrical stimulator supplies, 2 lead, per month, (e.g. Tens, nmes)
CIM: 45-25

SUPPLIES FOR OXYGEN AND RELATED RESPIRATORY EQUIPMENT

● A4604   Tubing with integrated heating element for use with positive airway pressure device

A4605   Tracheal suction catheter, closed system, each

A4606   Oxygen probe for use with oximeter device, replacement

A4608   Transtracheal oxygen catheter, each

(A4609)   Code deleted December 31, 2004; use A4605

(A4610)   Code deleted December 31, 2004; use A4605

A4611   Battery, heavy duty; replacement for patient-owned ventilator

A4612   Battery cables; replacement for patient-owned ventilator

A4613   Battery charger; replacement for patient-owned ventilator

A4614   Peak expiratory flow rate meter, hand held

A4615   Cannula, nasal
CIM: 60-4   MCM: 3312

A4616   Tubing (oxygen), per foot
CIM: 60-4   MCM: 3312

A4617   Mouth piece
CIM: 60-4   MCM: 3312

A4618   Breathing circuits
CIM: 60-4   MCM: 3312

A4619   Face tent
CIM: 60-4   MCM: 3312

A4620 Variable concentration mask
CIM: 60-4 MCM: 3312

A4623 Tracheostomy, inner cannula
CIM: 65-16 MCM: 2130

A4624 Tracheal suction catheter, any type other than closed system, each

A4625 Tracheostomy care kit for new tracheostomy
MCM: 2130

A4626 Tracheostomy cleaning brush, each
MCM: 2130

NOTE: All of the descriptions for tracheostomy supplies, codes A4622-A4626 are "per item". The correct number of items purchased must be entered in the days or units field (box 24-G) on the CMS1500 claim form. The terms "items" and "units" are used interchangeably.

A4627 Spacer, bag or reservoir, with or without mask, for use with metered dose inhaler
MCM: 2100

A4628 Oropharyngeal suction catheter, each

A4629 Tracheostomy care kit for established tracheostomy
MCM: 2130

SUPPLIES FOR OTHER DURABLE MEDICAL EQUIPMENT

▲ **A4630** Replacement batteries, medically necessary, transcutaneous electrical stimulator, owned by patient
CIM: 65-8

A4632 Replacement battery for external infusion pump, any type, each

A4633 Replacement bulb/lamp for ultraviolet light therapy system, each

A4634 Replacement bulb for therapeutic light box, tabletop model

A4635 Underarm pad, crutch, replacement, each
CIM: 60-9

A4636   Replacement, handgrip, cane, crutch, or walker, each
CIM: 60-9

A4637   Replacement, tip, cane, crutch, walker, each
CIM: 60-9

A4638   Replacement battery for patient-owned ear pulse generator, each

A4639   Replacement pad for infrared heating pad system, each

A4640   Replacement pad for use with medically necessary alternating pressure pad owned by patient
CIM: 60-9   MCM: 4107.6

▲ A4641   Radiopharmaceutical, diagnostic, not otherwise classified
MCM: 15030

▲ A4642   Indium in-111 satumomab pendetide, diagnostic, per study dose, up to 6 millicuries
MCM: 15030

(A4643)   Code deleted December 31, 2005

(A4644)   Code deleted December 31, 2005

(A4645)   Code deleted December 31, 2005

(A4646)   Code deleted December 31, 2005

SUPPLIES FOR RADIOLOGICAL PROCEDURES

(A4647)   Code deleted December 31, 2005

A4649   Surgical supply, miscellaneous

SUPPLIES FOR ESRD

NOTE: For DME items for ESRD see procedure codes D1500-E1699. For dialysis Procedures, see M0900-M0999.

A4651   Calibrated microcapillary tube, each
MCM: 4270

● New code   ▲ Revised code   ( ) Deleted code

A4652 Microcapillary tube sealant
MCM: 4270

A4653 Peritoneal dialysis catheter anchoring device, belt, each

A4656 Needle, any size, each
MCM: 4270

A4657 Syringe, with or without needle, each
MCM: 4270

A4660 Sphygmomanometer/blood pressure apparatus with cuff and stethoscope
MCM: 4270

A4663 Blood pressure cuff only
MCM: 4270

A4670 Automatic blood pressure monitor
CIM: 50-42 MCM: 4270

A4671 Disposable cycler set used with cycler dialysis machine, each
MCM: 4270

A4672 Drainage extension line, sterile, for dialysis, each
MCM: 4270

A4673 Extension line with easy lock connectors, used with dialysis
MCM: 4270

A4674 Chemicals/antiseptics solution used to clean/sterilize dialysis equipment, per 8 oz.
MCM: 4270

A4680 Activated carbon filter for hemodialysis, each
CIM: 55-1 MCM: 4270

A4690 Dialyzer (artificial kidneys), all types, all sizes, for hemodialysis, each
MCM: 4270

A4706 Bicarbonate concentrate, solution, for hemodialysis, per gallon
MCM: 4270

A4707 Bicarbonate concentrate, powder, for hemodialysis, per packet
MCM: 4270

Not valid for Medicare Non-covered by Medicare Special coverage instructions Carrier discretion

A4708   Acetate concentrate solution, for hemodialysis, per gallon
MCM: 4270

A4709   Acid concentrate solution, for hemodialysis, per gallon
MCM: 4270

A4714   Treated water (deionized, distilled, or reverse osmosis) for peritoneal dialysis, per gallon
CIM: 55-1 MCM: 4270

A4719   Y set tubing for peritoneal dialysis
MCM: 4270

A4720   Dialysate solution, any concentration of dextrose, fluid volume greater than 249cc, but less than or equal to 999cc, for peritoneal dialysis
MCM: 4270

A4721   Dialysate solution, any concentration of dextrose, fluid volume greater than 999cc, but less than or equal to 1999cc, for peritoneal dialysis
MCM: 4270

A4722   Dialysate solution, any concentration of dextrose, fluid volume greater than 1999cc, but less than or equal to 2999cc, for peritoneal dialysis
MCM: 4270

A4723   Dialysate solution, any concentration of dextrose, fluid volume greater than 2999cc, but less than or equal to 3999cc, for peritoneal dialysis
MCM: 4270

A4724   Dialysate solution, any concentration of dextrose, fluid volume greater than 3999cc, but less than or equal to 4999cc, for peritoneal dialysis
MCM: 4270

A4725   Dialysate solution, any concentration of dextrose, fluid volume greater than 4999cc, but less than or equal to 5999cc, for peritoneal dialysis
MCM: 4270

A4726   Dialysate solution, any concentration of dextrose, fluid volume greater than 5999cc, for peritoneal dialysis
MCM: 4270

A4728   Dialysate solution, non-dextrose containing, 500 ml

A4730   Fistula cannulation set for hemodialysis, each
MCM: 4270

● New code   ▲ Revised code   ( ) Deleted code

A4736   Topical anesthetic, for dialysis, per gram
MCM: 4270

A4737   Injectable anesthetic, for dialysis, per 10 ml
MCM: 4270

A4740   Shunt accessory, for hemodialysis, any type, each
MCM: 4270

A4750   Blood tubing, arterial or venous, for hemodialysis, each
MCM: 4270

A4755   Blood tubing, arterial and venous combined, for hemodialysis, each
MCM: 4270

A4760   Dialysate solution test kit, for peritoneal dialysis, any type, each
MCM: 4270

A4765   Dialysate concentrate, powder, additive for peritoneal dialysis, per packet
MCM: 4270

A4766   Dialysate concentrate, solution, additive for peritoneal dialysis, per 10 ml
MCM: 4270

A4770   Blood collection tube, vacuum, for dialysis, per 50
MCM: 4270

A4771   Serum clotting time tube, for dialysis, per 50
MCM: 4270

A4772   Blood glucose test strips, for dialysis, per 50
MCM: 4270

A4773   Occult blood test strips, for dialysis, per 50
MCM: 4270

A4774   Ammonia test strips, for dialysis, per 50
MCM: 4270

A4802   Protamine sulfate, for hemodialysis, per 50 mg
MCM: 4270

A4860   Disposable catheter tips for peritoneal dialysis, per 10
MCM: 4270

A4870   Plumbing and/or electrical work for home hemodialysis equipment
MCM: 4270

A4890   Contracts, repair and maintenance, for hemodialysis equipment
MCM: 2100.4

NOTE: The above procedure includes the following: scale, scissors, stopwatch, surgical brush, thermometer, tool kit, tourniquet, tube occluding forceps/clamps.

A4911   Drain bag/bottle, for dialysis, each

A4913   Miscellaneous dialysis supplies, not otherwise specified

A4918   Venous pressure clamp, for hemodialysis, each

A4927   Gloves, non-sterile, per 100

A4928   Surgical mask, per 20

A4929   Tourniquet for dialysis, each

A4930   Gloves, sterile, per pair

A4931   Oral thermometer, reusable, any type, each

A4932   Rectal thermometer, reusable, any type, each

ADDITIONAL OSTOMY SUPPLIES

A5051   Ostomy pouch, closed; with barrier attached (1 piece), each
MCM: 2130

A5052   without barrier attached (1 piece), each
MCM: 2130

A5053   for use on faceplate, each
MCM: 2130

A5054   for use on barrier with flange (2 piece), each
MCM: 2130

A5055   Stoma cap
MCM: 2130

● New code   ▲ Revised code   ( ) Deleted code

A5061 Ostomy pouch, drainable; with barrier attached (1 piece), each

A5062 without barrier attached (1 piece), each
MCM: 2130

A5063 for use on barrier with flange (2-piece system), each
MCM: 2130

A5071 Ostomy pouch, urinary; with barrier attached (1 piece), each
MCM: 2130

A5072 without barrier attached (1 piece), each
MCM: 2130

A5073 for use on barrier with flange (2 piece), each
MCM: 2130

A5081 Continent device; plug for continent stoma
MCM: 2130

A5082 catheter for continent stoma
MCM: 2130

A5093 Ostomy accessory; convex insert
MCM: 2130

ADDITIONAL INCONTINENCE APPLIANCES/SUPPLIES

A5102 Bedside drainage bottle with or without tubing, rigid or expandable, each
MCM: 2130

A5105 Urinary suspensory; with leg bag, with or without tube
MCM: 2130

A5112 Urinary leg bag; latex
MCM: 2130

A5113 Leg strap; latex, replacement only, per set
MCM: 2130

A5114 foam or fabric, replacement only, per set
MCM: 2130

SUPPLIES FOR EITHER INCONTINENCE OR OSTOMY APPLIANCES

(A5119)   Code deleted December 31, 2005

● **A5120**   Skin barrier, wipes or swabs, each
MCM: 2130

A5121   solid, 6 x 6 or equivalent, each
MCM: 2130

A5122   solid, 8 x 8 or equivalent, each
MCM: 2130

A5126   Adhesive or non-adhesive; disk or foam pad
MCM: 2130

A5131   Appliance cleaner, incontinence and ostomy appliances, per 16 oz.
MCM: 2130

A5200   Percutaneous catheter/tube anchoring device, adhesive skin attachment
MCM: 2130

SHOE SUPPLIES FOR DIABETICS

A5500   For diabetics only, fitting (including follow-up), custom preparation and supply of off-the-shelf depth-inlay shoe manufactured to accommodate multi-density insert(s), per shoe
MCM: 2134

A5501   For diabetics only, fitting (including follow-up), custom preparation and supply of shoe molded from cast(s) of patient's foot (custom molded shoe), per shoe
MCM: 2134

A5503   For diabetics only, modification (including fitting) of off-the-shelf depth-inlay shoe or custom-molded shoe with roller or rigid rocker bottom, per shoe
MCM: 2134

A5504   For diabetics only, modification (including fitting) of off-the-shelf depth-inlay shoe or custom-molded shoe with wedge(s), per shoe
MCM: 2134

A5505 For diabetics only, modification (including fitting) of off-the-shelf depth-inlay shoe or custom-molded shoe with metatarsal bar, per shoe
MCM: 2134

A5506 For diabetics only, modification (including fitting) of off-the-shelf depth-inlay shoe or custom-molded shoe with off-set heel(s), per shoe
MCM: 2134

A5507 For diabetics only, not otherwise specified modification (including fitting) of off-the-shelf depth-inlay shoe or custom-molded shoe, per shoe
MCM: 2134

A5508 For diabetics only, deluxe feature of off-the-shelf depth-inlay shoe or custom-molded shoe, per shoe
MCM: 2134

(A5509) Code deleted December 31, 2005

A5510 For diabetics only, direct formed, compression molded to patient's foot without external heat source, multiple-density insert(s), prefabricated, per shoe
MCM: 2134

(A5511) Code deleted December 31, 2005

● **A5512** For diabetics only, multiple density insert, direct formed, molded to foot after external heat source of 230 degrees fahrenheit or higher, total contact with patient's foot, including arch, base layer minimum of 1/4 inch material of shore a 35 durometer or 3/16 inch material of shore a 40 durometer (or higher), prefabricated, each

● **A5513** For diabetics only, multiple density insert, custom molded from model of patient's foot, total contact with patient's foot, including arch, base layer minimum of 1/4 inch material of shore a 35 durometer or 3/16 inch material of shore a 40 durometer (or higher), includes arch filler and other shaping material, custom fabricated, each

WOUND DRESSINGS

A6000 Non-contact wound warming wound cover for use with the non-contact wound warming device and warming card
MCM: 2303

A6010 Collagen based wound filler, dry form, per gram of collagen
MCM: 2079

A6011 Collagen based wound filler, gel/paste, per gram of collagen
MCM: 2079

A6021 Collagen dressing, pad size 16 sq. in. or less, each
MCM: 2079

A6022 Collagen dressing, pad size more than 16 sq. in. but less than or equal to 48 sq. in., each
MCM: 2079

A6023 Collagen dressing, pad size more than 48 sq. in., each
MCM: 2079

A6024 Collagen dressing wound filler, per 6 inches
MCM: 2079

A6025 Gel sheet for dermal or epidermal application, (eg., silicone, hydrogel, other), each

A6154 Wound pouch, each
MCM: 2079

A6196 Alginate or other fiber gelling dressing, wound cover, pad size 16 sq. in. or less, each dressing
MCM: 2079

A6197 Alginate or other fiber gelling dressing, wound cover, pad size more than 16 sq. in. but less than or equal to 48 sq. in., each dressing
MCM: 2079

A6198 Alginate or other fiber gelling dressing, wound cover, pad size more than 48 sq. in., each dressing
MCM: 2079

A6199 Alginate or other fiber gelling dressing, wound filler, per 6 inches
MCM: 2079

A6200 Composite dressing, pad size 16 sq. in. or less, without adhesive border, each dressing
MCM: 2079

A6201 Composite dressing, pad size more than 16 sq. in. but less than or equal to 48 sq. in., without adhesive border, each dressing
MCM: 2079

A6202 Composite dressing, pad size more than 48 sq. in., without adhesive border, each dressing
MCM: 2079

A6203 Composite dressing, pad size 16 sq. in. or less, with any size adhesive border, each dressing
MCM: 2079

A6204 Composite dressing, pad size more than 16 sq. in. but less than or equal to 48 sq. in., with any size adhesive border, each dressing
MCM: 2079

A6205 Composite dressing, pad size more than 48 sq. in., with any size adhesive border, each dressing
MCM: 2079

A6206 Contact layer, 16 sq. in. or less, each dressing
MCM: 2079

A6207 Contact layer, more than 16 sq. in. but less than or equal to 48 sq. in., each dressing
MCM: 2079

A6208 Contact layer, more than 48 sq. in., each dressing
MCM: 2079

A6209 Foam dressing, wound cover, pad size 16 sq. in. or less, without adhesive border, each dressing
MCM: 2079

A6210 Foam dressing, wound cover, pad size more than 16 sq. in. but less than or equal to 48 sq. in., without adhesive border, each dressing
MCM: 2079

A6211 Foam dressing, wound cover, pad size more than 48 sq. in., without adhesive border, each dressing
MCM: 2079

A6212 Foam dressing, wound cover, pad size 16 sq. in. or less, with any size adhesive border, each dressing
MCM: 2079

A6213   Foam dressing, wound cover, pad size more than 16 sq. in. but less than or equal to 48 sq. in., with any size adhesive border, each dressing
MCM: 2079

A6214   Foam dressing, wound cover, pad size more than 48 sq. in., with any size adhesive border, each dressing
MCM: 2079

A6215   Foam dressing, wound filler, per gram
MCM: 2079

A6216   Gauze, non-impregnated, non-sterile, pad size 16 sq. in. or less, without adhesive border, each dressing
MCM: 2079

A6217   Gauze, non-impregnated, non-sterile, pad size more than 16 sq. in. but less than or equal to 48 sq. in., without adhesive border, each dressing
MCM: 2079

A6218   Gauze, non-impregnated, non-sterile, pad size more than 48 sq. in., without adhesive border, each dressing
MCM: 2079

A6219   Gauze, non-impregnated, pad size 16 sq. in. or less, with any size adhesive border, each dressing
MCM: 2079

A6220   Gauze, non-impregnated, pad size more than 16 sq. in. but less than or equal to 48 sq. in., with any size adhesive border, each dressing
MCM: 2079

A6221   Gauze, non-impregnated, pad size more than 48 sq. in., with any size adhesive border, each dressing
MCM: 2079

A6222   Gauze, impregnated with other than water, normal saline, or hydrogel, pad size 16 sq. in. or less, without adhesive border, each dressing
MCM: 2079

A6223   Gauze, impregnated with other than water, normal saline, or hydrogel, pad size more than 16 sq. in. but less than or equal to 48 sq. in., without adhesive border, each dressing
MCM: 2079

A6224 Gauze, impregnated with other than water, normal saline, or hydrogel, pad size more than 48 sq. in., without adhesive border, each dressing
MCM: 2079

A6228 Gauze, impregnated, water or normal saline, pad size 16 sq. in. or less, without adhesive border, each dressing
MCM: 2079

A6229 Gauze, impregnated, water or normal saline, pad size more than 16 sq. in. but less than or equal to 48 sq. in., without adhesive border, each dressing
MCM: 2079

A6230 Gauze, impregnated, water or normal saline, pad size more than 48 sq. in., without adhesive border, each dressing
MCM: 2079

A6231 Gauze, impregnated, hydrogel, for direct wound contact, pad size 16 sq. in. or less, each dressing
MCM: 2079

A6232 Gauze, impregnated, hydrogel, for direct wound contact, pad size greater than 16 sq. in., but less than or equal to 48 sq. in., each dressing
MCM: 2079

A6233 Gauze, impregnated, hydrogel, for direct wound contact, pad size more than 48 sq. in., each dressing
MCM: 2079

A6234 Hydrocolloid dressing, wound cover, pad size 16 sq. in. or less, without adhesive border, each dressing
MCM: 2079

A6235 Hydrocolloid dressing, wound cover, pad size more than 16 sq. in. but less than or equal to 48 sq. in., without adhesive border, each dressing
MCM: 2079

A6236 Hydrocolloid dressing, wound cover, pad size more than 48 sq. in., without adhesive border, each dressing
MCM: 2079

A6237 Hydrocolloid dressing, wound cover, pad size 16 sq. in. or less, with any size adhesive border, each dressing
MCM: 2079

A6238   Hydrocolloid dressing, wound cover, pad size more than 16 sq. in. but less than or equal to 48 sq. in., with any size adhesive border, each dressing
MCM: 2079

A6239   Hydrocolloid dressing, wound cover, pad size more than 48 sq. in., with any size adhesive border, each dressing
MCM: 2079

A6240   Hydrocolloid dressing, wound filler, paste, per fluid ounce
MCM: 2079

A6241   Hydrocolloid dressing, wound filler, dry form, per gram
MCM: 2079

A6242   Hydrogel dressing, wound cover, pad size 16 sq. in. or less, without adhesive border, each dressing
MCM: 2079

A6243   Hydrogel dressing, wound cover, pad size more than 16 sq. in. but less than or equal to 48 sq. in., without adhesive border, each dressing
MCM: 2079

A6244   Hydrogel dressing, wound cover, pad size more than 48 sq. in., without adhesive border, each dressing
MCM: 2079

A6245   Hydrogel dressing, wound cover, pad size 16 sq. in. or less, with any size adhesive border, each dressing
MCM: 2079

A6246   Hydrogel dressing, wound cover, pad size more than 16 sq. in. but less than or equal to 48 sq. in., with any size adhesive border, each dressing
MCM: 2079

A6247   Hydrogel dressing, wound cover, pad size more than 48 sq. in., with any size adhesive border, each dressing
MCM: 2079

A6248   Hydrogel dressing, wound filler, gel, per fluid ounce
MCM: 2079

A6250   Skin sealants, protectants, moisturizers, ointments, any type, any size
MCM: 2079

A6251   Specialty absorptive dressing, wound cover, pad size 16 sq. in. or less, without adhesive border, each dressing
MCM: 2079

A6252 Specialty absorptive dressing, wound cover, pad size more than 16 sq. in. but less than or equal to 48 sq. in., without adhesive border, each dressing
MCM: 2079

A6253 Specialty absorptive dressing, wound cover, pad size more than 48 sq. in., without adhesive border, each dressing
MCM: 2079

A6254 Specialty absorptive dressing, wound cover, pad size 16 sq. in. or less, with any size adhesive border, each dressing
MCM: 2079

A6255 Specialty absorptive dressing, wound cover, pad size more than 16 sq. in. but less than or equal to 48 sq. in., with any size adhesive border, each dressing
MCM: 2079

A6256 Specialty absorptive dressing, wound cover, pad size more than 48 sq. in., with any size adhesive border, each dressing
MCM: 2079

A6257 Transparent film, 16 sq. in. or less, each dressing
MCM: 2079

A6258 Transparent film, more than 16 sq. in. but less than or equal to 48 sq. in., each dressing
MCM: 2079

A6259 Transparent film, more than 48 sq. in., each dressing
MCM: 2079

A6260 Wound cleansers, any type, any size
MCM: 2079

A6261 Wound filler, gel/paste, per fluid ounce, not elsewhere classified
MCM: 2079

A6262 Wound filler, dry form, per gram, not elsewhere classified
MCM: 2079

A6266 Gauze, impregnated, other than water, normal saline or zinc paste, any width, per linear yard
MCM: 2079

A6402 Gauze, non-impregnated, sterile, pad size 16 sq. in. or less, without adhesive border, each dressing
MCM: 2079

A6403   Gauze, non-impregnated, sterile, pad size more than 16 sq. in. but less than or equal to 48 sq. in., without adhesive border, each dressing
MCM: 2079

A6404   Gauze, non-impregnated, sterile, pad size more than 48 sq. in., without adhesive border, each dressing
MCM: 2079

A6407   Packing strips, non-impregnated, up to 2 inches in width, per linear yard

A6410   Eye pad, sterile, each
MCM: 2079

A6411   Eye pad, non-sterile, each
MCM: 2079

A6412   Eye patch, occlusive, each

A6441   Padding bandage, non-elastic, non-woven/non-knitted, width greater than or equal to three inches and less than five inches, per yard

A6442   Conforming bandage, non-elastic, knitted-woven, non-sterile, width less than three inches, per yard

A6443   Conforming bandage, non-elastic, knitted/woven, non-sterile, width greater than or equal to three inches and less than five inches, per yard

A6444   Conforming bandage, non-elastic, knitted/woven, non-sterile, width greater than or equal to 5 inches, per yard

A6445   Conforming bandage, non-elastic, knitted/woven, sterile, width less than three inches, per yard

A6446   Conforming bandage, non-elastic, knitted/woven, sterile, width greater than or equal to three inches and less than five inches, per yard

A6447   Conforming bandage, non-elastic, knitted/woven, sterile, width greater than or equal to five inches, per yard

A6448   Light compression bandage, elastic, knitted/woven, width less than three inches, per yard

A6449 Light compression bandage, elastic, knitted/woven, width greater than or equal to three inches and less than five inches, per yard

A6450 Light compression bandage, elastic, knitted/woven, width greater than or equal to five inches, per yard

A6451 Moderate compression bandage, elastic, knitted/woven, load resistance of 1.25 to 1.34 foot pounds at 50% maximum stretch, width greater than or equal to three inches and less than five inches, per yard

A6452 High compression bandage, elastic, knitted/woven, load resistance greater than or equal to 1.35 foot pounds at 50% maximum stretch, width greater than or equal to three inches and less than five inches, per yard

A6453 Self-adherent bandage, elastic, non-knitted/non-woven, width less than three inches, per yard

A6454 Self-adherent bandage, elastic, non-knitted/non-woven, width greater than or equal to three inches and less than five inches, per yard

A6455 Self-adherent bandage, elastic, non-knitted/non-woven, width greater than or equal to five inches, per yard

A6456 Zinc paste impregnated bandage, non-elastic, knitted/woven, width greater than or equal to three inches and less than five inches, per yard

● **A6457** Tubular dressing with or without elastic, any width, per linear yard

A6501 Compression burn garment, bodysuit (head to foot), custom fabricated
MCM: 2079

A6502 Compression burn garment, chin strap, custom fabricated
MCM: 2079

A6503 Compression burn garment, facial hood, custom fabricated
MCM: 2079

A6504 Compression burn garment, glove to wrist, custom fabricated
MCM: 2079

A6505   Compression burn garment, glove to elbow, custom fabricated
MCM: 2079

A6506   Compression burn garment, glove to axilla, custom fabricated
MCM: 2079

A6507   Compression burn garment, foot to knee length, custom fabricated
MCM: 2079

A6508   Compression burn garment, foot to thigh length, custom fabricated
MCM: 2079

A6509   Compression burn garment, upper trunk to waist including arm openings (vest), custom fabricated
MCM: 2079

A6510   Compression burn garment, trunk, including arms down to leg openings (leotard), custom fabricated
MCM: 2079

A6511   Compression burn garment, lower trunk including leg openings (panty), custom fabricated
MCM: 2079

A6512   Compression burn garment, not otherwise classified
MCM: 2079

● **A6513**   Compression burn mask, face and/or neck, plastic or equal, custom fabricated

● **A6530**   Gradient compression stocking, below knee, 18-30 mmhg, each
CIM: 60-9

● **A6531**   Gradient compression stocking, below knee, 30-40 mmhg, each
MCM: 2079

● **A6532**   Gradient compression stocking, below knee, 40-50 mmhg, each
MCM: 2079

● **A6533**   Gradient compression stocking, thigh length, 18-30 mmhg, each
CIM: 60-9 MCM: 2133

● **A6534**   Gradient compression stocking, thigh length, 30-40 mmhg, each
CIM: 60-9 MCM: 2133

● **A6535**   Gradient compression stocking, thigh length, 40-50 mmhg, each
CIM: 60-9 MCM: 2133

● **A6536**   Gradient compression stocking, full length/chap style, 18-30 mmhg, each
CIM: 60-9 MCM: 2133

● **A6537**   Gradient compression stocking, full length/chap style, 30-40 mmhg, each
CIM: 60-9 MCM: 2133

● **A6538**   Gradient compression stocking, full length/chap style, 40-50 mmhg, each
CIM: 60-9 MCM: 2133

● **A6539**   Gradient compression stocking, waist length, 18-30 mmhg, each
CIM: 60-9 MCM: 2133

● **A6540**   Gradient compression stocking, waist length, 30-40 mmhg, each
CIM: 60-9 MCM: 2133

● **A6541**   Gradient compression stocking, waist length, 40-50 mmhg, each
CIM: 60-9 MCM: 2133

● **A6542**   Gradient compression stocking, custom made
CIM: 60-9 MCM: 2133

● **A6543**   Gradient compression stocking, lymphedema
CIM: 60-9 MCM: 2133

● **A6544**   Gradient compression stocking, garter belt
CIM: 60-9 MCM: 2133

● **A6549**   Gradient compression stocking, not otherwise specified
CIM: 60-9 MCM: 2133

▲ **A6550**   Wound care set, for negative pressure wound therapy electrical pump, includes all supplies and accessories

(A6551) Code deleted December 31, 2005

A7000 Canister, disposable, used with suction pump, each

A7001 Canister, non-disposable, used with suction pump, each

A7002 Tubing, used with suction pump, each

A7003 Administration set, with small volume nonfiltered pneumatic nebulizer, disposable

A7004 Small volume nonfiltered pneumatic nebulizer, disposable

A7005 Administration set, with small volume nonfiltered pneumatic nebulizer, non-disposable

A7006 Administration set, with small volume filtered pneumatic nebulizer

A7007 Large volume nebulizer, disposable, unfilled, used with aerosol compressor

A7008 Large volume nebulizer, disposable, prefilled, used with aerosol compressor

A7009 Reservoir bottle, non-disposable, used with large volume ultrasonic nebulizer

A7010 Corrugated tubing, disposable, used with large volume nebulizer, 100 feet

A7011 Corrugated tubing, non-disposable, used with large volume nebulizer, 10 feet

A7012 Water collection device, used with large volume nebulizer

A7013 Filter, disposable, used with aerosol compressor

A7014 Filter, non-disposable, used with aerosol compressor or ultrasonic generator

A7015 Aerosol mask, used with DME nebulizer

A7016 Dome and mouthpiece, used with small volume ultrasonic nebulizer

---

● New code   ▲ Revised code   ( ) Deleted code

A7017 Nebulizer, durable, glass or autoclavable plastic, bottle type, not used with oxygen
CIM: 60-9

A7018 Water, distilled, used with large volume nebulizer, 1000 ml

A7025 High frequency chest wall oscillation system vest, replacement for use with patient owned equipment, each

A7026 High frequency chest wall oscillation system hose, replacement for use with patient owned equipment, each

A7030 Full face mask used with positive airway pressure device, each

A7031 Face mask interface, replacement for full face mask, each

▲**A7032** Cushion for use on nasal mask interface, replacement only, each

▲**A7033** Pillow for use on nasal cannula type interface, replacement only, pair

A7034 Nasal interface (mask or cannula type) used with positive airway pressure device, with or without head strap

A7035 Headgear used with positive airway pressure device

A7036 Chinstrap used with positive airway pressure device

A7037 Tubing used with positive airway pressure device

A7038 Filter, disposable, used with positive airway pressure device

A7039 Filter, non-disposable, used with positive airway pressure device

A7040 One way chest drain valve

A7041 Water seal drainage container and tubing for use with implanted chest tube

A7042 Implanted pleural catheter, each

A7043 Vacuum drainage bottle and tubing for use with implanted catheter

A7044 Oral interface used with positive airway pressure device, each

A7045 Exhalation port with or without swivel used with accessories for positive airway devices, replacement only
CIM: 60-17

A7046 Water chamber for humidifier, used with positive airway pressure device, replacement, each
CIM: 60-17

A7501 Tracheostoma valve, including diaphram, each
MCM: 2130

A7502 Replacement diaphram/faceplate for tracheostoma valve, each
MCM: 2130

A7503 Filter holder or filter cap, reusable, for use in a tracheostoma heat and moisture exchange system, each
MCM: 2130

A7504 Filter for use in a tracheostoma heat and moisture exchange system, each
MCM: 2130

A7505 Housing, reusable without adhesive, for use in a heat and moisture exchange system and/or with a tracheostoma valve, each
MCM: 2130

A7506 Adhesive disc for use in a heat and moisture exchange system and/or with tracheostoma valve, any type, each
MCM: 2130

A7507 Filter holder and integrated filter without adhesive, for use in a tracheostoma heat and moisture exchange system, each
MCM: 2130

A7508 Housing and integrated adhesive, for use in a tracheostoma heat and moisture exchange system and/or with a tracheostoma valve, each
MCM: 2130

A7509 Filter holder and integrated filter housing, and adhesive, for use as a tracheostoma heat and moisture exchange system, each
MCM: 2130

A7520 Tracheostomy/laryngectomy tube, non-cuffed, polyvinylchloride (PVC), silicone or equal, each

A7521 Tracheostomy/laryngectomy tube, cuffed, polyvinylchloride (PVC), silicone or equal, each

A7522 Tracheostomy/laryngectomy tube, stainless steel or equal (sterilizable and reusable), each

A7523 Tracheostomy shower protector, each

A7524 Tracheostoma stent/stud/button, each

A7525 Tracheostomy mask, each

A7526 Tracheostomy tube collar/holder, each

A7527 Tracheostomy/laryngectomy tube plug/stop, each

● New code ▲ Revised code ( ) Deleted code

ADMINISTRATIVE, MISCELLANEOUS AND INVESTIGATIONAL

NOTE: The following codes do not imply that codes in other sections are necessarily covered.

Guidelines

In addition to the information presented in the INTRODUCTION, several other items unique to this section are defined or identified here:

1. SPECIAL REPORT: A service, material or supply that is rarely provided, unusual, variable or new may require a special report in determining medical appropriateness for reimbursement purposes. Pertinent information should include an adequate definition or description of the nature, extent, and need for the service, material or supply.

2. CPT CODE CROSS-REFERENCE: Unless specified otherwise, there is no equivalent CPT code for listings in this section.

Miscellaneous and Experimental

A9150   Non-prescription drugs
MCM: 2050.5

A9152   Single vitamin/mineral/trace element, oral, per dose, not otherwise specified

A9153   Multiple vitamins, with or without minerals and trace elements, oral, per dose, not otherwise specified

A9180   Pediculosis (lice infestation) treatment, topical, for administration by patient/caretaker

A9270   Non-covered item or service
MCM: 2303

● **A9275**   Home glucose disposable monitor, includes test strips

A9280   Alert or alarm device, not otherwise classified

■ Not valid   ■ Non-covered   Special   ■ Carrier   **57**
for Medicare   by Medicare   coverage   discretion
                                   instructions

● A9281   Reaching/grabbing device, any type, any length, each

● A9282   Wig, any type, each

A9300   Exercise equipment
CIM: 60-9 MCM: 2100.1

▲ A9500   Technetium TC-99m sestamibi, diagnostic, per study dose, up to 40 millicuries
MCM: 15022

▲ A9502   Technetium TC-99m tetrofosmin, diagnostic, per study dose, up to 40 millicuries
MCM: 15022

▲ A9503   Technetium TC-99m medronate, diagnostic, per study dose, up to 30 millicuries
MCM: 15022

▲ A9504   Technetium TC-99m apcitide, diagnostic, per study dose, up to 20 millicuries
MCM: 15022

▲ A9505   Thallium TL-201 thallous chloride, diagnostic, per millicurie
MCM: 15022

▲ A9507   Indium IN-111 capromablue pendetide, diagnostic, per study dose, up to 10 millicuries
MCM: 15022

▲ A9508   Iodine I-131 ioblueenguane sulfate, diagnostic, per 0.5 millicurie
MCM: 15030

▲ A9510   Technetium TC-99m disofenin, diagnostic, per study dose, up to 15 millicuries
MCM: 15030

(A9511)   Code deleted December 31, 2005

▲ A9512   Technetium TC-99m pertechnetate, diagnostic, per millicurie

(A9513)   Code deleted December 31, 2005

(A9514)   Code deleted December 31, 2005

(A9515)   Code deleted December 31, 2005

▲**A9516** Iodine I-123 sodium iodide capsule(s), diagnostic, per 100 microcuries

▲**A9517** Iodine I-131 sodium iodide capsule(s), therapeutic, per millicurie

(A9519) Code deleted December 31, 2005

(A9520) Code deleted December 31, 2005

▲**A9521** Technetium TC-99m exametazime, diagnostic, per study dose, up to 25 millicuries

(A9522) Code deleted December 31, 2005

(A9523) Code deleted December 31, 2005

▲**A9524** Iodine I-131 iodinated serum alblueumin, diagnostic, per 5 microcuries
MCM: 15022

(A9525) Code deleted December 31, 2005

▲**A9526** Nitrogen n-13 ammonia, diagnostic, per study dose, up to 40 millicuries
CIM: 50-36

▲**A9528** Iodine I-131 sodium iodide capsule(s), diagnostic, per millicurie

▲**A9529** Iodine I-131 sodium iodide solution, diagnostic, per millicurie

▲**A9530** Iodine I-131 sodium iodide solution, therapeutic, per millicurie

▲**A9531** Iodine I-131 sodium iodide, diagnostic, per microcurie (up to 100 microcuries)

▲**A9532** Iodine I-125 serum alblueumin, diagnostic, per 5 microcuries

(A9533) Code deleted December 31, 2005

(A9534) Code deleted December 31, 2005

●**A9535** Injection, methylene blue, 1 ml

● **A9536** Technetium tc-99m depreotide, diagnostic, per study dose, up to 35 millicuries

● **A9537** Technetium tc-99m mebrofenin, diagnostic, per study dose, up to 15 millicuries

● **A9538** Technetium tc-99m pyrophosphate, diagnostic, per study dose, up to 25 millicuries

● **A9539** Technetium tc-99m pentetate, diagnostic, per study dose, up to 25 millicuries

● **A9540** Technetium tc-99m macroaggregated albumin, diagnostic, per study dose, up to 10 millicuries

● **A9541** Technetium tc-99m sulfur colloid, diagnostic, per study dose, up to 20 millicuries

● **A9542** Indium in-111 ibritumomab tiuxetan, diagnostic, per study dose, up to 5 millicuries

● **A9543** Yttrium y-90 ibritumomab tiuxetan, therapeutic, per treatment dose, up to 40 millicuries

● **A9544** Iodine i-131 tositumomab, diagnostic, per study dose

● **A9545** Iodine i-131 tositumomab, therapeutic, per treatment dose

● **A9546** Cobalt co-57/58, cyanocobalamin, diagnostic, per study dose, up to 1 microcurie

● **A9547** Indium in-111 oxyquinoline, diagnostic, per 0.5 millicurie

● **A9548** Indium in-111 pentetate, diagnostic, per 0.5 millicurie

● **A9549** Technetium tc-99m arcitumomab, diagnostic, per study dose, up to 25 millicuries

● **A9550** Technetium tc-99m sodium gluceptate, diagnostic, per study dose, up to 25 millicuries

● **A9551** Technetium tc-99m succimer, diagnostic, per study dose, up to 10 millicuries

● **A9552** Fluorodeoxyglucose f-18 fdg, diagnostic, per study dose, up to 45 millicuries

● **A9553** Chromium cr-51 sodium chromate, diagnostic, per study dose, up to 250 microcuries

● **A9554** Iodine i-125 sodium iothalamate, diagnostic, per study dose, up to 10 microcuries

● **A9555** Rubidium rb-82, diagnostic, per study dose, up to 60 millicuries

● **A9556** Gallium ga-67 citrate, diagnostic, per millicurie

● **A9557** Technetium tc-99m bicisate, diagnostic, per study dose, up to 25 millicuries

● **A9558** Xenon xe-133 gas, diagnostic, per 10 millicuries

● **A9559** Cobalt co-57 cyanocobalamin, oral, diagnostic, per study dose, up to 1 microcurie

● **A9560** Technetium tc-99m labeled red blood cells, diagnostic, per study dose, up to 30 millicuries

● **A9561** Technetium tc-99m oxidronate, diagnostic, per study dose, up to 30 millicuries

● **A9562** Technetium tc-99m mertiatide, diagnostic, per study dose, up to 15 millicuries

● **A9563** Sodium phosphate p-32, therapeutic, per millicurie

● **A9564** Chromic phosphate p-32 suspension, therapeutic, per millicurie

● **A9565** Indium in-111 pentetreotide, diagnostic, per millicurie

● **A9566** Technetium tc-99m fanolesomab, diagnostic, per study dose, up to 25 millicuries

● **A9567** Technetium tc-99m pentetate, diagnostic, aerosol, per study dose, up to 75 millicuries

▲ **A9600** Strontium SR-89 chloride, therapeutic, per millicurie

▲ **A9605** Samarium SM-153 lexidronamm, therapeutic, per 50 millicuries

● **A9698**   Non-radioactive contrast imaging material, not otherwise classified, per study
MCM: 15022

▲ **A9699**   Radiopharmaceutical, therapeutic, not otherwise classified

A9700   Supply of injectable contrast material for use in echocardiography, per study
MCM: 15360

A9900   Miscellaneous DME supply, accessory, and/or service component of another HCPCS code

A9901   DME delivery, set up, and/or dispensing service component of another HCPCS code

A9999   Miscellaneous DME supply or accessory, not otherwise specified

ENTERAL AND PARENTERAL THERAPY

Guidelines

In addition to the information presented in the INTRODUCTION, several other items unique to this section are defined or identified here:

1. SUBSECTION INFORMATION: Some of the listed subheadings or subsections have special needs or instructions unique to that section. Where these are indicated, special "notes" will be presented preceding or following the listings. Those subsections within the ENTERAL AND PARENTERAL THERAPY section that have "notes" are as follows:

Subsection	Code Numbers
Enteral formulae and enteral medical supplies	B4034-B5200

2. UNLISTED SERVICE OR PROCEDURE: A service or procedure may be provided that is not listed in this edition of HCPCS. When reporting such a service, the appropriate "unlisted procedure" code may be used to indicate the service, identifying it by "special report" as defined below. HCPCS terminology is inconsistent in defining unlisted procedures. The procedure definition may include the term(s) "unlisted", "not otherwise classified", "unspecified", "unclassified", "other" and "miscellaneous". Prior to using these codes, try to determine if a Local Level III code or CPT code is available. The "unlisted procedures" and accompanying codes for ENTERAL AND PARENTERAL THERAPY are as follows:

B9998	NOC for enteral supplies
B9999	NOC for parenteral supplies

3. SPECIAL REPORT: A service, material or supply that is rarely provided, unusual, variable or new may require a special report in determining medical appropriateness for reimbursement purposes. Pertinent information should include an adequate definition or description of the nature, extent, and need for the service, material or supply.

4. MODIFIERS: Listed services may be modified under certain circumstances. When appropriate, the modifying circumstance is identified by adding a modifier to the basic procedure code. CPT and HCPCS National Level II modifiers may be used with CPT and

---

HCPCS National Level II procedure codes. Modifiers commonly used with ENTERAL AND PARENTERAL THERAPY are as follows:

-CC   Procedure code change (used when the procedure code submitted was changed either for administrative reasons or because an incorrect code was filed)

5.   CPT CODE CROSS-REFERENCE: Unless specified otherwise, the equivalent CPT code for all listings in this section is 99070.

Enteral Formulae and Enteral Medical Supplies

B4034   Enteral feeding supply kit; syringe, per day
CIM: 65-10   MCM: 2130, 4450

B4035   pump fed, per day
CIM: 65-10   MCM: 2130, 4450

B4036   gravity fed, per day
CIM: 65-10   MCM: 2130, 4450

B4081   Nasogastric tubing; with stylet
CIM: 65-10   MCM: 2130, 4450

B4082   without stylet
CIM: 65-10   MCM: 2130, 4450

B4083   Stomach tube - levine type
CIM: 65-10   MCM: 2130, 4450

B4086   Gastrostomy/jejunostomy tube, any material, any type, (standard or low profile), each

B4100   Food thickener, administered orally, per ounce

B4102   Enteral formula, for adults, used to replace fluids and electrolytes (e.g. clear liquids), 500 ml = 1 unit
CIM: 65-10

B4103   Enteral formula, for pediatrics, used to replace fluids and electrolytes (e.g. clear liquids), 500 ml = 1 unit
CIM: 65-10

B4104   Additive for enteral formula (e.g. fiber)
CIM: 65-10

▲**B4149**   Enteral formula, manufactured bluelenderized natural
foods with intact nutrients, includes proteins, fats,
carblueohydrates, vitamins and minerals, may include
fiblueer, administered through an enteral feeding tube, 100
calories = 1 unit
CIM: 65-10 MCM: 2130, 4450

B4150   Enteral formula, nutritionally complete with intact
nutrients, includes proteins, fats, carbohydrates, vitamins
and minerals, may include fiber, administered through an
enteral feeding tube, 100 calories = 1 unit
CIM: 65-10 MCM: 2130, 4450

(B4151)   Code deleted December 31, 2004; use CPT

B4152   Enteral formula, nutritionally complete, calorically dense
(equal to or greater than 1.5 Kcal/ml) with intact
nutrients, includes proteins, fats, carbohydrates, vitamins
and minerals, may include fiber, administered through an
enteral feeding tube, 100 calories = 1 unit
CIM: 65-10 MCM: 2130, 4450

B4153   Enteral formula, nutritionally complete, hydrolyzed
proteins (amino acids and peptide chain), includes fats,
carbohydrates, vitamins and minerals, may include fiber,
administered through an enteral feeding tube, 100 calories
= 1 unit
CIM: 65-10 MCM: 2130, 4450

B4154   Enteral formula, nutritionally complete, for special
metabolic needs, excludes inherited disease of
metabolism, includes altered composition of proteins, fats,
carbohydrates, vitamins and/or minerals, may include
fiber, administered through an enteral feeding tube, 100
calories = 1 unit
CIM: 65-10 MCM: 2130, 4450

B4155   Enteral formula, nutritionally incomplete/modular
nutrients, includes specific nutrients, carbohydrates (e.g.
glucose polymers), proteins/amino acids (e.g. glutamine,
arginine), fat (e.g. medium chain triglycerides) or
combination, administered through an enteral feeding
tube, 100 calories = 1 unit
CIM: 65-10 MCM: 2130, 4450

(B4156)   Code deleted December 31, 2004; use CPT

Not valid   Non-covered   Special   Carrier   **65**
for Medicare   by Medicare   coverage   discretion
instructions

B4157   Enteral formula, nutritionally complete, for special metabolic needs for inherited disease of metabolism, includes proteins, fats, carbohydrates, vitamins and minerals, may include fiber, administered through an enteral feeding tube, 100 calories = 1 unit
CIM: 65-10

B4158   Enteral formula, for pediatrics, nutritionally complete with intact nutrients, includes proteins, fats, carbohydrates, vitamins and minerals, may include fiber and/or iron, administered through an enteral feeding tube, 100 calories = 1 unit
CIM: 65-10

B4159   Enteral formula, for pediatrics, nutritionally complete soy based with intact nutrients, includes proteins, fats, carbohydrates, vitamins and minerals, may include fiber and/or iron, administered through an enteral feeding tube, 100 calories = 1 unit
CIM: 65-10

B4160   Enteral formula, for pediatrics, nutritionally complete calorically dense (equal to or greater than 0.7 Kcal/ml) with intact nutrients, includes proteins, fats, carbohydrates, vitamins and minerals, may include fiber, administered through an enteral feeding tube, 100 calories = 1 unit
CIM: 65-10

B4161   Enteral formula, for pediatrics, hydrolyzed/amino acids and peptide chain proteins, includes fats, carbohydrates, vitamins and minerals, may include fiber, administered through an enteral feeding tube, 100 calories = 1 unit
CIM: 65-10

B4162   Enteral formula, for pediatrics, special metabolic needs for inherited disease of metabolism, includes proteins, fats, carbohydrates, vitamins and minerals, may include fiber, administered through an enteral feeding tube, 100 calories = 1 unit
CIM: 65-10

NOTE: For solution codes for other than parenteral nutrition therapy use, see J7060, J7070 and J7042.

PARENTERAL NUTRITION

B4164   Parenteral nutrition solution; carbohydrates (dextrose), 50% or less (500 ml = 1 unit)—homemix
CIM: 65-10   MCM: 2130, 4450

B4168   amino acid, 3.5% (500 ml = 1 unit)—homemix
CIM: 65-10   MCM: 2130, 4450

B4172   amino acid, 5.5% Thru 7%, (500 ml = 1 unit)—
homemix
CIM: 65-10   MCM: 2130, 4450

B4176   amino acid, 7% thru 8.5% (500 ml = 1 unit)—
homemix
CIM: 65-10   MCM: 2130, 4450

B4178   amino acid, greater than 8.5% (500 ml = 1 unit)—
homemix
CIM: 65-10   MCM: 2130, 4450

B4180   carbohydrates (dextrose), greater than 50% (500 ml =
1 unit)—homemix
CIM: 65-10   MCM: 2130, 4450

(B4184)   Code deleted December 31, 2005

● **B4185**   Parenteral nutrition solution, per 10 grams lipids

(B4186)   Code deleted December 31, 2005

B4189   compounded amino acids and carbohydrates with
electrolytes, trace elements, and vitamins, including
preparation, any strength, 10 to 51 grams of
protein-premix
CIM: 65-10   MCM: 2130, 4450

B4193   compounded amino acid and carbohydrates with
electrolytes, trace elements, and vitamins, including
preparation, any strength, 52 to 73 grams of
protein-premix
CIM: 65-10   MCM: 2130, 4450

B4197   compounded amino acid and carbohydrates with
electrolytes, trace elements and vitamins, including
preparation, any strength, 74 to 100 grams of protein -
premix
CIM: 65-10   MCM: 2130, 4450

B4199   compounded amino acid and carbohydrates with
electrolytes, trace elements and vitamins, including
preparation, any strength, over 100 grams of protein -
premix
CIM: 65-10   MCM: 2130, 4450

| | Not valid for Medicare | | Non-covered by Medicare | | Special coverage instructions | | Carrier discretion |

B4216 Parenteral nutrition; additives (vitamins, trace elements, heparin, electrolytes) homemix per day
CIM: 65-10   MCM: 2130, 4450

B4220 Parenteral nutrition supply kit; premix, per day
CIM: 65-10   MCM: 2130, 4450

B4222   home mix, per day
CIM: 65-10   MCM: 2130, 4450

B4224 Parenteral nutrition administration kit, per day
CIM: 65-10   MCM: 2130, 4450

B5000 Parenteral nutrition solution: compounded amino acid and carbohydrates with electrolytes, trace elements, and vitamins, including preparation, any strength; renal - amirosyn RF, nephramine, renamine - premix
CIM: 65-10   MCM: 2130, 4450

B5100   hepatic - freamine HBC, hepatamine - premix
CIM: 65-10   MCM: 2130, 4450

B5200   stress - branch chain amino acids - premix
CIM: 65-10   MCM: 2130, 4450

ENTERAL AND PARENTERAL PUMPS

B9000 Enteral nutrition infusion pump; without alarm
CIM: 65-10   MCM: 2130, 4450

B9002   with alarm
CIM: 65-10   MCM: 2130, 4450

B9004 Parenteral nutrition infusion pump; portable
CIM: 65-10   MCM: 2130, 4450

B9006   stationary
CIM: 65-10   MCM: 2130, 4450

B9998 NOC for enteral supplies
CIM: 65-10   MCM: 2130, 4450

B9999 NOC for parenteral supplies
CIM: 65-10   MCM: 2130, 4450

HOSPITAL OUTPATIENT PPS CODES

Guidelines

The "C" codes are unique temporary codes established by CMS for use under the Hospital Outpatient Prospective Payment System (OPPS). Non-OPPS use of these codes for Medicare is not valid.

The purpose of the "C" codes is to provide hospitals with a list of codes and long descriptors for drugs, biologicals and devices eligible for transitional pass-through payments, and for items classified in "new technology" ambulatory payment classifications (APCs) under the new Hospital Outpatient Prospective Payment System (OPPS).

The listing of HCPCS codes in this section does not assure coverage of the specific item or service in a given case. To be eligible for pass-through and new technology payments, the items reported with "C" codes must be considered reasonable and necessary.

All of the "C" codes are used exclusively for services paid under the Hospital Outpatient Prospective Payment System and may not be used to bill for services paid under other Medicare payment systems.

In addition to the information presented above, several other items unique to this section are defined here:

1. SPECIAL REPORT: A service, material or supply that is rarely provided, unusual, variable or new may require a special report in determining medical appropriateness for reimbursement purposes. Pertinent information should include an adequate definition or description of the nature, extent, and need for the service, material or supply.

2. MODIFIERS: Listed services may be modified under certain circumstances. When appropriate, the modifying circumstance is identified by adding a modifier to the basic procedure code. CPT and HCPCS National Level II modifiers may be used with CPT and HCPCS National Level II procedure codes.

69

Not valid
for Medicare

Non-covered
by Medicare

Special
coverage
instructions

Carrier
discretion

Hospital Outpatient PPS Codes

(C1079) Code deleted December 31, 2005; use A9546

(C1080) Code deleted December 31, 2005; use A9544

(C1081) Code deleted December 31, 2005; use A9545

(C1082) Code deleted December 31, 2005; use A9542

(C1083) Code deleted December 31, 2005; use A9543

(C1091) Code deleted December 31, 2005; use A9547

(C1092) Code deleted December 31, 2005; use A9548

(C1093) Code deleted December 31, 2005; use A9566

(C1122) Code deleted December 31, 2005; use A9549

C1178 Injection, busulfan, per 6 mg

(C1200) Code deleted December 31, 2005

(C1201) Code deleted December 31, 2005; use A9551

C1300 Hyperbaric oxygen under pressure, full body chamber, per 30 minute interval

(C1305) Code deleted December 31, 2005; use J7340

C1713 Anchor/screw for opposing bone-to-bone or soft tissue-to-bone (implantable)

C1714 Catheter, transluminal atherectomy, directional

C1715 Brachytherapy needle

C1716 Brachytherapy source, gold 198, per source

C1717 Brachytherapy seed, high dose rate iridium 192, per source

C1718 Brachytherapy source, iodine 125, per source

C1719   Brachytherapy source, non-high dose rate iridium 192, per source

C1720   Brachytherapy source, palladium 103, per source

C1721   Cardioverter-defibrillator, dual chamber (implantable)

C1722   Cardioverter-defibrillator, single chamber (implantable)

C1724   Catheter, transluminal atherectomy, rotational

C1725   Cathcter, transluminal angioplasty, non-laser (may include guidance, infusion/perfusion capability)

C1726   Catheter, balloon dilatation, non-vascular

C1727   Catheter, balloon tissue dissector, non-vascular (insertable)

C1728   Catheter, brachytherapy seed administration

C1729   Catheter, drainage

C1730   Catheter, electrophysiology, diagnostic, other than 3d mapping (19 or fewer electrodes)

C1731   Catheter, electrophysiology, diagnostic, other than 3d mapping (20 or more electrodes)

C1732   Catheter, electrophysiology, diagnostic/ablation, 3d or vector mapping

C1733   Catheter, electrophysiology, diagnostic/ablation, other than 3d or vector mapping, other than cool-tip

C1750   Catheter, hemodialysis, long-term

C1751   Catheter, infusion, inserted peripherally, centrally or midline (other than hemodialysis)

C1752   Catheter, hemodialysis, short-term

C1753   Catheter, intravascular ultrasound

C1754   Catheter, intradiscal

C1755   Catheter, intraspinal

Not valid   Non-covered   Special   Carrier   **71**
for Medicare   by Medicare   coverage   discretion
                                    instructions

C1756 Catheter, pacing, transesophageal

C1757 Catheter, thrombectomy/embolectomy

C1758 Catheter, ureteral

C1759 Catheter, intracardiac echocardiography

C1760 Closure device, vascular (implantable/insertable)

C1762 Connective tissue, human (includes fascia lata)

C1763 Connective tissue, non-human (includes synthetic)

C1764 Event recorder, cardiac (implantable)

C1765 Adhesion barrier

C1766 Introducer/sheath, guiding, intracardiac electrophysiological, steerable, other than peel-away

C1767 Generator, neurostimulator (implantable)

C1768 Graft, vascular

C1769 Guide wire

C1770 Imaging coil, magnetic resonance (insertable)

C1771 Repair device, urinary, incontinence, with sling graft

C1772 Infusion pump, programmable (implantable)

C1773 Retrieval device, insertable (used to retrieve fractured medical devices)

(C1775) Code deleted December 31, 2005; use A9552

C1776 Joint device (implantable)

C1777 Lead, cardioverter-defibrillator, endocardial single coil (implantable)

C1778 Lead, neurostimulator (implantable)

C1779 Lead, pacemaker, transvenous vdd single pass

C1780 Lens, intraocular (new technology)

C1781 Mesh (implantable)

C1782 Morcellator

C1783 Ocular implant, aqueous drainage assist device

C1784 Ocular device, intraoperative, detached retina

C1785 Pacemaker, dual chamber, rate-responsive (implantable)

C1786 Pacemaker, single chamber, rate-responsive (implantable)

C1787 Patient programmer, neurostimulator

C1788 Port, indwelling (implantable)

C1789 Prosthesis, breast (implantable)

C1813 Prosthesis, penile, inflatable

C1814 Retinal tamponade device, silicone oil

C1815 Prosthesis, urinary sphincter (implantable)

C1816 Receiver and/or transmitter, neurostimulator (implantable)

C1817 Septal defect implant system, intracardiac

C1818 Integrated keratoprosthesis

C1819 Surgical tissue localization and excision device (implantable)

C1874 Stent, coated/covered, with delivery system

C1875 Stent, coated/covered, without delivery system

C1876 Stent, non-coated/non-covered, with delivery system

C1877 Stent, non-coated/non-covered, without delivery system

C1878 Material for vocal cord medialization, synthetic (implantable)

C1879   Tissue marker (implantable)

C1880   Vena cava filter

C1881   Dialysis access system (implantable)

C1882   Cardioverter-defibrillator, other than single or dual chamber (implantable)

C1883   Adaptor/extension, pacing lead or neurostimulator lead (implantable)

C1884   Embolization protective system

C1885   Catheter, transluminal angioplasty, laser

C1887   Catheter, guiding (may include infusion/perfusion capability)

C1888   Catheter, ablation, non-cardiac, endovascular (implantable)

C1891   Infusion pump, non-programmable, permanent (implantable)

C1892   Introducer/sheath, guiding, intracardiac electrophysiological, fixed-curve, peel-away

C1893   Introducer/sheath, guiding, intracardiac electrophysiological, fixed-curve, other than peel-away

C1894   Introducer/sheath, othe than guiding, intracardiac electrophysiological, non-laser

C1895   Lead, cardioverter-defibrillator, endocardial dual coil (implantable)

C1896   Lead, cardioverter-defibrillator, other than endocardial single or dual coil (implantable)

C1897   Lead, neurostimulator test kit (implantable)

C1898   Lead, pacemaker, other than transvenous vdd single pass

C1899   Lead, pacemaker/cardioverter-defibrillator combination (implantable)

C1900   Lead, left ventricular coronary venous system

C2614   Probe, percutaneous lumbar discectomy

C2615   Sealant, pulmonary, liquid

C2616   Brachytherapy source, yttrium-90, per source

C2617   Stent, non-coronary, temporary, without delivery system

C2618   Probe, cryoablation

C2619   Pacemaker, dual chamber, non rate-responsive (implantable)

C2620   Paccmaker, single chamber, non rate-responsive (implantable)

C2621   Pacemaker, other than single or dual chamber (implantable)

C2622   Prosthesis, penile, non-inflatable

C2625   Stent, non-coronary, temporary, with delivery system

C2626   Infusion pump, non-programmable, temporary (implantable)

C2627   Catheter, suprapubic/cystoscopic

C2628   Catheter, occlusion

C2629   Introducer/sheath, other than guiding, intracardiac electrophysiological, laser

C2630   Catheter, electrophysiology, diagnostic/ablation, other than 3d or vector mapping, cool-tip

C2631   Repair device, urinary, incontinence, without sling graft

C2632   Brachytherapy solution, iodine-125, per MCI

C2633   Brachytherapy source, cesium-131, per source

▲**C2634**   Brachytherapy source, high activity, iodine-125, greater than 1.01 mci (nist), per source

Not valid for Medicare   Non-covered by Medicare   Special coverage instructions   Carrier discretion

▲ **C2635** Brachytherapy source, high activity, paladium-103, greater than 2.2 mci (nist), per source

C2636 Brachytherapy linear source, paladium-103, per 1mm

● **C2637** Brachytherapy source, ytterbium-169, per source

C8900 Magnetic resonance angiography with contrast, abdomen

C8901 Magnetic resonance angiography without contrast, abdomen

C8902 Magnetic resonance angiography without contrast followed by with contrast, abdomen

C8903 Magnetic resonance imaging with contrast, breast; unilateral

C8904 Magnetic resonance imaging without contrast, breast; unilateral

C8905 Magnetic resonance imaging without contrast followed by with contrast, breast; unilateral

C8906 Magnetic resonance imaging with contrast, breast; bilateral

C8907 Magnetic resonance imaging without contrast, breast; bilateral

C8908 Magnetic resonance imaging without contrast followed by with contrast, breast; bilateral

C8909 Magnetic resonance angiography with contrast, chest (excluding myocardium)

C8910 Magnetic resonance angiography without contrast, chest (excluding myocardium)

C8911 Magnetic resonance angiography without contrast followed by with contrast, chest (excluding myocardium)

C8912 Magnetic resonance angiography with contrast, lower extremity

C8913 Magnetic resonance angiography without contrast, lower extremity

C8914   Magnetic resonance angiography without contrast followed by with contrast, lower extremity

C8918   Magnetic resonance angiography with contrast, pelvis

C8919   Magentic resonance angiography without contrast, pelvis

C8920   Magnetic resonance angiography without contrast followed by with contrast, pelvis

(C9000)   Code deleted December 31, 2005; use A9553

C9003   Palivizumab-rsv-igm, per 50 mg

(C9007)   Code deleted December 31, 2005; use J0476

(C9008)   Code deleted December 31, 2005; use J0475

(C9009)   Code deleted December 31, 2005; use J0475

(C9013)   Code delcted December 31, 2005

(C9102)   Code deleted December 31, 2005; use A9553

(C9103)   Code deleted December 31, 2005; use A9554

(C9105)   Code deleted December 31, 2005; use 90371

(C9109)   Code deleted December 31, 2004; use J3246

(C9112)   Code deleted December 31, 2005; use Q9957

C9113   Injection, pantoprazole sodium, per vial

C9121   Injection, argatroban, per 5 mg

(C9123)   Code deleted December 31, 2005

(C9124)   Code deleted December 31, 2004; use J0878

(C9125)   Code deleted December 31, 2004; use J2794

(C9200)   Code deleted December 31, 2005; use J7340

(C9201)   Code deleted December 31, 2005; use J7342

(**C9202**) Code deleted December 31, 2005; use Q9956

(**C9203**) Code deleted December 31, 2005; use Q9955

(**C9205**) Code deleted December 31, 2005; use J9263

(**C9207**) Code deleted December 31, 2004; use J9041

(**C9208**) Code deleted December 31, 2004; use J0180

(**C9209**) Code deleted December 31, 2004; use J1931

(**C9210**) Code deleted December 31, 2004; use J2469

(**C9211**) Code deleted December 31, 2005; use J0215

(**C9212**) Code deleted December 31, 2005; use J0215

(**C9213**) Code deleted December 31, 2004; use J9305

(**C9214**) Code deleted December 31, 2004; use J9035

(**C9215**) Code deleted December 31, 2004; use J9055

(**C9216**) Code deleted December 31, 2004; use J0128

(**C9217**) Code deleted December 31, 2004; use J2357

(**C9218**) Code deleted December 31, 2005; use J9025

(**C9219**) Code deleted December 31, 2004; use J7518

● **C9224** Injection, galsulfase, per 5 mg

● **C9225** Injection, fluocinolone acetonide intravitreal implant, per 0.59 mg

C9399 Unclassified drugs or biologicals

(**C9400**) Code deleted December 31, 2005; use A9505

(**C9401**) Code deleted December 31, 2005; use A9600

(**C9402**) Code deleted December 31, 2005; use A9517

(**C9403**) Code deleted December 31, 2005; use A9528

(C9404)   Code deleted December 31, 2005; use A9529

(C9405)   Code deleted December 31, 2005; use A9530

(C9410)   Code deleted December 31, 2005; use J1190

(C9411)   Code deleted December 31, 2005; use J2430

(C9412)   Code deleted December 31, 2004; use J7310

(C9413)   Code deleted December 31, 2005; use J7317

(C9414)   Code deleted December 31, 2005; use J8560

(C9415)   Code deleted December 31, 2005; use J9000

(C9417)   Code deleted December 31, 2005; use J9040

(C9418)   Code deleted December 31, 2005; use J9060

(C9419)   Code deleted December 31, 2005; use J9065

(C9420)   Code deleted December 31, 2005; use J9070

(C9421)   Code deleted December 31, 2005; use J9093

(C9422)   Code deleted December 31, 2005; use J9100

(C9423)   Code deleted December 31, 2005; use J9130

(C9424)   Code deleted December 31, 2005; use J9150

(C9425)   Code deleted December 31, 2005; use J9181

(C9426)   Code deleted December 31, 2005; use J9200

(C9427)   Code deleted December 31, 2005; use J9208

(C9428)   Code deleted December 31, 2005; use J9209

(C9429)   Code deleted December 31, 2005; use J9211

(C9430   Code deleted December 31, 2005; use J9218

(C9431)   Code deleted December 31, 2005; use J9265

Not valid
for Medicare

Non-covered
by Medicare

Special
coverage
instructions

Carrier
discretion

79

(C9432)   Code deleted December 31, 2005; use J9280

(C9433)   Code deleted December 31, 2005; use J9340

(C9438)   Code deleted December 31, 2005; use J7502

(C9701)   Code deleted December 31, 2004; use CPT

(C9703)   Code deleted December 31, 2004; use CPT

(C9704)   Code deleted December 31, 2005; use 0133T

(C9712)   Code deleted December 31, 2004; use 91035

(C9713)   Code deleted December 31, 2005; use 52648

(C9714)   Code deleted December 31, 2004; use 19297

(C9715)   Code deleted December 31, 2004; use 19296

C9716   Creations of thermal anal lesions by radiofrequency energy

(C9717)   Code deleted December 31, 2004; use 46947

● C9723   Dynamic infrared blood perfusion imaging (diri)

● C9724   Endoscopic full-thickness plication in the gastric cardia using endoscopic plication system (eps); includes endoscopy

● C9725   Placement of endorectal intracavitary applicator for high intensity brachytherapy

DENTAL PROCEDURES

Guidelines

In addition to the information presented in the INTRODUCTION, several other items unique to this section are defined or identified here:

1. SUBSECTION INFORMATION: Some of the listed subheadings or subsections have special needs or instructions unique to that section. Where these are indicated, special "notes" will be presented preceding or following the listings. Those subsections within the DENTAL PROCEDURES section that have "notes" are as follows:

Subsection	Code Numbers
Root canal therapy	D3310-D3350
Surgical services	D4210-D4274
Complete dentures	D5110-D5140
Partial dentures	D5211-D5281
Extraoral prostheses	D5911-D5921
Prosthodontics, fixed	D6200-D6999
Oral surgery	D7000-D7999
Complicated suturing	D7911-D7912
Professional consultation	D9310

2. UNLISTED SERVICE OR PROCEDURE: A service or procedure may be provided that is not listed in this edition of HCPCS. When reporting such a service, the appropriate "unlisted procedure" code may be used to indicate the service, identifying it by "special report" as defined below. HCPCS terminology is inconsistent in defining unlisted procedures. The procedure definition may include the term(s) "unlisted", "not otherwise classified", "unspecified", "unclassified", "other" and "miscellaneous". Prior to using these codes, try to determine if a Local Level III code or CPT code is available. The "unlisted procedures" and accompanying codes for DENTAL PROCEDURES are as follows:

D0502	Other oral pathology procedures, by report
D0999	Unspecified diagnostic procedure, by report
D2999	Unspecified restorative procedure, by report
D3999	Unspecified endodontic procedure, by report
D4999	Unspecified periodontal procedure, by report
D5899	Unspecified removable prosthodontic procedure, by report
D5999	Unspecified maxillofacial prosthesis, by report
D6199	Unspecified implant procedure, by report
D6999	Unspecified, fixed prosthodontic procedure, by report

Not valid for Medicare   Non-covered by Medicare   Special coverage instructions   Carrier discretion

D7899	Unspecified TMD therapy, by report
D7999	Unspecified oral surgery procedure, by report
D8999	Unspecified orthodontic procedure, by report
D9999	Unspecified adjunctive procedure, by report

3. SPECIAL REPORT: A service, material or supply that is rarely provided, unusual, variable or new may require a special report in determining medical appropriateness for reimbursement purposes. Pertinent information should include an adequate definition or description of the nature, extent, and need for the service, material or supply.

4. MODIFIERS: Listed services may be modified under certain circumstances. When appropriate, the modifying circumstance is identified by adding a modifier to the basic procedure code. CPT and HCPCS National Level II modifiers may be used with CPT and HCPCS National Level II procedure codes. Modifiers commonly used with DENTAL PROCEDURES are as follows:

-CC Procedure code change (use "CC" when the procedure code submitted was changed either for administrative reasons or because an incorrect code was filed)

-ET Emergency services (dental procedures performed in emergency situations should show the modifier -ET)

-LT Left side (used to identify procedures performed on the left side of the body)

(-QB) Code deleted December 31, 2005

(-QU) Code deleted December 31, 2005

-RT Right side (used to identify procedures performed on the right side of the body)

-TC Technical component. Under certain circumstances, a charge may be made for the technical component alone. Under these circumstances, the technical component charge is identified by adding the modifier -TC to the usual procedure number. Technical component charges are institutional charges and not billed separately by physicians. However, portable x-ray suppliers only bill for technical component and should utilize modifier -TC. The charge data from portable x-ray suppliers will then be used to build customary and prevailing profiles.

5. CPT CODE CROSS-REFERENCE: Unless specified otherwise, there are no equivalent CPT codes for listings in this section.

6. CDT CODES: Dental procedures are reported to non-Medicare carriers using Common Dental Terminology (CDT), published by the American Dental Association (ADA).

Dental Procedures

I. DIAGNOSTIC PROCEDURES (D0100-D0999)

CLINICAL ORAL EXAMINATIONS

D0120 Periodic oral evaluation

D0140 Limited oral evaluation - problem focused

D0150 Comprehensive oral evaluation - new or established patient
CIM: 50-26 MCM: 2136, 2336

D0160 Detailed and extensive oral evaluation - problem focused, by report

D0170 Re-evaluation - limited, problem focused (established patient; not post-operative visit)

D0180 Comprehensive periodontal evaluation - new or established patient

RADIOGRAPHS/DIAGNOSTIC IMAGING

D0210 Intraoral; complete series (including bitewings)

D0220 periapical - first film

D0230 periapical - each additional film

D0240 occlusal film
MCM: 2136, 2336

D0250 Extraoral; first film
MCM: 2136, 2336

D0260 each additional film
MCM: 2136, 2336

D0270   Bitewing(s); single film
MCM: 2136, 2336

D0272   two films
MCM: 2136, 2336

D0274   four films
MCM: 2136, 2336

D0277   Vertical bitewings; 7 to 8 films
MCM: 2136, 2336

D0290   Posterior-anterior or lateral skull and facial bone, survey film

D0310   Sialography

D0320   Temporomandibular joint arthrogram, including injection

D0321   Other temporomandibular joint films, by report

D0322   Tomographic survey
CIM: 50-26

D0330   Panoramic film

D0340   Cephalometric film

D0350   Oral/facial photographic images

TESTS AND LABORATORY EXAMINATIONS

D0415   Collection of microorganisms for culture and sensitivity

D0416   Viral culture

D0421   Genetic test for susceptibility to oral diseases

D0425   Caries susceptibility tests

D0431   Adjunctive pre-diagnostic test that aids in detection of mucosal abnormalities including premalignant and malignant lesions, not to include cytology or biopsy procedures

D0460   Pulp vitality tests
CIM: 50-26   MCM: 2136, 2336

D0470 Diagnostic casts

ORAL PATHOLOGY LABORATORY
(USE CODES D0472-D0474)

D0472 Accession of tissue; gross examination, preparation and transmission of written report
CIM: 50-26   MCM: 2136, 2336

D0473 gross and microscopic examination, preparation and transmission of written report
CIM: 50-26   MCM: 2136, 2336

D0474 gross and microscopic examination, including assessment of surgical margins for presence of disease, preparation and transmission of written report
CIM: 50-26   MCM: 2136, 2336

D0475 Decalcification procedure

D0476 Special stains for microorganisms

D0477 Special stains, not for microorganisms

D0478 Immunohistochemical stains

D0479 Tissue in-situ hybridization, including interpretation

D0480 Processing and interpretation of exfoliative cytologic smears, including the preparation and transmission of written report
CIM: 50-26   MCM: 2136, 2336

D0481 Electron microscopy - diagnostic

D0482 Direct immunofluorescence

D0483 Indirect immunofluorescence

D0484 Consultation on slides prepared elsewhere

D0485 Consultation, including preparation of slides from biopsy material supplied by referring source

D0502 Other oral pathology procedures, by report
CIM: 50-26   MCM: 2136, 2336

Not valid for Medicare   Non-covered by Medicare   Special coverage instructions   Carrier discretion

D0999 Unspecified diagnostic procedure, by report
CIM: 50-26   MCM: 2136, 2336

II. PREVENTIVE (D1000-D1999)

DENTAL PROPHYLAXIS

D1110 Prophylaxis; adult

D1120   child

TOPICAL FLUORIDE TREATMENT (OFFICE PROCEDURE)

D1201 Topical application of fluoride (including prophylaxis); child

D1203 Topical application of fluoride (prophylaxis not included); child

D1204   adult

D1205 Topical application of fluoride (including prophylaxis); adult

OTHER PREVENTIVE SERVICES

D1310 Nutritional counseling for control of dental disease
MCM: 2300

D1320 Tobacco counseling for the control and prevention of oral disease
MCM: 2300

D1330 Oral hygiene instructions
MCM: 2300

D1351 Sealant - per tooth

SPACE MAINTENANCE (PASSIVE APPLIANCES)

D1510 Space maintainer; fixed-unilateral
MCM: 2336

D1515   fixed-bilateral
MCM: 2336, 2136

D1520   removable-unilateral
MCM: 2336, 2136

D1525   removable-bilateral
MCM: 2336, 2136

D1550   Recementation of space maintainer
MCM: 2336, 2136

III. RESTORATIVE PROCEDURES (D2000-D2999)

AMALGAM RESTORATIONS (INCLUDING POLISHING)

D2140   Amalgam; one surface, primary or permanent

D2150   two surfaces, primary or permanent

D2160   three surfaces, primary or permanent

D2161   four or more surfaces, primary or permanent

RESIN-BASED COMPOSITE RESTORATIONS

D2330   Resin-based composite; one surface, anterior

D2331   two surfaces, anterior

D2332   three surfaces, anterior

D2335   four or more surfaces or involving incisal angle (anterior)

D2390   Resin-based composite crown, anterior

D2391   Resin-based composite - one surface, posterior

D2392   Resin-based composite - two surfaces, posterior

D2393   Resin-based composite - three surfaces, posterior

D2394   Resin-based composite - four or more surfaces, posterior

GOLD FOIL RESTORATIONS

D2410   Gold foil; one surface

D2420   two surfaces

| | Not valid for Medicare | | Non-covered by Medicare | Special coverage instructions | | Carrier discretion | **87** |

D2430	three surfaces

INLAY/ONLAY RESTORATIONS

D2510	Inlay - metallic; one surface
D2520	two surfaces
D2530	three or more surfaces
D2542	Onlay - metallic; two surfaces
D2543	three surfaces
D2544	four or more surfaces
D2610	Inlay - porcelain/ceramic; one surface
D2620	two surfaces
D2630	three or more surfaces
D2642	Onlay - porcelain/ceramic; two surfaces
D2643	three surfaces
D2644	four or more surfaces
D2650	Inlay - resin-based composite; one surface
D2651	two surfaces
D2652	three or more surfaces
D2662	Onlay - resin-based composite; two surfaces
D2663	three surfaces
D2664	four or more surfaces

CROWNS - SINGLE RESTORATIONS ONLY

D2710	Crown - resin-based composite (indirect)
D2712	Crown - 3/4 resin-based composite (indirect)

D2720	resin with high noble metal
D2721	resin with predominantly base metal
D2722	resin with noble metal
D2740	porcelain/ceramic substrate
D2750	porcelain fused to high noble metal
D2751	porcelain fused to predominantly base metal
D2752	porcelain fused to noble metal
D2780	3/4 cast high noble metal
D2781	3/4 cast predominantly base metal
D2782	3/4 cast noble metal
D2783	3/4 porcelain/ceramic
D2790	full cast high noble metal
D2791	full cast predominantly base metal
D2792	full cast noble metal
D2794	Crown-titanium
D2799	Provisional crown

OTHER RESTORATIVE SERVICES

D2910	Recement inlay, onlay or partial coverage restoration
D2915	Recement cast or prefabricated post and core
D2920	Recement crown
D2930	Prefabricated stainless steel crown; primary tooth
D2931	permanent tooth
D2932	Prefabricated resin crown

Not valid for Medicare   Non-covered by Medicare   Special coverage instructions   Carrier discretion

D2933   Prefabricated stainless steel crown with resin window

D2934   Prefabricated esthetic coated stainless steel crown - primary tooth

D2940   Sedative filling

D2950   Crown build-up, including any pins

D2951   Pin retention - per tooth, in addition to restoration

D2952   Cast post and core in addition to crown

D2953   Each additional cast post - same tooth

D2954   Prefabricated post and core in addition to crown

D2955   Post removal (not in conjunction with endodontic therapy)

D2957   Each additional prefabricated post — same tooth (to be used with D2954)

D2960   Labial veneer (resin laminate); chairside

D2961   Labial veneer (resin laminate); laboratory

D2962   Labial veneer (porcelain laminate); laboratory

(D2970)   Code deleted December 31, 2004; use CPT

D2971   Additional procedures to construct new crown under existing partial denture framework

D2975   Coping

D2980   Crown repair, by report

D2999   Unspecified restorative procedure, by report
MCM: 2336, 2136

IV. ENDODONTICS (D3000-D3999)

PULP CAPPING

D3110   Pulp cap; direct (excluding final restoration)

   ●   New code   ▲   Revised code   ( )   Deleted code

D3120   indirect (excluding final restoration)

PULPOTOMY

D3220   Therapeutic pulpotomy (excluding final restoration); removal of pulp coronal to the dentinocemental junction and application of medicament

D3221   Pulpal debridement, primary and permanent teeth

ENDODONTIC THERAPY ON PRIMARY TEETH

D3230   Pulpal therapy (resorbable filling); anterior, primary tooth (excluding final restoration)

D3240   posterior, primary tooth (excluding final restoration)

ENDODONTIC THERAPY (INCLUDING TREATMENT PLAN, CLINICAL PROCEDURES AND FOLLOW-UP CARE)

D3310   Anterior (excluding final restoration)

D3320   Bicuspid (excluding final restoration)

D3330   Molar (excluding final restoration)

D3331   Treatment of root canal obstruction; non-surgical access

D3332   Incomplete endodontic therapy; inoperable, unrestorable or fractured tooth

D3333   Internal root repair of perforation defects

ENDODONTIC RETREATMENT

D3346   Retreatment of previous root canal therapy; anterior

D3347   bicuspid

D3348   molar

APEXICATION/RECALCIFICATION PROCEDURES

D3351   Apexification/recalcification; initial visit (apical closure/calcific repair of perforations, root resorption, etc.)

D3352	interim medication replacement (apical closure/calcific repair of perforations, root resorption, etc.)
D3353	final visit (includes completed root canal therapy, apical closure/calcific repair of perforations, root resorption, etc.)

APICOECTOMY/PERIRADICULAR SERVICES

D3410	Apicoectomy/periradicular surgery; anterior
D3421	bicuspid (first root)
D3425	molar (first root)
D3426	(each additional root)
D3430	Retrograde filling - per root
D3450	Root amputation - per root
D3460	Endodontic endosseous implant MCM: 2336, 2136
D3470	Intentional reimplantation (including necessary splinting)

OTHER ENDODONTIC PROCEDURES

D3910	Surgical procedure for isolation of tooth with rubber dam
D3920	Hemisection (including any root removal), not including root canal therapy
D3950	Canal preparation and fitting of preformed dowel or post
D3999	Unspecified endodontic procedure, by report MCM: 2336, 2136

V. PERIODONTICS (D4000-D4999)

SURGICAL SERVICES (INCLUDING USUAL POSTOPERATIVE CARE)

D4210	Gingivectomy or gingivoplasty - four or more contiguous teeth or bounded teeth spaces per quadrant

D4211 one to three contiguous teeth or bounded teeth spaces per quadrant

D4240 Gingival flap procedure, including root planing - four or more contiguous teeth or bounded teeth spaces, per quadrant

D4241 one to three contiguous teeth or bounded teeth spaces, per quadrant

D4245 Apically positioned flap

D4249 Clinical crown lengthening; hard tissue

D4260 Osseous surgery (including flap entry and closure) - four or more contiguous teeth or bounded teeth spaces, per quadrant
MCM: 2136, 2336

D4261 Osseous surgery (including flap entry and closure) - one to three contiguous teeth or bounded teeth spaces per quadrant

D4263 Bone replacement graft; first site in quadrant
CIM: 50-26 MCM: 2336, 2136

D4264 each additional site in quadrant
CIM: 50-26 MCM: 2336, 2136

D4265 Biologic materials to aid in soft and osseous tissue regeneration

D4266 Guided tissue regeneration; resorbable barrier, per site

D4267 non-resorbable barrier, per site (includes membrane removal)

D4268 Surgical revision procedure, per tooth
MCM: 2136, 2336

D4270 Pedicle soft tissue graft procedure
MCM: 2336, 2136

D4271 Free soft tissue graft procedure (including donor site surgery)
MCM: 2336, 2136

D4273 Subepithelial connective tissue graft procedures, per tooth
CIM: 50-26 MCM: 2136, 2336

| Not valid for Medicare | Non-covered by Medicare | Special coverage instructions | Carrier discretion |

D4274 Distal or proximal wedge procedure (when not performed in conjunction with surgical procedures in the same anatomical area)

D4275 Soft tissue allograft

D4276 Combined connective tissue and double pedicle graft, per tooth

NON-SURGICAL PERIODONTAL SERVICES

D4320 Provisional splinting; intracoronal

D4321 extracoronal

D4341 Periodontal scaling and root planing - four or more teeth per quadrant

D4342 Periodontal scaling and root planing - one to three teeth, per quadrant

D4355 Full mouth debridement to enable comprehensive evaluation and diagnosis
CIM: 50-26   MCM: 2136, 2336

D4381 Localized delivery of antimicrobial agents via a controlled release vehicle into diseased crevicular tissue, per tooth, by report
CIM: 50-26   MCM: 2136, 2336

OTHER PERIODONTIC SERVICES

D4910 Periodontal maintenance

D4920 Unscheduled dressing change (by someone other than treating dentist)

D4999 Unspecified periodontal procedure, by report

VI. PROSTHODONTICS (REMOVABLE) (D5000-D5899)

COMPLETE DENTURES (INCLUDING ROUTINE POST-DELIVERY CARE)

D5110 Complete denture; maxillary

D5120 mandibular

● New code   ▲ Revised code   ( ) Deleted code

D5130   Immediate denture; maxillary

D5140   mandibular

PARTIAL DENTURES (INCLUDING ROUTINE POST-DELIVERY CARE)

D5211   Maxillary (upper) partial denture; resin base (including any conventional clasps, rests and teeth)

D5212   Mandibular (lower) partial denture; resin base (including any conventional clasps, rests and teeth)

D5213   Maxillary partial denture; cast metal framework with resin denture bases (including any conventional clasps, rests and teeth)

D5214   Mandibular partial denture; cast metal framework with resin denture bases (including any conventional clasps, rests and teeth)

D5225   Maxillary partial denture - flexible base (including any clasps, rests and teeth)

D5226   Mandibular partial denture - flexible base (including any clasps, rests and teeth)

D5281   Removable unilateral partial denture; one piece cast metal (including clasps and teeth)

ADJUSTMENTS TO DENTURES

D5410   Adjust complete denture; maxillary

D5411   mandibular

D5421   Adjust partial denture; maxillary

D5422   mandibular

REPAIRS TO COMPLETE DENTURES

D5510   Repair broken complete denture base

D5520   Replace missing or broken teeth - complete denture (each tooth)

Not valid for Medicare   Non-covered by Medicare   Special coverage instructions   Carrier discretion

REPAIRS TO PARTIAL DENTURES

D5610 Repair resin denture base

D5620 Repair cast framework

D5630 Repair or replace broken clasp

D5640 Replace broken teeth - per tooth

D5650 Add tooth to existing partial denture

D5660 Add clasp to existing partial denture

D5670 Replace all teeth and acrylic on cast metal framework (maxillary)

D5671 Replace all teeth and acrylic on cast metal framework (mandibular)

DENTURE REBASE PROCEDURES

D5710 Rebase complete maxillary denture

D5711 Rebase complete mandibular denture

D5720 Rebase maxillary partial denture

D5721 Rebase mandibular partial denture

DENTURE RELINE PROCEDURES

D5730 Reline complete maxillary denture (chairside)

D5731 Reline complete mandibular denture (chairside)

D5740 Reline maxillary partial denture (chairside)

D5741 Reline mandibular partial denture (chairside)

D5750 Reline complete maxillary denture (laboratory)

D5751 Reline complete mandibular denture (laboratory)

D5760 Reline maxillary partial denture (laboratory)

D5761   Reline mandibular partial denture (laboratory)

INTERIM PROSTHESIS

D5810   Interim complete denture (maxillary)

D5811   Interim complete denture (mandibular)

D5820   Interim partial denture (maxillary)

D5821   Interim partial denture (mandibular)

OTHER REMOVABLE PROSTHETIC SERVICES

D5850   Tissue conditioning; maxillary

D5851   mandibular

D5860   Overdenture; complete, by report

D5861   partial, by report

D5862   Precision attachment, by report

D5867   Replacement of replaceable part of semi-precision or precision attachment (male or female component)

D5875   Modification of removable prosthesis following implant surgery

D5899   Unspecified removable prosthodontic procedure, by report

VII. MAXILLOFACIAL PROSTHETICS (D5900-D5999)

D5911   Facial moulage (sectional)
MCM: 2130.A, 2136

D5912   Facial moulage (complete)
MCM: 2130.A

D5913   Nasal prosthesis

D5914   Auricular prosthesis

D5915   Orbital prosthesis

D5916   Ocular prosthesis

Not valid   Non-covered   Special   Carrier   **97**
for Medicare   by Medicare   coverage   discretion
                                    instructions

D5919 Facial prosthesis

D5922 Nasal septal prosthesis

D5923 Ocular prosthesis, interim

D5924 Cranial prosthesis

D5925 Facial augmentation implant prosthesis

D5926 Nasal prosthesis, replacement

D5927 Auricular prosthesis, replacement

D5928 Orbital prosthesis, replacement

D5929 Facial prosthesis, replacement

D5931 Obturator prosthesis; surgical

D5932 definitive

D5933 modification

D5934 Mandibular resection prosthesis with guide flange

D5935 Mandibular resection prosthesis without guide flange

D5936 Obturator prosthesis, interim

D5937 Trismus appliance (not for TM treatment)
MCM: 2130

D5951 Feeding aid
MCM: 2336, 2130

D5952 Speech aid prosthesis; pediatric

D5953 adult

D5954 Palatal augmentation prosthesis

D5955 Palatal lift prosthesis, definitive

D5958 interim

D5959 modification

● New code ▲ Revised code ( ) Deleted code

D5960 Speech aid prosthesis, modification

D5982 Surgical stent

D5983 Radiation carrier
MCM: 2336, 2136

D5984 Radiation shield
MCM: 2336, 2136

D5985 Radiation cone locator
MCM: 2336, 2136

D5986 Fluoride gel carrier
MCM: 2136, 2336

D5987 Commissure splint

D5988 Surgical splint

D5999 Unspecified maxillofacial prosthesis, by report

VIII. IMPLANT SERVICES (D6000-D6199)

D6010 Surgical placement of implant body: endosteal implant

(D6020) Code deleted December 31, 2004; use 21248

D6040 Surgical placement: eposteal implant

D6050 Surgical placement: transosteal implant

IMPLANT SUPPORTED PROSTHETICS

D6053 Implant/abutment supported removable denture for completely edentulous arch
MCM: 2136

D6054 Implant/abutment supported removable denture for partially edentulous arch
MCM: 2136

D6055 Dental implant supported connection bar
MCM: 2136

D6056 Prefabricated abutment - includes placement
MCM: 2136

| | Not valid for Medicare | | Non-covered by Medicare | | Special coverage instructions | | Carrier discretion | **99** |

D6057 Custom abutment - includes placement
MCM: 2136

D6058 Abutment supported porcelain/ceramic crown
MCM: 2136

D6059 Abutment supported porcelain fused to metal crown (high noble metal)
MCM: 2136

D6060 Abutment supported porcelain fused to metal crown (predominantly base metal)
MCM: 2136

D6061 Abutment supported porcelain fused to metal crown (noble metal)
MCM: 2136

D6062 Abutment supported cast metal crown (high noble metal)
MCM: 2136

D6063 Abutment supported cast metal crown (predominantly base metal)
MCM: 2136

D6064 Abutment supported cast metal crown (noble metal)
MCM: 2136

D6065 Implant supported porcelain/ceramic crown
MCM: 2136

D6066 Implant supported porcelain fused to metal crown (titanium, titanium alloy, high noble metal)
MCM: 2136

D6067 Implant supported metal crown (titanium, titanium alloy, high noble metal)
MCM: 2136

D6068 Abutment supported retainer for porcelain/ceramic FPD
MCM: 2136

D6069 Abutment supported retainer for porcelain fused to metal FPD (high noble metal)
MCM: 2136

D6070 Abutment supported retainer for porcelain fused to metal FPD (predominantly base metal)
MCM: 2136

D6071 Abutment supported retainer for porcelain fused to metal FPD (noble metal)
MCM: 2136

D6072 Abutment supported retainer for cast metal FPD (high noble metal)
MCM: 2136

D6073 Abutment supported retainer for cast metal FPD (predominantly base metal)
MCM: 2136

D6074 Abutment supported retainer for cast metal FPD (noble metal)
MCM: 2136

D6075 Implant supported retainer for ceramic FPD
MCM: 2136

D6076 Implant supported retainer for porcelain fused to metal FPD (titanium, titanium alloy, or high noble metal)
MCM: 2136

D6077 Implant supported retainer for cast metal FPD (titanium, titanium alloy, or high noble metal)
MCM: 2136

D6078 Implant/abutment supported fixed denture for completely edentulous arch
MCM: 2136

D6079 Implant/abutment supported fixed denture for partially edentulous arch
MCM: 2136

OTHER IMPLANT SERVICES

D6080 Implant maintenance procedures, including; removal of prosthesis, cleansing of prosthesis and abutment reinsertion of prosthesis
MCM: 2136

D6090 Repair implant supported prosthesis, by report

D6094 Abutment supported crown - (titanium)

D6095 Repair implant abutment, by report

D6100 Implant removal, by report

Not valid for Medicare   Non-covered by Medicare   Special coverage instructions   Carrier discretion

D6190	Radiographic/surgical implant index, by report
D6194	Abutment supported retainer crown for fpd - (titanium)
D6199	Unspecified implant procedure, by report

IX. PROSTHODONTICS, FIXED (EACH RETAINER AND EACH PONTIC CONSTITUTES A UNIT IN A FIXED PARTIAL DENTURE) (D6200-D6999)

FIXED PARTIAL DENTURE PONTICS

D6205	Pontic - indirect resin based composite
D6210	Pontic; cast high noble metal
D6211	cast predominantly base metal
D6212	cast noble metal
D6214	Pontic - titanium
D6240	porcelain fused to high noble metal
D6241	porcelain fused to predominantly base metal
D6242	porcelain fused to noble metal
D6245	porcelain/ceramic MCM: 2136
D6250	resin with high noble metal
D6251	resin base predominantly base metal
D6252	resin with noble metal
D6253	Provisional pontic

FIXED PARTIAL DENTURE RETAINERS - INLAYS/ONLAYS

D6545	Retainer; cast metal for resin bonded fixed prosthesis
D6548	porcelain/ceramic for resin bonded fixed prosthesis MCM: 2136

D6600 Inlay - porcelain/ceramic, two surfaces
MCM: 2136

D6601 Inlay - porcelain/ceramic, three or more surfaces
MCM: 2136

D6602 Inlay - cast high noble metal, two surfaces
MCM: 2136

D6603 Inlay - cast high noble metal, three or more surfaces
MCM: 2136

D6604 Inlay - cast predominantly base metal, two surfaces
MCM: 2136

D6605 Inlay - cast predominantly base metal, three or more surfaces
MCM: 2136

D6606 Inlay - cast noble metal, two surfaces
MCM: 2136

D6607 Inlay - cast noble metal, three or more surfaces
MCM: 2136

D6608 Onlay - porcelain/ceramic, two surfaces
MCM: 2136

D6609 Onlay - porcelain/ceramic, three or more surfaces
MCM: 2136

D6610 Onlay - cast high noble metal, two surfaces
MCM: 2136

D6611 Onlay - cast high noble metal, three or more surfaces
MCM: 2136

D6612 Onlay - cast predominantly base metal, two surfaces
MCM: 2136

D6613 Onlay - cast predominantly base metal, three or more surfaces
MCM: 2136

D6614 Onlay - cast noble metal, two surfaces
MCM: 2136

D6615 Onlay - cast noble metal, three or more surfaces
MCM: 2136

D6624 Inlay - titanium

Not valid   Non-covered   Special   Carrier
for Medicare   by Medicare   coverage   discretion
                                        instructions

D6634   Onlay - titanium

FIXED PARTIAL DENTURE RETAINERS - CROWNS

D6710   Crown - indirect resin based composite

D6720   Crown; resin with high noble metal

D6721   resin with predominantly base metal

D6722   resin with noble metal

D6740   porcelain/ceramic
MCM: 2136

D6750   porcelain fused to high noble metal

D6751   porcelain fused to predominantly base metal

D6752   porcelain fused to noble metal

D6780   3/4 cast high noble metal

D6781   3/4 cast predominantly base metal
MCM: 2136

D6782   3/4 cast noble metal
MCM: 2136

D6783   3/4 porcelain/ceramic
MCM: 2136

D6790   full cast high noble metal

D6791   full cast predominantly base metal

D6792   full cast noble metal

D6793   Provisional retainer crown

D6794'   Crown - titanium

OTHER FIXED PARTIAL DENTURE SERVICES

D6920   Connector bar
CIM: 50-26 MCM: 2336, 2136

D6930   Recement fixed partial denture

D6940   Stress breaker

D6950   Precision attachment

D6970   Cast post and core in addition to fixed partial denture retainer

D6971   Cast post as part of fixed partial denture retainer

D6972   Prefabricated post and core in addition to fixed partial denture retainer

D6973   Core build up for retainer, including any pins

D6975   Coping; metal

D6976   Each additional cast post - same tooth
MCM: 2136

D6977   Each additional prefabricated post - same tooth
MCM: 2136

D6980   Fixed partial denture repair, by report

D6985   Pediatric partial denture, fixed

D6999   Unspecified, fixed prosthodontic procedure, by report

X. ORAL AND MAXILLOFACIAL SURGERY (D7000- D7999)

EXTRACTIONS (INCLUDES LOCAL ANESTHESIA, SUTURING, IF NEEDED, AND ROUTINE POSTOPERATIVE CARE)

D7111   Extraction, coronal remnants - deciduous tooth
MCM: 2336

D7140   Extraction, erupted tooth or exposed root (elevation and/or forceps removal)
MCM: 2336

	Not valid for Medicare		Non-covered by Medicare		Special coverage instructions		Carrier discretion

SURGICAL EXTRACTIONS (INCLUDES LOCAL ANESTHESIA, SUTURING, IF NEEDED, AND ROUTINE POSTOPERATIVE CARE)

D7210 Surgical removal of erupted tooth requiring elevation of mucoperiosteal flap and removal of bone and/or section of tooth
MCM: 2336, 2136

D7220 Removal of impacted tooth; soft tissue
MCM: 2336, 2136

D7230 partially bony
MCM: 2336, 2136

D7240 completely bony
MCM: 2336, 2136

D7241 completely bony, with unusual surgical complications
MCM: 2336, 2136

D7250 Surgical removal of residual tooth roots (cutting procedure)
MCM: 2336, 2136

OTHER SURGICAL PROCEDURES

D7260 Oroantral fistula closure
MCM: 2336, 2136

D7261 Primary closure of a sinus perforation
MCM: 2336

D7270 Tooth reimplantation and/or stabilization of accidentally evulsed or displaced tooth

D7272 Tooth transplantation (includes reimplantation from one site to another and splinting and/or stabilization)

D7280 Surgical access of an unerupted tooth

(D7281) Code deleted December 31, 2004; use CPT

D7282 Mobilization of erupted or malpositioned tooth to aid eruption

D7283 Placement of device to facilitate eruption of impacted tooth

---

● New code ▲ Revised code ( ) Deleted code

D7285 Biopsy of oral tissue; hard (bone, tooth)

D7286 soft

D7287 Exfoliative cytological sample collection

D7288 Brush biopsy - transepithelial sample collection

D7290 Surgical repositioning of teeth

D7291 Transseptal fiberotomy/supra crestal fiberotomy, by report
MCM: 2136, 2336

ALVEOLOPLASTY - SURGICAL PREPARATION OF RIDGE FOR DENTURES

D7310 Alveoloplasty in conjunction with extractions - per quadrant

D7311 Alveoloplasty in conjunction with extractions - one to three teeth or tooth spaces, per quadrant

D7320 Alveoloplasty not in conjunction with extractions - per quadrant

D7321 Alveoloplasty not in conjunction with extractions - one to three teeth or tooth spaces, per quadrant

VESTIBULOPLASTY

D7340 Vestibuloplasty; ridge extension (secondary epithelialization)

D7350 ridge extension (including soft tissue grafts, muscle reattachments, revision of soft tissue attachment and management of hypertrophied and hyperplastic tissue)

SURGICAL EXCISION OF REACTIVE INFLAMMATORY LESIONS (SCAR TISSUE OR LOCALIZED CONGENITAL LESIONS)

D7410 Excision of benign lesion up to 1.25 cm

D7411 Excision of benign lesion greater than 1.25 cm

D7412 Excision of benign lesion, complicated

D7413 Excision of malignant lesion up to 1.25 cm

D7414 Excision of malignant lesion greater than 1.25 cm

D7415 Excision of malignant lesion, complicated

REMOVAL OF TUMORS, CYSTS, AND NEOPLASMS

D7440 Excision of malignant tumor; lesion diameter up to 1.25 cm

D7441 lesion diameter greater than 1.25 cm

D7450 Removal of benign odontogenic cyst or tumor; lesion diameter up to 1.25 cm

D7451 lesion diameter greater than 1.25 cm

D7460 Removal of benign nonodontogenic cyst or tumor; lesion diameter up to 1.25 cm

D7461 lesion diameter greater than 1.25 cm

D7465 Destruction of lesion(s) by physical methods, by report

EXCISION OF BONE TISSUE

D7471 Removal of lateral exostosis (maxilla or mandible)

D7472 Removal of torus palatinus

D7473 Removal of torus mandibularis

D7485 Surgical reduction of osseous tuberosity

D7490 Radical resection of maxilla or mandible

SURGICAL INCISION

D7510 Incision and drainage of abscess; intraoral soft tissue

D7511 Incision and drainage of abscess - intraoral soft tissue - complicated (includes drainage of multiple fascial spaces)

D7520 extraoral soft tissue

D7521 Incision and drainage of abscess - extraoral soft tissue - complicated (includes drainage of multiple fascial spaces)

D7530 Removal of foreign body from mucosa, skin, or subcutaneous alveolar tissue

D7540 Removal of reaction-producing foreign bodies, musculoskeletal system

D7550 Partial ostectomy/sequestrectomy for removal of non-vital bone

D7560 Maxillary sinusotomy for removal of tooth fragment or foreign body

TREATMENT OF FRACTURES - SIMPLE

D7610 Maxilla; open reduction (teeth immobilized, if present)

D7620 closed reduction (teeth immobilized, if present)

D7630 Mandible; open reduction (teeth immobilized, if present)

D7640 closed reduction (teeth immobilized, if present)

D7650 Malar and/or zygomatic arch; open reduction

D7660 closed reduction

D7670 Alveolus - closed reduction, may include stabilization of teeth

D7671 Alveolus - open reduction, may include stabilization of teeth

D7680 Facial bones - complicated reduction with fixation and multiple surgical approaches

TREATMENT OF FRACTURES - COMPOUND

D7710 Maxilla; open reduction

D7720 closed reduction

D7730 Mandible; open reduction

| Not valid for Medicare | Non-covered by Medicare | Special coverage instructions | Carrier discretion |

D7740 closed reduction

D7750 Malar and/or zygomatic arch; open reduction

D7760 closed reduction

D7770 Alveolus - open reduction stabilization of teeth

D7771 Alveolus - closed reduction stabilization of teeth

D7780 Facial bones - complicated reduction with fixation and multiple surgical approaches

REDUCTION OF DISLOCATION AND MANAGEMENT OF OTHER TEMPOROMANDIBULAR JOINT DYSFUNCTIONS

D7810 Open reduction of dislocation

D7820 Closed reduction of dislocation

D7830 Manipulation under anesthesia

D7840 Condylectomy

D7850 Surgical discectomy, with/without implant

D7852 Disc repair

D7854 Synovectomy

D7856 Myotomy

D7858 Joint reconstruction

D7860 Arthrotomy
MCM: 2336, 2136

D7865 Arthroplasty

D7870 Arthrocentesis

D7871 Non-arthroscopic lysis and lavage

D7872 Arthroscopy - diagnosis, with or without biopsy

D7873 Arthroscopy - surgical; lavage and lysis of adhesions

D7874 disc repositioning and stabilization

D7875 synovectomy

D7876 discectomy

D7877 debridement

D7880 Occlusal orthotic device, by report

D7899 Unspecified TMD therapy, by report

REPAIR OF TRAUMATIC WOUNDS

D7910 Suture of recent small wounds up to 5 cm

COMPLICATED SUTURING (RECONSTRUCTION REQUIRING DELICATE HANDLING OF TISSUES AND WIDE UNDERMINING FOR METICULOUS CLOSURE)

D7911 Complicated suture; up to 5 cm

D7912 greater than 5 cm

OTHER REPAIR PROCEDURES

D7920 Skin graft (identify defect covered, location, and type of graft)

D7940 Osteoplasty - for orthognathic deformities
MCM: 2336, 2136

D7941 Osteotomy; mandibular rami

D7943 Osteotomy; mandibular rami with bone graft; includes obtaining the graft

D7944 segmented or subapical - per sextant or quadrant

D7945 body of mandible

D7946 LeFort I (maxilla - total)

D7947 LeFort I (maxilla - segmented)

D7948 LeFort II or LeFort III (osteoplasty of facial bones for midface hypoplasia or retrusion); without bone graft

D7949 LeFort II or LeFort III; with bone graft

D7950 Osseous, osteoperiosteal, or cartilage graft of the mandible or facial bones - autogeneous or nonautogeneous, by report

D7953 Bone replacement graft for ridge preservation - per site

D7955 Repair of maxillofacial soft and/or hard tissue defect

D7960 Frenulectomy (frenectomy or frenotomy) - separate procedure

D7963 Frenuloplasty

D7970 Excision of hyperplastic tissue - per arch

D7971 Excision of pericoronal gingiva

D7972 Surgical reduction of fibrous tuberosity

D7980 Sialolithotomy

D7981 Excision of salivary gland, by report

D7982 Sialodochoplasty

D7983 Closure of salivary fistula

D7990 Emergency tracheotomy

D7991 Coronoidectomy

D7995 Synthetic graft - mandible or facial bones, by report

D7996 Implant-mandible for augmentation purposes (excluding alveolar ridge), by report

D7997 Appliance removal (not by dentist who placed appliance), includes removal of archbar

D7999 Unspecified oral surgery procedure, by report

XI. ORTHODONTICS (D8000-D8999)

LIMITED ORTHODONTIC TREATMENT

D8010 Limited orthodontic treatment; of the primary dentition

D8020 of the transitional dentition

D8030 of the adolescent dentition

D8040 of the adult dentition

INTERCEPTIVE ORTHODONTIC TREATMENT

D8050 Interceptive orthodontic treatment; of the primary dentition

D8060 of the transitional dentition

COMPREHENSIVE ORTHODONTIC TREATMENT

D8070 Comprehensive orthodontic treatment; of the transitional dentition

D8080 of the adolescent dentition

D8090 of the adult dentition

MINOR TREATMENT TO CONTROL HARMFUL HABITS

D8210 Removable appliance therapy

D8220 Fixed appliance therapy

OTHER ORTHODONTIC SERVICES

D8660 Pre-orthodontic visit

D8670 Periodic orthodontic treatment visit (as part of contract)

D8680 Orthodontic retention (removal of appliances, construction and placement of retainer(s))

D8690 Orthodontic treatment (alternative billing to a contract fee)

D8691 Repair of orthodontic appliance

D8692 Replacement of lost or broken retainer

D8999 Unspecified orthodontic procedure, by report

XII. ADJUNCTIVE GENERAL SERVICES (D9000-D9999)

UNCLASSIFIED TREATMENT

D9110 Palliative (emergency) treatment of dental pain - minor procedures
MCM: 2336, 2136

ANESTHESIA

D9210 Local anesthesia not in conjunction with operative or surgical procedures

D9211 Regional block anesthesia

D9212 Trigeminal division block anesthesia

D9215 Local anesthesia

D9220 Deep sedation/general anesthesia; first 30 minutes

D9221 each additional 15 minutes
MCM: 2136, 2336

D9230 Analgesia, anxiolysis, inhalation of nitrous oxide
MCM: 2136, 2336

D9241 Intravenous conscious sedation/analgesia; first 30 minutes

D9242 each additional 15 minutes

D9248 Non-intravenous conscious sedation

PROFESSIONAL CONSULTATION

D9310 Consultation (diagnostic service provided by dentist or physician other than practitioner providing treatment)

PROFESSIONAL VISITS

D9410 House/extended care facility call

D9420 Hospital call

D9430 Office visit for observation (during regularly scheduled hours) - no other services performed

D9440 Office visit - after regularly scheduled hours

D9450 Case presentation, detailed and extensive treatment planning

DRUGS

D9610 Therapeutic drug injection, by report

D9630 Other drugs and/or medicaments, by report
MCM: 2336, 2136

MISCELLANEOUS SERVICES

D9910 Application of desensitizing medicament

D9911 Application of desensitizing resin for cervical and/or root surface, per tooth

D9920 Behavior management, by report

D9930 Treatment of complications (post-surgical) - unusual circumstances, by report
MCM: 2336, 2136

D9940 Occlusal guard, by report
MCM: 2336, 2136

D9941 Fabrication of athletic mouthguards

D9942 Repair and/or reline of occlusal guard

D9950 Occlusion analysis; mounted case
MCM: 2336, 2136

D9951 Occlusal adjustment; limited
MCM: 2336, 2136

D9952 complete
MCM: 2336, 2136

D9970 Enamel microabrasion

D9971 Odontoplasty 1-2 teeth; includes removal of enamel projections

D9972 External bleaching; per arch

D9973 per tooth

D9974 Internal bleaching; per tooth

D9999 Unspecified adjunctive procedure, by report

NOTE: The Noble Metal Classification System has been adopted as a more precise method of reporting various alloys used in dentistry. The alloys are defined on the basis of the percentage of Noble Metal Content.

DURABLE MEDICAL EQUIPMENT

Guidelines

In addition to the information presented in the INTRODUCTION, several other items unique to this section are defined or identified here:

1. DEFINITION OF DURABLE MEDICAL EQUIPMENT: Durable medical equipment (DME) can withstand repeated use and is used primarily to serve a medical purpose. It generally is not useful in the absence of an illness or injury, and is appropriate for use in the home. Expendable medical supplies, such as incontinent pads, lamb's wool pads, catheters, ace bandages, elastic stockings, surgical face masks, irrigating kits, sheets and bags, are not considered to be DME.

2. REASONABLE AND NECESSARY: DME may not be covered in every instance. The equipment must be reasonable and necessary for the illness or injury being treated or for improving the functioning of a malformed body part. A physician's prescription is normally sufficient to establish that the equipment is necessary. To determine reasonableness, the following conditions must be met: the expense must be proportionate to the therapeutic benefits of using the equipment; the cost must not substantially exceed a medically appropriate care plan; and, the item must not serve the same purpose as equipment already available to the patient. Claims for items that are not reasonable will be denied except when it is determined that no alternative plan of care is available for which payment could be made.

3. SUBSECTION INFORMATION: Some of the listed subheadings or subsections have special needs or instructions unique to that section. Where these are indicated, special "notes" will be presented preceding or following the listings. Those subsections within the DURABLE MEDICAL EQUIPMENT section that have "notes" are as follows:

Subsection	Code Numbers
Artificial kidney machines and accessories	E1510-E1699

4. UNLISTED SERVICE OR PROCEDURE: A service or procedure may be provided that is not listed in this edition of HCPCS. When reporting such a service, the appropriate "unlisted procedure" code may be used to indicate the service, identifying it by "special report" as defined below. HCPCS terminology is inconsistent in defining

Not valid for Medicare   Non-covered by Medicare   Special coverage instructions   Carrier discretion

unlisted procedures. The procedure definition may include the term(s) "unlisted", "not otherwise classified", "unspecified", "unclassified", "other" and "miscellaneous". Prior to using these codes, try to determine if a Local Level III code or CPT code is available. The "unlisted procedures" and accompanying codes for DURABLE MEDICAL EQUIPMENT are as follows:

E1399   Durable medical equipment, miscellaneous
E1699   Dialysis equipment, not otherwise specified

5. SPECIAL REPORT: A service, material or supply that is rarely provided, unusual, variable or new may require a special report in determining medical appropriateness for reimbursement purposes. Pertinent information should include an adequate definition or description of the nature, extent, and need for the service, material or supply.

6. MODIFIERS: Listed services may be modified under certain circumstances. When appropriate, the modifying circumstance is identified by adding a modifier to the basic procedure code. CPT and HCPCS National Level II modifiers may be used with CPT and HCPCS National Level II procedure codes. Modifiers commonly used with DURABLE MEDICAL EQUIPMENT are as follows:

-CC   Procedure code change (use "CC" when the procedure code submitted was changed either for administrative reasons or because an incorrect code was filed)

-LL   Lease/rental (used the "LL" modifier when DME rental is to be applied against the purchase price)

-LT   Left side (used to identify procedures performed on the left sideof the body)

-MS   Six-month maintenance and servicing fee for reasonable and necessary parts and labor which are not covered under any manufacturer or supplier warranty

-NR   New when rented (use the "NR" modifier when DME which was new at the time of rental is subsequently purchased)

-NU   New equipment

-QE   Prescribed amount of oxygen is less than 1 liter per minute (LPM)

-QF   Prescribed amount of oxygen exceeds 4 liters per minute (LPM) and portable oxygen is prescribed

-QG   Prescribed amount of oxygen is greater than 4 liters per minute (LPM)

-QH   Oxygen conserving device is being used with an oxygen delivery system

-QT   Recording and storage on tape by an analog tape recorder

-RP   Replacement and repair (may be used to indicate replacement of DME, orthotic and prosthetic devices which have been in use for some time. The claim shows the code for the part, followed by the "RP" modifier and the charge for the part.)

-RR   Rental (used when DME is to be rented)

-RT   Right side (used to identify procedures performed on the right side of the body)

-TC   Technical component. Under certain circumstances, a charge may be made for the technical component alone. Under those circumstances, the technical component charge is identified by adding modifier -TC to the usual procedure code. Technical component charges are institutional charges and are not billed separately by physicians. However, portable x-ray suppliers bill only for technical component and should utilize modifier -TC. The charge data from portable x-ray suppliers will then be used to build customary and prevailing profiles.

-UE   Used durable medical equipment

7. CPT CODE CROSS-REFERENCE: Unless otherwise specified, the equivalent CPT code for all listings in this section is 99070.

8. DURABLE MEDICAL EQUIPMENT REGIONAL CARRIERS (DMERCS): Effective October 1, 1993 claims for durable medical equipment (DME) must be billed to one of four regional carriers depending upon the residence of the beneficiary. The transition dates for DMERC claims is from November 1, 1993 to March 1, 1994 depending upon the state you practice in. See the Introduction for a complete discussion of DMERCs.

DURABLE MEDICAL EQUIPMENT

CANES

E0100   Cane, includes canes of all materials, adjustable or fixed, with tip
CIM: 60-3, 60-9   MCM: 2100.1

E0105   Cane, quad or three prong, includes canes of all materials, adjustable or fixed, with tips
CIM: 60-15, 60-9   MCM: 2100.1

CRUTCHES

E0110   Crutches, forearm, includes crutches of various materials, adjustable or fixed; pair, complete with tips and handgrip
CIM: 60-9   MCM: 2100.1

E0111   each, with tip and handgrip
CIM: 60-9   MCM: 2100.1

E0112   Crutches, underarm, wood, adjustable or fixed; pair, with pads, tips and handgrip
CIM: 60-9   MCM: 2100.1

E0113   each, with pad, tip and handgrip
CIM: 60-9   MCM: 2100.1

E0114   Crutches, underarm, other than wood, adjustable or fixed; pair, with pads, tips and handgrips
CIM: 60-9   MCM: 2100.1

▲ **E0116**   Crutch, underarm, other than wood, adjustable or fixed, with pad, tip, handgrip, with or without shock absorber, each
CIM: 60-9   MCM: 2100.1

E0117   Crutch, underarm, articulating, spring assisted, each
MCM: 2100.1

E0118   Crutch substitute, lower leg platform, with or without wheels, each

WALKERS

E0130   Walker, rigid (pickup), adjustable or fixed height
CIM: 60-9   MCM: 2100.1

E0135   Walker, folding (pickup), adjustable or fixed height
CIM: 60-9   MCM: 2100.1

E0140 Walker, with trunk support, adjustable or fixed height, any type
CIM: 60-9   MCM: 2100.1

E0141 Walker, rigid, wheeled, adjustable or fixed height
CIM: 60-9   MCM: 2100.1

E0143 Walker, folding, wheeled, adjustable or fixed height
CIM: 60-9   MCM: 2100.1

E0144 Walker, enclosed, four-sided frame, rigid or folding, wheeled with posterior seat
CIM: 60-9   MCM: 2100.1

E0147 Walker, heavy duty, multiple braking system, variable wheel resistance
CIM: 60-15   MCM: 2100.1

E0148 Walker, heavy duty, without wheels, rigid or folding, any type, each

E0149 Walker, heavy duty, wheeled, rigid or folding, any type

ATTACHMENTS

E0153 Platform attachment; forearm crutch, each

E0154   walker, each

E0155 Wheel attachment, rigid pick-up walker, per pair

E0156 Seat attachment, walker

E0157 Crutch attachment, walker, each

E0158 Leg extensions for a walker, per set of four (4)

E0159 Brake attachment for wheeled walker, replacement, each

COMMODES

E0160 Sitz type bath or equipment, portable, used with or without commode;
CIM: 60-9

E0161   with faucet attachments
CIM: 60-9

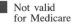 Not valid
for Medicare
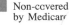 Non-covered
by Medicare
Special
coverage
instructions
 Carrier
discretion
121

E0162   Sitz bath chair
CIM: 60-9

E0163   Commode chair; stationary, with fixed arms
CIM: 60-9   MCM: 2100.1

E0164   mobile, with fixed arms
CIM: 60-9   MCM: 2100.1

E0165   Commode chair, stationary, with detachable arms
CIM: 60-9   MCM: 2100.1

E0166   Commode chair, mobile, with detachable arms
CIM: 60-9   MCM: 2100.1

E0167   Pail or pan for use with commode chair
CIM: 60-9

E0168   Commode chair, extra wide and/or heavy duty, stationary or mobile, with or without arms, any type, each

(E0169)   Code deleted December 31, 2005

● **E0170**   Commode chair with integrated seat lift mechanism, electric, any type

● **E0171**   Commode chair with integrated seat lift mechanism, non-electric, any type

● **E0172**   Seat lift mechanism placed over or on top of toilet, any type

E0175   Foot rest, for use with commode chair, each

(E0176)   Code deleted December 31, 2004; use CPT

(E0177)   Code deleted December 31, 2004; use CPT

(E0178)   Code deleted December 31, 2004; use CPT

(E0179)   Code deleted December 31, 2004; use CPT

DECUBITUS CARE EQUIPMENT

E0180   Pressure pad, alternating with pump;
CIM: 60-9   MCM: 4107.6

E0181   heavy duty
CIM: 60-9   MCM: 4107.6

E0182 Pump for alternating pressure pad
CIM: 60-9 MCM: 4107.6

E0184 Dry pressure mattress
CIM: 60-9 MCM: 4107.6

E0185 Gel or gel-like pressure pad for mattress, standard mattress length and width
CIM: 60-9 MCM: 4107.6

E0186 Air pressure mattress
CIM: 60-9

E0187 Water pressure mattress
CIM: 60-9

E0188 Synthetic sheepskin pad
CIM: 60-9 MCM: 4107.6

E0189 Lambswool sheepskin pad, any size
CIM: 60-9 MCM: 4107.6

E0190 Positioning cushion/pillow/wedge, any shape or size
MCM: 2100.1

E0191 Heel or elbow protector, each

(E0192) Code deleted December 31, 2004; use CPT

E0193 Powered air floatation bed (low air loss therapy)

E0194 Air fluidized bed
CIM: 60-19

E0196 Gel pressure mattress
CIM: 60-9

E0197 Air pressure pad for mattress, standard mattress length and width
CIM: 60-9

E0198 Water pressure pad for mattress, standard mattress length and width
CIM: 60-9

E0199 Dry pressure pad for mattress, standard mattress length and width
CIM: 60-9

HEAT/COLD APPLICATION

E0200 Heat lamp, without stand (table model), includes bulb, or infrared element
CIM: 60-9 MCM: 2100.1

E0202 Phototherapy (bilirubin) light with photometer

E0203 Therapeutic lightbox, minimum 10,000 lux, table top model

E0205 Heat lamp, with stand, includes bulb, or infrared element
CIM: 60-9 MCM: 2100.1

E0210 Electric heat pad; standard
CIM: 60-9

E0215 moist
CIM: 60-9

E0217 Water circulating heat pad with pump
CIM: 60-9

E0218 Water circulating cold pad with pump
CIM: 60-9

E0220 Hot water bottle

E0221 Infrared heating pad system
CIM: 60-25

E0225 Hydrocollator unit, includes pads
CIM: 60-9 MCM: 2210.3

E0230 Ice cap or collar

E0231 Non-contact wound warming device (temperature control unit, AC adapter and power cord) for use with warming card and wound cover
MCM: 2303

E0232 Warming card for use with the non-contact wound warming device and non-contact wound warming wound cover
MCM: 2303

E0235 Paraffin bath unit, portable (see medical supply code A4265 for paraffin)
CIM: 60-9 MCM: 2210.3

E0236 Pump for water circulating pad
CIM: 60-9

E0238 Non-electric heat pad, moist
CIM: 60-9

E0239 Hydrocollator unit, portable
CIM: 60-9 MCM: 2210.3

BATH AND TOILET AIDS

E0240 Bath/shower chair, with or without wheels, any size
CIM: 60-9

E0241 Bath tub wall rail, each
CIM: 60-9 MCM: 2100.1

E0242 Bath tub rail, floor base
CIM: 60-9 MCM: 2100.1

E0243 Toilet rail, each
CIM: 60-9 MCM: 2100.1

E0244 Raised toilet seat
CIM: 60-9

E0245 Tub stool or bench
CIM: 60-9

E0246 Transfer tub rail attachment

E0247 Transfer bench for tub or toilet with or without commode opening
CIM: 60-9

E0248 Transfer bench, heavy duty, for tub or toilet with or without commode opening
CIM: 60-9

E0249 Pad for water circulating heat unit
CIM: 60-9

HOSPITAL BEDS AND ACCESSORIES

E0250 Hospital bed, fixed height, with any type side rails; with mattress
CIM: 60-18 MCM: 2100.1

E0251 without mattress
CIM: 60-18 MCM: 2100.1

Not valid for Medicare   Non-covered by Medicare   Special coverage instructions   Carrier discretion

E0255   Hospital bed, variable height, hi-lo, with any type side rails; with mattress
CIM: 60-18   MCM: 2100.1

E0256   without mattress
CIM: 60-18   MCM: 2100.1

E0260   Hospital bed, semi-electric (head and foot adjustment), with any type side rails; with mattress
CIM: 60-18   MCM: 2100.1

E0261   without mattress
CIM: 60-18   MCM: 2100.1

E0265   Hospital bed, total electric (head, foot and height adjustments), with any type side rails; with mattress
CIM: 60-18   MCM: 2100.1

E0266   without mattress
CIM: 60-18   MCM: 2100.1

E0270   Hospital bed, institutional type includes: oscillating, circulating and stryker frame, with mattress
CIM: 60-9

E0271   Mattress; innerspring
CIM: 60-18, 60-9

E0272   foam rubber
CIM: 60-18, 60-9

E0273   Bed board
CIM: 60-9

E0274   Over-bed table
CIM: 60-9

E0275   Bed pan; standard, metal or plastic
CIM: 60-9

E0276   fracture, metal or plastic
CIM: 60-9

E0277   Powered pressure-reducing air mattress
CIM: 60-9

E0280   Bed cradle, any type

E0290   Hospital bed; fixed-height, without side rails; with mattress
CIM: 60-18   MCM: 2100.1

E0291   without mattress
CIM: 60-18   MCM: 2100.1

E0292   Hospital variable height, hi-lo, without side rails; with mattress
CIM: 60-18   MCM: 2100.1

E0293   without mattress
CIM: 60-18   MCM: 2100.1

E0294   Hospital bed, semi-electric (head and foot adjustment), without side rails; with mattress
CIM: 60-18   MCM: 2100.1

E0295   without mattress
CIM: 60-18   MCM: 2100.1

E0296   Hospital bed, total electric (head, foot and height adjustments), without side rails; with mattress
CIM: 60-18   MCM: 2100.1

E0297   without mattress
CIM: 60-18   MCM: 2100.1

HOSPITAL BED ACCESSORIES

E0300   Pediatric crib, hospital grade, fully enclosed

E0301   Hospital bed, heavy duty, extra wide, with weight capacity greater than 350 pounds, but less than or equal to 600 pounds, with any type side rails, without mattress
CIM: 60-18

E0302   Hospital bed, extra heavy duty, extra wide, with weight capacity greater than 600 pounds, with any type side rails, without mattress
CIM: 60-18

E0303   Hospital bed, heavy duty, extra wide, with weight capacity greater than 350 pounds, but less than or equal to 600 pounds, with any type side rails, with mattress
CIM: 60-18

E0304   Hosptial bed, extra heavy duty, extra wide, with weight capacity greater than 600 pounds, with any type side rails, with mattress
CIM: 60-18

E0305   Bed side rails; half length
CIM: 60-18

Not valid   Non-covered   Special   Carrier
for Medicare   by Medicare   coverage   discretion
                                        instructions

E0310   full length
CIM: 60-18

E0315   Bed accessory: board, table, or support device, any type
CIM: 60-9

E0316   Safety enclosure frame/canopy for use with hospital bed, any type

E0325   Urinal; male, jug/type, any material
CIM: 60-9

E0326   female, jug/type, any material
CIM: 60-9

E0350   Control unit for electronic bowel irrigation/evacuation system

E0352   Disposable pack (water reservoir bag, speculum, valving mechanism and collection bag/box) for use with the electronic bowel irrigation/evacuation system

E0370   Air pressure elevator for heel

E0371   Nonpowered advanced pressure reducing overlay for mattress, standard mattress length and width

E0372   Powered air overlay for mattress, standard mattress length and width

E0373   Nonpowered advanced pressure reducing mattress

OXYGEN AND RELATED RESPIRATORY EQUIPMENT

E0424   Stationary compressed gaseous oxygen system, rental; includes container, contents, regulator, flowmeter, humidifier, nebulizer, cannula or mask, and tubing
CIM: 60-4 MCM: 4107.9

E0425   Stationary compressed gas system, purchase; includes regulator, flowmeter, humidifier, nebulizer, cannula or mask, and tubing
CIM: 60-4 MCM: 4107.9

E0430   Portable gaseous oxygen system, purchase; includes regulator flowmeter, humidifier, cannula or mask, and tubing
CIM: 60-4 MCM: 4107.9

● New code   ▲ Revised code   ( ) Deleted code

E0431   Portable gaseous oxygen system, rental; includes portable container, regulator, flowmeter, humidifier, cannula or mask, and tubing
CIM: 60-4   MCM: 4107.9

E0434   Portable liquid oxygen system, rental; includes portable container, supply reservoir, humidifier, flowmeter, refill adaptor, contents gauge, cannula or mask, and tubing
CIM: 60-4   MCM: 4107.9

E0435   Portable liquid oxygen system, purchase; includes portable container, supply reservoir, flowmeter, humidifier, contents gauge, cannula or masks, tubing and refill adaptor
CIM: 60-4   MCM: 4107.9

E0439   Stationary liquid oxygen system; rental, includes container, contents, regulator, flowmeter, humidifier, nebulizer, cannula or mask, and tubing
CIM: 60-4   MCM: 4107.9

E0440   purchase, includes use of reservoir, contents indicator, regulator, flowmeter, humidifier, nebulizer, cannula or mask, and tubing
CIM: 60-4   MCM: 4107.9

E0441   Oxygen contents, gaseous (for use with owned gaseous stationary systems or when both a stationary and portable gaseous system are owned), 1 month's supply = 1 unit
CIM: 60-4   MCM: 4107.9

E0442   Oxygen contents, liquid (for use with owned liquid stationary systems or when both a stationary and portable liquid system are owned), 1 month's supply = 1 unit
CIM: 60-4   MCM: 4107.9

E0443   Portable oxygen contents, gaseous (for use only with portable gaseous systems when no stationary gas or liquid system is used), 1 month's supply = 1 unit
CIM: 60-4   MCM: 4107.9

E0444   Portable oxygen contents, liquid (for use only with portable liquid systems when no stationary gas or liquid system is used), 1 month's supply = 1 unit
CIM: 60-4   MCM: 4107.9

E0445   Oximeter device for measuring blood oxygen levels non-invasively

Not valid   Non-covered   Special   Carrier
for Medicare   by Medicare   coverage   discretion
                                        instructions

E0450 Volume control ventilator, without pressure support mode, may include pressure control mode, used with invasive interface (e.g., tracheostomy tube)
CIM: 60-9

(E0454) Code deleted December 31, 2004; use CPT

E0455 Oxygen tent, excluding croup or pediatric tents
CIM: 60-4 MCM: 4107.9

E0457 Chest shell (cuirass)

E0459 Chest wrap

E0460 Negative pressure ventilator, portable or stationary
CIM: 60-9

E0461 Volume control ventilator, without pressure support mode, may include pressure control mode, used with non-invasive interface (e.g. mask)
CIM: 60-9

E0462 Rocking bed with or without side rails

E0463 Pressure support ventilator with volume control mode, may include pressure control mode, used with invasive interface (e.g. tracheostomy tube)

E0464 Pressure support ventilator with volume control mode, may include pressure control mode, used with non-invasive interface (e.g. mask)

E0470 Respiratory assist device, bi-level pressure capability, without backup rate feature, used with noninvasive interface, eg., nasal or facial mask (intermittent assist device with continuous positive airway pressure device)
CIM: 60-9

E0471 Respiratory assist device, bi-level pressure capability, with backup rate feature, used with noninvasive interface, eg., nasal or facial mask (intermittent assist device with continuous positive airway pressure device)
CIM: 60-9

E0472 Respiratory assist device, bi-level pressure capability, with backup rate feature, used with invasive interface, eg., tracheostomy tube (intermittent assist device with continuous positive airway pressure device
CIM: 60-9

● New code ▲ Revised code ( ) Deleted code

E0480 Percussor, electric or pneumatic, home model
CIM: 60-9

E0481 Intrapulmonary percussive ventilation system and related accessories
CIM: 60-21

E0482 Cough stimulating device, alternating positive and negative airway pressure

E0483 High frequency chest wall oscillation air-pulse generator system, (includes hoses and vest), each

E0484 Oscillatory positive expiratory pressure device, non-electric, any type, each

● **E0485** Oral device/appliance used to reduce upper airway collapsibility, adjustable or non-adjustable, prefabricated, includes fitting and adjustment

● **E0486** Oral device/appliance used to reduce upper airway collapsibility, adjustable or non-adjustable, custom fabricated, includes fitting and adjustment

IPPB MACHINES

E0500 IPPB machine, all types, with built-in nebulization; manual or automatic valves; internal or external power source
CIM: 60-9

HUMIDIFIERS/NEBULIZERS FOR USE WITH OXYGEN IPPB EQUIPMENT

COMPRESSORS

E0550 Humidifier, durable for extensive supplemental humidification during IPPB treatments or oxygen delivery
CIM: 60-9

E0555 Humidifier, durable, glass or autoclavable plastic bottle type, for use with regulator or flowmeter
CIM: 60-9   MCM: 4107.9

E0560 Humidifier, durable for supplemental humidification during IPPB treatment or oxygen delivery
CIM: 60-9

Not valid for Medicare   Non-covered by Medicare   Special coverage instructions   Carrier discretion

E0561 Humidifier, non-heated, used with positive airway pressure device

E0562 Humidifier, heated, used with positive airway pressure device

E0565 Compressor, air power source for equipment which is not self-contained or cylinder driven

E0570 Nebulizer; with compressor
CIM: 60-9   MCM: 4107.9

E0571 Aerosol compressor, battery powered, for use with small volume nebulizer
CIM: 60-9

E0572 Aerosol compressor, adjustable pressure, light duty for intermittent use

E0574 Ultrasonic/electronic aerosol generator with small volume nebulizer

E0575 Nebulizer, ultrasonic, large volume
CIM: 60-9

E0580 Nebulizer, with compressor, durable, glass or autoclavable plastic, bottle type, for use with regulator or flowmeter
CIM: 60-9   MCM: 4107.9

E0585 Nebulizer with compressor and heater
CIM: 60-9   MCM: 4107.9

E0590 Dispensing fee covered drug administered through DME nebulizer

SUCTION PUMP/ROOM VAPORIZERS

E0600 Respiratory suction pump, home model, portable or stationary, electric
CIM: 60-9

E0601 Continuous airway pressure (CPAP) device
CIM: 60-17

E0602 Breast pump, manual, any type

E0603 Breast pump, electric (AC and/or DC), any type

E0604 Breast pump, heavy duty, hospital grade, piston operated, pulsatile vacuum suction/release cycles, vacuum regulator, supplies, transformer, electric (AC and/or DC)

E0605 Vaporizer, room type
CIM: 60-9

E0606 Postural drainage board
CIM: 60-9

MONITORING EQUIPMENT

E0607 Home blood glucose monitor
CIM: 60-11

PACEMAKER MONITOR

E0610 Pacemaker monitor, self-contained; (checks battery depletion, included audible and visible check systems)
CIM: 60-7, 50-1

E0615 (checks battery depletion and other pacemaker components, includes digital/visible check systems)
CIM: 60-7, 50-1

E0616 Implantable cardiac event recorder with memory, activator and programmer

E0617 External defibrillator with integrated electrocardiogram analysis

E0618 Apnea monitor, without recording feature

E0619 Apnea monitor, with recording feature

E0620 Skin piercing device for collection of capillary blood, laser, each

PATIENT LIFTS

E0621 Sling or seat, patient lift, canvas or nylon
CIM: 60-9

E0625 Patient lift, bathroom or toilet, not otherwise classified
CIM: 60-9

E0627 Seat lift mechanism incorporated into a combination lift-chair mechanism
CIM: 60-8 MCM: 4107.8

Not valid for Medicare   Non-covered by Medicare   Special coverage instructions   Carrier discretion

E0628 Separate seat life mechanism for use with patient owned furniture; electric
CIM: 60-8   MCM: 4107.8

E0629 non-electric
MCM: 4107.8

E0630 Patient lift; hydraulic, with seat or sling
CIM: 60-9

E0635 electric, with seat or sling
CIM: 60-9

E0636 Multipositional patient support system, with integrated lift, patient accessible controls

▲**E0637** Combination sit to stand system, any size including pediatric, with seatlift feature, with or without wheels
CIM: 60-9

▲**E0638** Standing frame system, one position (e.g. Upright, supine or prone stander), any size including pediatric, with or without wheels
CIM: 60-9

E0639 Patient lift, moveable from room to room with disassembly and reassembly, includes all components/accessories

E0640 Patient lift, fixed system, includes all components/accessories

●**E0641** Standing frame system, multi-position (e.g. Three-way stander), any size including pediatric, with or without wheels
CIM: 60-9

●**E0642** Standing frame system, mobile (dynamic stander), any size including pediatric
CIM: 60-9

PNEUMATIC COMPRESSOR AND APPLIANCES (LYMPHEDEMA PUMP)

E0650 Pneumatic compressor; non-segmental home model
CIM: 60-16

E0651   segmental home model without calibrated gradient
pressure
CIM: 60-16

E0652   segmental home model with calibrated gradient
pressure
CIM: 60-16

E0655   Non-segmental pneumatic appliance for use with
pneumatic compressor; half arm
CIM: 60-16

E0660   full leg
CIM: 60-16

E0665   full arm
CIM: 60-16

E0666   half leg
CIM: 60-16

E0667   Segmental pneumatic appliance for use with pneumatic
compressor; full leg
CIM: 60-16

E0668   full arm
CIM: 60-16

E0669   half leg
CIM: 60-16

E0671   Segmental gradient pressure pneumatic appliance, full leg
CIM: 60-16

E0672   full arm
CIM: 60-16

E0673   half leg
CIM: 60-16

E0675   Pneumatic compression device, high pressure, rapid
inflation/deflation cycle, for arterial insufficiency
(unilateral or bilateral system)

ULTRAVIOLET CABINET

E0691   Ultraviolet light therapy system panel, includes
bulbs/lamps, timer and eye protection; treatment area 2
square feet or less

| Not valid for Medicare | Non-covered by Medicare | Special coverage instructions | Carrier discretion |

E0692   Ultraviolet light therapy system panel, includes bulbs/lamps, timer and eye protection, 4 foot panel

E0693   Ultraviolet light therapy system panel, includes bulbs/lamps, timer and eye protection, 6 foot panel

E0694   Ultraviolet multidirectional light therapy system in 6 foot cabinet, includes bulbs/lamps, timer and eye protection

SAFETY EQUIPMENT

E0700   Safety equipment (e.g., belt, harness or vest)

E0701   Helmet with face guard and soft interface material, prefabricated

RESTRAINTS

● E0705   Transfer board or device, any type, each

E0710   Restraints, any type (body, chest, wrist or ankle)

TRANSCUTANEOUS AND/OR NEUROMUSCULAR ELECTRICAL NERVE STIMULATORS - TENS

E0720   TENS; two lead, localized stimulation
CIM: 35-20, 35-46   MCM: 4107.6

E0730   four or more leads, for multiple nerve stimulation
CIM: 35-20, 35-46   MCM: 4107.6

E0731   Form fitting conductive garment for delivery of TENS or NMES (with conductive fibers separated from the patient's skin by layers of fabric)
CIM: 45-25

E0740   Incontinence treatment system, pelvic floor stimulator, monitor, sensor and/or trainer
CIM: 60.24

E0744   Neuromuscular stimulator for scoliosis

E0745   Neuromuscular stimulator, electronic shock unit
CIM: 35-77

E0746   Electromyography (EMG), biofeedback device
CIM: 35-27

E0747   Osteogenesis stimulator; electrical, non-invasive, other than spinal applications
CIM: 35-48

E0748   Osteogenesis stimulator; electrical, noninvasive, spinal applications
CIM: 35-48

E0749   Osteogenesis stimulator, electrical, surgically implanted
CIM: 35-48

(E0752   Code deleted December 31, 2005; use L8680

(E0754)   Code deleted December 31, 2005; use L8681

E0755   Electronic salivary reflex stimulator (intra-oral/non-invasive)

(E0756)   Code deleted December 31, 2005

(E0757)   Code deleted December 31, 2005; use L8682

(E0758)   Code deleted December 31, 2005; use L8683

(E0759)   Code deleted December 31, 2005; use L8684

E0760   Ostogenesis stimulator, low intensity ultrasound, non-invasive
MCM: 35-48

E0761   Non-thermal pulsed high frequency radiowaves, high peak power electromagnetic energy treatment device

● **E0762**   Transcutaneous electrical joint stimulation device system, includes all accessories

● **E0764**   Functional neuromuscular stimulator, transcutaneous stimulation of muscles of ambulation with computer control, used for walking by spinal cord injured, entire system, after completion of training program
CIM: 35-77

E0765   FDA approved nerve stimulator with replaceable batteries for treatment of nausea and vomiting

E0769   Electrical stimulation or electromagnetic wound treatment device, not otherwise classified
CIM: 35-102

E0776   IV pole

E0779   Ambulatory infusion pump, mechanical, reusable, for
         infusion 8 hours or greater

E0780   Ambulatory infusion pump, mechanical, reusable, for
         infusion less than 8 hours

E0781   Ambulatory infusion pump, single or multiple channels,
         electric or battery operated, with administrative
         equipment, worn by patient
         CIM: 60-14

E0782   Infusion pump, implantable, non-programmable (includes
         all components, e.g., pump, catheter, connectors, etc.)
         CIM: 60-14

E0783   Infusion pump system, implantable, programmable
         (includes all components, e.g., pump, catheter, connectors,
         etc.)
         CIM: 60-14

E0784   External ambulatory infusion pump, insulin
         CIM: 60-14

E0785   Implantable intraspinal (epidural/intrathecal) catheter used
         with implantable infusion pump, replacement
         MCM: 60-14

E0786   Implantable programmable infusion pump, replacement
         (excludes implantable intraspinal catheter)
         CIM: 60-14

E0791   Parenteral infusion pump, stationary, single or
         multi-channel
         CIM: 65-10   MCM: 2130, 4450

TRACTION EQUIPMENT

TRACTION - CERVICAL

E0830   Ambulatory traction device, all types, each
         CIM: 60-9

E0840   Traction frame, attached to headboard, cervical traction
         CIM: 60-9

E0849   Traction equipment, cervical, free-standing stand/frame,
         pneumatic, applying traction force to other than mandible

E0850   Traction stand, free standing, cervical traction
CIM: 60-9

E0855   Cervical traction equipment not requiring additional stand or frame

TRACTION - OVERDOOR

E0860   Traction equipment, overdoor, cervical
CIM: 60-9

TRACTION - EXTREMITY

E0870   Traction frame, attached to footboard, extremity traction, (e.g., Buck's)
CIM: 60-9

E0880   Traction stand, free standing, extremity traction, (e.g., Buck's)
CIM: 60-9

TRACTION - PELVIC

E0890   Traction frame, attached to footboard, pelvic traction
CIM: 60-9

E0900   Traction stand, free standing, pelvic traction (e.g., Buck's)
CIM: 60-9

TRAPEZE EQUIPMENT, FRACTURE FRAME, AND OTHER ORTHOPEDIC DEVICES

E0910   Trapeze bars, A/K/A patient helper, attached to bed, with grab bar
CIM: 60-9

● **E0911**   Trapeze bar, heavy duty, for patient weight capacity greater than 250 pounds, attached to bed, with grab bar
CIM: 60-9

● **E0912**   Trapeze bar, heavy duty, for patient weight capacity greater than 250 pounds, free standing, complete with grab bar
CIM: 60-9

E0920   Fracture frame; attached to bed, includes weights
CIM: 60-9

E0930   free standing, includes weights
CIM: 60-9

▲**E0935** Continuous passive motion exercise device for use on knee only
CIM: 60-9

E0940 Trapeze bar, free standing, complete with grab bar
CIM: 60-9

E0941 Gravity assisted traction device, any type
CIM: 60-9

E0942 Cervical head harness/halter

E0944 Pelvic belt/harness/boot

E0945 Extremity belt/harness

E0946 Fracture frame; dual with cross bars, attached to bed, (e.g., Balken, 4 poster)
CIM: 60-9

E0947 attachments for complex pelvic traction
CIM: 60-9

E0948 attachments for complex cervical traction
CIM: 60-9

WHEELCHAIRS AND WHEELCHAIR ACCESSORIES

E0950 Wheelchair accessory, tray, each
CIM: 60-9

E0951 Heel loop/holder, any type, with or without ankle strap, each

E0952 Toe loop/holder, any type, each
CIM: 60-9

(E0953) Code deleted December 31, 2005; use E2211

(E0954) Code deleted December 31, 2005; use E2219

E0955 Wheelchair accessory, headrest, cushioned, any type, including fixed mounting hardware, each

E0956 Wheelchair accessory, lateral trunk or hip support, any type, including fixed mounting hardware, each

E0957 Wheelchair accessory, medial thigh support, any type, including fixed mounting hardware, each

E0958 Manual wheelchair accessory, one-arm drive attachment, each
CIM: 60-9

E0959 Manual wheelchair accessory, adapter for amputee, each
CIM: 60-9

E0960 Wheelchair accessory, shoulder harness/straps or chest strap, including any type mounting hardware

E0961 Manual wheelchair accessory, wheel lock brake extension (handle), each
CIM: 60-9

(E0962) Code deleted December 31, 2004; use CPT

(E0963) Code deleted December 31, 2004; use CPT

(E0964) Code deleted December 31, 2004; use CPT

(E0965) Code deleted December 31, 2004; use CPT

E0966 Manual wheelchair accessory, headrest extension, e..
CIM: 60-9

E0967 Manual wheelchair accessory, hand rim with projections, any type, replacement only, each
CIM: 60-9

E0968 Commode seat, wheelchair
CIM: 60-9

E0969 Narrowing device, wheelchair
CIM: 60-9

E0970 No. 2 Footplates, except for elevating leg rest
CIM: 60-9

▲ **E0971** Manual wheelchair accessory, anti-tipping device, each
CIM: 60-9

(E0972) Code deleted December 31, 2005

E0973 Wheelchair accessory, adjustable height, detachable armrest, complete assembly, each
CIM: 60-9

E0974 Manual wheelchair accessory, anti-rollback device, each
CIM: 60-9

E0977 Wedge cushion, wheelchair

E0978 Wheelchair accessory, positioning belt/safety belt/pelvic strap, each

E0980 Safety vest, wheelchair

E0981 Wheelchair accessory, seat upholstery, replacement only, each

E0982 Wheelchair accessory, back upholstery, replacement only, each

E0983 Manual wheelchair accessory, power add-on to convert manual wheelchair to motorized wheelchair, joystick control

E0984 Manual wheelchair accessory, power add-on to convert manual wheelchair to motorized wheelchair, tiller control

E0985 Wheelchair accessory, seat lift mechanism

E0986 Manual wheelchair accessory, push activated power assist, each

E0990 Wheelchair accessory, elevating leg rest, complete assembly, each
CIM: 60-9

E0992 Manual wheelchair accessory, solid seat insert

E0994 Arm rest, each
CIM: 60-9

E0995 Wheelchair accessory, calf rest/pad, each
CIM: 60-9

(E0996) Code deleted December 31, 2005; use E2220

E0997 Caster with a fork
CIM: 60-9

E0998 Caster without fork
CIM: 60-9

E0999 Pneumatic tire with wheel
CIM: 60-9

(E1000) Code deleted December 31, 2005; use E2214

(E1001) Code deleted December 31, 2005; use E2224

E1002 Wheelchair accessory, power seating system, tilt only

E1003 Wheelchair accessory, power seating system, recline only, without shear reduction

E1004 Wheelchair accessory, power seating system, recline only, with mechanical shear reduction

E1005 Wheelchair accessory, power seating system, recline only, with power shear reduction

E1006 Wheelchair accessory, power seating system, combination tilt and recline, without shear reduction

E1007 Wheelchair accessory, power seating system, combination tilt and recline, with mechanical shear reduction

E1008 Wheelchair accessory, power seating system, combination tilt and recline, with power shear reduction

E1009 Wheelchair accessory, addition to power seating system, mechanically linked leg elevation system, including pushrod and leg rest, each

E1010 Wheelchair accessory, addition to power seating system, power leg elevation system, including leg rest, pair

E1011 Modification to pediatric size wheelchair, width adjustment package (not to be dispensed with initial chair)
CIM: 60-9

(E1012) Code deleted December 31, 2004; use CPT

(E1013) Code deleted December 31, 2004; use CPT

E1014 Reclining back, addition to pediatric size wheelchair
CIM: 60-9

E1015 Shock absorber for manual wheelchair, each
MCM: 60.9

E1016 Shock absorber for power wheelchair, each
MCM: 60.9

E1017   Heavy duty shock absorber for heavy duty or extra heavy duty manual wheelchair, each
MCM: 60.9

E1018   Heavy duty shock absorber for heavy duty or extra heavy duty power wheelchair, each
MCM: 60.9

(E1019)   Code deleted December 31, 2005

E1020   Residual limb support system for wheelchair
MCM: 60-6

(E1021)   Code deleted December 31, 2005

(E1025)   Code deleted December 31, 2005

(E1026)   Code deleted December 31, 2005

(E1027)   Code deleted December 31, 2005

E1028   Wheelchair accessory, manual swingaway, retractable or removable mounting hardware for joystick, other control interface or positioning accessory

E1029   Wheelchair accessory, ventilator tray, fixed

E1030   Wheelchair accessory, ventilator tray, gimbaled

ROLLABOUT CHAIR

E1031   Rollabout chair, any and all types with castors 5 inches or greater
CIM: 60-9

E1035   Multi-positional patient transfer system, with integrated seat, operated by care giver
MCM: 2100

E1037   Transport chair, pediatric size
CIM: 60-9

▲**E1038**   Transport chair, adult size, patient weight capacity up to and including 300 pounds
CIM: 60-9

▲**E1039**   Transport chair, adult size, heavy duty, patient weight capacity greater than 300 pounds

144   ● New code   ▲ Revised code   ( ) Deleted code

WHEELCHAIR - FULLY-RECLINING

E1050   Fully-reclining wheelchair; fixed full length arms, swing away detachable elevating leg rests
CIM: 60-9

E1060   Fully-reclining wheelchair; detachable arms, desk or full length, swing away detachable elevating leg rests
CIM: 60-9

E1070   Fully-reclining wheelchair, detachable arms (desk or full length) swing away detachable footrest
CIM: 60-9

E1083   Hemi-wheelchair; fixed full length arms, swing away detachable elevating leg rest
CIM: 60-9

E1084   detachable arms desk or full length arms, swing away detachable elevating leg rests
CIM: 60-9

E1085   fixed full length arms, swing away detachable footrests
CIM: 60-9

E1086   detachable arms desk or full length, swing away detachable footrests
CIM: 60-9

E1087   High strength lightweight wheelchair; fixed full length arms, swing away detachable elevating leg rests
CIM: 60-9

E1088   detachable arms desk or full length, swing away detachable elevating leg rests
CIM: 60-9

E1089   fixed length arms, swing away detachable footrest
CIM: 60-9

E1090   detachable arms desk or full length, swing away detachable footrests
CIM: 60-9

E1092   Wide heavy duty wheelchair, detachable arms (desk or full length); swing away detachable elevating leg rests
CIM: 60-9

E1093   swing away detachable footrests
CIM: 60-9

WHEELCHAIR - SEMI-RECLINING

E1100   Semi-reclining wheelchair; fixed full length arms, swing away detachable elevating leg rests
CIM: 60-9

E1110   detachable arms (desk or full length), elevating leg rest
CIM: 60-9

WHEELCHAIR - STANDARD

E1130   Standard wheelchair, fixed full length arms, fixed or swing away detachable footrests
CIM: 60-9

E1140   Wheelchair, detachable arms, desk or full length; swing away detachable footrests
CIM: 60-9

E1150   swing away detachable elevating leg rests
CIM: 60-9

E1160   Wheelchair, fixed full length arms, swing away detachable elevating leg rests
CIM: 60-9

E1161   Manual adult size wheelchair, includes tilt in space

WHEELCHAIR - AMPUTEE

E1170   Amputee wheelchair; fixed full length arms, swing away detachable elevating leg rests
CIM: 60-9

E1171   fixed full length arms, without foot rests or leg rest
CIM: 60-9

E1172   detachable arms (desk or full length), without foot rests or leg rest
CIM: 60-9

E1180   detachable arms (desk or full length), swing away detachable foot rests
CIM: 60-9

E1190   detachable arms (desk or full length), swing away detachable elevating leg rests
CIM: 60-9

E1195   Heavy duty wheelchair, fixed full length arms, swing
away detachable elevating leg rests
CIM: 60-9

E1200   Amputee wheelchair, fixed full length arms, swing away
detachable foot rest
CIM: 60-9

WHEELCHAIR - POWER

(E1210)   Code deleted December 31, 2005

(E1211)   Code deleted December 31, 2005

(E1212)   Code deleted December 31, 2005; use K0010

(E1213)   Code deleted December 31, 2005; use K0010

WHEELCHAIR - SPECIAL SIZE

E1220   Wheelchair specially sized or constructed (indicate brand
name, model number, if any, and justification)
CIM: 60-6

E1221   Wheelchair with fixed arm; footrests
CIM: 60-6

E1222   elevating leg rests
CIM: 60-6

E1223   Wheelchair with detachable arms; foot rests
CIM: 60-6

E1224   elevating leg rests
CIM: 60-6

E1225   Wheelchair accessory, manual semi-reclining back,
(recline greater than 15 degrees, but less than 80 degrees),
each
CIM: 60-6

E1226   Wheelchair accessory, manual fully reclining back,
(recline greater than 80 degrees), each
CIM: 60-9

E1227   Special height arms for wheelchair
CIM: 60-6

E1228   Special back height for wheelchair
CIM: 60-6

Not valid   Non-covered   Special   Carrier   **147**
for Medicare   by Medicare   coverage   discretion
                                        instructions

E1229   Wheelchair, pediatric size, not otherwise specified

POWER OPERATED VEHICLE

E1230   Power operated vehicle (3 or 4 wheel non-highway)
          specify brand name and model number
          CIM: 60-5   MCM: 4107.6

E1231   Wheelchair, pediatric size, tilt-in-space, rigid, adjustable,
          with seating system
          CIM: 60-9

E1232   Wheelchair, pediatric size, tilt-in-space, folding,
          adjustable, with seating system
          CIM: 60-9

E1233   Wheelchair, pediatric size, tilt-in-space, rigid, adjustable,
          without seating system
          CIM: 60-9

E1234   Wheelchair, pediatric size, tilt-in-space, folding,
          adjustable, without seating system
          CIM: 60-9

E1235   Wheelchair, pediatric size, rigid, adjustable, with seating
          system
          CIM: 60-9

E1236   Wheelchair, pediatric size, folding, adjustable, with
          seating system
          CIM: 60-9

E1237   Wheelchair, pediatric size, rigid, adjustable, without
          seating system
          CIM: 60-9

E1238   Wheelchair, pediatric size, folding, adjustable, without
          seating system
          CIM: 60-9

(E1239)   Code deleted December 31, 2005

WHEELCHAIR - LIGHTWEIGHT

E1240   Lightweight wheelchair; detachable arms, (desk or full
          length) swing away detachable, elevating leg rest
          CIM: 60-9

E1250   fixed full length arms, swing away detachable footrest
          CIM: 60-9

● New code   ▲ Revised code   ( ) Deleted code

E1260   detachable arms (desk or full length) swing away
detachable footrest
CIM: 60-9

E1270   fixed full length arms, swing away detachable
elevating leg rests
CIM: 60-9

WHEELCHAIR - HEAVY DUTY

E1280   Heavy duty wheelchair; detachable arms (desk or full
length) elevating leg rests
CIM: 60-9

E1285   fixed full length arms, swing away detachable foot rest
CIM: 60-9

E1290   detachable arms (desk or full length) swing away
detachable foot rest
CIM: 60-9

E1295   fixed full length arms, elevating leg rest
CIM: 60-9

E1296   Special wheelchair; seat height from floor
CIM: 60-6

E1297   seat depth, by upholstery
CIM: 60-6

E1298   seat depth and/or width, by construction
CIM: 60-6

WHIRLPOOL EQUIPMENT

E1300   Whirlpool; portable (overtub type)
CIM: 60-9

E1310   non-portable (built-in type)
CIM: 60-9

REPAIRS AND REPLACEMENT SUPPLIES

E1340   Repair or nonroutine service for DME requiring the skill
of a technician, labor component, per 15 minutes
MCM: 2100.4

Not valid   Non-covered   Special   Carrier
for Medicare   by Medicare   coverage   discretion
                                    instructions

ADDITIONAL OXYGEN RELATED SUPPLIES AND EQUIPMENT

E1353 Regulator
CIM: 60-4 MCM: 4107.9

E1355 Stand/Rack
CIM: 60-4

E1372 Immersion external heater for nebulizer
CIM: 60-4

E1390 Oxygen concentrator, single delivery port, capable of delivering 85 percent or greater oxygen concentration at the prescribed flow rate
CIM: 60-4

E1391 Oxygen concentrator, dual delivery port, capable of delivering 85 percent or greater oxygen concentration at the prescribed flow rate
CIM: 60-4

● **E1392** Portable oxygen concentrator, rental
CIM: 60-4

E1399 Durable medical equipment, miscellaneous

E1405 Oxygen and water vapor enriching system; with heated delivery
CIM: 60-4 MCM: 4107

E1406 without heated delivery
CIM: 60-4 MCM: 4107

ARTIFICIAL KIDNEY MACHINES AND ACCESSORIES

NOTE: For supplies for ESRD, see codes A4650-A4999.

E1500 Centrifuge, for dialysis

E1510 Kidney dialysate delivery system; kidney machine, pump recirculating, air removal system, flowrate meter, power off, heater and temp control with alarm, I.V. poles, pressure gauge, concentrate container

E1520 Heparin infusion pump for hemodialysis

E1530 Air bubble detector for hemodialysis, each, replacement

E1540   Pressure alarm for hemodialysis, each, replacement

E1550   Bath conductivity meter for hemodialysis, each

E1560   Blood leak detector for hemodialysis, each, replacement

E1570   Adjustable chair, for ESRD patients

E1575   Transducer protectors/fluid barriers, for hemodialysis, any size, per 10

E1580   Unipuncture control system for hemodialysis

E1590   Hemodialysis machine

E1592   Automatic intermittent peritoneal dialysis system

E1594   Cycler dialysis machine for peritoneal dialysis

E1600   Delivery and/or installation charges for hemodialysis equipment

E1610   Reverse osmosis water purification system, for hemodialysis
CIM: 55-1A

E1615   Deionizer water purification system, for hemodialysis
CIM: 55-1A

E1620   Blood pump for hemodialysis, replacement

E1625   Water softening system, for hemodialysis
CIM: 55-1B

E1630   Reciprocating peritoneal dialysis system

E1632   Wearable artificial kidney, each

E1634   Peritoneal dialysis clamps, each
MCM: 4270

E1635   Compact (portable) travel hemodialyzer system

E1636   Sorbent cartridges, for hemodialysis, per 10

E1637   Hemostats, each

E1639   Scale, each

E1699   Dialysis equipment, not otherwise specified

E1700   Jaw motion rehabilitation system

E1701   Replacement cushions for jaw motion rehabilitation system, pkg. of 6

E1702   Replacement measuring scales for jaw motion rehabilitation system, pkg. of 200

E1800   Dynamic adjustable elbow extension/flexion device, includes soft interface material

E1801   Bi-directional static progressive stretch elbow device with range of motion adjustment, includes cuffs

E1802   Dynamic adjustable forearm pronation/supination device, includes soft interface material

E1805   Dynamic adjustable wrist extension/flexion device, includes soft interface material

E1806   Bi-directional static progressive stretch wrist device with range of motion adjustment, includes cuffs

E1810   Dynamic adjustable knee extension/flexion device, includes soft interface material

E1811   Bi-directional static progressive stretch knee device with range of motion adjustment, includes cuffs

● **E1812**   Dynamic knee, extension/flexion device with active resistance control

E1815   Dynamic adjustable ankle extension/flexion device, includes soft interface material

E1816   Bi-directional static progressive stretch ankle device with range of motion adjustment, includes cuffs

E1818   Bi-directional static progressive stretch forearm pronation/supination device with range of motion adjustment, includes cuffs

E1820   Replacement soft interface material, dynamic adjustable extension/flexion device

E1821   Replacement soft interface material/cuffs for bi-directional static progressive stretch device

E1825   Dynamic adjustable finger extension/flexion device, includes soft interface material

E1830   Dynamic adjustable toe extension/flexion device, includes soft interface material

E1840   Dynamic adjustable shoulder flexion/abduction/rotation device, includes soft interface material

E1841   Multi-directional static progressive stretch shoulder device, with range of motion adjustability, includes cuffs

E1902   Communication board, non-electronic augmentative or alternative communication device

E2000   Gastric suction pump, home model, portable or stationary, electric

E2100   Blood glucose monitor with integrated voice synthesizer
CIM: 60-11

E2101   Blood glucose monitor with integrated lancing/blood sample
CIM: 60-11

E2120   Pulse generator system for tympanic treatment of inner ear endolymphatic fluid

WHEELCHAIR ACCESSORIES

E2201   Manual wheelchair accessory, nonstandard seat frame, width greater than or equal to 20 inches and less than 24 inches

E2202   Manual wheelchair accessory, nonstandard seat frame width, 24-27 inches

E2203   Manual wheelchair accessory, nonstandard seat frame depth, 20 to less than 22 inches

E2204   Manual wheelchair accessory, nonstandard seat frame depth, 22 to 25 inches

E2205   Manual wheelchair accessory, hand rim without projections, any type, replacement only, each

E2206   Manual wheelchair accessory, wheel lock assembly, complete, each

● E2207   Wheelchair accessory, crutch and cane holder, each

● E2208   Wheelchair accessory, cylinder tank carrier, each

● E2209   Wheelchair accessory, arm trough, each

● E2210   Wheelchair accessory, bearings, any type, replacement only, each

● E2211   Manual wheelchair accessory, pneumatic propulsion tire, any size, each

● E2212   Manual wheelchair accessory, tube for pneumatic propulsion tire, any size, each

● E2213   Manual wheelchair accessory, insert for pneumatic propulsion tire (removable), any type, any size, each

● E2214   Manual wheelchair accessory, pneumatic caster tire, any size, each

● E2215   Manual wheelchair accessory, tube for pneumatic caster tire, any size, each

● E2216   Manual wheelchair accessory, foam filled propulsion tire, any size, each

● E2217   Manual wheelchair accessory, foam filled caster tire, any size, each

● E2218   Manual wheelchair accessory, foam propulsion tire, any size, each

● E2219   Manual wheelchair accessory, foam caster tire, any size, each

● E2220   Manual wheelchair accessory, solid (rubber/plastic) propulsion tire, any size, each

● E2221   Manual wheelchair accessory, solid (rubber/plastic) caster tire (removable), any size, each

● **E2222**   Manual wheelchair accessory, solid (rubber/plastic) caster tire with integrated wheel, any size, each

● **E2223**   Manual wheelchair accessory, valve, any type, replacement only, each

● **E2224**   Manual wheelchair accessory, propulsion wheel excludes tire, any size, each

● **E2225**   Manual wheelchair accessory, caster wheel excludes tire, any size, replacement only, each

● **E2226**   Manual wheelchair accessory, caster fork, any size, replacement only, each

E2291   Back, planar, for pediatric size wheelchair including fixed attaching hardware

E2292   Seat, planar, for pediatric size wheelchair including fixed attaching hardware

E2293   Back, contoured, for pediatric size wheelchair including fixed attaching hardware

E2294   Seat, contoured, for pediatric size wheelchair including fixed attaching hardware

E2300   Power wheelchair accessory, power seat elevation system

E2301   Power wheelchair accessory, power standing system

E2310   Power wheelchair accessory, electronic connection between wheelchair controller and one power seating system motor, including all related electronics, indicator feature, mechanical function selection switch, and fixed mounting hardware

E2311   Power wheelchair accessory, electronic connection between wheelchair controller and two or more power seating system motors, including all related electronics, indicator feature, mechanical function selection switch, and fixed mounting hardware

E2320   Power wheelchair accessory, hand or chin control interface, remote joystick or touchpad, proportional, including all related electronics, and fixed mounting hardware

E2321 Power wheelchair accessory, hand control interface, remote joystick, nonproportional, including all related electronics, mechanical stop switch, and fixed mounting hardware

E2322 Power wheelchair accessory, hand control interface, multiple mechanical switches, nonproportional, including all related electronics, mechanical stop switch, and fixed mounting hardware

E2323 Power wheelchair accessory, specialty joystick handle for hand control interface, prefabricated

E2324 Power wheelchair accessory, chin cup for chin control interface

E2325 Power wheelchair accessory, sip and puff interface, nonproportional, including all related electronics, mechanical stop switch, and manual swingaway mounting hardware

E2326 Power wheelchair accessory, breath tube kit for sip and puff interface

E2327 Power wheelchair accessory, head control interface, mechanical, proportional, including all related electronics, mechanical direction change switch, and fixed mounting hardware

E2328 Power wheelchair accessory, head control or extremity control interface, electronic, proportional, including all related electronics and fixed mounting hardware

E2329 Power wheelchair accessory, head control interface, contact switch mechanism, nonproportional, including all related electronics, mechanical stop switch, mechanical direction change switch, head array, and fixed mounting hardware

E2330 Power wheelchair accessory, head control interface, proximity switch mechanism, nonproportional, including all related electronics, mechanical stop switch, mehcanical direction change switch, head array, and fixed mounting hardware

E2331 Power wheelchair accessory, attendant control, proportional, including all related electronics and fixed mounting hardware

E2340   Power wheelchair accessory, nonstandard seat frame width, 20-23 inches

E2341   Power wheelchair accessory, nonstandard seat frame width, 24-27 inches

E2342   Power wheelchair accessory, nonstandard seat frame depth, 20 or 21 inches

E2343   Power wheelchair accessory, nonstandard seat frame depth, 22-25 inches

E2351   Power wheelchair accessory, electronic interface to operate speech generating device using power wheelchair control interface

E2360   Power wheelchair accessory, 22 NF non-sealed lead acid battery, each

E2361   Power wheelchair accessory, 22 NF sealed lead acid battery, each (eg., gel cell, absorbed glassmat)

E2362   Power wheelchair accessory, group 24 non-sealed lead acid battery, each

E2363   Power wheelchair accessory, group 24 sealed lead acid battery, each (eg., gel cell, absorbed glassmat)

E2364   Power wheelchair accessory, U-1 non-sealed lead acid battery, each

E2365   Power wheelchair accessory, U-1 sealed lead acid battery, each (eg., gel cell, absorbed glassmat)

E2366   Power wheelchair accessory, battery charger, single mode, for use with only one battery type, sealed or non-sealed, each

E2367   Power wheelchair accessory, battery charger, dual mode, for use with either battery type, sealed or non-sealed, each

E2368   Power wheelchair component, motor, replacement only

E2369   Power wheelchair component, gear box, replacement only

Not valid for Medicare   Non-covered by Medicare   Special coverage instructions   Carrier discretion

E2370   Power wheelchair component, motor and gear box combination, replacement only

● **E2371**   Power wheelchair accessory, group 27 sealed lead acid battery, (e.g. Gel cell, absorbed glassmat), each

● **E2372**   Power wheelchair accessory, group 27 non-sealed lead acid battery, each

E2399   Power wheelchair accessory, not otherwise classified interface, including all related electronics and any type mounting hardware

E2402   Negative pressure wound therapy electrical pump, stationary or portable

E2500   Speech generating device, digitized speech, using pre-recorded messages, less than or equal to 8 minutes recording time
CIM: 60-23

E2502   Speech generating device, digitized speech, using pre-recorded messages, greater than 8 minutes but less than or equal to 20 minutes recording time
CIM: 60-23

E2504   Speech generating device, digitized speech, using pre-recorded messages, greater than 20 minutes but less than or equal to 40 minutes recording time
CIM: 60-23

E2506   Speech generating device, digitized speech, using pre-recorded messages, greater than 40 minutes recording time
CIM: 60-23

E2508   Speech generating device, synthesized speech, requiring message formulation by spelling and access by physical contact with the device
CIM: 60-23

E2510   Speech generating device, synthesized speech, permitting multiple methods of message formulation and multiple methods of device access
CIM: 60-23

E2511   Speech generating software program, for personal computer or personal digital assistant
CIM: 60-23

E2512   Accessory for speech generating device, mounting system
CIM: 60-23

E2599   Accessory for speech generating device, not otherwise classified
CIM: 60-23

E2601   General use wheelchair seat cushion, width less than 22 inches, any depth

E2602   General use wheelchair seat cushion, width 22 inches or greater, any depth

E2603   Skin protection wheelchair seat cushion, width less than 22 inches, any depth

E2604   Skin protection wheelchair seat cushion, width 22 inches or greater, any depth

E2605   Positioning wheelchair seat cushion, width less than 22 inches, any depth

E2606   Positioning wheelchair seat cushion, width 22 inches or greater, any depth

E2607   Skin protection and positioning wheelchair seat cushion, width less than 22 inches, any depth

E2608   Skin protection and positioning wheelchair seat cushion, width 22 inches or greater, any depth

E2609   Custom fabricated wheelchair seat cushion, any size

E2610   Wheelchair seat cushion, powered

E2611   General use wheelchair back cushion, width less than 22 inches, any height, including any type mounting hardware

E2612   General use wheelchair back cushion, width 22 inches or greater, any height, including any type mounting hardware

E2613   Positioning wheelchair back cushion, posterior, width less than 22 inches, any height, including any type mounting hardware

Not valid for Medicare   Non-covered by Medicare   Special coverage instructions   Carrier discretion

E2614 Positioning wheelchair back cushion, posterior, width 22 inches or greater, any height, including any type mounting hardware

E2615 Positioning wheelchair back cushion, posterior-lateral, width less than 22 inches, any height, including any type mounting hardware

E2616 Positioning wheelchair back cushion, posterior-lateral, width 22 inches or greater, any height, including any type mounting hardware

E2617 Custom fabricated wheelchair back cushion, any size, including any type mounting hardware

E2618 Wheelchair accessory, solid seat support base (replaces sling seat), for use with manual wheelchair or lightweight power wheelchair, includes any type mounting hardware

E2619 Replacement cover for wheelchair seat cushion or back cushion, each

E2620 Positioning wheelchair back cushion, planar back with lateral supports, width less than 22 inches, any height, including any type mounting hardware

E2621 Positioning wheelchair back cushion, planar back with lateral supports, width 22 inches or greater, any height, including any type mounting hardware

GAIT TRAINER

E8000 Gait trainer, pediatric size, posterior support, includes all accessories and components

E8001 Gait trainer, pediatric size, upright support, includes all accessories and components

E8002 Gait trainer, pediatric size, anterior support, includes all accessories and components

PROCEDURES AND PROFESSIONAL SERVICES

Guidelines

In addition to the information presented in the INTRODUCTION, several other items unique to this section are defined or identified here:

1. TEMPORARY CODES: The codes listed in this section are assigned by CMS on a temporary basis to identify procedures/services.

PROCEDURES/PROFESSIONAL SERVICES

(G0001)   Code deleted December 31, 2004; use CPT

G0008   Administration of influenza virus vaccine

G0009   Administration of pneumococcal vaccine

G0010   Administration of hepatitis B vaccine

G0027   Semen analysis; presence and/or motility of sperm excluding huhner

(G0030)   Code deleted March 31, 2005

(G0031)   Code deleted March 31, 2005

(G0032)   Code deleted March 31, 2005

(G0033)   Code deleted March 31, 2005
CIM: 50-36

(G0034)   Code deleted March 31, 2005

(G0035)   Code deleted March 31, 2005

(G0036)   Code deleted March 31, 2005

(G0037)   Code deleted March 31, 2005

G-H CODES

(G0038)   Code deleted March 31, 2005

(G0039)   Code deleted March 31, 2005

(G0040)   Code deleted March 31, 2005

(G0041)   Code deleted March 31, 2005

(G0042)   Code deleted March 31, 2005

(G0043)   Code deleted March 31, 2005

(G0044)   Code deleted March 31, 2005

(G0045)   Code deleted March 31, 2005

(G0046)   Code deleted March 31, 2005

(G0047)   Code deleted March 31, 2005

G0101   Cervical or vaginal cancer screening; pelvic and clinical breast examination

G0102   Prostate cancer screening; digital rectal examination
CIM: 50-55   MCM: 4182

G0103   Prostate cancer screening; prostate specific antigen test (PSA), total
CIM: 50-55   MCM: 4182

G0104   Colorectal cancer screening; flexible sigmoidoscopy

G0105   colonoscopy on individual at high risk

G0106   alternative to G0104, screening sigmoidoscopy, barium enema

G0107   fecal-occult blood test, 1-3 simultaneous determinations

G0108   Diabetes outpatient self-management training services, individual, per 30 minutes

G0109   Diabetes outpatient self-management training services, group session (2 or more), per 30 minutes

(G0110)   Code deleted December 31, 2005

(G0111)   Code deleted December 31, 2005

(G0112)   Code deleted December 31, 2005

(G0113)   Code deleted December 31, 2005

(G0114)   Code deleted December 31, 2005

(G0115)   Code deleted December 31, 2005

(G0116)   Code deleted December 31, 2005

G0117   Glaucoma screening for high risk patients furnished by an optometrist or ophthalmologist

G0118   Glaucoma screening for high risk patient furnished under the direct supervision of an optometrist or ophthalmologist

G0120   Colorectal cancer screening; alternative to G0105, screening colonoscopy, barium enema

G0121   colonoscopy on individual not meeting criteria for high risk

G0122   barium enema

G0123   Screening cytopathology, cervical or vaginal (any reporting system), collected in preservative fluid, automated thin layer preparation; screening by cytotechnologist under physician supervision
CIM: 50-20

G0124   requiring interpretation by physician
CIM: 50-20

(G0125)   Code deleted March 31, 2005

G0127   Trimming of dystrophic nails, any number
MCM: 2323, 4120

G0128   Direct (fact-to-face with patient) skilled nursing services of a registered nurse provided in a comprehensive outpatient rehabilitation facility, each 10 minutes beyond the first 5 minutes

G0129 Occupational therapy requiring the skills of a qualified occupational therapist, furnished as a component of a partial hospitalization treatment program, per day

G0130 Single energy X-ray absorptiometry (sexa) bone density study, one or more sites; appendicular skeleton (peripheral) (e.g., radius, wrist, heel)
CIM: 50-44

G0141 Screening cytopathology smears, cervical or vaginal, performed by automated system, with manual rescreening, requiring interpretation by physician

G0143 Screening cytopathology, cervical or vaginal (any reporting system), collected in preservative fluid, automated thin layer preparation; with manual screening and rescreening by cytotechnologist under physician supervision

G0144 with screening by automated system, under physician supervision

G0145 with screening by automated system and manual rescreening under physician supervision

G0147 Screening cytopathology smears, cervical or vaginal; performed by automated system under physician supervision

G0148 performed by automated system with manual rescreening

G0151 Services of physical therapist in home or health setting, each 15 minutes

G0152 Services of occupational therapist in home health setting, each 15 minutes

G0153 Services of speech and language pathologist in home health setting, each 15 minutes

G0154 Services of skilled nurse in home health setting, each 15 minutes

G0155 Services of clinical social worker in home health setting, each 15 minutes

G0156 Services of home health aide in home health setting, each 15 minutes

G0166 External counterpulsation, per treatment session
CIM: 35-74

G0168 Wound closure utilizing tissue adhesive(s) only

G0173 Linear accelerator based stereotactic radiosurgery, complete course of therapy in one session

G0175 Scheduled interdisciplinary team conference (minimum of three exclusive of patient care nursing staff) with patient present

G0176 Activity therapy, such as music, dance, art or play therapies not for recreation, related to the care and treatment of patient's disabling mental health problems, per session (45 minutes or more)

G0177 Training and education services related to the care and treatment of patient's disabling mental health problems per session (45 minutes or more)

G0179 Physician recertification services for Medicare-covered services provided by a participating home health agency (patient not present) including review of subsequent reports of patient status, review of patient's responses to the Oasis assessment instrument, contact with the home health agency to ascertain the follow-up implementation plan of care, and documentation in the patient's office record, per certification period

G0180 Physician certification services for Medicare-covered services provided by a participating home health agency (patient not present), including review of initial or subsequent reports of patient status, review of patient's responses to the oasis assessment instrument, contact with the home health agency to ascertain the initial implementation plan of care, and documentation in the patient's office record, per certification period

■■■ Not valid   ■■■ Non-covered   Special   ■■■ Carrier   **165**
for Medicare   by Medicare   coverage   discretion
instructions

G0181   Physician supervision of a patient receiving Medicare-covered services provided by a participating home health agency (patient not present), requiring complex and multidisciplinary care modalities involving regular physician development and/or revision of care plans, review of subsequent reports of patient status, review of laboratory and other studies, communication (including telephone calls) with other health care professionals involved in the patient's care, integration of new information into the medical treatment plan and/or adjustment of medical therapy, within a calendar month, 30 minutes or more

G0182   Physician supervision of a patient under a Medicare-approved hospice (patient not present) requiring complex and multidisciplinary care modalities involving regular physician development and/or revision of care plans, review of subsequent reports of patient status, review of laboratory and other studies, communication (including telephone calls) with other health care professionals involved in the patient's care, integration of new information into the medical treatment plan and/or adjustment of medical therapy, within a calendar month, 30 minutes or more

G0186   Destruction of localized lesion of choroid (for example, choroidal neovascularization); photocoagulation, feeder vessel technique (one or more sessions)

G0202   Screening mammography, producing direct digital image, bilateral, all views

G0204   Diagnostic mammography, producing direct digital image, bilateral, all views

G0206   Diagnostic mammography, producing direct digital image, unilateral, all views

(G0210)   Code deleted March 31, 2005

(G0211)   Code deleted March 31, 2005

(G0212)   Code deleted March 31, 2005

(G0213)   Code deleted March 31, 2005

(G0214)   Code deleted March 31, 2005

(G0215)   Code deleted March 31, 2005

(G0216)   Code deleted March 31, 2005

(G0217)   Code deleted March 31, 2005

(G0218)   Code deleted March 31, 2005

G0219   PET imaging whole body; full and partial ring PET scanners only, for non-covered indications
CIM: 50-36   MCM: 4173

(G0220)   Code deleted March 31, 2005

(G0221)   Code deleted March 31, 2005

(G0222)   Code deleted March 31, 2005

(G0223)   Code deleted March 31, 2005

(G0224)   Code deleted March 31, 2005

(G0225)   Code deleted March 31, 2005

(G0226)   Code deleted March 31, 2005

(G0227)   Code deleted March 31, 2005

(G0228)   Code deleted March 31, 2005

(G0229)   Code deleted March 31, 2005

(G0230)   Code deleted March 31, 2005

(G0231)   Code deleted March 31, 2005

(G0232)   Code deleted March 31, 2005

(G0233)   Code deleted March 31, 2005

(G0234)   Code deleted March 31, 2005

● **G0235**   Pet imaging, any site, not otherwise specified
CIM: 50-36

Not valid   Non-covered   Special   Carrier   **167**
for Medicare   by Medicare   coverage   discretion
                                    instructions

G0237   Therapeutic procedures to increase strength or endurance of respiratory muscles, face to face, one on one, each 15 minutes (includes monitoring)

G0238   Therapeutic procedures to improve respiratory function, other than described by G0237, one on one, face to face, per 15 minutes (includes monitoring)

G0239   Therapeutic procedures to improve respiratory function or increase strength or endurance of respiratory muscles, two or more individuals (includes monitoring)

(G0242)   Code deleted December 31, 2005

G0243   Multi-source photon stereotactic radiosurgery, delivery including collimator changes and custom plugging, complete course of treatment, all lesions

(G0244)   Code deleted December 31, 2005

G0245   Initial physician evaluation of a diabetic patient with diabetic sensory neuropathy resulting in a loss of protective sensation (LOPS) which must include the diagnosis of LOPS; a patient history; a physical examination that consists of at least the following elements: (a) visual inspection of the forefoot, hindfoot and toe web spaces, (b) evaluation of a protective sensation, (c) evaluation of foot structure and biomechanics, (d) evaluation of vascular status and skin integrity, (e) evaluation and recommendation of footwear, (f) patient education
CIM: 50.81

G0246   Follow up evaluation of a diabetic patient with diabetic sensory neuropathy resulting in a loss of protective sensation (LOPS) to include at least the following, a patient history and physical examination that includes: (a) visual inspection of the forefoot, hindfoot and toe web spaces, (b) evaluation of protective sensation, (c) evaluation of foot structure and biomechanics, (d) evaluation of vascular status and skin integrity, (e) evaluation and recommendation of footwear, (f) patient education
CIM: 50.81

G0247   Routine foot care by a physician of a diabetic patient with diabetic sensory neuropathy resulting in a loss of protective sensation (LOPS) to include, the local care of superficial wounds (i.e., superficial to muscle and fascia) and at least the following if present: (1) local care of superficial wounds, (2) debridement of corns and callouses, and (3) trimming and debridement of nails
CIM: 50.81

G0248   Demonstration, at initial use, of home INR (international normalized ratio) monitoring for patient with mechanical heart valve(s) who meets Medicare coverage criteria, under the direction of a physician; includes: demonstrating use and care of the INR monitor, obtaining at least one blood sample, provision of instructions for reporting home INR test results, and documentation of patient ability to perform testing.
CIM: 50.55

G0249   Provision of test materials and equipment for home INR monitoring to patient with mechanical heart valve(s) who meets Medicare coverage criteria. Includes provision of materials for use in the home and reporting of test results to physician; per 8 tests.
CIM: 50.55

G0250   Physician review, interpretation and patient management of home INR testing for a patient with mechanical heart valve(s) who meets other coverage criteria; per 8 tests (does not require face-to-face service)
CIM: 50.55

G0251   Linear accelerator based stereotactic radiosurgery, delivery including collimator changes and custom plugging, fractionated treatment, all lesions, per session, maximum five sessions per course of treatment

(G0252)   Code deleted March 31, 2005

(G0253)   Code deleted March 31, 2005

(G0254)   Code deleted March 31, 2005

G0255   Current perception threshold/sensory nerve conduction test, (SNCT) per limb, any nerve
CIM: 50-57

███ - Not valid for Medicare   ███ Non-covered by Medicare   Special coverage instructions   ███ Carrier discretion

G0257   Unscheduled or emergency dialysis treatment for an ESRD patient in a hospital outpatient department that is not certified as an ESRD facility

(G0258)   Code deleted December 31, 2005

G0259   Injection procedure for sacroiliac joint; arthrography

G0260   Injection procedure for sacroiliac joint; provision of anesthetic, steroid and/or other therapeutic agent, with or without arthrography

(G0263)   Code deleted December 31, 2005

(G0264)   Code deleted December 31, 2005

G0265   Cryopreservation, freezing and storage of cells for therapeutic use, each cell line

G0266   Thawing and expansion of frozen cells for therapeutic use, each aliquot

G0267   Bone marrow or peripheral stem cell harvest, modification or treatment to eliminate cell type(s) (e.g. T-cells, metastatic carcinoma)

G0268   Removal of impacted cerumen (one or both ears) by physician on same date of service as audiologic function testing

G0269   Placement of occlusive device into either a venous or arterial access site, post surgical or interventional procedure (e.g. angioseal plug, vascular plug)

G0270   Medical nutrition therapy; reassessment and subsequent intervention(s) following second referral in same year for change in diagnosis, medical condition or treatment regimen (including additional hours needed for renal disease), individual, face to face with the patient, each 15 minutes

G0271   Medical nutrition therapy, reassessment and subsequent intervention(s) following second referral in same year for change in diagnosis, medical condition, or treatment regimen (including additional hours needed for renal disease), group (2 or more individuals), each 30 minutes

G0275 Renal artery angiography (unilateral or bilateral) performed at the time of cardiac catheterization, includes catheter placement, injection of dye, flush aortogram, and radiologic supervision and interpretation, and production of images (list separately in addition to primary procedure)

G0278 Iliac artery angiography performed at the same time of cardiac catheterization, includes catheter placement, injection of dye, radiologic supervision and interpretation, and production of images (list separately in addition to primary procedure)

(G0279) Code deleted December 31, 2005

(G0280) Code deleted December 31, 2005

G0281 Electrical stimulation, (unattended), to one or more areas, for chronic stage iii and stage iv pressure ulcers, arterial ulcers, diabetic ulcers, and venous stasis ulcers not demonstrating measurable signs of healing after 30 days of conventional care, as part of a therapy plan of care

G0282 Electrical stimulation, (unattended), to one or more areas, for wound care other than described in G0281
MCM: 35-98

G0283 Electrical stimulation (unattended), to one or more areas for indication(s) other than wound care, as part of a therapy plan of care

G0288 Reconstruction, computed tomographic angiography of aorta for surgical planning for vascular surgery

G0289 Arthroscopy, knee, surgical, for removal of loose body, foreign body, debridement/shaving of articular cartilage (chondroplasty) at the time of other surgical knee arthroscopy in a different compartment of the same knee

G0290 Transcatheter placement of a drug eluting intracoronary stent(s), percutaneous, with or without other therapeutic intervention, any method; single vessel

G0291 Transcatheter placement of a drug eluting intracoronary stent(s), percutaneous, with or without other therapeutic intervention, any method; each additional vessel

(G0292) Code deleted December 31, 2004; use CPT

G0293   Noncovered surgical procedure(s) using conscious sedation, regional, general or spinal anesthesia in a Medicare qualifying clinical trial, per day

G0294   Noncovered procedure(s) using either no anesthesia or local anesthesia only, in a Medicare qualifying clinical trial, per day

G0295   Electromagnetic therapy, to one or more areas, for wound care other than described in G0329 or for other uses
CIM: 35-98

(G0296)   Code deleted March 31, 2005

G0297   Insertion of single chamber pacing cardioverter defibrillator pulse generator

G0298   Insertion of dual chamber pacing cardioverter defibrillator pulse generator

G0299   Insertion or repositioning of electronic lead for single chamber pacing cardioverter defibrillator and insertion of pulse generator

G0300   Insertion or repositioning of electrode lead(s) for dual chamber pacing cardioverter defibrillator and insertion of pulse generator

G0302   Pre-operative pulmonary surgery services for preparation for LVRS, complete course of services, to include a minimum of 16 days of services

G0303   Pre-operative pulmonary surgery services for preparation for LVRS, 10 to 15 days of services

G0304   Pre-operative pulmonary surgery services for preparation for LVRS, 1 to 9 days of services

G0305   Post-discharge pulmonary surgery services after LVRS, minimum of 6 days of services

G0306   Complete CBC, automated (HGB, HCT, RBC, WBC, without platelet count) and automated WBC differential count

G0307   Complete (CBC), automated (HGB, HCT, RBC, WBC, without platelet count)

G0308   End stage renal disease (ESRD) related services during the course of treatment, for patients under 2 years of age to include monitoring for the adequacy of nutrition, assessment of growth and development, and counseling of parents; with 4 or more face-to-face physician visits per month
MCM: 2230

G0309   End stage renal disease (ESRD) related services during the course of treatment for patients under 2 years of age to include monitoring for the adequacy of nutrition, assessment of growth and development, and counseling of parents; with 2 or 3 face-to-face physician visits per month
MCM: 2230

G0310   End stage renal disease (ESRD) related services during the course of treatment, for patients under 2 years of age to include monitoring for the adequacy of nutrition, assessment of growth and development, and counseling of parents; with 1 face-to-face physician visit per month
MCM: 2230

G0311   End stage renal disease (ESRD) related services during the course of treatment, for patients between 2 and 11 years of age to include monitoring for the adequacy of nutrition, assessment of growth and development, and counseling of parents; with 4 or more face-to-face physician visits per month
MCM: 2230

G0312   End stage renal disease (ESRD) related services during the course of treatment, for patients between 2 and 11 years of age to include monitoring for the adequacy of nutrition, assessment of growth and development, and counseling of parents; with 2 or 3 face-to-face physician visits per month
MCM: 2230

G0313   End stage renal disease (ESRD) related services during the course of treatment, for patients between 2 and 11 years of age to include monitoring for the adequacy of nutrition, assessment of growth and development, and counseling of parents; with 1 face-to-face physician visit per month
MCM: 2230

G0314   End stage renal disease (ESRD) related services, during the course of treatment, for patients between 12 and 19 years of age to include monitoring for the adequacy of nutrition, assessment of growth and development, and counseling of parents; with 4 or more face-to-face physician visits per month
MCM: 2230

G0315   End stage renal disease (ESRD) related services during the course of treatment, for patients between 12 and 19 years of age to include monitoring for the adequacy of nutrition, assessment of growth and development, and counseling of parents; with 2 or 3 face-to-face physician visits per month
MCM: 2230

G0316   End stage renal disease (ESRD) related services during the course of treatment, for patients between 12 and 19 years of age to include monitoring for the adequacy of nutrition, assessment of growth and development, and counseling of parents; with 1 face-to-face physician visit per month
MCM: 2230

G0317   End stage renal disease (ESRD) related services during the course of treatment, for patients 20 years of age and over; with 4 or more face-to-face physician visits per month
MCM: 2230

G0318   End stage renal disease (ESRD) related services during the course of treatment, for patients 20 years of age and over; with 2 or 3 face-to-face physician visits per month
MCM: 2230

G0319   End stage renal disease (ESRD) related services during the course of treatment, for patients 20 years of age and over; with 1 face-to-face physician visit per month
MCM: 2230

G0320   End stage renal disease (ESRD) related services for home dialysis patients per full month; for patients under two years of age to include monitoring for adequacy of nutrition, assessment of growth and development, and counseling of parents
MCM: 2230

G0321 End stage renal disease (ESRD) related services for home dialysis patients per full month; for patients two to eleven years of age to include monitoring for adequacy of nutrition, assessment of growth and development, and counseling of parents
MCM: 2230

G0322 End stage renal disease (ESRD) related services for home dialysis patients per full month; for patients twelve to nineteen years of age to include monitoring for adequacy of nutrition, assessment of growth and development, and counseling of parents
MCM: 2230

G0323 End stage renal disease (ESRD) related services for home dialysis patients per full month; for patients twenty years of age and older
MCM: 2230

G0324 End stage renal disease (ESRD) related services for home dialysis (less than full month), per day; for patients under two years of age
MCM: 2230

G0325 End stage renal disease (ESRD) related services for home dialysis (less than full month), per day; for patients between two and eleven years of age
MCM: 2230

G0326 End stage renal disease (ESRD) related services for home dialysis (less than full month), per day; for patients between twelve and nineteen years of age
MCM: 2230

G0327 End stage renal disease (ESRD) related services for home dialysis (less than full month), per day; for patients twenty years of age and over
MCM: 2230

G0328 Colorectal cancer screening; fecal occult blood test, immunoassay, 1-3 simultaneous

G0329 Electromagnetic therapy, to one or more areas for chronic stage III and stage IV pressure ulcers, arterial ulcers, diabetic ulcers and venous stasis ulcers not demonstrating measurable signs of healing after 30 days of conventional care as part of a therapy plan of care

(G0336) Code deleted March 31, 2005

G0337   Hospice evaluation and counseling services, pre-election

(G0338)   Code deleted December 31, 2005

G0339   Image-guided robotic linear accelerator-based stereotactic radiosurgery, complete course of therapy in one session or first session of fractionated treatment

G0340   Image-guided robotic linear accelerator-based sterotactic radiosurgery, delivery including collimator changes and custom plugging, fractionated treatment, all lesions, per session, second through fifth sessions, maximum five sessions per course of treatment

G0341   Percutaneous islet cell transplant, includes portal vein catheterization and infusion
CIM: 260.3, 35-82

G0342   Laparoscopy for islet cell transplant, includes portal vein catheterization and infusion
CIM: 35-82

G0343   Laparotomy for islet cell transplant, includes portal vein catheterization and infusion
CIM: 35-82

G0344   Initial preventive physical examination; face-to-face visit, services limited to new beneficiary during the first six months of medicare enrollment

(G0345)   Code deleted December 31, 2005

(G0346)   Code deleted December 31, 2005

(G0347)   Code deleted December 31, 2005

(G0348)   Code deleted December 31, 2005

(G0349)   Code deleted December 31, 2005

(G0350)   Code deleted December 31, 2005

(G0351)   Code deleted December 31, 2005

(G0353)   Code deleted December 31, 2005

(G0354)   Code deleted December 31, 2005

(G0355) Code deleted December 31, 2005

(G0356) Code deleted December 31, 2005

(G0357) Code deleted December 31, 2005

(G0358) Code deleted December 31, 2005

(G0359) Code deleted December 31, 2005

(G0360) Code deleted December 31, 2005

(G0361) Code deleted December 31, 2005

(G0362) Code deleted December 31, 2005

(G0363) Code deleted December 31, 2005

G0364 Bone marrow aspiration performed with bone marrow biopsy through the same incision on the same date of service

G0365 Vessel mapping of vessels for hemodialysis access (services for preoperative vessel mapping prior to creation of hemodialysis access using an autogenous hemodialysis conduit, including arterial inflow and venous outflow)

G0366 Electrocardiogram, routine ECG with at least 12 leads; with interpretation and report, performed as a component of the initial preventive physical examination

G0367 Tracing only, without interpretation and report, performed as a component of the initial preventive physical examination

G0368 Interpretation and report only, performed as a component of the initial preventive physical examination

● **G0372** Physician service required to establish and document the need for a power mobility device (use in addition to primary evaluation and management code)

● **G0375** Smoking and tobacco use cessation counseling visit; intermediate, greater than 3 minutes up to 10 minutes

● **G0376** Smoking and tobacco use cessation counseling visit; intensive, greater than 10 minutes

● **G0378**   Hospital observation service, per hour

● **G0379**   Direct admission of patient for hospital observation care

G3001   Administration and supply of Tositumomab, 450 mg

G9001   Coordinated care fee; initial rate

G9002   maintenance rate

G9003   risk adjusted high, initial

G9004   risk adjusted low, initial

G9005   risk adjusted maintenance

G9006   home monitoring

G9007   scheduled team conference

G9008   physician coordinated care oversight services

G9009   risk adjusted maintenance, level 3

G9010   risk adjusted maintenance, level 4

G9011   risk adjusted maintenance, level 5

G9012   Other specified case management service not elsewhere classified

G9013   ESRD demo basic bundle level I

G9014   ESRD demo expanded bundle including venous access and related services

G9016   Smoking cessation counseling, individual, in the absence of or in addition to any other evaluation and management service, per session (6-10 minutes) [DEMO PROJECT CODE ONLY]

G9017   Amantadine hydrochloride, oral, per 100 mg (for use as a Medicare approved demonstration project)

G9018 Zanamivir, inhalation powder administered through inhaler, per 10 mg (for use as a Medicare approved demonstration project)

G9019 Oseltamivir phosphate, oral, per 75 mg (for use as a Medicare approved demonstration project)

G9020 Rimantadine hydrochloride, oral, per 100 mg (for use as a Medicare approved demonstration project)

● **G9033** Amantadine hydrochloride, oral brand, per 100 mg (for use in a Medicare-approved demonstration project)

● **G9041** Sensory integrative techniques to enhance sensory processing and promote adaptive responses to environmental demands, self care/home management training (e.g. Activities of daily living (adl) and compensatory training, meal preparation, safety procedures, and instructions in use of assistive technology devices/adaptive equipment), community/work reintegration training (e.g. shopping, transportation, money management, avocational activities and/or work environment modification analysis, work task analysis), direct one-on-one contact by the provider, each 15 minutes

● **G9042** Sensory integrative techniques to enhance sensory processing and promote adaptive responses to environmental demands, self care/home management training (e.g. Activities of daily living (adl) and compensatory training, meal preparation, safety procedures, and instructions in use of assistive technology devices/adaptive equipment), community/work reintegration training (e.g. shopping, transportation, money management, avocational activities and/or work environment modification analysis, work task analysis), direct one-on-one contact by the provider, each 15 minutes

● G9043   Sensory integrative techniques to enhance sensory processing and promote adaptive responses to environmental demands, self care/home management training (e.g. Activities of daily living (adl) and compensatory training, meal preparation, safety procedures, and instructions in use of assistive technology devices/adaptive equipment), community/work reintegration training (e.g. shopping, transportation, money management, avocational activities and/or work environment modification analysis, work task analysis), direct one-on-one contact by the provider, each 15 minutes

● G9044   Sensory integrative techniques to enhance sensory processing and promote adaptive responses to environmental demands, self care/home management training (e.g. Activities of daily living (adl) and compensatory training, meal preparation, safety procedures, and instructions in use of assistive technology devices/adaptive equipment), community/work reintegration training (e.g. shopping, transportation, money management, avocational activities and/or work environment modification analysis, work task analysis), direct one-on-one contact by the provider, each 15 minutes

REHABILITATIVE SERVICES

Rehabilitative Services

H0001 Alcohol and/or drug assessment

H0002 Behavioral health screening to determine eligibility for admission to treatment program

H0003 Alcohol and/or drug screening; laboratory analysis of specimens for presence of alcohol and/or drugs

H0004 Behavioral health counseling and therapy, per 15 minutes

H0005 Alcohol and/or drug services; group counseling by a clinician

H0006 Alcohol and/or drug services; case management

H0007 Alcohol and/or drug services; crisis intervention (outpatient)

H0008 Alcohol and/or drug services; sub-acute detoxification (hospital inpatient)

H0009 Alcohol and/or drug services; acute detoxification (hospital inpatient)

H0010 Alcohol and/or drug services; sub-acute detoxification (residential addiction program inpatient)

H0011 Alcohol and/or drug services; acute detoxification (residential addiction program inpatient)

H0012 Alcohol and/or drug services; sub-acute detoxification (residential addiction program outpatient)

H0013 Alcohol and/or drug services; acute detoxification (residential addiction program outpatient)

H0014 Alcohol and/or drug services; ambulatory detoxification

H0015 Alcohol and/or drug services; intensive outpatient (treatment program that operates at least 3 hours/day and at least 3 days/week and is based on an individualized treatment plan), including assessment, counseling, crisis intervention, and activity therapies or education

H0016 Alcohol and/or drug services; medical/somatic (medical intervention in ambulatory setting)

H0017 Behavioral health; residential (hospital residential treatment program), without room and board, per diem

H0018 Behavioral health; short-term residential (non-hospital residential treatment program), without room and board, per diem

H0019 Behavioral health; long-term residential (non-medical, non-acute care in residential treatment program where stay is typically longer than 30 days), without room and board, per diem

H0020 Alcohol and/or drug services; methadone administration and/or service (provision of the drug by a licensed program)

H0021 Alcohol and/or drug training service (for staff and personnel not employed by providers)

H0022 Alcohol and/or drug intervention service (planned facilitation)

H0023 Behavioral health outreach service (planned approach to reach a targeted population)

H0024 Behavioral health prevention information dissemination service (one-way direct or non-direct contact with service audiences to affect knowledge and attitude)

H0025 Behavioral health prevention education service (delivery of services with target population to affect knowledge, attitude and/or behavior)

H0026 Alcohol and/or drug prevention process services, community-based (delivery of services to develop skills of impactors)

H0027 Alcohol and/or drug prevention environmental services (broad range of external activities geared toward modifying systems in order to mainstream prevention through policy and law)

H0028 Alcohol and/or drug prevention problem identification and referral service (e.g., student assistance and employee assistance programs), does not include assessment

H0029 Alcohol and/or drug prevention alternatives service (services for populations that exclude alcohol and other drug use, e.g. alcohol-free social events)

H0030 Behavioral health hotline service

H0031 Mental health assessment, by non-physician

H0032 Mental health service plan development by non-physician

H0033 Oral medication administration, direct observation

H0034 Medication training and support, per 15 minutes

H0035 Mental health partial hospitalization, treatment, less than 24 hours

H0036 Community psychiatric supportive treatment, face-to-face, per 15 minutes

H0037 Community psychiatric supportive treatment program, per diem

H0038 Self-help/peer services, per 15 minutes

H0039 Assertive community treatment, face-to-face, per 15 minutes

H0040 Assertive community treatment program, per diem

H0041 Foster care, child, non-therapeutic, per diem

H0042 Foster care, child, non-therapeutic, per month

H0043 Supported housing, per diem

H0044 Supported housing, per month

H0045 Respite care services, not in the home, per diem

H0046 Mental health services, not otherwise specified

H0047 Alcohol and/or other drug abuse services, not otherwise specified

H0048 Alcohol and/or other drug testing: collection and handling only, specimens other than blood

H1000 Prenatal care, at-risk assessment

H1001 Prenatal care, at-risk enhanced service; antepartum management

H1002 Prenatal care, at-risk enhanced service; care coordination

H1003 Prenatal care, at-risk enhanced service; education

H1004 Prenatal care, at-risk enhanced service; follow-up home visit

H1005 Prenatal care, at-risk enhanced service package (includes H1001-H1004)

H1010 Non-medical family planning education, per session

H1011 Family assessment by licensed behavioral health professional for state defined purposes

H2000 Comprehensive multidisciplinary evaluation

H2001 Rehabilitation program, per 1/2 day

H2010 Comprehensive medication services, per 15 minutes

H2011 Crisis intervention service, per 15 minutes

H2012 Behavioral health day treatment, per hour

H2013 Psychiatric health facility service, per diem

H2014 Skills training and development, per 15 minutes

H2015 Comprehensive community support services, per 15 minutes

H2016 Comprehensive community support services, per diem

H2017 Psychosocial rehabilitation services, per 15 mintues

H2018 Psychosocial rehabilitation services, per diem

H2019 Therapeutic behavioral services, per 15 minutes

H2020 Therapeutic behavioral services, per diem

H2021 Community-based wrap-around services, per 15 minutes

H2022 Community-based wrap-around services, per diem

H2023 Supported employment, per 15 minutes

H2024 Supported employment, per diem

H2025 Ongoing support to maintain employment, per 15 minutes

H2026 Ongoing support to maintain employment, per diem

H2027 Psychoeducational service, per 15 minutes

H2028 Sexual offender treatment service, per 15 minutes

H2029 Sexual offender treatment service, per diem

H2030 Mental health clubhouse services, per 15 minutes

H2031 Mental health clubhouse services, per diem

H2032 Activity therapy, per 15 minutes

H2033 Multisystemic therapy for juveniles, per 15 minutes

H2034 Alcohol and/or drug abuse halfway house services, per diem

H2035 Alcohol and/or other drug treatment program, per hour

H2036 Alcohol and/or other drug treatment program, per diem

H2037 Developmental delay prevention activities, dependent child of client, per 15 minutes

● New code ▲ Revised code ( ) Deleted code

DRUGS ADMINISTERED OTHER THAN ORAL METHOD

(EXCEPTION: ORAL IMMUNOSUPPRESSIVE DRUGS)

Guidelines

In addition to the information presented in the INTRODUCTION, several other items unique to this section are defined or identified here:

1. EXCEPTION: Oral immunosuppressive drugs are not included in this section.

2. ROUTE OF ADMINISTRATION: Unless otherwise specified, the drugs listed in this section may be injected either subcutaneously, intramuscularly or intravenously.

3. SUBSECTION INFORMATION: Some of the listed subheadings or subsections have special needs or instructions unique to that section. Where these are indicated, special "notes" will be presented preceding or following the listings. Those subsections within the DRUGS ADMINISTERED OTHER THAN ORAL METHOD section that have "notes" are as follows:

Subsection	Code Numbers
Drugs administered other than oral method	J0000-J8999
Immunosuppressive drugs	J7500-J7506
Chemotherapy drugs	J9000-J9999

4. UNLISTED SERVICE OR PROCEDURE: A service or procedure may be provided that is not listed in this edition of HCPCS. When reporting such a service, the appropriate "unlisted procedure" code may be used to indicate the service, identifying it by "special report" as defined below. HCPCS terminology is inconsistent in defining unlisted procedures. The procedure definition may include the term(s) "unlisted", "not otherwise classified", "unspecified", "unclassified", "other" and "miscellaneous". Prior to using these codes, try to determine if a Local Level III code or CPT code is available. The "unlisted procedures" and accompanying codes for DRUGS ADMINISTERED OTHER THAN ORAL METHOD are as follows:

J CODES

J3490   Unclassified drugs
J9999   Not otherwise classified, antineoplastic drugs

5. SPECIAL REPORT: A service, material or supply that is rarely
    provided, unusual, variable or new may require a special report in
    determining medical appropriateness for reimbursement purposes.
    Pertinent information should include an adequate definition or
    description of the nature, extent, and need for the service, material or
    supply.

6. MODIFIERS: Listed services may be modified under certain
    circumstances. When appropriate, the modifying circumstance is
    identified by adding a modifier to the basic procedure code. CPT and
    HCPCS National Level II modifiers may be used with CPT and
    HCPCS National Level II procedure codes. Modifiers commonly
    used with DRUGS ADMINISTERED OTHER THAN ORAL
    METHOD are as follows:

    -AA   Anesthesia services performed personally by anesthesiologist

    -AD   Medical supervision by a physician: more than four
          concurrent anesthesia procedures.

    -CC   Procedure code change (use "CC" when the procedure code
          submitted was changed either for administrative reasons or
          because an incorrect code was filed)

    -G8   Monitored anesthesia care (MAC) for deep complex,
          complicated, or markedly invasive surgical procedure

    -G9   Monitored anesthesia care (MAC) for patient who has history
          of severe cardio-pulmonary condition

    -TC   Technical component. Under certain circumstances, a charge
          may be made for the technical component alone. Under those
          circumstances, the technical component charge is identified by
          adding modifier -TC to the usual procedure code. Technical
          component charges are institutional charges and are not billed
          separately by physicians. However, portable x-ray suppliers
          bill only for the technical component and should use modifier
          -TC. The charge data from portable x-ray suppliers will then
          be used to build customary and prevailing profiles.

7. CPT CODE CROSS-REFERENCE: Unless otherwise specified, the
    equivalent CPT codes for all listings in this section fall within the
    range 90701-90799.

Drugs Administered Other Than Oral Method

The following list of drugs can be injected either subcutaneous, intramuscular, or intravenous. The brand name(s) of the drugs has been included as bold-type in brackets [ ] in some cases.

NOTE: Third party payers may wish to determine a threshold and pay up to a certain dollar limit before developing for the drug. Use procedure code J0110 for processing these cases.

J0120   Injection, tetracycline, up to 250 mg
MCM: 2049

J0128   Injection, abarelix, 10 mg

J0130   Injection abciximab, 10 mg
MCM: 2049

● **J0132**   Injection, acetylcysteine, 100 mg

● **J0133**   Injection, acyclovir, 5 mg

J0135   Injection, adalimumab, 20 mg

J0150   Injection, adenosine for therapeutic use, 6 mg (not to be used to report any adenosine phosphate compounds, instead use A9270)
MCM: 2049

J0152   Injection, adenosine for diagnostic use, 30 mg (not to be used to report any adenosine phosphate compounds; instead use A9270)

J0170   Injection, adrenalin, epinephrine, up to 1 ml ampul
MCM: 2049

J0180   Injection, agalsidase beta, 1 mg

J0190   Injection, biperiden lactate, per 5 mg
MCM: 2049

J0200   Injection, alatrofloxacin mesylate, 100 mg
MCM: 2049.5

J0205   Injection, alglucerase, per 10 units
MCM: 2049

J0207   Injection, amifostine, 500 mg
MCM: 2049

J0210   Injection, methyldopa HCl, [Aldomet], up to 250 mg
MCM: 2049

J0215   Injection, alefacept, 0.5 mg

J0256   Injection, alpha 1—proteinase inhibitor—human, 10 mg
MCM: 2049

J0270   Injection, alprostadil, 1.25 mcg (code may be used for
Medicare when drug administered under the direct
supervision of a physician, not for use when drug is self
administered)
MCM: 2049

J0275   Alprostadil urethral suppository (code may be used for
Medicare when drug administered under the direct
supervision of a physician, not for use when drug is self
administered)
MCM: 2049

● **J0278**   Injection, amikacin sulfate, 100 mg

J0280   Injection, aminophylline, up to 250 mg
MCM: 2049

J0282   Injection, amiodarone hydrochloride, 30 mg
MCM: 2049

J0285   Injection, amphotericin B, 50 mg
MCM: 2049

J0287   Injection, amphotericin b lipid complex, 10 mg
MCM: 2049

J0288   Injection, amphotericin b cholesteryl sulfate complex, 10
mg
MCM: 2049

J0289   Injection, amphotericin b liposome, 10 mg
MCM: 2049

J0290   Injection, ampicillin sodium, 500 mg
MCM: 2049

J0295   Injection, ampicillin sodium/sulbactam sodium, per 1.5
gram
MCM: 2049

J0300   Injection, amobarbital, up to 125 mg
MCM: 2049

J0330   Injection, succinylcholine chloride, [Anectine], up to 20 mg
MCM: 2049

J0350   Injection, anistreplase, per 30 units
MCM: 2049

J0360   Injection, hydralazine HCl, [Apresoline], up to 20 mg
MCM: 2049

● **J0365**   Injection, aprotonin, 10,000 kiu
MCM: 2049

J0380   Injection, metaraminol bitartrate, per 10 mg
MCM: 2049

J0390   Injection, chloroquine HCl, [Aralen HCl], up to 250 mg
MCM: 2049

J0395   Injection, arbutamine HCl, 1 mg
MCM: 2049

J0456   Injection, azithromycin, 500 mg
MCM: 2049.5

J0460   Injection, atropine sulfate, up to 0.3 mg
MCM: 2049

J0470   Injection, dimercaprol, per 100 mg
MCM: 2049

J0475   Injection, baclofen, 10 mg
MCM: 2049

J0476   Injection, baclofen, 50 mcg for intrathecal trial
MCM: 2049

● **J0480**   Injection, basiliximab, 20 mg
MCM: 2049

J0500   Injection, dicyclomine HCl, [Bentyl, Spasmoject], up to 20 mg
MCM: 2049

J0515   Injection, benztropine mesylate, [Cogentin], per 1 mg
MCM: 2049

Not valid
for Medicare   Non-covered
by Medicare   Special
coverage
instructions   Carrier
discretion   **191**

J0520   Injection, bethanechol chloride, myotonachol or
urecholine, up to 5 mg
MCM: 2049

J0530   Injection, penicillin G benzathine and penicillin G
procaine, [Bicillin C-R]; up to 600,000 units
MCM: 2049

J0540   up to 1,200,000 units
MCM: 2049

J0550   up to 2,400,000 units
MCM: 2049

J0560   Injection, penicillin G benzathine, [Bicillin long-acting];
up to 600,000 units
MCM: 2049

J0570   up to 1,200,000 units
MCM: 2049

J0580   up to 2,400,000 units
MCM: 2049

J0583   Injection, bivalirudin, 1 mg

J0585   Botulinum toxin type A, per unit
MCM: 2049

J0587   Botulinum toxin type B, per 100 units
MCM: 2049

J0592   Injection, buprenorphine hydrochloride, 0.1 mg
MCM: 2049

J0595   Injection, butorphanol tartrate, 1 mg

J0600   Injection, edetate calcium disodium, [calcium disodium
versenate], up to 1,000 mg
MCM: 2049

J0610   Injection, calcium gluconate, per 10 ml
MCM: 2049

J0620   Injection, calcium glycerophosphate and calcium lactate,
per 10 ml
MCM: 2049

J0630   Injection, calcitonin salmon, up to 400 units
MCM: 2049

J0636 Injection, calcitriol, 0.1 mcg
MCM: 2049

J0637 Injection, caspofungin acetate, 5 mg

J0640 Injection, leucovorin calcium, per 50 mg
MCM: 2049

J0670 Injection, mepivacaine HCl, [Carbocaine], per 10 ml
MCM: 2049

J0690 Injection, cefazolin sodium, 500 mg
MCM: 2049

J0692 Injection, cefepime hydrochloride, 500 mg

J0694 Injection, cefoxitin sodium, [Mefoxin], 1 gram
MCM: 2049

J0696 Injection, ceftriaxone sodium, [Rocephin], per 250 mg
MCM: 2049

J0697 Injection sterile cefuroxime sodium, [Ceftin, Kefurox, Zihacef injection], per 750 mg
MCM: 2049

J0698 Injection, cefotaxime sodium, [Claforan], per gram
MCM: 2049

J0702 Injection, betamethasone acetate and betamethasone sodium phosphate, per 3 mg
MCM: 2049

J0704 Injection, betamethasone sodium phosphate, per 4 mg
MCM: 2049

J0706 Injection, caffeine citrate, 5 mg

J0710 Injection, cephapirin sodium, [Cefadyl], up to 1 gram
MCM: 2049

J0713 Injection, ceftazidime, per 500 mg
MCM: 2049

J0715 Injection, ceftizoxime sodium, per 500 mg
MCM: 2049

J0720 Injection, chloramphenicol sodium succinate, [Chloromycetin Sodium Succinate], up to 1 gram
MCM: 2049

Not valid | Non-covered | Special | Carrier
for Medicare | by Medicare | coverage | discretion
| | instructions |

J0725   Injection, chorionic gonadotropin, per 1,000 USP units
MCM: 2049

J0735   Injection, clonidine hydrochloride, 1 mg
MCM: 2049

J0740   Injection, cidofovir, 375 mg
MCM: 2049

J0743   Injection, cilastatin sodium/imipenem, [Primaxin], per 250 mg
MCM: 2049

J0744   Injection, ciprofloxacin for intravenous infusion, 200 mg

J0745   Injection, codeine phosphate, per 30 mg
MCM: 2049

J0760   Injection, colchicine, per 1 mg
MCM: 2049

J0770   Injection, colistimethate sodium, [Coly-Mycin M], up to 150 mg
MCM: 2049

J0780   Injection, prochlorperazine, [Compazine], up to 10 mg
MCM: 2049

● **J0795**   Injection, corticorelin ovine triflutate, 1 microgram
MCM: 2049

J0800   Injection, corticotropin, up to 40 units
MCM: 2049

J0835   Injection, cosyntropin, per 0.25 mg
MCM: 2049

J0850   Injection, cytomegalovirus immune globulin intravenous (human), per vial
MCM: 2049

J0878   Injection, daptomycin, 1 mg

(J0880)   Code deleted December 31, 2005

● **J0881**   Injection, darbepoetin alfa, 1 microgram (non-esrd use)
MCM: 4273.1

● **J0882**   Injection, darbepoetin alfa, 1 microgram (for esrd on dialysis)
MCM: 4273.1

● **J0885** Injection, epoetin alfa, (for non-esrd use), 1000 units
MCM: 2049

● **J0886** Injection, epoetin alfa, 1000 units (for esrd on dialysis)
MCM: 4273.1

J0895 Injection, deferoxamine mesylate, [Desferal] 500 mg
MCM: 2049

J0900 Injection, testosterone enanthate and estradiol valerate, up to 1 cc
MCM: 2049

J0945 Injection, brompheniramine maleate, per 10 mg
MCM: 2049

J0970 Injection, estradiol valerate, up to 40 mg
MCM: 2049

J1000 Injection, depo-estradiol cypionate, up to 5 mg
MCM: 2049

J1020 Injection, methylprednisolone acetate; 20 mg
MCM: 2049

J1030 40 mg
MCM: 2049

J1040 80 mg
MCM: 2049

J1051 Injection, medroxyprogesterone acetate, 50 mg
MCM: 2049

J1055 Injection, medroxyprogesterone acetate for contraceptive use, 150 mg

J1056 Injection, medroxyprogesterone acetate/estradiol cypionate, 5 mg/25 mg

J1060 Injection, testosterone cypionate and estradiol cypionate, up to 1 ml
MCM: 2049

J1070 Injection, testosterone cypionate, up to 100 mg
MCM: 2049

J1080 Injection, testosterone cypionate, 1 cc, 200 mg
MCM: 2049

Not valid
for Medicare   Non-covered
by Medicare   Special
coverage
instructions   Carrier
discretion

J1094   Injection, dexamethasone acetate, 1 mg
MCM: 2049

J1100   Injection, dexamethasone sodium phosphate, 1mg
MCM: 2049

J1110   Injection, dihydroergotamine mesylate, per 1 mg
MCM: 2049

J1120   Injection, acetazolamide sodium, [Diamox Sodium], up to 500 mg
MCM: 2049

J1160   Injection, digoxin, up to 0.5 mg
MCM: 2049

● **J1162**   Injection, digoxin immune fab (ovine), per vial
MCM: 2049

J1165   Injection, phenytoin sodium, [Dilantin], per 50 mg
MCM: 2049

J1170   Injection, hydromorphone, up to 4 mg
MCM: 2049

J1180   Injection, dyphylline, [Dilor, Lufyllin], up to 500 mg
MCM: 2049

J1190   Injection, dexrazoxane hydrochloride, per 250 mg
MCM: 2049

J1200   Injection, diphenhydramine HCl, [Benadryl], up to 50 mg
MCM: 2049

J1205   Injection, chlorothiazide sodium [Diuril], per 500 mg
MCM: 2049

J1212   Injection, DMSO, dimethyl sulfoxide, 50%, 50 ml
CIM: 45-23 MCM: 2049

J1230   Injection, methadone HCl, [Dolophine HCl], up to 10 mg
MCM: 2049

J1240   Injection, dimenhydrinate, [Dramamine], up to 50 mg
MCM: 2049

J1245   Injection, dipyridamole, per 10 mg
MCM: 15030, 2049

J1250   Injection, dobutamine hydrochloride, per 250 mg
MCM: 2049

J1260   Injection, dolasetron mesylate, 10 mg
MCM: 2049

●**J1265**   Injection, dopamine hcl, 40 mg

J1270   Injection, doxercalciferol, 1 mcg

J1320   Injection, amitriptyline HCl, [Elavil HCl], up to 20 mg
MCM: 2049

J1325   Injection, epoprostenol, 0.5 mg
MCM: 2049

J1327   Injection, eptifibatide, 5 mg
MCM: 2049

J1330   Injection, ergonovine maleate, up to 0.2 mg
MCM: 2049

J1335   Injection, ertapenem sodium, 500 mg

J1364   Injection, erythromycin lactobionate, per 500 mg
MCM: 2049

J1380   Injection, estradiol valerate, up to 10 mg
MCM: 2049

J1390   Injection, estradiol valerate, up to 20 mg
MCM: 2049

J1410   Injection, estrogen conjugated, per 25 mg
MCM: 2049

●**J1430**   Injection, ethanolamine oleate, 100 mg
MCM: 2049

J1435   Injection, estrone, per 1 mg
MCM: 2049

J1436   Injection, etidronate disodium per 300 mg
MCM: 2049

J1438   Injection, etanercept, 25 mg (code may be used for Medicare when drug administered under the direct supervision of a physician, not for use when drug is self administered)
MCM: 2049

J1440   Injection, filgrastim (G-CSF); 300 mcg
MCM: 2049

J1441   480 mcg
MCM: 2049

J1450   Injection, fluconazole, 200 mg
MCM: 2049.5

● **J1451**   Injection, fomepizole, 15 mg
MCM: 2049

J1452   Injection, fomivirsen sodium, intraocular, 1.65 mg
MCM: 2049.3

J1455   Injection, foscarnet sodium, [Foscavir], per 1000 mg
MCM: 2049

J1457   Injection, gallium nitrate, 1 mg

J1460   Injection, gamma globulin; intramuscular 1 cc
MCM: 2049

J1470   intramuscular 2 cc
MCM: 2049

J1480   intramuscular 3 cc
MCM: 2049

J1490   intramuscular 4 cc
MCM: 2049

J1500   intramuscular 5 cc
MCM: 2049

J1510   intramuscular 6 cc
MCM: 2049

J1520   intramuscular 7 cc
MCM: 2049

J1530   intramuscular 8 cc
MCM: 2049

J1540   intramuscular 9 cc
MCM: 2049

J1550   intramuscular 10 cc
MCM: 2049

J1560   intramuscular over 10 cc
MCM: 2049

(J1563)   Code deleted December 31, 2005

(J1564)   Code deleted December 31, 2005

J1565   Injection, respiratory syncytial virus immune globulin,
intravenous, 50 mg
MCM: 2049

● **J1566**   Injection, immune globulin, intravenous, lyophilized (e.g.
Powder), 500 mg
MCM: 2049

● **J1567**   Injection, immune globulin, intravenous, non-lyophilized
(e.g. Liquid), 500 mg
MCM: 2049

J1570   Injection, ganciclovir sodium, [Cytovene], 500 mg
MCM: 2049

J1580   Injection, garamycin, gentamicin, up to 80 mg
MCM: 2049

J1590   Injection, gatifloxacin, 10 mg

J1595   Injection, glatiramer acetate, 20 mg
MCM: 2049

J1600   Injection, gold sodium thiomalate, up to 50 mg
MCM: 2049

J1610   Injection, glucagon hydrochloride, per 1 mg
MCM: 2049

J1620   Injection, gonadorelin hydrochloride, per 100 mcg
MCM: 2049

J1626   Injection, granisetron hydrochloride, 100 mcg
MCM: 2049

J1630   Injection, haloperidol, up to 5 mg
MCM: 2049

J1631   Injection, haloperidol decanoate, per 50 mg
MCM: 2049

● **J1640**   Injection, hemin, 1 mg
MCM: 2049

J1642   Injection, heparin sodium, (heparin lock flush), per 10
units
MCM: 2049

J1644   Injection, heparin sodium, per 1,000 units
MCM: 2049

J1645   Injection, dalteparin sodium, per 2500 IU
MCM: 2049

J1650   Injection, enoxaparin sodium, 10 mg

J1652   Injection, fondaparinux sodium, 0.5 mg
MCM: 2049

J1655   Injection, tinzaparin sodium, 1000 IU

J1670   Injection, tetanus immune globulin, human, up to 250
units
MCM: 2049

● **J1675**   Injection, histrelin acetate, 10 micrograms
MCM: 2049

J1700   Injection, hydrocortisone acetate, [Analpram HC,
Hydrocortone Acetate], up to 25 mg
MCM: 2049

J1710   Injection, hydrocortisone sodium phosphate,
[Hydrocortone Phosphate], up to 50 mg
MCM: 2049

J1720   Injection, hydrocortisone sodium succinate, [Solu-Cortef],
up to 100 mg
MCM: 2049

J1730   Injection, diazoxide, [Hyperstat], up to 300 mg
MCM: 2049

J1742   Injection, ibutilide fumarate, 1 mg
MCM: 2049

J1745   Injection, infliximab, 10 mg
MCM: 2049

(J1750)   Code deleted December 31, 2005

● **J1751**   Injection, iron dextran 165, 50 mg

● **J1752**   Injection, iron dextran 267, 50 mg

J1756   Injection, iron sucrose, 1 mg

J1785 Injection, imiglucerase, per unit
MCM: 2049

J1790 Injection, droperidol, [Inapsine], up to 5 mg
MCM: 2049

J1800 Injection, propranolol HCl, [Inderal], up to 1 mg
MCM: 2049

J1810 Injection, droperidol and fentanyl citrate, [Innovar], up to 2 ml ampule
MCM: 2049

J1815 Injection, insulin, per 5 units
CIM: 60-14 MCM: 2049

J1817 Insulin for administration through DME (i.e., Insulin pump) per 50 units

J1825 Injection, interferon beta-1a, 33 mcg

J1830 Injection, interferon beta-1b, 0.25 mg (code may be used for Medicare when drug administered under the direct supervision of a physician, not for use when drug is self administered)
MCM: 2049

J1835 Injection, itraconazole, 50 mg

J1840 Injection, kanamycin sulfate, [Kantrex], up to 500 mg
MCM: 2049

J1850 Injection, kanamycin sulfate, [Kantrex Pediatric], up to 75 mg
MCM: 2049

J1885 Injection, ketorolac tromethamine, [Toradol IM], per 15 mg
MCM: 2049

J1890 Injection, cephalothin sodium, [Keflin], up to 1 gram
MCM: 2049

J1931 Injection, laronidase, 0.1 Mg

J1940 Injection, furosemide, [Lasix], up to 20 mg
MCM: 2049

● **J1945** Injection, lepirudin, 50 mg
MCM: 2049

J1950   Injection, leuprolide acetate (for depot suspension), per
3.75 mg
MCM: 2049

J1955   Injection, levocarnitine, per 1 gram
MCM: 2049

J1956   Injection, levofloxacin, 250 mg
MCM: 2049

J1960   Injection, levorphanal tartrate, up to 2 mg
MCM: 2049

J1980   Injection, hyoscyamine sulfate, [Levsin], up to 0.25 mg
MCM: 2049

J1990   Injection, chlordiazepoxide HCl, [Librium], up to 100 mg
MCM: 2049

J2001   Injection, lidocaine HCl for intravenous infusion, 10 mg
MCM: 2049

J2010   Injection, lincomycin HCl, up to 300 mg
MCM: 2049

J2020   Injection, linezolid, 200 mg

J2060   Injection, lorazepam, [Ativan], 2 mg
MCM: 2049

J2150   Injection, mannitol, 25% in 50 ml
MCM: 2049

J2175   Injection, meperidine HCl, per 100 mg
MCM: 2049

J2180   Injection, meperidine and promethazine HCl, [Mepergan],
up to 50 mg
MCM: 2049

J2185   Injection, meropenem, 100 mg

J2210   Injection, methylergonovine maleate, [Methergine
Maleate], up to 0.2 mg
MCM: 2049

J2250   Injection, midazolam hydrochloride, per 1 mg
MCM: 2049

J2260   Injection, milrinone lactate, 5 mg
MCM: 2049

J2270   Injection, morphine sulfate, up to 10 mg
MCM: 2049

J2271   Injection, morphine sulfate, 100 mg
CIM: 60-14A MCM: 2049

J2275   Injection, morphine sulfate (preservative-free sterile solution), per 10 mg
CIM: 60-14B MCM: 2049

● **J2278**   Injection, ziconotide, 1 microgram

J2280   Injection, moxifloxacin, 100 mg

J2300   Injection, nalbuphine HCl, per 10 mg
MCM: 2049

J2310   Injection, naloxone hydrochloride, per 1 mg
MCM: 2049

J2320   Injection, nandrolone deconoate; up to 50 mg
MCM: 2049

J2321   up to 100 mg
MCM: 2049

J2322   up to 200 mg
MCM: 2049

(J2324)   Code deleted December 31, 2005

● **J2325**   Injection, nesiritide, 0.1 mg
MCM: 2049

J2353   Injection, octreotide, depot form for intramuscular injection, 1 mg

J2354   Injection, octreotide, non-depot form for subcutaneous or intravenous injection, 25 mcg

J2355   Injection, oprelvekin, 5 mg
MCM: 2049

J2357   Injection, omalizumab, 5 mg

J2360   Injection, orphenadrine citrate, [Norflex, Norgesic], up to 60 mg
MCM: 2049

J2370   Injection, phenylephrine HCl, [Neo-Synephrine], up to 1 ml
MCM: 2049

J2400   Injection, chloroprocaine HCl [Nesacaine and Nesacaine-MPF], per 30 ml
MCM: 2049

J2405   Injection, ondansetron hydrochloride, per 1 mg
MCM: 2049

J2410   Injection, oxymorphone HCl [Numorphan], up to 1 mg
MCM: 2049

● **J2425**   Injection, palifermin, 50 micrograms

J2430   Injection, pamidronate disodium, per 30 mg
MCM: 2049

J2440   Injection, papaverine HCl, up to 60 mg
MCM: 2049

J2460   Injection, oxytetracycline HCl, up to 50 mg
MCM: 2049

J2469   Injection, palonosetron hcl, 25 mcg

J2501   Injection, paricalcitol, 1 mcg
MCM: 2049

● **J2503**   Injection, pegaptanib sodium, 0.3 mg

● **J2504**   Injection, pegademase bovine, 25 iu
MCM: 2049

J2505   Injection, pegfilgrastim, 6 mg

J2510   Injection, penicillin G procaine, aqueous, up to 600,000 units
MCM: 2049

● **J2513**   Injection, pentastarch, 10% solution, 100 ml
MCM: 2049

J2515   Injection, pentobarbital sodium, per 50 mg
MCM: 2049

J2540   Injection, penicillin G potassium, [Pfizerpen], up to 600,000 units
MCM: 2049

J2543 Injection, piperacillin sodium/tazobactam sodium,
1 gram/0.125 grams (1.125 grams)
MCM: 2049

J2545 Pentamidine isethionate, inhalation solution, per 300 mg,
administered through a DME
MCM: 2049

J2550 Injection, promethazine HCl, [Phenergan], up to 50 mg
MCM: 2049

J2560 Injection, phenobarbital sodium, [Phenobarbital], up to
120 mg
MCM: 2049

J2590 Injection, oxytocin, [Pitocin], up to 10 units
MCM: 2049

J2597 Injection, desmopressin acetate, per 1 mcg
MCM: 2049

J2650 Injection, prednisolone acetate, up to 1 ml
MCM: 2049

J2670 Injection, tolazoline HCl, [Priscoline HCl], up to 25 mg
MCM: 2049

J2675 Injection, progesterone, per 50 mg
MCM: 2049

J2680 Injection, fluphenazine deconoate, [Prolixin Deconoate],
up to 25 mg
MCM: 2049

J2690 Injection, procainamide HCl, [Proenstyl], up to 1 gram
MCM: 2049

J2700 Injection, oxacillin sodium, [Prostaphlin], up to 250 mg
MCM: 2049

J2710 Injection, neostigmine methylsulfate, [Prostigmin
Methylsulfate], up to 0.5 mg
MCM: 2049

J2720 Injection, protamine sulfate, per 10 mg
MCM: 2049

J2725 Injection, protirelin, per 250 mcg
MCM: 2049

Not valid
for Medicare

Non-covered
by Medicare

Special
coverage
instructions

Carrier
discretion

205

J2730   Injection, pralidoxime chloride, [Protopam Chloride], up
to 1 gram
MCM: 2049

J2760   Injection, phentolamine mesylate, [Regitine], up to 5 mg
MCM: 2049

J2765   Injection, metoclopramide HCl [Reglan], up to 10 mg
MCM: 2049

J2770   Injection, quinupristin/dalfopristin, 500 mg (150/350)
MCM: 2049

J2780   Injection, ranitidine hydrochloride, 25 mg
MCM: 2049

J2783   Injection, rasburicase, 0.5 mg

J2788   Injection, RHo (D) immune globulin, human, minidose,
50 mcg
MCM: 2049

J2790   Injection, RHo(D) immune globulin, human, full dose,
300 mcg
MCM: 2049

J2792   Injection, RHo(D) immune globulin, intravenous, human,
solvent detergent, 100 IU
MCM: 2049

J2794   Injection, risperidone, long acting, 0.5 Mg

J2795   Injection, ropivacaine hydrochloride, 1 mg

J2800   Injection, methocarbamol, [Robaxin], up to 10 ml
MCM: 2049

● **J2805**   Injection, sincalide, 5 micrograms

J2810   Injection, theophylline, per 40 mg
MCM: 2049

J2820   Injection, sargramostim (GM-CSF), 50 mcg
MCM: 2049

● **J2850**   Injection, secretin, synthetic, human, 1 microgram
MCM: 2049

J2910   Injection, aurothioglucose, [Solganal], up to 50 mg
MCM: 2049

J2912   Injection, sodium chloride, 0.9%, per 2 ml
MCM: 2049

J2916   Injection, sodium ferric gluconate complex in sucrose injection, 12.5 mg
MCM: 2049.2, 2049.4

J2920   Injection, methylprednisolone sodium succinate, [Solu-Medrol], up to 40 mg
MCM: 2049

J2930   Injection, methylprednisolone sodium succinate, [Solu-Medrol], up to 125 mg
MCM: 2049

J2940   Injection, somatrem, 1 mg
MCM: 2049

J2941   Injection, somatropin, 1 mg
MCM: 2049

J2950   Injection, promazine HCl, [Prozine, Sparine], up to 25 mg
MCM: 2049

J2993   Injection, reteplase, 18.1 mg
MCM: 2049

J2995   Injection, streptokinase, per 250,000 IU
MCM: 2049

J2997   Injection, alteplase recombinant, 1 mg
MCM: 2049

J3000   Injection, streptomycin, up to 1 gram
MCM: 2049

J3010   Injection, fentanyl citrate, 0.1 mg
MCM: 2049

J3030   Injection, sumatriptan succinate, 6 mg (code may be used for Medicare when drug administered under the direct supervision of a physician, not for use when drug is self administered)
MCM: 2049

J3070   Injection, pentazocine, 30 mg
MCM: 2049

J3100   Injection, tenecteplase, 50 mg

J3105   Injection, terbutaline sulfate, up to 1 mg
MCM: 2049

J3110   Injection, teriparatide, 10 mcg

J3120   Injection, testosterone enanthate; up to 100 mg
MCM: 2049

J3130   up to 200 mg
MCM: 2049

J3140   Injection, testosterone suspension, up to 50 mg
MCM: 2049

J3150   Injection, testosterone propionate, up to 100 mg
MCM: 2049

J3230   Injection, chlorpromazine HCl, [Thorazine], up to 50 mg
MCM: 2049

J3240   Injection, thyrotropin alpha, 0.9 mg, provided in 1.1 mg vial
MCM: 2049

(J3245)   Code deleted December 31, 2004; use CPT

J3246   Injection, tirofiban HCl, 0.25 Mg

J3250   Injection, trimethobenzamide HCl, up to 200 mg
MCM: 2049

J3260   Injection, tobramycin sulfate, [Nebcin], up to 80 mg
MCM: 2049

J3265   Injection, torsemide, 10 mg/ml
MCM: 2049

J3280   Injection, thiethylperazine maleate, up to 10 mg
MCM: 2049

● **J3285**   Injection, treprostinil, 1 mg

J3301   Injection, triamcinolone acetonide, [Kenalog], per 10 mg
MCM: 2049

J3302   Injection, triamcinolone diacetate, [Aristocort], per 5 mg
MCM: 2049

J3303 Injection, triamcinolone hexacetonide, [Aristospan], per 5 mg
MCM: 2049

J3305 Injection, trimetrexate glucoronate, per 25 mg
MCM: 2049

J3310 Injection, perphenazine, [Trilafon], up to 5 mg
MCM: 2049

J3315 Injection, triptorelin pamoate, 3.75 mg
MCM: 2049

J3320 Injection, spectinomycin hydrochloride, [Trobicin], up to 2 gram
MCM: 2049

J3350 Injection, urea, [Ureaphil], up to 40 grams
MCM: 2049

● **J3355** Injection, urofollitropin, 75 iu
MCM: 2049

J3360 Injection, diazepam, [Valium], up to 5 mg
MCM: 2049

J3364 Injection, urokinase, 5000 IU vial
MCM: 2049

J3365 Injection, IV, urokinase, 250,000 IU vial
MCM: 2049

J3370 Injection, vancomycin HCl, 500 mg
CIM: 60-14 MCM: 2049

(J3395) Code deleted December 31, 2004; use CPT

J3396 Injection, verteporfin, 0.1 Mg
MCM: 35-100, 45-30

J3400 Injection, triflupromazine HCl, [Vesprin], up to 20 mg
MCM: 2049

J3410 Injection, hydroxyzine HCl, [Vistaril], up to 25 mg
MCM: 2049

J3411 Injection, thiamine HCl, 100 mg

J3415 Injection, pyridoxine HCl, 100 mg

J3420   Injection, vitamin B-12 cyanocobalamin, up to 1000 mcg
CIM: 45-4   MCM: 2049

J3430   Injection, phytonadione (vitamin K), per 1 mg
MCM: 2049

J3465   Injection, voriconazole, 10 mg
MCM: 2049

J3470   Injection, hyaluronidase, [Wydase], up to 150 units
MCM: 2049

● **J3471**   Injection, hyaluronidase, ovine, preservative free, per 1 usp unit (up to 999 USP units)

● **J3472**   Injection, hyaluronidase, ovine, preservative free, per 1000 usp units

J3475   Injection, magnesium sulfate, per 500 mg
MCM: 2049

J3480   Injection, potassium chloride, per 2 mEq
MCM: 2049

J3485   Injection, zidovudine, 10 mg
MCM: 2049

J3486   Injection, ziprasidone mesylate, 10 mg

J3487   Injection, zoledronic acid, 1 mg

J3490   Unclassified drugs
MCM: 2049

J3520   Edetate disodium, per 150 mg
CIM: 35-64, 45-20

J3530   Nasal vaccine inhalation
MCM: 2049

J3535   Drug administered through a metered dose inhaler
MCM: 2050.5

J3570   Laetrile, amygdalin, vitamin B17
CIM: 45-10

J3590   Unclassified biologics

● New code   ▲ Revised code   ( ) Deleted code

MISCELLANEOUS DRUGS AND SOLUTIONS

J7030   Infusion, normal saline solution, 1000 cc
MCM: 2049

J7040   Infusion, normal saline solution, sterile (500 ml = 1 unit)
MCM: 2049

J7042   5% dextrose/normal saline solution (500 ml = 1 unit)
MCM: 2049

J7050   Infusion, normal saline solution, 250 cc
MCM: 2049

(J7051)   Code deleted December 31, 2005

J7060   5% dextrose/water (500 ml = 1 unit)
MCM: 2049

J7070   Infusion, D5W, 1000 cc
MCM: 2049

J7100   Infusion, dextran 40, 500 ml
MCM: 2049

J7110   Infusion, dextran 75, 500 ml
MCM: 2049

J7120   Ringers lactate infusion, up to 1000 cc
MCM: 2049

J7130   Hypertonic saline solution, 50 or 100 mEq, 20 cc vial
MCM: 2049

● **J7188**   Injection, von willebrand factor complex, human, iu
CIM: 35.30 MCM: 2049.5

● **J7189**   Factor VIIA (antihemophilic factor, recombinant), per 1 microgram
MCM: 2049

J7190   Factor VIII (antihemophilic factor, human), per IU
MCM: 2049

J7191   Factor VIII (antihemophilic factor (porcine)), per IU
MCM: 2049

J7192   Factor VIII (antihemophilic factor, recombinant), per IU
MCM: 2049

J7193 Factor IX (antihemophilic factor, purified, non-recombinant) per IU
MCM: 2049

J7194 Factor IX, complex, per IU
MCM: 2049

J7195 Factor IX (antihemophilic factor, recombinant) per IU
MCM: 2049

J7197 Antithrombin III (human), per IU
MCM: 2049

J7198 Anti-inhibitor, per IU
CIM: 45-24 MCM: 2049

J7199 Hemophilia clotting factor, not otherwise classified
CIM: 45-24 MCM: 2049

J7300 Intrauterine copper contraceptive

J7302 Levonorgestrel-releasing intrauterine contraceptive system, 52 mg

J7303 Contraceptive supply, hormone containing vaginal ring, each

J7304 Contraceptive supply, hormone containing patch, each

● **J7306** Levonorgestrel (contraceptive) implant system, including implants and supplies

J7308 Aminolevulinic acid HCL for topical administration, 20%, single unit dosage form (354 mg)

J7310 Ganciclovir, 4.5 mg, long-acting implant
MCM: 2049

(J7317) Code deleted December 31, 2005

● **J7318** Hyaluronan (sodium hyaluronate) or derivative, intra-articular injection, 1 mg

(J7320) Code deleted December 31, 2005

J7330 Autologous cultured chondrocytes, implant

● New code ▲ Revised code ( ) Deleted code

▲ **J7340** Dermal and epidermal, (substitute) tissue of human origin, with or without bioengineered or processed elements, with metabolically active elements, per square centimeter

● **J7341** Dermal (substitute) tissue of non-human origin, with or without other bioengineered or processed elements, with metabolically active elements, per square centimeter

▲ **J7342** Dermal (substitute) tissue of human origin, with or without other bioengineered or processed elements, with metabolically active elements, per square centimeter

▲ **J7343** Dermal and epidermal, (substitute) tissue of non-human origin, with or without other bioengineered or processed elements, without metabolically active elements, per square centimeter

▲ **J7344** Dermal (substitute) tissue of human origin, with or without other Bioengineered or processed elements, without metabolically active elements, per square centimeter

▲ **J7350** Dermal (substitute) tissue of human origin, injectable, with or without other bioengineered or processed elements, but without metabolized active elements, per 10 mg

IMMUNOSUPPRESSIVE DRUGS (INCLUDES NON-INJECTIBLES)

J7500 Azathioprine, oral, 50 mg
MCM: 2049.5

J7501 Azathioprine, parenteral, 100 mg
MCM: 2049

J7502 Cyclosporine, oral, 100 mg
MCM: 2049.5

J7504 Lymphocyte immune globulin, antithymocyte globulin, equine, parenteral, 250 mg
CIM: 45-22 MCM: 2049

J7505 muromonab-CD3, parenteral, 5 mg
MCM: 2049

J7506 Prednisone, oral, per 5 mg
MCM: 2049.5

J7507   Tacrolimus, oral; per 1 mg
MCM: 2049.5

J7509   Methylprednisolone, oral, per 4 mg
MCM: 2049.5

J7510   Prednisolone, oral, per 5 mg
MCM: 2049.5

J7511   Lymphocyte immune globulin, antithymocyte globulin, rabbit, parenteral, 25 mg

J7513   Daclizumab, parenteral, 25 mg
MCM: 2049.5

J7515   Cyclosporine, oral, 25 mg

J7516   Cyclosporine, parenteral, 250 mg

J7517   Mycophenolate mofetil, oral, 250 mg

J7518   Mycophenolic acid, oral, 180 mg
MCM: 2050.5, 4471, 5249

J7520   Sirolimus, oral, 1 mg
MCM: 2049.5

J7525   Tacrolimus, parenteral, 5 mg
MCM: 2049.5

J7599   Immunosuppressive drug, not otherwise classified
MCM: 2049.5

J7608   Acetylcysteine, inhalation solution administered through DME, unit dose form, per gram
MCM: 2100.5

J7611   Albuterol, inhalation solution, administered through DME, concentrated form, 1 mg
MCM: 2100.5

J7612   Levalbuterol, inhalation solution, administered through DME, concentrated form, 0.5 Mg
MCM: 2100.5

J7613   Albuterol, inhalation solution, administered through DME, unit dose, 1 mg
MCM: 2100.5

J7614 Levalbuterol, inhalation solution, administered through DME, unit dose, 0.5 Mg
MCM: 2100.5

(J7616) Code deleted December 31, 2005

(J7617) Code deleted December 31, 2005

(J7618) Code deleted December 31, 2004; use CPT

(J7619) Code deleted December 31, 2004; use CPT

● **J7620** Albuterol, up to 2.5 mg and ipratropium bromide, up to 0.5 mg, non-compounded Inhalation solution, administered through DME
MCM: 2100.5

(J7621) Code deleted December 31, 2004; use CPT

J7622 Beclomethasone, inhalation solution administered through DME, unit dose form, per milligram

J7624 Betamethasone, inhalation solution administered through DME, unit dose form, per milligram

▲ **J7626** Budesonide inhalation solution, non-compounded, administered through DME, unit dose form, up to 0.5 mg

● **J7627** Budesonide, powder, compounded for inhalation solution, administered through DME, unit dose form, up to 0.5 mg

J7628 Bitolterol mesylate, inhalation solution administered through DME, concentrated form, per mg
MCM: 2100.5

J7629 Bitolterol mesylate, inhalation solution administered through DME, unit dose form, per mg
MCM: 2100.5

J7631 Cromolyn sodium, inhalation solution administered through DME, unit dose form, per 10 mg
MCM: 2100.5

J7633 Budesonide, inhalation solution administered through dme, concentrated form, per 0.25 mg

J7635   Atropine, inhalation solution administered through DME, concentrated form, per mg
MCM: 2100.5

J7636   Atropine, inhalation solution administered through DME, unit dose form, per mg
MCM: 2100.5

J7637   Dexamethasone, inhalation solution administered through DME, concentrated form, per mg
MCM: 2100.5

J7638   Dexamethasone, inhalation solution administered through DME, unit dose form, per mg
MCM: 2100.5

J7639   Dornase alpha, inhalation solution administered through DME, unit dose form, per mg
MCM: 2100.5

● **J7640**   Formorterol, inhalation solution administered through DME, unit dose form, 12 micrograms

J7641   Flunisolide, inhalation solution administered through DME, unit dose, per milligram

J7642   Glycopyrrolate, inhalation solution administered through DME, concentrated form, per mg
MCM: 2100.5

J7643   Glycopyrrolate, inhalation solution administered through DME, unit dose form, per mg
MCM: 2100.5

J7644   Ipratropium bromide, inhalation solution administered through DME, unit dose form, per mg
MCM: 2100.5

J7648   Isoetharine HCl, inhalation solution administered through DME, concentrated form, per mg
MCM: 2100.5

J7649   Isoetharine HCl, inhalation solution administered through DME, unit dose form, per mg
MCM: 2100.5

J7658   Isoproterenol HCl, inhalation solution administered through DME, concentrated form, per mg
MCM: 2100.5

J7659   Isoproterenol HCl, inhalation solution administered through DME, unit dose form, per mg
MCM: 2100.5

J7668   Metaproterenol sulfate, inhalation solution administered through DME, concentrated form, per 10 mg
MCM: 2100.5

J7669   Metaproterenol sulfate, inhalation solution administered through DME, unit dose form, per 10 mg
MCM: 2100.5

J7674   Methacholine chloride administered as inhalation solution through a nebulizer, per 1 mg

J7680   Terbutaline sulfate, inhalation solution administered through DME, concentrated form, per mg
MCM: 2100.5

J7681   Terbutaline sulfate, inhalation solution administered through DME, unit dose form, per mg
MCM: 2100.5

J7682   Tobramycin, unit dose form, 300 mg, inhalation solution, administered through DME
MCM: 2100.5

J7683   Triamcinolone, inhalation solution administered through DME, concentrated form, per mg
MCM: 2100.5

J7684   Triamcinolone, inhalation solution administered through DME, unit dose form, per mg
MCM: 2100.5

J7699   NOC drugs, inhalation solution administered through DME
MCM: 2100.5

J7799   NOC drugs, other than inhalation drugs, administered through DME
MCM: 2100.5

● **J8498**   Antiemetic drug, rectal/suppository, not otherwise specified
MCM: 2049.5

J8499   Prescription drug, oral, non-chemotherapeutic, NOS
MCM: 2049

J8501   Aprepitant, oral, 5 mg

J8510   Busulfan, oral, 2 mg
MCM: 2049.5

● **J8515**   Cabergoline, oral, 0.25 mg
MCM: 2049.5

J8520   Capecitabine, oral, 150 mg
MCM: 2049.5

J8521   Capecitabine, oral, 500 mg
MCM: 2049.5

J8530   Cyclophosphamide, oral, 25 mg
MCM: 2049.5

● **J8540**   Dexamethasone, oral, 0.25 mg

J8560   Etoposide, oral, 50 mg
MCM: 2049.5

J8565   Gefitinib, oral, 250 mg

● **J8597**   Antiemetic drug, oral, not otherwise specified

J8600   Melphalan, oral, 2 mg
MCM: 2049.5

J8610   Methotrexate, oral, 2.5 mg
MCM: 2049.5

J8700   Temozolmide, oral, 5 mg
MCM: 2049.5C

J8999   Prescription drug, oral, chemotherapeutic, NOS
MCM: 2049.5

CHEMOTHERAPY DRUGS

Guidelines

In addition to the information presented in the INTRODUCTION, several other items unique to this section are defined or identified here:

1. EXCEPTION: Oral immunosuppressive drugs are not included in this section.

2. ROUTE OF ADMINISTRATION: Unless otherwise specified, the drugs listed in this section may be injected either subcutaneously, intramuscularly or intravenously.

3. DRUG COST ONLY: The codes listed in this section include the cost of the chemotherapy drug only and do not include the administration of the drug.

4. SUBSECTION INFORMATION: Some of the listed subheadings or subsections have special needs or instructions unique to that section. Where these are indicated, special "notes" will be presented preceding or following the listings. Those subsections within the CHEMOTHERAPY DRUGS section that have "notes" are as follows:

Subsection	Code Numbers
Chemotherapy drugs	J9000-J9999

5. UNLISTED SERVICE OR PROCEDURE: A service or procedure may be provided that is not listed in this edition of HCPCS. When reporting such a service, the appropriate "unlisted procedure" code may be used to indicate the service, identifying it by "special report" as defined below. HCPCS terminology is inconsistent in defining unlisted procedures. The procedure definition may include the term(s) "unlisted", "not otherwise classified", "unspecified", "unclassified", "other" and "miscellaneous". Prior to using these codes, try to determine if a Local Level III code or CPT code is available. The "unlisted procedures" and accompanying codes for CHEMOTHERAPY DRUGS are as follows:

J9999   Not otherwise classified, antineoplastic drugs

---

6. SPECIAL REPORT: A service, material or supply that is rarely provided, unusual, variable or new may require a special report in determining medical appropriateness for reimbursement purposes. Pertinent information should include an adequate definition or description of the nature, extent, and need for the service, material or supply.

7. MODIFIERS: Listed services may be modified under certain circumstances. When appropriate, the modifying circumstance is identified by adding a modifier to the basic procedure code. CPT and HCPCS National Level II modifiers may be used with CPT and HCPCS National Level II procedure codes. Modifiers commonly used with CHEMOTHERAPY DRUGS are as follows:

-CC Procedure code change (used when the procedure code submitted was changed either for administrative reasons or because an incorrect code was filed)

(-QB) Code deleted December 31, 2005

(-QU) Code deleted December 31, 2005

-TC Technical component. Under certain circumstances, a charge may be made for the technical component alone. Under these circumstances, the technical component charge is identified by adding the modifier -TC to the usual procedure code. Technical component charges are institutional charges and are not billed separately by physicians. Portable x-ray suppliers bill only for the technical component however, and should use modifier -TC.

8. CPT CODE CROSS-REFERENCE: Unless otherwise specified, the equivalent CPT code for all listings in this section is 96545.

Chemotherapy Drugs

J9000 Doxorubicin HCl, [Adriamycin], 10 mg
MCM: 2049

J9001 Doxorubicin HCl, all lipid formulations, 10 mg
MCM: 2049

J9010 Alemtuzumab, 10 mg

J9015 Aldesleukin, per single use vial
MCM: 2049

● New code ▲ Revised code ( ) Deleted code

J9017   Arsenic trioxide, 1 mg

J9020   Asparaginase, 10,000 units
MCM: 2049

● **J9025**   Injection, azacitidine, 1 mg

● **J9027**   Injection, clofarabine, 1 mg

J9031   BCG (intravesical), per installation
MCM: 2049

J9035   Injection, bevacizumab, 10 mg

J9040   Bleomycin sulfate, [Blenoxane], 15 units
MCM: 2049

J9041   Injection, bortezomib, 0.1 Mg

J9045   Carboplatin, [Paraplatin], 50 mg
MCM: 2049

J9050   Carmustine, [BiCNU], 100 mg
MCM: 2049

J9055   Injection, cetuximab, 10 mg

J9060   Cisplatin, [Platinol], powder or solution, per 10 mg
MCM: 2049

J9062   Cisplatin, 50 mg
MCM: 2049

J9065   Injection, cladribine, [Leustatin], per 1 mg
MCM: 2049

J9070   Cyclophosphamide, [Cytoxan]; 100 mg
MCM: 2049

J9080   200 mg
MCM: 2049

J9090   500 mg
MCM: 2049

J9091   1.0 gram
MCM: 2049

J9092   2.0 gram
MCM: 2049

■ Not valid   ■ Non-covered   Special   ■ Carrier   **221**
for Medicare   by Medicare   coverage   discretion
instructions

J9093   Cyclophosphamide, lyophilized, [Lyophilized Cytoxan];
100 mg
MCM: 2049

J9094   200 mg
MCM: 2049

J9095   500 mg
MCM: 2049

J9096   1.0 gram
MCM: 2049

J9097   2.0 gram
MCM: 2049

J9098   Cytarabine liposome, 10 mg

J9100   Cytarabine, [Cytarabine Hydrochloride]; 100 mg
MCM: 2049

J9110   500 mg
MCM: 2049

J9120   Dactinomycin, 0.5 mg
MCM: 2049

J9130   Dacarbazine, 100 mg
MCM: 2049

J9140   200 mg
MCM: 2049

J9150   Daunorubicin, 10 mg
MCM: 2049

J9151   Daunorubicin citrate, liposomal formulation, 10 mg
MCM: 2049

J9160   Denileukin diftitox, 300 mcg

J9165   Diethylstilbestrol diphosphate, [Stilphostrol], 250 mg
MCM: 2049

J9170   Docetaxel, 20 mg
MCM: 2049

● **J9175**   Injection, Elliott's' b solution, 1 ml
MCM: 2049

J9178   Injection, epirubicin HCl, 2 mg

J9181 Etoposide, [VePesid]; 10 mg
MCM: 2049

J9182 100 mg
MCM: 2049

J9185 Fludarabine phosphate, 50 mg
MCM: 2049

J9190 Fluorouracil, 500 mg
MCM: 2049

J9200 Floxuridine, 500 mg
MCM: 2049

J9201 Gemcitabine HCl, 200 mg
MCM: 2049

J9202 Goserelin acetate implant, [Zoladex], per 3.6 mg
MCM: 2049

J9206 Irinotecan, 20 mg
MCM: 2049

J9208 Ifosfomide, 1 gram
MCM: 2049

J9209 Mesna, [Mcsnex], 200 mg
MCM: 2049

J9211 Idarubicin hydrochloride, 5 mg
MCM: 2049

J9212 Injection, interferon alfacon-1, recombinant, 1 mcg
MCM: 2049

J9213 Interferon, alfa-2A, recombinant, 3 million units
MCM: 2049

J9214 Interferon, alfa-2B, recombinant, 1 million units
MCM: 2049

J9215 Interferon, alfa-N3, (human leukocyte derived), 250,000 IU
MCM: 2049

J9216 Interferon, gamma 1-B, 3 million units
MCM: 2049

J9217   Leuprolide acetate, [Lupron Depot], (for depot suspension), 7.5 mg
MCM: 2049

J9218   Leuprolide acetate, [Lupron], per 1 mg
MCM: 2049

J9219   Leuprolide acetate implant, 65 mg
MCM: 2049

● **J9225**   Histrelin implant, 50 mg
MCM: 2049

J9230   Mechlorethamine HCl, (nitrogen mustard), [Mustargen], 10 mg
MCM: 2049

J9245   Injection, melphalan HCl, 50 mg
MCM: 2049

J9250   Methotrexate sodium; 5 mg
MCM: 2049

J9260   50 mg
MCM: 2049

J9263   Injection, oxaliplatin, 0.5 mg

● **J9264**   Injection, paclitaxel protein-bound particles, 1 mg

J9265   Paclitaxel, 30 mg
MCM: 2049

J9266   Pegaspargase, per single dose vial
MCM: 2049

J9268   Pentostatin, per 10 mg
MCM: 2049

J9270   Plicamycin, [Mithracin], 2.5 mg
MCM: 2049

J9280   Mitomycin; 5 mg
MCM: 2049

J9290   20 mg
MCM: 2049

J9291   40 mg
MCM: 2049

J9293   Injection, mitoxantrone HCl, per 5 mg
MCM: 2049

J9300   Gemtuzumab ozogamicin, 5 mg

J9305   Injection, pemetrexed, 10 mg

J9310   Rituximab, 100 mg
MCM: 2049

J9320   Streptozocin, 1 gram
MCM: 2049

J9340   Thiotepa, 15 mg
MCM: 2049

J9350   Topotecan, 4 mg
MCM: 2049

J9355   Trastuzumab, 10 mg

J9357   Valrubicin, intravesical, 200 mg
MCM: 2049

J9360   Vinblastine sulfate, [Velban], 1 mg
MCM: 2049

J9370   Vincristine sulfate, [Oncovin]; 1 mg
MCM: 2049

J9375   2 mg
MCM: 2049

J9380   5 mg
MCM: 2049

J9390   Vinorelbine tartrate, per 10 mg
MCM: 2049

J9395   Injection, fulvestrant, 25 mg

J9600   Porfimer sodium, [Photofrin], 75 mg
MCM: 2049

J9999   Not otherwise classified, antineoplastic drugs
CIM: 45-16 MCM: 2049

● New code ▲ Revised code ( ) Deleted code

K CODES: FOR DMERCs' USE ONLY

Guidelines

In addition to the information presented in the INTRODUCTION, several other items unique to this section are defined or identified here:

1. EXCLUSIVE USE BY DMERCs: The codes listed in this section are assigned by CMS on a temporary basis and are for the exclusive use of the Durable Medical Equipment Regional Carriers (DMERCs). These codes are not to be used by providers for reporting purposes unless specifically instructed to do so by the local carrier.

2. UNLISTED SERVICE OR PROCEDURE: A service or procedure may be provided that is not listed in this edition of HCPCS. When reporting such a service, the appropriate "unlisted procedure" code may be used to indicate the service, identifying it by "special report" as defined below. HCPCS terminology is inconsistent in defining unlisted procedures. The procedure definition may include the term(s) "unlisted", "not otherwise classified", "unspecified", "unclassified", "other" and "miscellaneous". Prior to using these codes, try to determine if a Local Level III code or CPT code is available.

3. SPECIAL REPORT: A service, material or supply that is rarely provided, unusual, variable or new may require a special report in determining medical appropriateness for reimbursement purposes. Pertinent information should include an adequate definition or description of the nature, extent, and need for the service, material or supply.

4. CPT CODE CROSS-REFERENCE: Unless otherwise specified, the equivalent CPT code for all listings in this section is 99070.

K CODES

Not valid for Medicare   Non-covered by Medicare   Special coverage instructions   Carrier discretion

Temporary Codes for DMERCS

WHEELCHAIRS

K0001 Standard wheelchair

K0002 Standard hemi (low seat) wheelchair

K0003 Lightweight wheelchair

K0004 High strength, lightweight wheelchair

K0005 Ultralightweight wheelchair

K0006 Heavy duty wheelchair

K0007 Extra heavy duty wheelchair

K0009 Other manual wheelchair/base

K0010 Standard - weight frame motorized/power wheelchair

K0011 Standard - weight frame motorized/power wheelchair with programmable control parameters for speed adjustment, tremor dampening, acceleration control and braking

K0012 Lightweight portable motorized/power wheelchair

K0014 Other motorized/power wheelchair base

K0015 Detachable, non-adjustable height armrest, each

K0017 Detachable, adjustable height armrest; base, each

K0018   upper portion each

K0019 Arm pad, each

K0020 Fixed, adjustable height armrest, pair

(K0023) Code deleted December 31, 2004; use CPT

(K0024) Code deleted December 31, 2004; use CPT

K0037 High mount flip-up foot rest, each

K0038   Leg strap, each

K0039   Leg strap, H style, each

K0040   Adjustable angle footplate, each

K0041   Large size footplate, each

K0042   Standard size footplate, each

K0043   Foot rest, lower extension tube, each

K0044   Foot rest, upper hanger bracket, each

K0045   Foot rest, complete assembly

K0046   Elevating leg rest; lower extension tube, each

K0047   upper hanger bracket, each

K0050   Ratchet assembly

K0051   Cam release assembly, foot rest or leg rest, each

K0052   Swingaway, detachable foot rests, each

K0053   Elevating foot rests, articulating (telescoping), each

K0056   Seat height less than 17" or equal to or greater than 21" for a high strength, lightweight, or ultralightweight wheelchair

(K0059)   Code deleted December 31, 2004; use CPT

(K0060)   Code deleted December 31, 2004; use CPT

(K0061)   Code deleted December 31, 2004; use CPT

(K0064)   Code deleted December 31, 2005; use E2213

K0065   Spoke protectors, each

(K0066)   Code deleted December 31, 2005; use E2220

(K0067)   Code deleted December 31, 2005; use E2211

Not valid for Medicare   Non-covered by Medicare   Special coverage instructions   Carrier discretion

(K0068) Code deleted December 31, 2005; use E2212

K0069 Rear wheel assembly, complete; with solid tire, spokes or molded, each

K0070 with pneumatic tire, spokes or molded, each

K0071 Front caster assembly, complete; with pneumatic tire, each

K0072 with semi-pneumatic tire, each

K0073 Caster pin lock, each

(K0074) Code deleted December 31, 2005; use E2214

(K0075) Code deleted December 31, 2005; use E2219

(K0076) Code deleted December 31, 2005; use E2221

K0077 Front caster assembly, complete, with solid tire, each

(K0078) Code deleted December 31, 2005; use E2215

(K0081) Code deleted December 31, 2004; use E2206

K0090 Rear wheel tire for power wheelchair, any size, each

K0091 Rear wheel tire tube other than zero pressure for power wheelchair, any size, each

K0092 Rear wheel assembly for power wheelchair, complete each

K0093 Rear wheel, zero pressure tire tube (flat free insert) for power wheelchair, any size, each

K0094 Wheel tire for power base, any size, each

K0095 Wheel tire tube other than zero pressure for each base, any size, each

K0096 Wheel assembly for power base, complete, each

K0097 Wheel zero pressure tire tube (flat free insert) for power base, any size, each

K0098 Drive belt for power wheelchair

K0099 Front caster for power wheelchair, each

(K0102) Code deleted December 31, 2005; use E2207

(K0104) Code deleted December 31, 2005; use E2208

K0105 IV hanger, each

(K0106) Code deleted December 31, 2005; use E2209

K0108 Wheelchair component or accessory, not otherwise specified

SPINAL ORTHOTICS

(K0114) Code deleted December 31, 2004; use CPT

(K0115) Code deleted December 31, 2004; use CPT

(K0116) Code deleted December 31, 2004; use CPT

TRACHEOSTOMY CARE SUPPLIES

K0195 Elevating leg rests, pair (for use with capped rental wheelchair base)
CIM: 60-9

(K0415) Code deleted December 31, 2005

(K0416) Code deleted December 31, 2005

(K0452) Code deleted December 31, 2005; use E2210

K0455 Infusion pump used for uninterrupted parenteral administration of medication, (eg., epoprostenol or treprostinol)
CIM: 60-14

K0462 Temporary replacement for patient owned equipment being repaired, any type
MCM: 5102.3

K0552 Supplies for external drug infusion pump, syringe type cartridge, sterile, each
CIM: 60-14

(K0600) Code deleted December 31, 2005; use E0762

Not valid for Medicare   Non-covered by Medicare   Special coverage instructions   Carrier discretion

K0601 Replacement battery for external infusion pump owned by patient, silver oxide, 1.5 volt, each

K0602 Replacement battery for external infusion pump owned by patient, silver oxide, 3 volt, each

K0603 Replacement battery for external infusion pump owned by patient, alkaline, 1.5 volt, each

K0604 Replacement battery for external infusion pump owned by patient, lithium, 3.6 volt, each

K0605 Replacement battery for external infusion pump owned by patient, lithium, 4.5 volt, each

K0606 Automatic external defibrillator, with integrated electrocardiogram analysis, garment type

K0607 Replacement battery for automated external defibrillator, garment type only, each

K0608 Replacement garment for use with automated external defibrillator, each

K0609 Replacement electrodes for use with automated external defibrillator, garment type only, each

(K0618) Code deleted December 31, 2005; use L0491

(K0619) Code deleted December 31, 2005; use L0492

(K0620) Code deleted December 31, 2005; use A6457

(K0627) Code deleted December 31, 2004; use E0849

(K0628) Code deleted December 31, 2005; use A5512

(K0629) Code deleted December 31, 2005; use A5513

(K0630) Code deleted December 31, 2005; use L0621

(K0631) Code deleted December 31, 2005; use L0622

(K0632) Code deleted December 31, 2005; use L0623

(K0633) Code deleted December 31, 2005; use L0624

● New code ▲ Revised code ( ) Deleted code

(K0634)   Code deleted December 31, 2005; use L0625

(K0635)   Code deleted December 31, 2005; use L0626

(K0636)   Code deleted December 31, 2005; use L0627

(K0637)   Code deleted December 31, 2005; use L0628

(K0638)   Code deleted December 31, 2005; use L0629

(K0639)   Code deleted December 31, 2005; use L0630

(K0640)   Code deleted December 31, 2005; use L0631

(K0641)   Code deleted December 31, 2005; use L0632

(K0642)   Code deleted December 31, 2005; use L0633

(K0643)   Code deleted December 31, 2005; use L0634

(K0644)   Code deleted December 31, 2005; use L0635

(K0645)   Code deleted December 31, 2005; use L0636

(K0646)   Code deleted December 31, 2005; use L0637

(K0647)   Code deleted December 31, 2005; use L0638

(K0648)   Code deleted December 31, 2005; use L0639

(K0649)   Code deleted December 31, 2005; use L0640

(K0650)   Code deleted December 31, 2004; use E2601

(K0651)   Code deleted December 31, 2004; use E2602

(K0652)   Code deleted December 31, 2004; use E2603

(K0653)   Code deleted December 31, 2004; use E2604

(K0654)   Code deleted December 31, 2004; use E2605

(K0655)   Code deleted December 31, 2004; use E2606

(K0656)   Code deleted December 31, 2004; use E2607

(K0657)   Code deleted December 31, 2004; use E2608

(K0658)   Code deleted December 31, 2004; use E2609

(K0659)   Code deleted December 31, 2004; use E2610

(K0660)   Code deleted December 31, 2004; use E2611

(K0661)   Code deleted December 31, 2004; use E2612

(K0662)   Code deleted December 31, 2004; use E2613

(K0663)   Code deleted December 31, 2004; use E2614

(K0664)   Code deleted December 31, 2004; use E2615

(K0665)   Code deleted December 31, 2004; use E2616

(K0666)   Code deleted December 31, 2004; use E2617

(K0667)   Code deleted December 31, 2004; use CPT

(K0668)   Code deleted December 31, 2004; use E2619

▲ **K0669**   Wheelchair accessory, wheelchair seat or back cushion, does not meet specific code criteria or no written coding verification from SADMERC

● **K0730**   Controlled dose inhalation drug delivery system

ORTHOTIC PROCEDURES

Guidelines

In addition to the information presented in the INTRODUCTION, several other items unique to this section are defined or identified here:

1. SUBSECTION INFORMATION: Some of the listed subheadings or subsections have special needs or instructions unique to that section. Where these are indicated, special "notes" will be presented preceding or following the listings. Those subsections within the ORTHOTIC PROCEDURES section that have "notes" are as follows:

Subsection	Code Numbers
Scoliosis procedures	L1000-L1499
Orthotic devices-lower limb	L1600-L2999
Lower limb-hip-knee-angle- foot (or any combination)	L2000-L2199
Orthotic devices-upper limb	L3650-L3999

2. UNLISTED SERVICE OR PROCEDURE: A service or procedure may be provided that is not listed in this edition of HCPCS. When reporting such a service, the appropriate "unlisted procedure" code may be used to indicate the service, identifying it by "special report" as defined below. HCPCS terminology is inconsistent in defining unlisted procedures. The procedure definition may include the term(s) "unlisted", "not otherwise classified", "unspecified", "unclassified", "other" and "miscellaneous". Prior to using these codes, try to determine if a Local Level III code or CPT code is available. The "unlisted procedures" and accompanying codes for ORTHOTIC PROCEDURES are as follows:

L0999	Addition to spinal orthosis, not otherwise specified
L1499	Spinal orthosis, not otherwise specified
L2999	Lower extremity orthosis, not otherwise specified
L3649	Orthopedic shoe, modification, addition or transfer, not otherwise specified
L3999	Upper limb orthosis, not otherwise specified

3. SPECIAL REPORT: A service, material or supply that is rarely provided, unusual, variable or new may require a special report in determining medical appropriateness for reimbursement purposes.

Pertinent information should include an adequate definition or description of the nature, extent, and need for the service, material or supply.

4. MODIFIERS: Listed services may be modified under certain circumstances. When appropriate, the modifying circumstance is identified by adding a modifier to the basic procedure code. CPT and HCPCS National Level II modifiers may be used with CPT and HCPCS National Level II procedure codes. Modifiers commonly used with ORTHOTIC PROCEDURES are as follows:

-CC   Procedure code change (use "CC" when the procedure code submitted was changed either for administrative reasons or because an incorrect code was filed)

-LT   Left side (used to identify procedures performed on the left side of the body)

-RT   Right side (used to identify procedures performed on the right side of the body)

-TC   Technical component. Under certain circumstances, a charge may be made for the technical component alone. Under those circumstances, the technical component charge is identified by adding modifier -TC to the usual procedure number. Technical component charges are institutional charges and are not billed separately by physicians. However, portable x-ray suppliers bill only for the technical component and should use modifier -TC. The change data from portable x-ray suppliers will then be used to build customary and prevailing profiles.

5. CPT CODE CROSS-REFERENCE: Unless otherwise specified, the equivalent CPT code for all listings in this section is 99070.

6. DURABLE MEDICAL EQUIPMENT REGIONAL CARRIERS (DMERCS): Effective October 1, 1993, claims orthotics must be billed to one of four regional carriers depending upon the residence of the beneficiary. The transition dates for DMERC claims is from November 1, 1993 to March 1, 1994, depending upon the state you practice in. See the Introduction for a complete discussion of DMERCs.

Orthotic Procedures

ORTHOTIC DEVICES

SPINAL - CERVICAL

L0100 Cranial orthosis (helmet), with or without soft-interface, molded to patient model

L0110 Cranial orthosis (helmet), with or without soft-interface, non-molded

L0112 Cranial cervical orthosis, congenital torticollis type, with or without soft interface material, adjustable range of motion joint, custom fabricated

L0120 Cervical, flexible; non-adjustable (foam collar)

L0130 thermoplastic collar, molded to patient

L0140 Cervical, semi-rigid; adjustable (plastic collar)

L0150 adjustable molded chin cup (plastic collar with mandibular/occipital piece)

L0160 wire frame occipital/mandibular support

L0170 Cervical collar; molded to patient model

L0172 semi-rigid thermoplastic foam, two piece

L0174 semi-rigid, thermoplastic foam, two piece with thoracic extension

L0180 Cervical, multiple post collar, occipital/mandibular supports; adjustable

L0190 adjustable cervical bars (somi, guilford, taylor types)

L0200 adjustable cervical bars, and thoracic extension

SPINAL - THORACIC

L0210 Thoracic, rib belt;

L0220 custom fabricated

SPINAL - THORACIC-LUMBAR-SACRAL

FLEXIBLE

ANTERIOR-POSTERIOR CONTROL

ANTERIOR-POSTERIOR-LATERAL-ROTARY CONTROL

L0450 TLSO, flexible, provides trunk support, upper thoracic region, produces intracavitary pressure to reduce load on the intervertebral disks with rigid stays or panel(s), includes shoulder straps and closures, prefabricated, includes fitting and adjustment

L0452 TLSO, flexible, provides trunk support, upper thoracic region, produces intracavitary pressure to reduce load on the intervertebral disks with rigid stays or panel(s), includes shoulder straps and closures, custom fabricated

L0454 TLSO flexible, provides trunk support, extends from sacrococcygeal junction to above t-9 vertebra, restricts gross trunk motion in the sagittal plane, produces intracavitary pressure to reduce load on the intervertebral disks with rigid stays or panel(s), includes shoulder straps and closures, prefabricated, includes fitting and adjustment

L0456 TLSO, flexible, provides trunk support, thoracic region, rigid posterior panel and soft anterior apron, extends from the sacrococcygeal junction and terminates just inferior to the scapular spine, restricts gross trunk motion in the sagittal plane, produces intracavitary pressure to reduce load on the intervertebral disks, includes straps and closures, prefabricated, includes fitting and adjustment

L0458 TLSO, triplanar control, modular segmented spinal system, two rigid plastic shells, posterior extends from the sacrococcygeal junction and terminates just inferior to the scapular spine, anterior extends from the symphysis pubis to the xiphoid, soft liner, restricts gross trunk motion in the sagittal, coronal, and transverse planes, lateral strength is provided by overlapping plastic and stabilizing closures, includes straps and closures, prefabricated, includes fitting and adjustment

L0460 TLSO, triplanar control, modular segmented spinal system, two rigid plastic shells, posterior extends from the sacrococcygeal junction and terminates just inferior to the scapular spine, anterior extends from the symphysis pubis to the sternal notch, soft liner, restricts gross trunk motion in the sagittal, coronal, and transverse planes, lateral strength is provided by overlapping plastic and stabilizing closures, includes straps and closures, prefabricated, includes fitting and adjustment

L0462 TLSO, triplanar control, modular segmented spinal system, three rigid plastic shells, posterior extends from the sacrococcygeal junction and terminates just inferior to the scapular spine, anterior extends from the symphysis pubis to the sternal notch, soft liner, restricts gross trunk motion in the sagittal, coronal, and transverse planes, lateral strength is provided by overlapping plastic and stabilizing closures, includes straps and closures, prefabricated, includes fitting and adjustment

L0464 TLSO, triplanar control, modular segmented spinal system, four rigid plastic shells, posterior extends from sacrococcygeal junction and terminates just inferior to scapular spine, anterior extends from symphysis pubis to the sternal notch, soft liner, restricts gross trunk motion in sagittal, coronal, and transverse planes, lateral strength is provided by overlapping plastic and stabilizing closures, includes straps and closures, prefabricated, includes fitting and adjustment

L0466 TLSO, sagittal control, rigid posterior frame and flexible soft anterior apron with straps, closures and padding, restricts gross trunk motion in sagittal plane, produces intracavitary pressure to reduce load on intervertebral disks, includes fitting and shaping the frame, prefabricated, includes fitting and adjustment

L0468 TLSO, sagittal-coronal control, rigid posterior frame and flexible soft anterior apron with straps, closures and padding, extends from sacrococcygeal junction over scapulae, lateral strength provided by pelvic, thoracic, and lateral frame pieces, restricts gross trunk motion in sagittal, and coronal planes, produces intracavitary pressure to reduce load on intervertebral disks, includes fitting and shaping the frame, prefabricated, includes fitting and adjustment

L0470 TLSO, triplanar control, rigid posterior frame and flexible soft anterior apron with straps, closures and padding, extends from sacrococcygeal junction to scapula, lateral strength provided by pelvic, thoracic, and lateral frame pieces, rotational strength provided by subclavicular extensions, restricts gross trunk motion in sagittal, coronal, and transverse planes, produces intracavitary pressure to reduce load on the intervertebral disks, includes fitting and shaping the frame, prefabricated, includes fitting and adjustment

L0472 TLSO, triplanar control, hyperextension, rigid anterior and lateral frame extends from symphysis pubis to sternal notch with two anterior components (one pubic and one sternal), posterior and lateral pads with straps and closures, limits spinal flexion, restricts gross trunk motion in sagittal, coronal, and transverse planes, includes fitting and shaping the frame, prefabricated, includes fitting and adjustment

(L0476) Code deleted December 31, 2004; use CPT

(L0478) Code deleted December 31, 2004; use CPT

L0480 TLSO, triplanar control, one piece rigid plastic shell without interface liner, with multiple straps and closures, posterior extends from sacrococcygeal junction and terminates just inferior to scapular spine, anterior extends from symphysis pubis to sternal notch, anterior or posterior opening, restricts gross trunk motion in sagittal, coronal, and transverse planes, includes a carved plaster or cad-cam model, custom fabricated

L0482 TLSO, triplanar control, one piece rigid plastic shell with interface liner, multiple straps and closures, posterior extends from sacrococcygeal junction and terminates just inferior to scapular spine, anterior extends from symphysis pubis to sternal notch, anterior or posterior opening, restricts gross trunk motion in sagittal, coronal, and transverse planes, includes a carved plaster or cad-cam model, custom fabricated

L0484 TLSO, triplanar control, two piece rigid plastic shell without interface liner, with multiple straps and closures, posterior extends from sacrococcygeal junction and terminates just inferior to scapular spine, anterior extends from symphysis pubis to sternal notch, lateral strength is enhanced by overlapping plastic, restricts gross trunk motion in the sagittal, coronal, and transverse planes, includes a carved plaster or cad-cam model, custom fabricated

L0486 TLSO, triplanar control, two piece rigid plastic shell with interface liner, multiple straps and closures, posterior extends from sacrococcygeal junction and terminates just inferior to scapular spine, anterior extends from symphysis pubis to sternal notch, lateral strength is enhanced by overlapping plastic, restricts gross trunk motion in the sagittal, coronal, and transverse planes, includes a carved plaster or cad-cam model, custom fabricated

L0488 TLSO, triplanar control, one piece rigid plastic shell with interface liner, multiple straps and closures, posterior extends from sacrococcygeal junction and terminates just inferior to scapular spine, anterior extends from symphysis pubis to sternal notch, anterior or posterior opening, restricts gross trunk motion in sagittal, coronal, and transverse planes, prefabricated, includes fitting and adjustment

L0490 TLSO, sagittal-coronal control, one piece rigid plastic shell, with overlapping reinforced anterior, with multiple straps and closures, posterior extends from sacrococcygeal junction and terminates at or before the t-9 vertebra, anterior extends from symphysis pubis to xiphoid, anterior opening, restricts gross trunk motion in sagittal and coronal planes, prefabricated, includes fitting and adjustment

● **L0491** TLSO, sagittal-coronal control, modular segmented spinal system, two rigid plastic shells, posterior extends from the sacrococcygeal junction and terminates just inferior to the scapular spine, anterior extends from the symphysis pubis to the xiphoid, soft liner, restricts gross trunk motion in the sagittal and coronal planes, lateral strength is provided by overlapping plastic and stabilizing closures, includes straps and closures, prefabricated, includes fitting and adjustment

● **L0492**   TLSO, sagittal-coronal control, modular segmented spinal system, three rigid plastic shells, posterior extends from the sacrococcygeal junction and terminates just inferior to the scapular spine, anterior extends from the symphysis pubis to the xiphoid, soft liner, restricts gross trunk motion in the sagittal and coronal planes, lateral strength is provided by overlapping plastic and stabilizing closures, includes straps and closures, prefabricated, includes fitting and adjustment

SPINAL - LUMBAR-SACRAL

FLEXIBLE

(L0500)   Code deleted December 31, 2004; use CPT

(L0510)   Code deleted December 31, 2004; use CPT

(L0515)   Code deleted December 31, 2004; use CPT

ANTERIOR-POSTERIOR-LATERAL CONTROL

(L0520)   Code deleted December 31, 2004; use CPT

ANTERIOR-POSTERIOR CONTROL

(L0530)   Code deleted December 31, 2004; use CPT

LUMBAR FLEXION

(L0540)   Code deleted December 31, 2004; use CPT

ANTERIOR-POSTERIOR-LATERAL CONTROL (BODY JACKET)

(L0550)   Code deleted December 31, 2004; use CPT

(L0560   Code deleted December 31, 2004; use CPT

(L0561)   Code deleted December 31, 2004; use CPT

(L0565)   Code deleted December 31, 2004; use CPT

SPINAL - SACROILIAC

FLEXIBLE

(L0600) Code deleted December 31, 2004; use CPT

(L0610) Code deleted December 31, 2004; use CPT

SEMI-RIGID

(L0620) Code deleted December 31, 2004; use CPT

● **L0621** Sacroiliac orthosis, flexible, provides pelvic-sacral support, reduces motion about the sacroiliac joint, includes straps, closures, may include pendulous abdomen design, prefabricated, includes fitting and adjustment

● **L0622** Sacroiliac orthosis, flexible, provides pelvic-sacral support, reduces motion about the sacroiliac joint, includes straps, closures, may include pendulous abdomen design, custom fabricated

● **L0623** Sacroiliac orthosis, provides pelvic-sacral support, with rigid or semi-rigid panels over the sacrum and abdomen, reduces motion about the sacroiliac joint, includes straps, closures, may include pendulous abdomen design, prefabricated, includes fitting and adjustment

● **L0624** Sacroiliac orthosis, provides pelvic-sacral support, with rigid or semi-rigid panels placed over the sacrum and abdomen, reduces motion about the sacroiliac joint, includes straps, closures, may include pendulous abdomen design, custom fabricated

● **L0625** Lumbar orthosis, flexible, provides lumbar support, posterior extends from L-1 to below L-5 vertebra, produces intracavitary pressure to reduce load on the intervertebral discs, includes straps, closures, may include pendulous abdomen design, shoulder straps, stays, prefabricated, includes fitting and adjustment

● **L0626** Lumbar orthosis, sagittal control, with rigid posterior panel(s), posterior extends from L-1 to below L-5 vertebra, produces intracavitary pressure to reduce load on the intervertebral discs, includes straps, closures, may include padding, stays, shoulder straps, pendulous abdomen design, prefabricated, includes fitting and adjustment

● **L0627** Lumbar orthosis, sagittal control, with rigid anterior and posterior panels, posterior extends from L-1 to below L-5 vertebra, produces intracavitary pressure to reduce load on the intervertebral discs, includes straps, closures, may include padding, shoulder straps, pendulous abdomen design, prefabricated, includes fitting and adjustment

● **L0628** Lumbar-sacral orthosis, flexible, provides lumbo-sacral support, posterior extends from sacrococcygeal junction to T-9 vertebra, produces intracavitary pressure to reduce load on the intervertebral discs, includes straps, closures, may include stays, shoulder straps, pendulous abdomen design, prefabricated, includes fitting and adjustment

● **L0629** Lumbar-sacral orthosis, flexible, provides lumbo-sacral support, posterior extends from sacrococcygeal junction to T-9 vertebra, produces intracavitary pressure to reduce load on the intervertebral discs, includes straps, closures, may include stays, shoulder straps, pendulous abdomen design, custom fabricated

● **L0630** Lumbar-sacral orthosis, sagittal control, with rigid posterior panel(s), posterior extends from sacrococcygeal junction to T-9 vertebra, produces intracavitary pressure to reduce load on the intervertebral discs, includes straps, closures, may include padding, stays, shoulder straps, pendulous abdomen design, prefabricated, includes fitting and adjustment

● **L0631** Lumbar-sacral orthosis, sagittal control, with rigid anterior and posterior panels, posterior extends from sacrococcygeal junction to T-9 vertebra, produces intracavitary pressure to reduce load on the intervertebral discs, includes straps, pendulous abdomen design, prefabricated, includes fitting and adjustment

● **L0632** Lumbar-sacral orthosis, sagittal control, with rigid anterior and posterior panels, posterior extends from sacrococcygeal junction to T-9 vertebra, produces intracavitary pressure to reduce load on the intervertebral discs, includes straps, closures, may include padding, shoulder straps, pendulous abdomen design, custom fabricated

● **L0633** Lumbar-sacral orthosis, sagittal-coronal control, with rigid posterior frame/panel(s), posterior extends from sacrococcygeal junction to T-9 vertebra, lateral strength provided by rigid lateral frame/panels, produces intracavitary pressure to reduce load on intervertebral discs, includes straps, closures, may include padding, stays, shoulder straps, pendulous abdomen design, prefabricated, includes fitting and adjustment

● **L0634** Lumbar-sacral orthosis, sagittal-coronal control, with rigid posterior frame/panel(s), posterior extends from sacrococcygeal junction to T-9 vertebra, lateral strength provided by rigid lateral frame/panel(s), produces intracavitary pressure to reduce load on intervertebral discs, includes straps, closures, may include padding, stays, shoulder straps, pendulous abdomen design, custom fabricated

● **L0635** Lumbar-sacral orthosis, sagittal-coronal control, lumbar flexion, rigid posterior frame/panel(s), lateral articulating design to flex the lumbar spine, posterior extends from sacrococcygeal junction to T-9 vertebra, lateral strength provided by rigid lateral frame/panel(s), produces intracavitary pressure to reduce load on intervertebral discs, includes straps, closures, may include padding, anterior panel, pendulous abdomen design, prefabricated, includes fitting and adjustment

● **L0636** Lumbar sacral orthosis, sagittal-coronal control, lumbar flexion, rigid posterior frame/panels, lateral articulating design to flex the lumbar spine, posterior extends from sacrococcygeal junction to T-9 vertebra, lateral strength provided by rigid lateral frame/panels, produces intracavitary pressure to reduce load on intervertebral discs, includes straps, closures, may include padding, anterior panel, pendulous abdomen design, custom fabricated

● **L0637** Lumbar-sacral orthosis, sagittal-coronal control, with rigid anterior and posterior frame/panels, posterior extends from sacrococcygeal junction to T-9 vertebra, lateral strength provided by rigid lateral frame/panels, produces intracavitary pressure to reduce load on intervertebral discs, includes straps, closures, may include padding, shoulder straps, pendulous abdomen design, prefabricated, includes fitting and adjustmentanel, pendulous abdomen design, custom fabricated

● **L0638** Lumbar-sacral orthosis, sagittal-coronal control, with rigid anterior and posterior frame/panels, posterior extends from sacrococcygeal junction to T-9 vertebra, lateral strength provided by rigid lateral frame/panels, produces intracavitary pressure to reduce load on intervertebral discs, includes straps, closures, may include padding, shoulder straps, pendulous abdomen design, custom fabricated

● **L0639** Lumbar-sacral orthosis, sagittal-coronal control, rigid shell(s)/panel(s), posterior extends from sacrococcygeal junction to T-9 vertebra, anterior extends from symphysis pubis to xyphoid, produces intracavitary pressure to reduce load on the intervertebral discs, overall strength is provided by overlapping rigid material and stabilizing closures, includes straps, closures, may include soft interface, pendulous abdomen design, prefabricated, includes fitting and adjustment

● **L0640** Lumbar-sacral orthosis, sagittal-coronal control, rigid shell(s)/panel(s), posterior extends from sacrococcygeal junction to T-9 vertebra, anterior extends from symphysis pubis to xyphoid, produces intracavitary pressure to reduce load on the intervertebral discs, overall strength is provided by overlapping rigid material and stabilizing closures, includes straps, closures, may include soft interface, pendulous abdomen design, custom fabricated

SPINAL - CERVICAL-THORACIC-LUMBAR-SACRAL-HALO PROCEDURE

ANTERIOR-POSTERIOR-LATERAL CONTROL

L0700 Cervical-thoracic-lumber-sacral-orthoses (CTLSO), anterior-posterior-lateral control, molded to patient model; (Minerva type)

L0710 with interface material, (Minerva type)

HALO PROCEDURE

L0810 Halo procedure; cervical halo incorporated into jacket vest

L0820 cervical halo incorporated into plaster body jacket

L0830 cervical halo incorporated into Milwaukee type orthosis

● **L0859**   Addition to halo procedure, magnetic resonance image compatible systems, rings and pins, any material

SPINAL - TORSO SUPPORTS

PTOSIS SUPPORTS

(L0860)   Code deleted December 31, 2005; use L0859

L0861   Addition to halo procedure, replacement liner/interface material

PENDULOUS ABDOMEN SUPPORT

POST SURGICAL SUPPORT

L0960   pads for post surgical support

ADDITIONS TO SPINAL ORTHOSES

L0970   TLSO, corset front

L0972   LSO, corset front

L0974   TLSO, full corset

L0976   LSO, full corset

L0978   Axillary crutch extension

L0980   Peroneal straps, pair

L0982   Stocking supporter grips, set of four (4)

L0984   Protective body sock, each

L0999   Addition to spinal orthosis, not otherwise specified

ORTHOTIC DEVICES - SCOLIOSIS PROCEDURES

NOTE: The orthotic care of scoliosis differs from other orthotic care in that the treatment is more dynamic in nature and utilizes ongoing, continual modification of the orthosis to the patient's changing condition. This coding structure uses the proper names or eponyms of the procedures because they have historic and universal acceptance in the profession. It should be recognized that variations to the basic procedures described by the founders/developers are accepted in various medical and orthotic practices throughout the country. All procedures include model of patient when indicated.

SCOLIOSIS - CERVICAL-THORACIC-LUMBAR-SACRAL (MILWAUKEE)

L1000 Cervical-thoracic-lumbar-sacral orthosis (CTLSO) (Milwaukee), inclusive of furnishing initial orthosis, including model

L1005 Tension based scoliosis orthosis and accessory pads, includes fitting and adjustment

CORRECTION PADS

L1010 Additions to cervical-thoracic-lumber-sacral orthosis (CTLSO) or scoliosis orthosis; axilla sling

L1020 kyphosis pad

L1025 kyphosis pad, floating

L1030 lumbar bolster pad

L1040 lumbar or lumbar rib pad

L1050 sternal pad

L1060 thoracic pad

L1070 trapezius sling

L1080 outrigger

L1085 outrigger, bilateral with vertical extensions

L1090	lumbar sling

L1100	ring flange, plastic or leather

L1110	ring flange, plastic or leather, molded to patient model

L1120	covers for upright, each

SCOLIOSIS - THORACIC-LUMBAR-SACRAL (LOW PROFILE)

L1200	Thoracic-lumbar-sacral-orthosis (TLSO), inclusive of furnishing initial orthosis only

L1210	Addition to TLSO, (low profile); lateral thoracic extension

L1220	anterior thoracic extension

L1230	Milwaukee type superstructure

L1240	lumbar derotation pad

L1250	anterior asis pad

L1260	anterior thoracic derotation pad

L1270	abdominal pad

L1280	rib gusset (elastic), each

L1290	lateral trochanteric pad

OTHER SCOLIOSIS PROCEDURES

L1300	Other scoliosis procedure; body jacket molded to patient model

L1310	post-operative body jacket

L1499	Spinal orthosis, not otherwise specified

Not valid for Medicare   Non-covered by Medicare   Special coverage instructions   Carrier discretion

THORACIC-HIP-KNEE-ANKLE

L1500 Thoracic-hip-knee-ankle, orthosis (THKAO), mobility frame (Newington, Parapodium types)

L1510 THKAO, standing frame, with or without tray and accessories

L1520 THKAO, swivel walker

ORTHOTIC DEVICES - LOWER LIMB

NOTE: The procedures L1600-L2999 are considered as "base" or the "basic procedures" and may be modified by listing other procedures from the "additions" (L2200-L2999) section and adding them to the base procedure.

LOWER LIMB-HIP

FLEXIBLE

L1600 Hip orthosis (HO), abduction control of hip joints, flexible, Frejka type with cover, prefabricated, includes fitting and adjustment

L1610 HO, abduction control of hip joints; flexible, (Frejka cover only), prefabricated, includes fitting and adjustment

L1620 HO, abduction control of hip joints; flexible, (Pavlik harness), prefabricated, includes fitting and adjustment

L1630 HO, abduction control of hip joints; semi-flexible (Von Rosen type), custom fabricated

L1640 HO, abduction control of hip joints; static, pelvic band or spreader bar, thigh cuffs, custom fabricated

L1650 HO, abduction control of hip joints; static, adjustable, (Ilfled type), prefabricated, includes fitting and adjustment

L1652 Hip orthosis, bilateral thigh cuffs with adjustable abductor spreader bar, adult size, prefabricated, includes fitting and adjustment, any type

L1660 HO, abduction control of hip joints; static, plastic, prefabricated, includes fitting and adjustment

---

L1680   HO, abduction control of hip joints; dynamic, pelvic control, adjustable hip motion control, thigh cuffs (Rancho hip action type), custom fabricated

L1685   HO, abduction control of hip joints; postoperative hip abduction type, custom fabricated

L1686   HO, abduction control of hip joints; postoperative hip abduction type, prefabricated, includes fitting and adjustment

L1690   Combination, bilateral, lumbo-sacral, hip, femur orthosis providing adduction and internal rotation control, prefabricated, includes fitting and adjustment

LOWER LIMB-LEGG PERTHES

L1700   Legg Perthes orthosis; (Toronto type), custom fabricated

L1710   (Newington type), custom fabricated

L1720   trilateral, (Tachidijan type), custom fabricated

L1730   (Scottish Rite type), custom fabricated

(L1750)   Code deleted December 31, 2005; use A4565

L1755   (Patten Bottom type), custom fabricated

LOWER LIMB-KNEE

L1800   Knee orthosis (KO); elastic with stays, prefabricated, includes fitting and adjustment

L1810   elastic with joints, prefabricated, includes fitting and adjustment

L1815   elastic or other elastic type material with condylar pad(s), prefabricated, includes fitting and adjustment

L1820   elastic with condylar pads and joints, with or without patellar control, prefabricated, includes fitting and adjustment

L1825   elastic knee cap, prefabricated, includes fitting and adjustment

L1830 immobilizer, canvas longitudinal, prefabricated, includes fitting and adjustment

L1831 Knee orthosis (KO); locking knee joint(s), positional orthosis, prefabricated, includes fitting and adjustment

▲L1832 adjustable knee joints (unicentric or polycentric), positional orthosis, rigid support, prefabricated, includes fitting and adjustment

L1834 without knee joint, rigid, custom fabricated

L1836 Knee orthosis, rigid, without joint(s), includes soft interface material, prefabricated, includes fitting and adjustment

L1840 derotation, medial-lateral, anterior cruciate ligament, custom fabricated

▲L1843 Knee orthosis, single upright, thigh and calf, with adjustable flexion and extension joint (unicentric or polycentric), medial-lateral and rotation control, with or without varus/valgus adjustment, prefabricated, includes fitting and adjustment

▲L1844 Knee orthosis, single upright, thigh and calf, with adjustable flexion and extension joint (unicentric or polycentric), medial-lateral and rotation control, with or without varus/valgus adjustment, custom fabricated

▲L1845 double upright, thigh and calf, with adjustable flexion and extension joint (unicentric or polycentric), medial-lateral and rotation control, with or without varus/valgus adjustment, prefabricated, includes fitting and adjustment

▲L1846 double upright, thigh and calf, with adjustable flexion and extension joint (unicentric or polycentric), medial-lateral and rotation control, with or without varus/valgus adjustment, custom fabricated

L1847 double upright with adjustable joint, with inflatable air support chamber(s), pre-fabricated, includes fitting and adjustment

L1850 Swedish type, pre-fabricated, includes fitting and adjustment

L1855   molded plastic, thigh and calf sections, with double upright knee joints, custom fabricated

L1858   molded plastic, polycentric knee joints, pneumatic knee pads (CTI), custom fabricated

L1860   modification of supracondylar prosthetic socket, custom fabricated (SK)

L1870   double upright, thigh and calf lacers with knee joint, custom fabricated

L1880   double upright, non-molded thigh and calf cuffs/lacers with knee joints, custom fabricated

LOWER LIMB-ANKLE-FOOT

L1900   Ankle-foot orthosis (AFO); spring wire, dorsiflexion assist calf band, custom fabricated

L1901   Ankle orthosis, elastic, prefabricated, includes fitting and adjustment (e.g. neoprene, Lycra)

L1902   AFO; ankle gauntlet, prefabricated, includes fitting and adjustment

L1904   molded ankle gauntlet, custom fabricated

L1906   multiligamentus ankle support, prefabricated, includes fitting and adjustment

L1907   supramalleolar with straps, with or without interface/ pads, custom fabricated

L1910   posterior, single bar, clasp attachment to shoe counter, prefabricated, includes fitting and adjustment

L1920   single upright with static or adjustable stop (Phelps or Perlstein type), custom fabricated

L1930   Ankle foot orthosis; plastic or other material, prefabricated, includes fitting and adjustment

L1932   AFO, rigid anterior tibial section, total carbon fiber or equal material, prefabricated, includes fitting and adjustment

L1940   Ankle foot orthosis; plastic or other material, custom-fabricated

L1945   plastic, rigid anterior tibial section (floor reaction), custom fabricated

L1950   spiral, (Institute of Rehabilitative Medicine type), plastic, custom-fabricated

L1951   spiral, (Institute of Rehabilitative Medicine type), plastic or other material, prefabricated, includes fitting and adjustment

L1960   posterior solid ankle, plastic, custom fabricated

L1970   plastic with ankle joint, custom fabricated

L1971   plastic or other material with ankle joint, prefabricated, includes fitting and adjustment

L1980   single upright free plantar dorsiflexion, solid stirrup, calf band/cuff (single bar "BK" orthosis), custom fabricated

L1990   double upright free plantar dorsiflexion, solid stirrup, calf band/cuff (double bar "BK" orthosis), custom fabricated

LOWER LIMB-HIP-KNEE-ANKLE-FOOT (OR ANY COMBINATION)

NOTE: L2000, L2020, and L2036 are base procedures to be used with any knee joint. L2010 and L2030 are to used only with no knee joint.

L2000   Knee-ankle-foot-orthosis (KAFO); single upright, free knee, free ankle, solid stirrup, thigh and calf bands/cuffs (single bar "AK" orthosis), custom fabricated

L2005   Knee ankle foot orthosis, any material, single or double upright, stance control, automatic lock and swing phase release, mechanical activation, includes ankle joint, any type, custom fabricated

L2010   single upright, free ankle, solid stirrup, thigh and calf bands/cuffs (single bar "AK" orthosis), without knee joint, custom fabricated

L2020   double upright, free ankle, solid stirrup, thigh and calf bands/cuffs (double bar "AK" orthosis), custom fabricated

L2030   double upright, free ankle, solid stirrup, thigh and calf bands/cuffs, (double bar "AK" orthosis), without knee joint, custom fabricated

● **L2034**   full plastic, single upright, with or without free motion knee, medial lateral rotation control, with or without free motion ankle, custom fabricated

L2035   full plastic, static (pediatric size), without free motion ankle, prefabricated, includes fitting and adjustment

▲ **L2036**   full plastic, double upright, with or without free motion knee, with or without free motion ankle, custom fabricated

▲ **L2037**   full plastic, single upright, with or without free motion knee, with or without free motion ankle, custom fabricated

▲ **L2038**   full plastic, with or without free motion knee, multiaxis ankle, custom fabricated

(L2039)   Code deleted December 31, 2005

TORSION CONTROL

L2040   Hip-knee-ankle-foot orthosis (HKAFO); torsion control, bilateral rotation straps, pelvic band/belt, custom fabricated

L2050   torsion control, bilateral torsion cables, hip joint, pelvic band/belt, custom fabricated

L2060   torsion control, bilateral torsion cables, ball bearing hip joint, pelvic band/belt, custom fabricated

L2070   torsion control, unilateral rotation straps, pelvic band/belt, custom fabricated

L2080   torsion control, unilateral torsion cable, hip joint, pelvic band/belt, custom fabricated

| L2090 | torsion control, unilateral torsion cable, ball bearing hip joint, pelvic band/belt, custom fabricated |

FRACTURE ORTHOSES

| L2106 | Ankle-foot-orthosis (AFO), fracture orthosis, tibial fracture cast orthosis; thermoplastic type casting material, custom fabricated |

| L2108 | custom fabricated |

| L2112 | soft, pre-fabricated, includes fitting and adjustment |

| L2114 | semi-rigid, pre-fabricated, includes fitting and adjustment |

| L2116 | rigid, pre-fabricated, includes fitting and adjustment |

| L2126 | Knee-ankle-foot-orthosis (KAFO), fracture orthosis, femoral fracture cast orthosis; thermoplastic type casting material, custom fabricated |

| L2128 | custom fabricated |

| L2132 | soft, prefabricated, includes fitting and adjustment |

| L2134 | semi-rigid, prefabricated, includes fitting and adjustment |

| L2136 | rigid, prefabricated, includes fitting and adjustment |

ADDITIONS TO FRACTURE ORTHOSIS

| L2180 | Addition to lower extremity fracture orthosis; plastic shoe insert with ankle joints |

| L2182 | drop lock knee joint |

| L2184 | limited motion knee joint |

| L2186 | adjustable motion knee joint, Lerman type |

| L2188 | quadrilateral brim |

| L2190 | waist belt |

L2192   hip joint, pelvic band, thigh flange, and pelvic belt

ADDITIONS TO LOWER EXTREMITY ORTHOSIS

ADDITIONS - SHOE-ANKLE-SHIN-KNEE

L2200   Addition to lower extremity; limited ankle motion, each joint

L2210   dorsiflexion assist (plantar flexion resist), each joint

L2220 .   dorsiflexion and plantar flexion assist/resist, each joint

L2230   split flat caliper stirrups and plate attachment

L2232   Addition to lower extremity orthosis, rocker bottom for total contact ankle foot orthosis, for custom fabricated orthosis only

L2240   round caliper and plate attachment

L2250   foot plate, molded to patient model, stirrup attachment

L2260   reinforced solid stirrup (Scott-Craig type)

L2265   long tongue stirrup

L2270   varus/valgus correction ("T") strap, padded/lined or malleolus pad

L2275   varus/valgus correction, plastic modification, padded/lined

L2280   molded inner boot

L2300   abduction bar (bilateral hip involvement), jointed, adjustable

L2310   abduction bar-straight

L2320   non-molded lacer, for custom fabricated orthosis only

L2330   lacer molded to patient model, for custom fabricated orthosis only

L2335   anterior swing band

L2340	pre-tibial shell, molded to patient model
L2350	prosthetic type, (BK) socket, molded to patient model, (used for "PTB" "AFO" orthoses)
L2360	extended steel shank
L2370	patten bottom
L2375	torsion control, ankle joint and half solid stirrup
L2380	torsion control, straight knee joint, each joint
L2385	straight knee joint, heavy duty, each joint
● **L2387**	Addition to lower extremity, polycentric knee joint, for custom fabricated knee ankle foot orthosis, each joint
L2390	offset knee joint, each joint
L2395	offset knee joint, heavy duty, each joint
L2397	Addition to lower extremity orthosis, suspension sleeve

ADDITIONS TO STRAIGHT OR OFFSET KNEE JOINTS

▲ **L2405**	Addition to knee joint, drop lock, each
L2415	Addition to knee lock with integrated release mechanism (bail, cable, or equal), any material, each joint
L2425	Addition to knee joint; disc or dial lock for adjustable knee flexion, each joint
L2430	ratchet lock for active and progressive knee extension, each joint
(L2435)	Code deleted December 31, 2004; use CPT
L2492	lift loop for drop lock ring

ADDITIONS - THIGH/WEIGHT BEARING

GLUTEAL/ISCHIAL WEIGHT

L2500 Addition to lower extremity, thigh/weight bearing; gluteal/ischial weight bearing, ring

L2510 quadrilateral brim, molded to patient model

L2520 quadrilateral brim, custom fitting

L2525 ischial containment/narrow M-L brim molded to patient model

L2526 ischial containment/narrow M-L brim, custom fitted

L2530 lacer, non-molded

L2540 lacer, molded to patient model

L2550 high roll cuff

ADDITIONS - PELVIC AND THORACIC CONTROL

L2570 Addition to lower extremity, pelvic control; hip joint, Clevis type two position joint; each

L2580 pelvic sling

L2600 hip joint, Clevis type, or thrust bearing, free, each

L2610 hip joint, Clevis or thrust bearing, lock, each

L2620 Addition to lower extremity, pelvic control, hip joint; heavy duty, each

L2622 adjustable flexion, each

L2624 adjustable flexion, extension, abduction control, each

L2627 Addition to lower extremity, pelvic control; plastic, molded to patient model, reciprocating hip joint and cables

L2628 metal frame, reciprocating hip joint and cables

L2630	band and belt, unilateral
L2640	band and belt, bilateral
L2650	Addition to lower extremity, pelvic and thoracic control, gluteal pad, each
L2660	Addition to lower extremity, thoracic control; thoracic band
L2670	paraspinal uprights
L2680	lateral support uprights

ADDITIONS - GENERAL

L2750	Addition to lower extremity orthosis; plating chrome or nickel, per bar
L2755	high strength, lightweight material, all hybrid lamination/prepreg composite, per segment, for custom fabricated orthosis only
L2760	extension, per extension, per bar (for lineal adjustment for growth)
L2768	orthotic side bar disconnect device, per bar
L2770	any material, per bar or joint
L2780	non-corrosive finish, per bar
L2785	drop lock retainer, each
L2795	knee control, full kneecap
L2800	knee control, knee cap, medial or lateral pull, for use with custom fabricated orthosis only
L2810	knee control, condylar pad
L2820	soft interface for molded plastic, below knee section
L2830	soft interface for molded plastic, above knee section
L2840	tibial length sock, fracture or equal, each

● New code ▲ Revised code ( ) Deleted code

L2850	femora...
L2860	Addition t... concentric...
L2999	Lower extremity ...

FOOT ORTHOPEDIC SHOES,...
TRANSFERS

FOOT, INSERT, REMOVABLE, MOLDED ...
MODEL

L3000	Foot, insert, removable, molded to patient model; '... type, Berkeley Shell, each MCM: 2323
L3001	Spenco, each MCM: 2323
L3002	plastazote or equal, each MCM: 2323
L3003	silicone gel, each MCM: 2323
L3010	longitudinal arch support, each MCM: 2323
L3020	longitudinal/metatarsal support, each MCM: 2323
L3030	Foot, insert, removable, formed to patient foot, each MCM: 2323
L3031	Foot, insert/plate, removable, addition to lower extremity orthosis, high strength, lightweight material, all hybrid lamination/prepreg composite, each

FOOT, ARCH SUPPORT, REMOVABLE, PREMOLDED

| L3040 | Foot, arch support, removable, premolded; longitudinal, each
MCM: 2323 |
| L3050 | metatarsal, each
MCM: 2323 |

Not valid for Medicare Non-covered by Medicare Special coverage instructions

al, each

, NONREMOVABLE, ATTACHED

L30

support, non-removable attached to shoe;
linal, each
MCM: 2323

metatarsal, each
MCM: 2323

90 longitudinal/metatarsal, each
MCM: 2323

L3100 Hallus-valgus night dynamic splint
MCM: 2323

ABDUCTION AND ROTATION BARS

L3140 Foot, abduction rotation bar, including shoes
MCM: 2323

L3150 Foot, abduction rotation bars, without shoes
MCM: 2323

L3160 Foot, adjustable shoe-styled positioning device

▲**L3170** Foot, plastic, silicone or equal, heel stabilizer, each
MCM: 2323

ORTHOPEDIC FOOTWEAR

L3201 Orthopedic shoe, oxford with supinator or pronator; infant
MCM: 2323

L3202 child
MCM: 2323

L3203 junior
MCM: 2323

L3204 Orthopedic shoe, hightop with supinator or pronator;
infant
MCM: 2323

3206 child
MCM: 2323

New code   ▲   Revised code   ( )   Deleted code

L2850   femoral length sock, fracture or equal, each

L2860   Addition to lower extremity joint, knee or ankle, concentric adjustable torsion style mechanism, each

L2999   Lower extremity orthosis, not otherwise specified

FOOT ORTHOPEDIC SHOES, SHOE MODIFICATIONS, TRANSFERS

FOOT, INSERT, REMOVABLE, MOLDED TO PATIENT MODEL

L3000   Foot, insert, removable, molded to patient model; "UCB" type, Berkeley Shell, each
MCM: 2323

L3001   Spenco, each
MCM: 2323

L3002   plastazote or equal, each
MCM: 2323

L3003   silicone gel, each
MCM: 2323

L3010   longitudinal arch support, each
MCM: 2323

L3020   longitudinal/metatarsal support, each
MCM: 2323

L3030   Foot, insert, removable, formed to patient foot, each
MCM: 2323

L3031   Foot, insert/plate, removable, addition to lower extremity orthosis, high strength, lightweight material, all hybrid lamination/prepreg composite, each

FOOT, ARCH SUPPORT, REMOVABLE, PREMOLDED

L3040   Foot, arch support, removable, premolded; longitudinal, each
MCM: 2323

L3050   metatarsal, each
MCM: 2323

L3060 longitudinal/metatarsal, each
MCM: 2323

FOOT, ARCH SUPPORT, NONREMOVABLE, ATTACHED TO SHOE

L3070 Foot, arch support, non-removable attached to shoe; longitudinal, each
MCM: 2323

L3080 metatarsal, each
MCM: 2323

L3090 longitudinal/metatarsal, each
MCM: 2323

L3100 Hallus-valgus night dynamic splint
MCM: 2323

ABDUCTION AND ROTATION BARS

L3140 Foot, abduction rotation bar, including shoes
MCM: 2323

L3150 Foot, abduction rotation bars, without shoes
MCM: 2323

L3160 Foot, adjustable shoe-styled positioning device

▲**L3170** Foot, plastic, silicone or equal, heel stabilizer, each
MCM: 2323

ORTHOPEDIC FOOTWEAR

L3201 Orthopedic shoe, oxford with supinator or pronator; infant
MCM: 2323

L3202 child
MCM: 2323

L3203 junior
MCM: 2323

L3204 Orthopedic shoe, hightop with supinator or pronator; infant
MCM: 2323

L3206 child
MCM: 2323

L3207 junior
MCM: 2323

L3208 Surgical boot, each; infant

L3209 child

L3211 junior

L3212 Benesch boot, pair; infant

L3213 child

L3214 junior

▲**L3215** Orthopedic footwear, ladies shoe, oxford, each

▲**L3216** depth inlay, each

▲**L3217** hightop, depth inlay, each

▲**L3219** Orthopedic footwear, mens shoe, oxford, each

▲**L3221** depth inlay, each

▲**L3222** hightop, depth inlay, each

L3224 Orthopedic footwear, woman's shoe, oxford, used as an integral part of a brace (orthosis)
MCM: 2323D

L3225 Orthopedic footwear, man's shoe, oxford, used as an integral part of a brace (orthosis)
MCM: 2323D

▲**L3230** Orthopedic footwear, custom shoe, depth inlay, each
MCM: 2323

L3250 Orthopedic footwear, custom molded shoe, removable inner mold, prosthetic shoe, each
MCM: 2323

L3251 Foot, shoe molded to patient model; silicone shoe, each
MCM: 2323

L3252 plastazote (or similar), custom fabricated, each
MCM: 2323

L3253 Foot, molded shoe plastazote (or similar) custom fitted, each
MCM: 2323

L3254 Non-standard size or width
MCM: 2323

L3255 Non-standard size or length
MCM: 2323

L3257 Orthopedic footwear, additional charge for split size
MCM: 2323

L3260 Surgical boot/shoe, each
MCM: 2079

L3265 Plastazote sandal, each

SHOE MODIFICATION

LIFTS

L3300 Lift, elevation; heel, tapered to metatarsal, per inch
MCM: 2323

L3310 heel and sole, neoprene, per inch
MCM: 2323

L3320 heel and sole, cork, per inch
MCM: 2323

L3330 metal extension (skate)
MCM: 2323

L3332 inside shoe, tapered, up to one-half inch
MCM: 2323

L3334 heel, per inch
MCM: 2323

WEDGES

L3340 Heel wedge, SACH
MCM: 2323

L3350 Heel wedge
MCM: 2323

L3360 Sole wedge; outside sole
MCM: 2323

● New code ▲ Revised code ( ) Deleted code

L3370   between sole
MCM: 2323

L3380   Clubfoot wedge
MCM: 2323

L3390   Outflare wedge
MCM: 2323

L3400   Metatarsal bar wedge; rocker
MCM: 2323

L3410   between sole
MCM: 2323

L3420   Full sole and heel wedge, between sole
MCM: 2323

HEELS

L3430   Heel; counter, plastic reinforced
MCM: 2323

L3440   counter, leather reinforced
MCM: 2323

L3450   SACH cushion type
MCM: 2323

L3455   new leather, standard
MCM: 2323

L3460   new rubber, standard
MCM: 2323

L3465   Thomas with wedge
MCM: 2323

L3470   Thomas extended to ball
MCM: 2323

L3480   pad and depression for spur
MCM: 2323

L3485   pad, removable for spur
MCM: 2323

ORTHOPEDIC SHOE ADDITIONS

L3500   Orthopedic shoe addition; insole, leather
MCM: 2323

L3510   insole, rubber
MCM: 2323

L3520   insole, felt covered with leather
MCM: 2323

L3530   sole, half
MCM: 2323

L3540   sole, full
MCM: 2323

L3550   toe tap, standard
MCM: 2323

L3560   toe tap, horseshoe
MCM: 2323

L3570   special extension to instep (leather with eyelets)
MCM: 2323

L3580   convert instep to velcro closure
MCM: 2323

L3590   convert firm shoe counter to soft counter
MCM: 2323

L3595   march bar
MCM: 2323

TRANSFER OR REPLACEMENT

L3600   Transfer of an orthosis from one shoe to another; caliper plate, existing
MCM: 2323

L3610   caliper plate, new
MCM: 2323

L3620   solid stirrup, existing
MCM: 2323

L3630   solid stirrup, new
MCM: 2323

L3640   Dennis Browne splint (Riveton), both shoes
MCM: 2323

L3649   Orthopedic shoe, modification, addition or transfer, not otherwise specified
MCM: 2323

ORTHOTIC DEVICES - UPPER LIMB

NOTE: The procedures in this section are considered as "base" or "basic" procedures and may be modified by listing other procedures from the "additions" section, and adding them to the base procedure.

UPPER LIMB-SHOULDER

L3650   Shoulder orthosis, (SO); figure of eight design abduction restrainer, prefabricated, includes fitting and adjusment

L3651   Shoulder orthosis, single shoulder, elastic, prefabricated, includes fitting and adjustment (e.g. neoprene, Lycra)

L3652   Shoulder orthosis, double shoulder, elastic, prefabricated, includes fitting and adjustment (e.g. neoprene, Lycra)

L3660   figure of eight design abduction restrainer, canvas and webbing, prefabricated, includes fitting and adjustment

L3670   acromio/clavicular (canvas and webbing type), prefabricated, includes fitting and adjustment

●**L3671**   Shoulder orthosis, shoulder cap design, without joints, may include soft interface, straps, custom fabricated, includes fitting and adjustment

●**L3672**   Shoulder orthosis, abduction positioning (airplane design), thoracic component and support bar, without joints, may include soft interface, straps, custom fabricated, includes fitting and adjustment

●**L3673**   Shoulder orthosis, abduction positioning (airplane design), thoracic component and support bar, includes nontorsion joint/turnbuckle, may include soft interface, straps, custom fabricated, includes fitting and adjustment

● **L3674**   Elbow wrist hand orthosis, includes one or more nontorsion joints, elastic bands, turnbuckles, may include soft interface, straps, custom fabricated, includes fitting and adjustment

L3675   vest type abduction restrainer, canvas webbing type, or equal, prefabricated, includes fitting and adjustment

L3677   hard plastic, shoulder stabilizer, pre-fabricated, includes fitting and adjustment
MCM: 2130

UPPER LIMB-ELBOW

L3700   Elbow orthosis (EO); elastic with stays, prefabricated, includes fitting and adjustment

L3701   Elbow orthosis; elastic, prefabricated, includes fitting and adjustment (e.g. neoprene, Lycra)

● **L3702**   without joints, may include soft interface, straps, custom fabricated, includes fitting and adjustment

L3710   elastic with metal joints, prefabricated, includes fitting and adjustment

L3720   double upright with forearm/arm cuffs, free motion, custom fabricated

L3730   double upright with forearm/arm cuffs, extension/flexion assist, custom fabricated

L3740   double upright with forearm/arm cuffs, adjustable position lock with active control, custom fabricated

L3760   with adjustable position locking joint(s), prefabricated, includes fitting and adjustment

L3762   Elbow orthosis, rigid, without joints, includes soft interface material, prefabricated, includes fitting and adjustment

● **L3763**   Elbow wrist hand orthosis; rigid, without joints, may include soft interface, straps, custom fabricated, includes fitting and adjustment

● **L3764** includes one or more nontorsion joints, elastic bands, turnbuckles, may include soft interface, straps, custom fabricated, includes fitting and adjustment

● **L3765** Elbow wrist hand finger orthosis, rigid, without joints, may include soft interface, straps, custom fabricated, includes fitting and adjustment

● **L3766** Elbow wrist hand finger orthosis, includes one or more nontorsion joints, elastic bands, turnbuckles, may include soft interface, straps, custom fabricated, includes fitting and adjustment

UPPER LIMB - WRIST-HAND-FINGER

L3800 Wrist-hand-finger-orthoses (WHFO); short opponens, no attachments, custom fabricated

L3805 long opponens, no attachment, custom fabricated

L3807 without joint(s), prefabricated, inlcudes fitting and adjustment

ADDITIONS

L3810 Wrist-hand-finger-orthosis, addition to short and long opponens; thumb abduction ("C") bar

L3815 second M.P. abduction assist

L3820 I.P. extension assist, with M.P. extension stop

L3825 M.P. extension stop

L3830 M.P. extension assist

L3835 M.P. spring extension assist

L3840 spring swivel thumb

L3845 thumb I.P. extension assist, with M.P. stop

L3850 action wrist, with dorsiflexion assist

L3855 adjustable M.P. flexion control

Not valid   Non-covered   Special   Carrier
for Medicare   by Medicare   coverage   discretion
                                        instructions

L3860   adjustable M.P. flexion control and I.P.

L3890   Addition to upper extremity joint, wrist or elbow, concentric adjustable torsion style mechanism, each

DYNAMIC FLEXOR HINGE, RECIPROCAL WRIST EXTENSION/FLEXION, FINGER FLEXION/EXTENSION

L3900   Wrist-hand-finger-orthosis, dynamic flexor hinge, reciprocal wrist extension/flexion, finger flexion/extension; wrist or finger driven, custom fabricated

L3901   cable driven, custom fabricated

EXTERNAL POWER

L3902   Wrist-hand-finger-orthosis, external powered; compressed gas, custom fabricated

L3904   electric, custom fabricated

OTHER WRIST-HAND-FINGER ORTHOSES - CUSTOM FITTED

● **L3905**   Wrist hand orthosis, includes one or more nontorsion joints, elastic bands, turnbuckles, may include soft interface, straps, custom fabricated, includes fitting and adjustment

▲ **L3906**   Wrist hand orthosis, without joints, may include soft interface, straps, custom fabricated, includes fitting and adjustment

L3907   Wrist-hand-finger-orthosis, wrist guantlet with thumb spica, custom fabricated

L3908   Wrist-hand-orthosis (WHO), wrist extension control cock-up, prefabricated, includes fitting and adjustment

L3909   Wrist orthosis, elastic, prefabricated, includes fitting and adjustment (e.g. neoprene, Lycra)

L3910   Wrist-hand-finger-orthosis (WHFO), Swanson design, prefabricated, includes fitting and adjustment

L3911 Wrist hand finger orthosis, elastic, prefabricated, includes fitting and adjustment (e.g. neoprene, Lycra)

L3912 Hand-finger-orthosis, flexion glove with elastic finger control, prefabricated, includes fitting and adjustment

●**L3913** Hand finger orthosis, without joints, may include soft interface, straps, custom fabricated, includes fitting and adjustment

L3914 Wrist-hand-orthosis (WHO), wrist extension cock-up, prefabricated, includes fitting and adjustment

L3916 Wrist-hand-finger-orthosis, wrist extension cock-up with outrigger, prefabricated, includes fitting and adjustment

L3917 Hand orthosis, metacarpal fracture orthosis, prefabricated, includes fitting and adjustment

L3918 Hand-finger-orthosis (HFO); knuckle bender, prefabricated, inlcudes fitting and adjustment

●**L3919** Hand orthosis, without joints, may include soft interface, straps, custom fabricated, includes fitting and adjustment

L3920 knuckle bender with outrigger, prefabricated, includes fitting and adjustment

●**L3921** Hand finger orthosis, includes one or more nontorsion joints, elastic bands, turnbuckles, may include soft interface, straps, custom fabricated, includes fitting and adjustment

L3922 knuckle bender, two segment to flex joints, prefabricated, includes fitting and adjustment

▲**L3923** Hand finger orthosis, without joints, may include soft interface, straps, prefabricated, includes fitting and adjustment

L3924 Wrist-hand-finger orthosis (WHFO); Oppenheimer, prefabricated, includes fitting and adjustment

L3926 Thomas suspension, prefabricated, includes fitting and adjustment

---

L3928 Hand-finger orthosis (HFO), finger extension, with clock spring, prefabricated, includes fitting and adjustment

L3930 Wrist-hand-finger orthosis, finger extension, with wrist support, prefabricated, includes fitting and adjustment

L3932 Finger orthosis (FO); safety pin, spring wire, prefabricated, includes fitting and adjustment

● **L3933** without joints, may include soft interface, custom fabricated, includes fitting and adjustment

L3934 safety pin, modified, prefabricated, includes fitting and adjustment

● **L3935** nontorsion joint, may include soft interface, custom fabricated, includes fitting and adjustment

L3936 Wrist-hand-finger orthosis (WHFO); Palmer, prefabricated, includes fitting and adjustment

L3938 dorsal wrist, prefabricated, includes fitting and adjustment

L3940 dorsal wrist, with outrigger attachment, prefabricated, includes fitting and adjustment

L3942 Hand-finger orthosis (HFO); reverse knuckle bender, prefabricated, includes fitting and adjustment

L3944 reverse knuckle bender, with outrigger, prefabricated, includes fitting and adjustment

L3946 composite elastic, prefabricated, includes fitting and adjustment

L3948 Finger orthosis (FO), finger knuckle bender, prefabricated, includes fitting and adjustment

L3950 Wrist-hand-finger orthosis (WHFO); combination Oppenheimer, with knuckle bender and two attachments, prefabricated, includes fitting and adjustment

L3952 combination Oppenheimer, with reverse knuckle and two attachments, prefabricated, includes fitting and adjustment

L3954   Hand-finger orthosis (HFO), spreading hand, prefabricated, includes fitting and adjustment

L3956   Addition of joint to upper extremity orthosis, any material; per joint

UPPER LIMB - SHOULDER-ELBOW-WRIST-HAND

ABDUCTION POSITIONING - CUSTOM FITTED

L3960   Shoulder-elbow-wrist-hand orthoses, (SEWHO); abduction positioning, airplane design, prefabricated, includes fitting and adjustment

● **L3961**   shoulder cap design, without joints, may include soft interface, straps, custom fabricated, includes fitting and adjustment

L3962   abduction positioning, Erbs palsey design, prefabricated, includes fitting and adjustment

(L3963)   Code deleted December 31, 2005

L3964   Shoulder-elbow orthosis (SEO), mobile arm support attached to wheelchair, balanced; adjustable, prefabricated, includes fitting and adjustment

L3965   adjustable rancho type, prefabricated, includes fitting and adjustment

L3966   reclining, prefabricated, includes fitting and adjustment

● **L3967**   Shoulder elbow wrist hand orthosis, abduction positioning (airplane design), thoracic component and support bar, without joints, may include soft interface, straps, custom fabricated, includes fitting and adjustment

L3968   friction arm support (friction dampening to proximal and distal joints), prefabricated, includes fitting and adjustment

L3969   Shoulder-elbow orthosis (SEO), mobile arm support, monosuspension arm and hand support, overhead elbow forearm hand sling support, yoke type suspension support, prefabricated, includes fitting and adjustment

ADDITIONS TO MOBILE ARM SUPPORTS

L3970 Shoulder-elbow orthosis (SEO), addition to mobile arm support; elevating proximal arm

● **L3971** Shoulder elbow wrist hand orthosis, shoulder cap design, includes one or more nontorsion joints, elastic bands, turnbuckles, may include soft interface, straps, custom fabricated, includes fitting and adjustment

L3972 offset or lateral rocker arm with elastic balance control

● **L3973** abduction positioning (airplane design), thoracic component and support bar, includes one or more nontorsion joints, elastic bands, turnbuckles, may include soft interface, straps, custom fabricated, includes fitting and adjustment

L3974 supinator

● **L3975** without joints, may include soft interface, straps, custom fabricated, includes fitting and adjustment

● **L3976** abduction positioning (airplane design), thoracic component and support bar, without joints, may include soft interface, straps, custom fabricated, includes fitting and adjustment

● **L3977** shoulder cap design, includes one or more nontorsion joints, elastic bands, turnbuckles, may include soft interface, straps, custom fabricated, includes fitting and adjustment

● **L3978** abduction positioning (airplane design), thoracic component and support bar, includes one or more nontorsion joints, elastic bands, turnbuckles, may include soft interface, straps, custom fabricated, includes fitting and adjustment

UPPER LIMB - FRACTURE ORTHOSES

L3980 Upper extremity fracture orthosis; humeral, prefabricated, includes fitting and adjustment

L3982 radius/ulnar, prefabricated, includes fitting and adjustment

L3984   wrist, prefabricated, includes fitting and adjustment

L3985   forearm, hand with wrist hinge, custom fabricated

L3986   combination of humeral, radius/ulnar, wrist, (example - Colles' fracture), custom fabricated

L3995   Addition to upper extremity orthosis, sock, fracture or equal, each

L3999   Upper limb orthosis, not otherwise specified

SPECIFIC REPAIR

L4000   Replace girdle for spinal orthosis (CTLSO or SO)

L4002   Replacement strap, any orthosis, includes all components, any length, any type

L4010   Replace trilateral socket brim

L4020   Replace quadrilateral socket brim; molded to patient model

L4030   custom fitted

L4040   Replace molded thigh lacer, for custom fabricated orthosis only

L4045   Replace non-molded thigh lacer, for custom fabricated orthosis only

L4050   Replace molded calf lacer, for custom fabricated orthosis only

L4055   Replace non-molded calf lacer, for custom fabricated orthosis only

L4060   Replace high roll cuff

L4070   Replace proximal and distal upright for KAFO

L4080   Replace metal bands KAFO, proximal thigh

L4090   Replace metal bands KAFO-AFO, calf or distal thigh

L4100   Replace leather cuff KAFO, proximal thigh

L4110   Replace leather cuff KAFO-AFO, calf or distal thigh

L4130   Replace pretibial shell

REPAIRS

L4205   Repair of orthotic device; labor component, per 15 minutes
MCM: 2100.4

L4210   repair or replace minor parts
MCM: 2133, 2100.4, 2130D

ANCILLARY ORTHOTIC SERVICES

L4350   Ankle control orthosis, stirrup style, rigid, includes any type interface (eg., pneumatic gel), prefabricated, includes fitting and adjustment

L4360   Walking boot, pneumatic, with or without joints, with or without interface material, prefabricated, includes fitting and adjustment

L4370   Pneumatic full leg splint, prefabricated, includes fitting and adjustment

L4380   Pneumatic knee splint, prefabricated, includes fitting and adjustment

L4386   Walking boot, non-pneumatic, with or without joints, with or without interface material, prefabricated, includes fitting and adjustment

L4392   Replacement, soft interface material; static AFO

L4394   foot drop splint

L4396   Static ankle foot orthosis, including soft interface material, adjustable for fit, for positioning, pressure reduction, may be used for minimal ambulation, prefabricated, includes fitting and adjustment

L4398   Foot drop splint, recumbent positioning device, prefabricated, includes fitting and adjustment

---

PROSTHETIC PROCEDURES

Guidelines

In addition to the information presented in the INTRODUCTION, several other items unique to this section are defined or identified here:

1. PROSTHETIC DEVICES: Prosthetic devices (other than dental) which replace all or part of an internal body organ (including contiguous tissue), or replace all or part of the function of a permanently inoperative or malfunctioning internal body organ, are covered when furnished upon a physician's order. This does not require a determination that there is no possibility that the patient's condition may improve in the future. If the medical record and the judgement of the attending physician indicate that the condition is of long and indefinite duration, the test of permanence is met. The device(s) may also be covered as a supply item when furnished incident to a physician's service.

2. SUBSECTION INFORMATION: Some of the listed subheadings or subsections have special needs or instructions unique to that section. Where these are indicated, special "notes" will be presented preceding or following the listings. Those subsections within the PROSTHETIC PROCEDURES section that have "notes" are as follows:

Subsection	Code Numbers
Prosthetic procedures-lower limb	L5000-L5999
Upper limb	L6000-L6590
Additions-upper limb	L6600-L6999

3. UNLISTED SERVICE OR PROCEDURE: A service or procedure may be provided that is not listed in this edition of HCPCS. When reporting such a service, the appropriate "unlisted procedure" code may be used to indicate the service, identifying it by "special report" as defined below. HCPCS terminology is inconsistent in defining unlisted procedures. The procedure definition may include the term(s) "unlisted", "not otherwise classified", "unspecified", "unclassified", "other" and "miscellaneous". Prior to using these codes, try to determine if a Local Level III code or CPT code is available. The "unlisted procedures" and accompanying codes for PROSTHETIC PROCEDURES are as follows:

L5999	Lower extremity prosthesis, not otherwise specified
L7499	Upper extremity prosthesis, not otherwise specified
L8039	Breast prosthesis, not otherwise specified
L8239	Gradient compression stocking, not otherwise specified
L8499	Unlisted procedure for miscellaneous prosthetic services
L8699	Prosthetic implant, not otherwise specified

4. SPECIAL REPORT: A service, material or supply that is rarely provided, unusual, variable or new may require a special report in determining medical appropriateness for reimbursement purposes. Pertinent information should include an adequate definition or description of the nature, extent, and need for the service, material or supply.

5. MODIFIERS: Listed services may be modified under certain circumstances. When appropriate, the modifying circumstance is identified by adding a modifier to the basic procedure code. CPT and HCPCS National Level II modifiers may be used with CPT and HCPCS National Level II procedure codes. Modifiers commonly used with PROSTHETIC PROCEDURES are as follows:

-CC   Procedure code change (use "CC" when the procedure code submitted was changed either for administrative reasons or because an incorrect code was filed)

-LT   Left side (used to identify procedures performed on the left side of the body)

(-QB)   Code deleted December 31, 2005

(-QU)   Code deleted December 31, 2005

-RT   Right side (used to identify procedures performed on the right side of the body)

-TC   Technical component. Under certain circumstances, a charge may be made for the technical component alone. Under those circumstances, the technical component charge is identified by adding modifier -TC to the usual procedure number. Technical component charges are institutional charges and are not billed separately by physicians. However, portable x-ray suppliers bill only for the technical component and should use modifier -TC. The charge data from portable x-ray suppliers will then be used to build customary and prevailing profiles.

6. CPT CODE CROSS-REFERENCE: Unless otherwise specified, the equivalent CPT code for all listings in this section is 99070.

7. DURABLE MEDICAL EQUIPMENT REGIONAL CARRIERS (DMERCS): Effective October 1, 1993 claims for prosthetics must be billed to one of four regional carriers depending upon the residence of the beneficiary. The transition dates for DMERC claims is from November 1, 1993 to March 1, 1994, depending upon the state you practice in. See the Introduction for a complete discussion of DMERCs.

Prosthetic Procedures

LOWER LIMB

NOTE: The procedures in this section are considered as "base" or "basic" procedures, and they may be modified by listing items, procedures or special materials from the "additions" section, and adding them to the base procedure.

LOWER LIMB-PARTIAL FOOT

L5000   Partial foot; shoe insert with longitudinal arch, toe filler
MCM: 2323

L5010   molded socket, ankle height, with toe filler
MCM: 2323

L5020   molded socket, tibial tubercle height, with toe filler
MCM: 2323

LOWER LIMB-ANKLE

L5050   Ankle, symes; molded socket, SACH foot

L5060   metal frame, molded leather socket, articulated ankle/ foot

LOWER LIMB-BELOW KNEE

L5100   Below knee; molded socket, shin, SACH foot

L5105   plastic socket, joints and thigh lacer, SACH foot

LOWER LIMB-KNEE DISARTICULATION

L5150   Knee disarticulation (or through knee), molded socket; external knee joints, shin, SACH foot

L5160   bent knee configuration, external knee joints, shin, SACH foot

LOWER LIMB-ABOVE KNEE

L5200   Above knee; molded socket, single axis constant friction knee, shin, SACH foot

L5210   short prosthesis, no knee joint ("stubbies"), with foot blocks, no ankle joints, each

L5220   short prosthesis, no knee joint ("stubbies"), with articulated ankle/foot, dynamically aligned, each

L5230   for proximal femoral focal deficiency, constant friction knee, shin, each foot

LOWER LIMB-HIP DISARTICULATION

L5250   Hip disarticulation; Canadian type, molded socket, hip joint, single axis constant friction knee, shin, SACH foot

L5270   tilt table type; molded socket, locking hip joint, single axis constant friction knee, shin, SACH foot

LOWER LIMB-HEMIPELVECTOMY

L5280   Hemipelvectomy, canadian type; molded socket, hip joint, single axis constant friction knee, shin, SACH foot

LOWER LIMB-ENDOSKELETAL-BELOW KNEE

L5301   Below knee, molded socket, shin, each foot, endoskeletal system

LOWER LIMB-ENDOSKELETAL-KNEE DISARTICULATION

L5311   Knee disarticulation (or through knee), molded socket, external knee joints, shin, sach foot, endoskeletal system

LOWER LIMB-ENDOSKELETAL-ABOVE KNEE

L5321   Above knee, molded socket, open end, sach foot, endoskeletal system, single axis knee

LOWER LIMB-ENDOSKELETAL-HIP DISARTICULATION

L5331   Hip disarticulation, Canadian type, molded socket, endoskeletal system, hip joint, single axis knee, sach foot

LOWER LIMB-ENDOSKELETAL-HEMIPELVECTOMY

L5341   Hemipelvectomy, Canadian type, molded socket, endoskeletal system, hip joint, single axis knee, sach foot

IMMEDIATE-EARLY-INITIAL-PREPARATORY PROCEDURES

IMMEDIATE POST SURGICAL OR EARLY FITTING PROCEDURES

L5400   Immediate post surgical or early fitting; application of initial rigid dressing, including fitting, alignment, suspension, and one cast change, below knee

L5410   application of initial rigid dressing, including fitting, alignment and suspension, below knee, each additional cast change and realignment

L5420   application of initial rigid dressing, including fitting, alignment and suspension and one cast change "AK" or knee disarticulation

L5430   application of initial rigid dressing, including fitting, alignment and suspension, "AK" or knee disarticulation, each additional cast change and realignment

L5450   application of non-weight bearing rigid dressing, below knee

L5460   application of non-weight bearing rigid dressing, above knee

▬ Not valid   ▬ Non-covered   Special   ▬ Carrier   **281**
for Medicare   by Medicare   coverage   discretion
                                   instructions

INITIAL PROSTHESIS

L5500 Initial, below knee "PTB" type socket, non-alignable system, pylon, no cover, SACH foot, plaster socket, direct formed

L5505 Initial, above knee - knee disarticulation, ischial level socket non-alignable system, pylon, no cover, SACH foot plaster socket, direct formed

PREPARATORY PROSTHESIS

L5510 Preparatory, below knee "PTB" type socket, non-alignable system, pylon, no cover, SACH foot; plaster socket, molded to model

L5520 thermoplastic or equal, direct formed

L5530 thermoplastic or equal, molded to model

L5535 Preparatory, below knee "PTB" type socket, non-alignable system, no cover, SACH foot, prefabricated, adjustable open end socket

L5540 Preparatory, below knee "PTB" type socket, non-alignable system, pylon, no cover, SACH foot, laminated socket, molded to model

L5560 Preparatory, above knee - knee disarticulation, ischial level socket, non-alignable system, pylon, no cover, SACH foot; plaster socket, molded to model

L5570 thermoplastic or equal, direct formed

L5580 thermoplastic or equal, molded to model

L5585 prefabricated adjustable open end socket

L5590 laminated socket, molded to model

L5595 Preparatory, hip disarticulation-hemipelvectomy, pylon, no cover, SACH foot; thermoplastic or equal, molded to patient model

L5600 laminated socket, molded to patient model

ADDITIONS TO LOWER EXTREMITY

L5610   Addition to lower extremity, endoskeletal system; above knee, hydracadence system

L5611   above knee - knee disarticulation, 4-bar linkage, with friction swing phase control

L5613   above knee-knee disarticulation, 4-bar linkage, with hydraulic swing phase control

L5614   above knee-knee disarticulation, 4-bar linkage, with pneumatic swing phase control

L5616   above knee, universal multiplex system, friction swing phase control

L5617   Addition to lower extremity, quick change self-aligning unit, above knee or below knee, each

ADDITIONS - TEST SOCKETS

L5618   Addition to lower extremity, test socket; Symes

L5620   below knee

L5622   knee disarticulation

L5624   above knee

L5626   hip disarticulation

L5628   hemipelvectomy

L5629   Addition to lower extremity, below knee, acrylic socket

ADDITIONS - SOCKET VARIATIONS

L5630   Addition to lower extremity, Symes type, expandable wall socket

L5631   Addition to lower extremity, above knee or knee disarticulation, acrylic socket

L5632   Addition to lower extremity, Symes type; "PTB" brim design socket

L5634　　posterior opening (Canadian) socket

L5636　　medial opening socket

L5637　Addition to lower extremity, below knee; total contact

L5638　　leather socket

L5639　　wood socket

L5640　Addition to lower extremity, knee disarticulation, leather socket

L5642　Addition to lower extremity, above knee, leather socket

L5643　Addition to lower extremity, hip disarticulation, flexible inner socket, external frame

L5644　Addition to lower extremity, above knee, wood socket

L5645　Addition to lower extremity, below knee; flexible inner socket, external frame

L5646　　air, fluid, gel or equal, cushion socket

L5647　　suction socket

L5648　Addition to lower extremity, above knee, air, fluid, gel or equal, cushion socket

L5649　Addition to lower extremity, ischial containment/narrow M-L socket

L5650　Addition to lower extremity, total contact, above knee or knee disarticulation socket

L5651　Addition to lower extremity, above knee, flexible inner socket, external frame

L5652　Addition to lower extremity, suction suspension, above knee or knee disarticulation socket

L5653　Addition to lower extremity, knee disarticulation, expandable wall socket

ADDITIONS - SOCKET INSERT AND SUSPENSION

L5654   Addition to lower extremity, socket insert; Symes, (Kemblo, Pelite, Aliplast, Plastazote or equal)

L5655   below knee (Kemblo, Pelite, Aliplast, Plastazote or equal)

L5656   knee disarticulation, (Kemblo, Pelite, Aliplast, Plastazote or equal)

L5658   above knee (Kemblo, Pelite, Aliplast, Plastazote or equal)

L5661   multi-durometer Symes

L5665   multi-durometer, below knee

L5666   Addition to lower extremity; below knee, cuff suspension

L5668   Addition to lower extremity; below knee, molded distal cushion

L5670   Addition to lower extremity; below knee, molded supracondylar suspension ("PTS" or similar)

L5671   Addition to lower extremity; below knee/above knee suspension locking mechanism (shuttle, lanyard or equal), excludes socket insert

L5672   below knee, removable medial brim suspension

L5673   below knee/above knee, custom fabricated from existing mold or prefabricated, socket insert, silicone gel, elastomeric or equal, for use with locking mechanism

(L5674)   Code deleted December 31, 2004; use L5685

(L5675)   Code deleted December 31, 2004; use L5685

L5676   below knee, knee joints, single axis, pair

L5677   below knee, knee joints, polycentric, pair

L5678   below knee, joint covers, pair

Not valid for Medicare   Non-covered by Medicare   Special coverage instructions   Carrier discretion   **285**

L5679   below knee/above knee, custom fabricated from existing mold or prefabricated, socket insert, silicone gel, elastomeric or equal, not for use with locking mechanism

L5680   below knee, thigh lacer, non-molded

L5681   below knee/above knee, custom fabricated socket insert for congenital or atypical traumatic amputee, silicone gel, elastomeric or equal, for use with or without locking mechanism, initial only (for other than initial, use code L5673 or L5679)

L5682   below knee, thigh lacer, gluteal/ischial, molded

L5683   below knee/above knee, custom fabricated socket insert for other than congenital or atypical traumatic amputee, silicone gel elastomeric or equal, for use with or without locking mechanism, initial only (for other than initial, use code L5673 or L5679)

L5684   below knee, fork strap

L5685   Addition to lower extremity prosthesis, below knee, suspension/sealing sleeve, with or without valve, any material, each

L5686   below knee, back check (extension control)

L5688   below knee, waist belt, webbing

L5690   below knee, waist belt, padded and lined

L5692   Addition to lower extremity, above knee; pelvic control belt, light

L5694   pelvic control belt, padded and lined

L5695   pelvic control, sleeve suspension, neoprene or equal, each

L5696   Addition to lower extremity, above knee or knee disarticulation; pelvic joint

L5697   pelvic band

---

286   ● New code   ▲ Revised code   ( ) Deleted code

L5698   silesian bandage

L5699   All lower extremity protheses, shoulder harness

L5700   Replacement, socket; below knee, molded to patient model

L5701   above knee/knee disarticulation, including attachment plate, molded to patient model

L5702   hip disarticulation, including hip joint, molded to patient model

● **L5703**   Ankle, symes, molded to patient model, socket without solid ankle cushion heel (Sach) foot, replacement only

L5704   Custom shaped protective cover, below knee

L5705   Custom shaped protective cover, above knee

L5706   Custom shaped protective cover, knee disarticulation

L5707   Custom shaped protective cover, hip disarticulation

ADDITIONS - KNEE-SHIN SYSTEM

EXOSKELETAL

L5710   Addition, exoskeletal knee-shin system, single axis; manual lock

L5711   manual lock, ultra-light material

L5712   friction swing and stance phase control (safety knee)

L5714   variable friction swing phase control

L5716   Addition, exoskeletal knee-shin system, polycentric; mechanical stance phase lock

L5718   friction swing and stance phase control

L5722   Addition, exoskeletal knee-shin system, single axis; pneumatic swing, friction stance phase control

L5724   fluid swing phase control

L5726   external joints fluid swing phase control

L5728   fluid swing and stance phase control

L5780   pneumatic/hydrapneumatic swing phase control

L5781   Addition to lower limb prosthesis, vacuum pump, residual limb volume management and moisture evacuation system

L5782   Addition to lower limb prosthesis, vacuum pump, residual limb volume management and moisture evacuation system, heavy duty

L5785   Addition, exoskeletal system, below knee, ultra-light material (titanium, carbon fiber or equal)

L5790   Addition, exoskeletal system, above knee, ultra-light material (titanium, carbon fiber or equal)

L5795   Addition, exoskeletal system, hip disarticulation, ultra-light material (titanium, carbon fiber or equal)

ENDOSKELETAL

L5810   Addition, endoskeletal knee-shin system, single axis; manual lock

L5811   manual lock, ultra-light material

L5812   friction swing and stance phase control (safety knee)

L5814   Addition, endoskeletal knee-shin system, polycentric; hydraulic swing phase control, mechanical stance phase lock

L5816   mechanical stance phase lock

L5818   friction swing and stance phase control

L5822   Addition, endoskeletal knee-shin system, single axis; pneumatic swing, friction stance phase control

L5824   fluid swing phase control

L5826   hydraulic swing phase control, with miniature high activity frame

L5828   fluid swing and stance phase control

L5830   pneumatic swing phase control

L5840   Addition, endoskeletal knee-shin system, 4-bar linkage or multiaxial, pneumatic swing phase control

L5845   Addition, endoskeletal, knee-shin system; stance flexion feature, adjustable

(L5846) Code deleted December 31, 2004; use CPT

(L5847) Code deleted December 31, 2004; use CPT

L5848   Addition to endoskeletal, knee-shin system, hydraulic stance extension, dampening feature, with or without adjustability

L5850   Addition, endoskeletal system; above knee or hip disarticulation, knee extension assist

L5855   hip disarticulation, mechanical hip extension assist

L5856   Addition to lower extremity prosthesis, endoskeletal knee-shin system, microprocessor control feature, swing and stance phase, includes electronic sensor(s), any type

L5857   Addition to lower extremity prosthesis, endoskeletal knee-shin system, microprocessor control feature, swing phase only, includes electronic sensor(s), any type

● **L5858**   Addition to lower extremity prosthesis, endoskeletal knee shin system, microprocessor control feature, stance phase only, includes electronic sensor(s), any type

L5910   below knee, alignable system

L5920   above knee or hip disarticulation, alignable system

L5925   above knee, knee disarticulation or hip disarticulation, manual lock

L5930   Addition, endoskeletal system; high activity knee control frame

L5940   below knee, ultra-light material (titanium, carbon fiber or equal)

L5950 above knee, ultra-light material (titanium, carbon fiber or equal)

L5960 hip disarticulation, ultra-light material (titanium, carbon fiber or equal)

L5962 below knee, flexible protective outer surface covering system

L5964 above knee, flexible protective outer surface covering system

L5966 hip disarticulation, flexible protective outer surface covering system

L5968 Addition to lower limb prosthesis, multiaxial ankle with swing phase active dorsiflexion feature

L5970 All lower extremity prostheses; foot, external keel, each foot

● **L5971** All lower extremity prosthesis, solid ankle cushion heel (sach) foot, replacement only

L5972 flexible keel foot (Safe, Sten, Bock Dynamic or equal)

L5974 foot, single axis ankle/foot

L5975 All lower extremity prosthesis; combination single axis ankle and flexible keel foot

L5976 energy storing foot (Seattle Carbon Copy II or equal)

L5978 foot, multiaxial ankle/foot

L5979 multiaxial ankle, dynamic response foot, one piece system

L5980 flex foot system

L5981 flex-walk system or equal

L5982 All exoskeletal lower extremity prostheses, axial rotation unit

L5984 All endoskeletal lower extremity prostheses, axial rotation unit, with or without adjustability

● New code ▲ Revised code ( ) Deleted code

L5985　All endoskeletal lower extremity prostheses, dynamic prosthetic pylon

L5986　All lower extremity prostheses, multi-axial rotation unit ("MCP" or equal)

L5987　All lower extremity prosthesis, shank foot system with vertical loading pylon

L5988　Addition to lower limb prosthesis, vertical shock reducing pylon feature

(L5989)　Code deleted December 31, 2004; use CPT

L5990　Addition to lower extremity prothesis, user adjustable heel height

L5995　Addition to lower extremity prosthesis, heavy duty feature (for patient weight > 300 lbs)

L5999　Lower extremity prosthesis, not otherwise specified

UPPER LIMB

NOTE:　The procedures in L6000-L6599 are considered as "base" or "basic" procedures and may be modified by listing procedures from the "additions" sections. The base procedures include only standard friction wrist and control cable system unless otherwise specified.

UPPER LIMB-PARTIAL HAND

L6000　Partial hand, Robin-aids; thumb remaining (or equal)

L6010　　little and/or ring ringer remaining (or equal)

L6020　　no finger remaining (or equal)

L6025　Transcarpal/metacarpal or partial hand disarticulation prosthesis, external power, self-suspended, inner socket with removable forearm section, electrodes and cables, two batteries, charger, myoelectric control of terminal device

UPPER LIMB-WRIST DISARTICULATION

L6050   Wrist disarticulation, molded socket, flexible elbow hinges, triceps pad

UPPER LIMB-BELOW ELBOW

L6055   Wrist disarticulation, molded socket with expandable interface, flexible elbow hinges, triceps pad

L6100   Below elbow, molded socket; flexible elbow hinge, triceps pad

L6110   (Muenster or Northwestern Suspension types)

L6120   Below elbow, molded double wall split socket; step-up hinges, half cuff

L6130   stump activated locking hinge, half cuff

UPPER LIMB-ELBOW DISARTICULATION

L6200   Elbow disarticulation, molded socket, outside locking hinge, forearm

UPPER LIMB-ABOVE ELBOW

L6205   Elbow disarticulation, molded socket with expandable interface, outside locking hinges, forearm

L6250   Above elbow, molded double wall socket, internal locking elbow, forearm

UPPER LIMB-SHOULDER DISARTICULATION

L6300   Shoulder disarticulation, molded socket, shoulder bulkhead, humeral section, internal locking elbow, forearm

L6310   Shoulder disarticulation, passive restoration; (complete prosthesis)

L6320   (shoulder cap only)

UPPER LIMB-INTERSCAPULAR THORACIC

L6350 Interscapular thoracic; molded socket, shoulder bulkhead, humeral section, internal locking elbow, forearm

L6360 passive restoration (complete prosthesis)

L6370 passive restoration (shoulder cap only)

UPPER LIMB-IMMEDIATE AND EARLY POST SURGICAL PROCEDURES

L6380 Immediate post surgical or early fitting, application of initial rigid dressing, including fitting alignment and suspension of components, and one cast change; wrist disarticulation or below elbow

L6382 elbow disarticulation or above elbow

L6384 shoulder disarticulation or interscapular thoracic

L6386 Immediate post surgical or early fitting; each additional cast change and realignment

L6388 application of rigid dressing only

UPPER LIMB-ENDOSKELETAL-BELOW ELBOW

L6400 Below elbow, molded socket endoskeletal system, including soft prosthetic tissue shaping

UPPER LIMB-ENDOSKELETAL-ELBOW DISARTICULATION

L6450 Elbow disarticulation, molded socket, endoskeletal system, including soft prosthetic tissue shaping

UPPER LIMB-ENDOSKELETAL-ABOVE ELBOW

L6500 Above elbow, molded socket, endoskeletal system, including soft prosthetic tissue shaping

UPPER LIMB-ENDOSKELETAL-SHOULDER DISARTICULATION

L6550 Shoulder disarticulation, molded socket, endoskeletal system, including soft prosthetic tissue shaping

UPPER LIMB-ENDOSKELETAL-INTERSCAPULAR THORACIC

L6570 Interscapular thoracic, molded socket, endoskeletal system, including soft prosthetic tissue shaping

L6580 Preparatory, wrist disarticulation or below elbow, single wall plastic socket, friction wrist, flexible elbow hinges, figure of eight harness, humeral cuff, Bowden cable control, USMC or equal pylon, no cover, molded to patient model

L6582 Preparatory, wrist disarticulation or below elbow, single wall socket, friction wrist, flexible elbow hinges, figure of eight harness, humeral cuff, bowden cable control, USMC or equal pylon, no cover, direct formed

L6584 Preparatory, elbow disarticulation or above elbow; single wall plastic socket, friction wrist, locking elbow, figure of eight harness, fair lead cable control, USMC or equal pylon, no cover, molded to patient model

L6586 single wall socket, friction wrist, locking elbow, figure of eight harness, fair lead cable control, USMC or equal pylon, no cover, direct formed

L6588 Preparatory shoulder disarticulation or interscapular thoracic; single wall plastic socket, shoulder joint, locking elbow, friction wrist, chest strap, fair lead cable control, USMC or equal pylon, no cover, molded to patient model

L6590 single wall socket, shoulder joint, locking elbow, friction wrist, chest strap, fair lead cable control, USMC or equal pylon, no cover, direct formed

ADDITIONS - UPPER LIMB

NOTE: The following procedures, modifications and/or components may be added to other base procedures. The items in this section should reflect the additional complexity of each modification procedure, in addition to base procedure, at the time of the original order.

L6600 Upper extremity additions; polycentric hinge, pair

L6605 single pivot hinge, pair

L6610 flexible metal hinge, pair

L6615 disconnect locking wrist unit

L6616 additional disconnect insert for locking wrist unit, each

L6620 flexion/extension wrist unit, with or without friction

● **L6621** flexion/extension wrist with or without friction, for use with external powered terminal device

L6623 spring assisted rotational wrist unit with latch release

L6625 rotation wrist unit with cable lock

L6628 quick disconnect hook adapter, Otto Bock or equal

L6629 quick disconnect lamination collar with coupling piece, Otto Bock or equal

L6630 stainless steel, any wrist

L6632 latex suspension sleeve, each

L6635 lift assist for elbow

L6637 nudge control elbow lock

L6638 Upper extremity addition to prosthesis, electric locking feature, only for use with manually powered elbow

L6640 shoulder abduction joint, pair

L6641 excursion amplifier, pulley type

| | Not valid for Medicare | | Non-covered by Medicare | Special coverage instructions | | Carrier discretion | **295** |

L6642	excursion amplifier, lever type
L6645	shoulder flexion - abduction joint, each
L6646	Upper extremity addition, shoulder joint, multipositional locking, flexion, adjustable abduction friction control, for use with body powered or external powered system
L6647	Upper extremity addition, shoulder lock mechanism, body powered actuator
L6648	Upper extremity addition; shoulder lock mechanism, external powered actuator
L6650	shoulder universal joint, each
L6655	standard control cable, extra
L6660	heavy duty control cable
L6665	teflon, or equal, cable lining
L6670	hook to hand, cable adapter
L6672	harness, chest or shoulder, saddle type
L6675	harness, (eg., figure of eight type), single cable design
L6676	harness, (eg., figure of eight type), dual cable design
●**L6677**	harness, triple control, simultaneous operation of terminal device and elbow
L6680	test socket, wrist disarticulation or below elbow
L6682	test socket, elbow disarticulation or above elbow
L6684	test socket, shoulder disarticulation or interscapular thoracic
L6686	suction socket
L6687	frame type socket, below elbow or wrist disarticulation
L6688	frame type socket, above elbow or elbow disarticulation

L6689   frame type socket, shoulder disarticulation

L6690   frame type socket, interscapular-thoracic

L6691   removable insert, each

L6692   silicone gel insert or equal, each

L6693   locking elbow, forearm counterbalance

L6694   Addition to upper extremity prosthesis, below elbow/above elbow, custom fabricated from existing mold or prefabricated, socket insert, silicone gel, elastomeric or equal, for use with locking mechanism

L6695   Addition to upper extremity prosthesis, below elbow/above elbow, custom fabricated from existing mold or prefabricated, socket insert, silicone gel, elastomeric or equal, not for use with locking mechanism

L6696   Addition to upper extremity prosthesis, below elbow/above elbow, custom fabricated socket insert for congenital or atypical traumatic amputee, silicone gel, elastomeric or equal, for use with or without locking mechanism, initial only (for other than initial, use code L6694 or L6695)

L6697   Addition to upper extremity prosthesis, below elbow/above elbow, custom fabricated socket insert for other than congenital or atypical traumatic amputee, silicone gel, elastomeric or equal, for use with or without locking mechanism, initial only (for other than initial, use code L6694 or L6695)

L6698   Addition to upper extremity prosthesis, below elbow/above elbow, lock mechanism, excludes socket insert

TERMINAL DEVICES

HOOKS

L6700   Terminal device, hook, Dorrance, or equal; model #3
MCM: 2133

L6705   model #5
MCM: 2133

L6710   model #5X
MCM: 2133

L6715   model #5XA
MCM: 2133

L6720   model #6
MCM: 2133

L6725   model #7
MCM: 2133

L6730   model #7LO
MCM: 2133

L6735   model #8
MCM: 2133

L6740   model #8X
MCM: 2133

L6745   model #88X
MCM: 2133

L6750   model #10P
MCM: 2133

L6755   model #10X
MCM: 2133

L6765   model #12P
MCM: 2133

L6770   model #99X
MCM: 2133

L6775   model #555
MCM: 2133

L6780   model #SS555
MCM: 2133

L6790   Terminal device; hook-Accu hook, or equal
MCM: 2133

L6795   hook-2 load, or equal
MCM: 2133

L6800   hook-APRL VC, or equal
MCM: 2133

L6805   modifier wrist flexion unit
MCM: 2133

L6806   Terminal device, hook; TRS grip, grip III, VC or equal
MCM: 2133

L6807   grip I, grip II, VC or equal
MCM: 2133

L6808   TRS adept, infant or child, VC or equal
MCM: 2133

L6809   TRS Super sport, passive
MCM: 2133

L6810   Terminal device; pincher tool, Otto Bock or equal
MCM: 2133

HANDS

L6825   Terminal device, hand; Dorrance, VO
MCM: 2133

L6830   Aprl, VC
MCM: 2133

L6835   Sierra, VO
MCM: 2133

L6840   Becker imperial
MCM: 2133

L6845   Becker lock grip
MCM: 2133

L6850   Becker plylite
MCM: 2133

L6855   Robin-aids, VO
MCM: 2133

L6860   Robin-aids, VO soft
MCM: 2133

L6865   passive hand
MCM: 2133

L6867   Detroit infant hand (mechanical)
MCM: 2133

Not valid   Non-covered   Special   Carrier   **299**
for Medicare   by Medicare   coverage   discretion
instructions

L6868   passive infant hand, (Steeper, Hosmer or equal)
MCM: 2133

L6870   child mitt
MCM: 2133

L6872   NYU child hand
MCM: 2133

L6873   mechanical infant hand, Steeper or equal
MCM: 2133

L6875   Bock, VC
MCM: 2133

L6880   Bock, VO
MCM: 2133

L6881 Automatic grasp feature, addition to upper limb prosthetic terminal device

L6882 Microprocessor control feature, addition to upper limb prosthetic terminal device
MCM: 2133

● **L6883** Replacement socket, below elbow/wrist disarticulation, molded to patient model, for use with or without external power

● **L6884** Replacement socket, above elbow disarticulation, molded to patient model, for use with or without external power

● **L6885** Replacement socket, shoulder disarticulation/interscapular thoracic, molded to patient model, for use with or without external power

GLOVES FOR ABOVE HANDS

L6890 Addition to upper extremity prosthesis, glove for terminal device, any material, prefabricated, includes fitting and adjustment

L6895 Addition to upper extremity prosthesis, glove for terminal device, any material, custom fabricated

HAND RESTORATION

L6900   Hand restoration (casts, shading and measurements included), partial hand; with glove, thumb or one finger remaining

L6905   with glove, multiple fingers remaining

L6910   with glove, no fingers remaining

L6915   Hand restoration (shading, and measurements included), replacement glove for above

EXTERNAL POWER - BASE DEVICES

L6920   Wrist disarticulation, external power, self-suspended inner socket, removable forearm shell, Otto Bock or equal; switch, cables, two batteries and one charger, switch control of terminal device

L6925   electrodes, cables, two batteries and one charger, myoelectronic control of terminal device

L6930   Below elbow, external power, self-suspended inner socket, removable forearm shell; Otto Bock or equal switch, cables, two batteries and one charger, switch control of terminal device

L6935   Otto Bock or equal electrodes, cables, two batteries and one charger, myoelectronic control of terminal device

L6940   Elbow disarticulation, external power, molded inner socket, removable humeral shell, outside locking hinges, forearm; Otto Bock or equal switch, cables, two batteries and one charger, switch control of terminal device

L6945   Otto Bock or equal electrodes, cables, two batteries and one charger, myoelectronic control of terminal device

L6950   Above elbow, external power, molded inner socket, removable humeral shell, internal locking elbow, forearm; Otto Bock or equal switch, cables two batteries and one charger, switch control of terminal device

L6955   Otto Bock or equal electrodes, cables, two batteries and one charger, myoelectronic control of terminal device

L6960 Shoulder disarticulation, external power, molded inner socket, removable shoulder shell, shoulder bulkhead, humeral section, mechanical elbow, forearm; Otto Bock or equal switch, cables, two batteries and one charger, switch control of terminal device

L6965 Otto Bock or equal electrodes, cables, two batteries and one charger, myoelectronic control of terminal device

L6970 Interscapular-thoracic, external power, molded inner socket removable shoulder shell, shoulder bulkhead, humeral section, mechanical elbow, forearm; Otto Bock or equal switch, cables, two batteries and one charger, switch control of terminal device

L6975 Otto Bock or equal electrodes cables, two batteries and one charger, myoelectronic control of terminal device

EXTERNAL POWER - TERMINAL DEVICES

L7010 Electronic hand; Otto Bock, Steeper or equal, switch controlled

L7015 System Teknik, Variety Village or equal, switch controlled

L7020 Electronic Greifer, Otto Bock or equal, switch controlled

L7025 Electronic hand; Otto Bock or equal, myoelectronically controlled

L7030 System Teknik, Variety Village or equal, myoelectronically controlled

L7035 Electronic Greifer, Otto Bock or equal, myoelectronically controlled

L7040 Prehensile actuator, Hosmer or equal, switch controlled

L7045 Electronic hook, child, Michigan or equal, switch controlled

EXTERNAL POWER - ELBOW

L7170 Electronic elbow; hosmer or equal, switch controlled

L7180   microprocessor sequential control of elbow and terminal device

L7181   Electronic elbow, microprocessor simultaneous control of elbow and terminal device

L7185   adolescent, Variety Village or equal, switch controlled

L7186   child, Variety Village or equal, switch controlled

L7190   adolescent, Variety Village or equal, myoelectronically controlled

L7191   child, Variety Village or equal, myoelectronically controlled

EXTERNAL POWER - CONTROL MODULES

L7260   Electronic wrist rotator; Otto Bock or equal

L7261   for Utah arm

L7266   Servo control, Steeper or equal

L7272   Analogue control, UNB or equal

L7274   Proportional control, 6-12 volt, Liberty, Utah or equal

EXTERNAL POWER - BATTERY COMPONENTS

L7360   Six volt battery, Otto Bock or equal, each

L7362   Battery charger, six volt, Otto Bock or equal

L7364   Twelve volt battery, Utah or equal, each

L7366   Battery charger, twelve volt, Utah or equal

L7367   Lithium ion battery, replacement

L7368   Lithium ion battery charger

● **L7400**   Addition to upper extremity prosthesis; below elbow/wrist disarticulation, ultralight material (titanium, carbon fiber or equal)

● **L7401**   above elbow disarticulation, ultralight material (titanium, carbon fiber or equal)

● **L7402**   shoulder disarticulation/interscapular thoracic, ultralight material (titanium, carbon fiber or equal)

● **L7403**   below elbow/wrist disarticulation, acrylic material

● **L7404**   above elbow disarticulation, acrylic material

● **L7405**   shoulder disarticulation/interscapular thoracic, acrylic material

L7499   Upper extremity prosthesis, not otherwise specified

REPAIRS

L7500   Repair of prosthetic device, hourly rate (excludes V5335 repair of oral or laryngeal prosthesis or artificial larynx)
MCM: 2100.4, 2130D, 2133

L7510   Repair of prosthetic device, repair or replace minor parts
MCM: 2100.4, 2130D, 2133

L7520   Repair prosthetic device, labor component, per 15 minutes

● **L7600**   Prosthetic donning sleeve, any material, each

L7900   Male vacuum erection system

GENERAL - BREAST PROSTHESES

L8000   Breast prosthesis; mastectomy bra
MCM: 2130.A

L8001   Breast prosthesis, mastectomy bra, with integrated breast prosthesis form, unilateral
MCM: 2130.A

L8002   Breast prosthesis, mastectomy bra, with integrated breast prosthesis form, bilateral
MCM: 2130.A

L8010   mastectomy sleeve
MCM: 2130.A

L8015 External breast prosthesis garment, with mastectomy form, post mastectomy
MCM: 2130

L8020 Breast prosthesis; mastectomy form
MCM: 2130.A

L8030 silicone or equal
MCM: 2130.A

L8035 Custom breast prosthesis, post mastectomy, molded to patient model
MCM: 2130

L8039 Breast prosthesis, not otherwise specified

L8040 Nasal prosthesis, provided by a non-physician

L8041 Midfacial prosthesis, provided by a non-physician

L8042 Orbital prosthesis, provided by a non-physician

L8043 Upper facial prosthesis, provided by a non-physician

L8044 Hemi-facial prosthesis, provided by a non-physician

L8045 Auricular prosthesis, provided by a non-physician

L8046 Partial facial prosthesis, provided by a non-physician

L8047 Nasal septal prosthesis, provided by a non-physician

L8048 Unspecified maxillofacial prosthesis, by report, provided by a non-physician

L8049 Repair or modification of maxillofacial prosthesis, labor component, 15 minute increments, provided by a non-physician

GENERAL - ELASTIC SUPPORTS

(L8100) Code deleted December 31, 2005; use A6530

(L8110) Code deleted December 31, 2005; use A6531

(L8120) Code deleted December 31, 2005; use A6532

(L8130) Code deleted December 31, 2005; use A6533
CIM: 60-9 MCM: 2133

(L8140) Code deleted December 31, 2005; use A6534

(L8150) Code deleted December 31, 2005; use A6535

(L8160) Code deleted December 31, 2005; use A6536

(L8170) Code deleted December 31, 2005; use A6537

(L8180) Code deleted December 31, 2005; use A6538

(L8190) Code deleted December 31, 2005; use A6539

(L8195) Code deleted December 31, 2005; use A6540

(L8200) Code deleted December 31, 2005; use A6541

(L8210) Code deleted December 31, 2005; use A6542

(L8220) Code deleted December 31, 2005; use A6543

(L8230) Code deleted December 31, 2005; use A6544

(L8239) Code deleted December 31, 2005; use A6549

GENERAL - TRUSSES

L8300 Truss; single with standard pad
CIM: 70-1, 70-2 MCM: 2133

L8310 double with standard pads
CIM: 70-1, 70-2 MCM: 2133

L8320 addition to standard pad, water pad
CIM: 70-1, 70-2 MCM: 2133

L8330 addition to standard pad, scrotal pad
CIM: 70-1, 70-2 MCM: 2133

PROSTHETIC SOCKS

L8400 Prosthetic sheath; below knee, each
MCM: 2133

L8410 above knee, each
MCM: 2133

L8415   upper limb, each
MCM: 2133

L8417   Prosthetic sheath/sock, including a gel cushion layer, below knee or above knee, each

L8420   Prosthetic sock, multiple ply; below knee, each
MCM: 2133

L8430   above knee, each
MCM: 2133

L8435   upper limb, each
MCM: 2133

L8440   Prosthetic shrinker; below knee, each
MCM: 2133

L8460   above knee, each
MCM: 2133

L8465   upper limb, each
MCM: 2133

L8470   Prosthetic sock, single ply, fitting; below knee, each
MCM: 2133

L8480   above knee, each
MCM: 2133

L8485   upper limb, each
MCM: 2133

(L8490) Code deleted December 31, 2004; use CPT

L8499   Unlisted procedure for miscellaneous prosthetic services

PROSTHETIC IMPLANTS

L8500   Artificial larynx, any type
CIM: 65-5 MCM: 2130

L8501   Tracheostomy speaking valve
CIM: 65-16

L8505   Artificial larynx replacement battery/accessory, any type

L8507   Tracheo-esophageal voice prosthesis, patient inserted, any type, each

L8509 Tracheo-esophageal voice prosthesis, inserted by a licensed health care provider, any type

L8510 Voice amplifier
CIM: 65-5

L8511 Insert for indwelling tracheoesophageal prosthesis, with or without valve, replacement only, each

L8512 Gelatin capsules or equivalent, for use with tracheo-esophageal voice prosthesis, replacement only, per 10

L8513 Cleaning device used with tracheoesophageal voice prosthesis, pipet, brush, or equal, replacement only, each

L8514 Tracheoesophageal puncture dilator, replacement only, each

L8515 Gelatin capsule, application device for use with tracheoesophageal voice prosthesis, each

INTEGUMENTARY SYSTEM

L8600 Implantable breast prosthesis, silicone or equal
CIM: 35-47   MCM: 2130

L8603 Injectable bulking agent, collagen implant, urinary tract, 2.5 ml syringe, includes shipping and necessary supplies
CIM: 65.9

L8606 Injectable bulking agent, synthetic implant, urinary tract, 1 ml syringe, includes shipping and necessary supplies
CIM: 65.9

HEAD (SKULL, FACIAL BONES, AND TEMPOROMANDIBULAR JOINT)

● L8609 Artificial cornea

L8610 Ocular implant
MCM: 2130

L8612 Aqueous shunt
MCM: 2130

L8613 Ossicula implant
MCM: 2130

L8614   Cochlear device/system
CIM: 65-14   MCM: 2130

L8615   Headset/headpiece for use with cochlear implant device, replacement
CIM: 65-14

L8616   Microphone for use with cochlear implant device, replacement
CIM: 65-14

L8617   Transmitting coil for use with cochlear implant device, replacement
CIM: 65-14

L8618   Transmitter cable for use with cochlear implant device, replacement
CIM: 65-14

L8619   Cochlear implant external speech processor, replacement
CIM: 65-14

(L8620)   Code deleted December 31, 2005

L8621   Zinc air battery for use with cochlear implant device, replacement, each

L8622   Alkaline battery for use with cochlear implant device, any size, replacement, each

●**L8623**   Lithium ion battery for use with cochlear implant device speech processor; other than ear level, replacement, each

●**L8624**   ear level, replacement, each

UPPER EXTREMITY

L8630   Metacarpophalangeal joint implant
MCM: 2130

L8631   Metacarpal phalangeal joint replacement, two or more pieces, metal (eg., stainless steel or cobalt chrome), ceramic-like material (eg., pyrocarbon), for surgical implantation (all sizes, includes entire system)
MCM: 2130

LOWER EXTREMITY (JOINT: KNEE, ANKLE, TOE)

L8641   Metatarsal joint implant
MCM: 2130

L8642   Hallux implant
MCM: 2130

MISCELLANEOUS MUSCULAR - SKELETAL

L8658   Interphalangeal joint spacer, silicone or equal, each
MCM: 2130

L8659   Interphalangeal finger joint replacement, 2 or more pieces, metal (eg., stainless steel or cobalt chrome), ceramic-like material (eg., pyrocarbon) for surgical implantation, any size
MCM: 2130

CARDIOVASCULAR SYSTEM

L8670   Vascular graft material, synthetic, implant
MCM: 2130

● **L8680**   Implantable neurostimulator electrode, each
CIM: 65-8

● **L8681**   Patient programmer (external) for use with implantable programmable neurostimulator pulse generator
CIM: 65-8

● **L8682**   Implantable neurostimulator radiofrequency receiver
CIM: 65-8

● **L8683**   Radiofrequency transmitter (external) for use with implantable neurostimulator radiofrequency receiver
CIM: 65-8

● **L8684**   Radiofrequency transmitter (external) for use with implantable sacral root neurostimulator receiver for bowel and bladder management, replacement
CIM: 65-8

● **L8685**   Implantable neurostimulator pulse generator, single array, rechargeable, includes extension
CIM: 65-8

● **L8686**   Implantable neurostimulator pulse generator, single array, non-rechargeable, includes extension
CIM: 65-8

● **L8687**   Implantable neurostimulator pulse generator, dual array, rechargeable, includes extension
CIM: 65-8

● **L8688**   Implantable neurostimulator pulse generator, dual array, non-rechargeable, includes extension
CIM: 65-8

● **L8689**   External recharging system for implanted neurostimulator, replacement only

OTHER

L8699   Prosthetic implant, not otherwise specified

L9900   Orthotic and prosthetic supply, accessory, and/or service component of another HCPCS "L" code

● New code ▲ Revised code ( ) Deleted code

MEDICAL SERVICES

Guidelines

In addition to the information presented in the INTRODUCTION, several other items unique to this section are defined or identified here:

1. SUBSECTION INFORMATION: Some of the listed subheadings or subsections have special needs or instructions unique to that section. Where these are indicated, special "notes" will be presented preceding or following the listings. Those subsections within the MEDICAL SERVICES section that have "notes" are as follows:

Subsection	Code Numbers
Office services	M0000-M0009
End-stage renal disease services	M0900-M0999

2. SPECIAL REPORT: A service, material or supply that is rarely provided, unusual, variable or new may require a special report in determining medical appropriateness for reimbursement purposes. Pertinent information should include an adequate definition or description of the nature, extent, and need for the service, material or supply.

3. MODIFIERS: Listed services may be modified under certain circumstances. When appropriate, the modifying circumstance is identified by adding a modifier to the basic procedure code. CPT and HCPCS National Level II modifiers may be used with CPT and HCPCS National Level II procedure codes. Modifiers commonly used with MEDICAL SERVICES are as follows:

   -AH   Clinical psychologist

   -AJ   Clinical social worker

   -CC   Procedure code change (use "CC" when the procedure code submitted was changed either for administrative reasons or because an incorrect code was filed)

   -EJ   Subsequent claims for a defined course of therapy (eg., EPO, sodium hyaluronate, infliximab)

   -EM   Emergency reserve supply (for ESRD benefit only)

█████ Not valid   █████ Non-covered   Special   █████ Carrier   **313**
for Medicare   by Medicare   coverage   discretion
                                                instructions

-EP   Service provided as part of Medicaid early periodic screening diagnosis and treatment (EPSDT) program

-FP   Service provided as part of Medicaid family planning program

-Q5   Service furnished by a substitute physician under a reciprocal billing arrangement

-Q6   Service furnished by a locum tenens physician

(-QB)   Code deleted December 31, 2005

-QC   Single channel monitoring

-QD   Recording and storage in solid state memory by a digital recorder

-QT   Recording and storage on tape by an analog tape recorder

(-QU)   Code deleted December 31, 2005

-SF   Second opinion ordered by a professional review organization (PRO) per section 9401, P.L. 99-272 (100 percent reimbursement; no Medicare deductible or coinsurance)

-TC   Technical component. Under certain circumstances, a charge may be made for the technical component alone. Under those circumstances, the technical component charge is identified by adding modifier -TC to the usual procedure number. Technical component charges are institutional charges and are not billed separately by physicians. However, portable x-ray suppliers bill only for the technical component and should use modifier -TC. The charge data from portable x-ray suppliers will then be used to build customary and prevailing profiles.

4. CPT CODE CROSS-REFERENCE: See sections for equivalent CPT code(s) for listings in this section.

Medical Services

ASC SERVICES

M0064 Brief office visit for the sole purpose of monitoring or changing drug prescriptions used in the treatment of mental psychoneurotic and personality disorders
MCM: 2476.3

OTHER MEDICAL SERVICES

M0075 Cellular therapy
CIM: 35-5

M0076 Prolotherapy
CIM: 35-13

M0100 Intragastric hypothermia using gastric freezing
CIM: 35-65

CARDIOVASCULAR SERVICES

M0300 IV chelation therapy (chemical endarterectomy)
CIM: 35-64

M0301 Fabric wrapping of abdominal aneurysm
CIM: 35-34

PHYSICAL MEDICINE SERVICES

OSTEOPATHIC MANIPULATION THERAPY (OMT)

NOTE: All OMT codes have been deleted; use CPT.

ESRD SERVICES

NOTE: For DME items for ESRD, see procedure codes E1500-E1699. For supplies for ESRD, see procedure codes A4650-A4999

● New code　　　　▲ Revised code　　　　( ) Deleted code

PATHOLOGY AND LABORATORY

Guidelines

In addition to the information presented in the INTRODUCTION, several other items unique to this section are defined or identified here:

1. SPECIAL REPORT: A service, material or supply that is rarely provided, unusual, variable or new may require a special report in determining medical appropriateness for reimbursement purposes. Pertinent information should include an adequate definition or description of the nature, extent, and need for the service, material or supply.

2. MODIFIERS: Listed services may be modified under certain circumstances. When appropriate, the modifying circumstance is identified by adding a modifier to the basic procedure code. CPT and HCPCS National Level II modifiers may be used with CPT and HCPCS National Level II procedure codes. Modifiers commonly used with PATHOLOGY AND LABORATORY SERVICES are as follows:

   -CC   Procedure code change (use "CC" when the procedure code submitted was changed either for administrative reasons or because an incorrect code was filed)

   -LR   Laboratory round trip

   -TC   Technical component. Under certain circumstances, a charge may be made for the technical component alone. Under these circumstances, the technical component charge is identified by adding the modifier -TC to the usual procedure code. Technical component charges are institutional charges and are not billed separately by physicians. Portable x-ray suppliers bill only for the technical component however, and should use modifier -TC. The charge data from portable x-ray suppliers will then be used to build customary and prevailing profiles.

3. CPT CODE CROSS-REFERENCE: See sections for equivalent CPT code(s) for all listings in this section.

■ Not valid   ■ Non-covered   Special   ■ Carrier   **317**
    for Medicare   by Medicare   coverage   discretion
                                               instructions

Pathology and Laboratory

CHEMISTRY AND TOXICOLOGY TESTS

P2028 Cephalin flocculation, blood
CIM: 50-34

P2029 Congo red, blood
CIM: 50-34

P2031 Hair analysis (excluding arsenic)
CIM: 50-24

P2033 Thymol turbidity, blood
CIM: 50-34

P2038 Mucoprotein, blood (seromucoid) (medical necessity procedure)
CIM: 50-34

PATHOLOGY SCREENING TESTS

P3000 Screening papanicolaou smear, cervical or vaginal, up to three smears; by technician under physician supervision
CIM: 50-20

P3001 requiring interpretation by physician
CIM: 50-20

MICROBIOLOGY TESTS

P7001 Culture, bacterial, urine; quantitative, sensitivity study

MISCELLANEOUS PATHOLOGY AND LABORATORY TESTS

P9010 Blood (whole), for transfusion, per unit
MCM: 2455.A

P9011 Blood (split unit), specify amount
MCM: 2455.A

P9012 Cryoprecipitate, each unit
MCM: 2455.B

P9016 Red blood cells, leukocytes reduced, each unit
MCM: 2455.B

● New code ▲ Revised code ( ) Deleted code

P9017   Fresh frozen plasma (single donor), frozen within eight hours of collection, each unit
MCM: 2455A.B

P9019   Platelets, each unit
MCM: 2455.B

P9020   Platelet rich plasma, each unit
MCM: 2455.B

P9021   Red blood cells, each unit
MCM: 2455.A

P9022   Red blood cells, washed, each unit
MCM: 2455.A

P9023   Plasma, pooled multiple donor, solvent/detergent treated, frozen, each unit
MCM: 2455.B

P9031   Platelets, leukocytes reduced, each unit
MCM: 2455

P9032   Platelets, irradiated, each unit
MCM: 2455

P9033   Platelets, leukocytes reduced, irradiated, each unit
MCM: 2455

P9034   Platelets, pheresis, each unit
MCM: 2455

P9035   Platelets, pheresis, leukocytes reduced, each unit
MCM: 2455

P9036   Platelets, pheresis, irradiated, each unit
MCM: 2455

P9037   Platelets, pheresis, leukocytes reduced, irradiated, each unit
MCM: 2455

P9038   Red blood cells, irradiated, each unit
MCM: 2455

P9039   Red blood cells, deglycerolized, each unit
MCM: 2455

P9040   Red blood cells, leukocytes reduced, irradiated, each unit
MCM: 2455

P9041 Infusion, albumin (human), 5%, 50 ml

P9043 Infusion, plasma protein fraction (human), 5%, 50 ml
MCM: 2455.B

P9044 Plasma, cryoprecipitate reduced, each unit
MCM: 2455.B

P9045 Infusion, albumin (human), 5%, 250 ml

P9046 Infusion, albumin (human), 25%, 20 ml

P9047 Infusion, albumin (human), 25%, 50 ml

P9048 Infusion, plasma protein fraction (human), 5%, 250 ml

P9050 Granulocytes, pheresis, each unit

P9051 Whole blood or red blood cells, leukocytes reduced, CMV-negative, each unit

P9052 Platelets, HLA-matched leukocytes reduced, apheresis/pheresis, each unit

P9053 Platelets, pheresis, leukocytes reduced, CMV-negative, irradiated, each unit

P9054 Whole blood or red blood cells, leukocytes reduced, frozen, deglycerol, washed, each unit

P9055 Platelets, leukocytes reduced, CMV-negative, apheresis/pheresis, each unit

P9056 Whole blood, leukocytes reduced, irradiated, each unit

P9057 Red blood cells, frozen/deglycerolized/washed, leukocytes reduced, irradiated, each unit

P9058 Red blood cells, leukocytes reduced, CMV-negative, irradiated, each unit

P9059 Fresh frozen plasma between 8-24 hours of collection, each unit

P9060 Fresh frozen plasma, donor retested, each unit

P9603   Travel allowance one way in connection with medically necessary laboratory specimen collection drawn from home bound or nursing home bound patient; prorated miles actually travelled
MCM: 5114.1K

P9604   prorated trip charge
MCM: 5114.1K

P9612   Catheterization for collection of specimen; single patient, all places of service
MCM: 5114.1D

P9615   multiple patients
MCM: 5114.1D

Not valid   Non-covered   Special   Carrier   **321**
for Medicare   by Medicare   coverage   discretion
instructions

TEMPORARY CODES

Guidelines

In addition to the information presented in the INTRODUCTION, several other items unique to this section are defined or identified here:

1. SUBSECTION INFORMATION: Some of the listed subheadings or subsections have special needs or instructions unique to that section. Where these are indicated, special "notes" will be presented preceding or following the listings. Those subsections within the TEMPORARY CODES section that have "notes" are as follows:

Subsection	Code Numbers
Temporary codes	Q0000-Q9999

2. SPECIAL REPORT: A service, material or supply that is rarely provided, unusual, variable or new may require a special report in determining medical appropriateness for reimbursement purposes. Pertinent information should include an adequate definition or description of the nature, extent, and need for the service, material or supply.

3. MODIFIERS: Listed services may be modified under certain circumstances. When appropriate, the modifying circumstance is identified by adding a modifier to the basic procedure code. CPT and HCPCS National Level II modifiers may be used with CPT and HCPCS National Level II procedure codes. Modifiers commonly used with TEMPORARY CODES are as follows.

   -CC   Procedure code change (use "CC" when the procedure code submitted was changed either for administrative reasons or because an incorrect code was filed)

   -LL   Lease/rental (used when DME equipment rental is to be applied against the purchase price)

   -LR   Laboratory round trip

   -QC   Single channel monitoring

   -QD   Recording and storage in solid state memory by a digital recorder

---

-QE   Prescribed amount of oxygen is less than 1 liter per minute (LPM)

-QF   Prescribed amount of oxygen exceeds 4 liters per minute (LPM) and portable oxygen is prescribed

-QG   Prescribed amount of oxygen is greater than 4 liters per minute (LPM)

-QH   Oxygen conserving device is being used with an oxygen delivery system

-QT   Recording and storage on tape by an analog tape recorder

-RP   Replacement and repair (may be used to indicate replacement of DME, orthotic and prosthetic devices that have been in use for some time. The claim shows the code for the part, followed by the "RP" modifier and the charge for the part.)

-RR   Rental (used when DME is to be rented)

-TC   Technical component. Under certain circumstances, a charge may be made for the technical component alone. Under these circumstances, the technical component charge is identified by adding the modifier -TC to the usual procedure code. Technical component charges are institutional charges and are not billed separately by physicians. Portable x-ray suppliers bill only for the technical component however, and should use modifier -TC. The charge data from portable x-ray suppliers will then be used to build customary and prevailing profiles.

-UE   Used durable medical equipment

4.   CPT CODE CROSS-REFERENCE: See sections for equivalent CPT code(s) for all listings in this section.

Temporary Codes

NOTE: Temporary codes are national codes given by CMS on a temporary basis. The list contains current codes, as well as those which have been superseded by permanent alphanumeric codes as indicated by the cross-reference.

Q0035 Cardiokymography
CIM: 50-50

Q0081 Infusion therapy, using other than chemotherapeutic drugs, per visit
CIM: 60-14

Q0083 Chemotherapy administration by other than infusion technique only (e.g., subcutaneous, intramuscular, push), per visit

Q0084 Chemotherapy administration by infusion technique only, per visit
CIM: 60-14

Q0085 Chemotherapy administration by both infusion technique and other technique(s) (e.g., subcutaneous, intramuscular, push), per visit

Q0091 Screening papanicolaou smear; obtaining, preparing and conveyance of cervical or vaginal smear to laboratory
CIM: 50-20

Q0092 Set up portable x-ray equipment
MCM: 2070.4

Q0111 Wet mounts, including preparations of vaginal, cervical or skin specimens

Q0112 All potassium hydroxide (koh) preparations

Q0113 Pinworm examinations

Q0114 Fern test

Q0115 Post-coital direct, qualitative examinations of vaginal or cervical mucous

(Q0136) Code deleted December 31, 2005; use J0885

Not valid for Medicare   Non-covered by Medicare   Special coverage instructions   Carrier discretion

(Q0137) Code deleted December 31, 2005; use J0881

Q0144 Azithromycin dihydrate, oral, capsules/powder, 1 gram

Q0163 Diphenhydramine HCl, 50 mg, oral, FDA approved prescription anti-emetic, for use as a complete therapeutic substitute for an IV anti-emetic at time of chemotherapy treatment not to exceed a 48 hour dosage regimen

Q0164 Prochlorperazine maleate, 5 mg, oral, FDA approved prescription anti-emetic, for use as a complete therapeutic substitute for an IV anti-emetic at the time of chemotherapy treatment, not to exceed a 48 hour dosage regimen

Q0165 Prochlorperazine maleate, 10 mg, oral, FDA approved prescription anti-emetic, for use as a complete therapeutic substitute for an IV anti-emetic at the time of chemotherapy treatment, not to exceed a 48 hour dosage regimen

Q0166 Granisetron HCl, 1 mg, oral, FDA approved prescription anti-emetic, for use as a complete therapeutic substitute for an IV anti-emetic at the time of chemotherapy treatment, not to exceed a 24 hour dosage regimen

Q0167 Dronabinol, 2.5 mg, oral, FDA approved prescription anti-emetic, for use as a complete therapeutic substitute for an IV anti-emetic at the time of chemotherapy treatment, not to exceed a 48 hour dosage regimen

Q0168 Dronabinol, 5 mg, oral, FDA approved prescription anti-emetic, for use as a complete therapeutic substitute for an IV anti-emetic at the time of chemotherapy treatment, not to exceed a 48 hour dosage regimen

Q0169 Promethazine HCl, 12.5 mg, oral, FDA approved prescription anti-emetic, for use as a complete therapeutic substitute for an IV anti-emetic at the time of chemotherapy treatment, not to exceed a 48 hour dosage regimen

Q0170 Promethazine HCl, 25 mg, oral, FDA approved prescription anti-emetic, for use as a complete therapeutic substitute for an IV anti-emetic at the time of chemotherapy treatment, not to exceed a 48 hour dosage regimen

Q0171   Chlorpromazine HCl, 10 mg, oral, FDA approved prescription anti-emetic, for use as a complete therapeutic substitute for an IV anti-emetic at the time of chemotherapy treatment, not to exceed a 48 hour dosage regimen

Q0172   Chlorpromazine HCl, 25 mg, oral, FDA approved prescription anti-emetic, for use as a complete therapeutic substitute for an IV anti-emetic at the time of chemotherapy treatment, not to exceed a 48 hour dosage regimen

Q0173   Trimethobenzamide HCl, 250 mg, oral, FDA approved prescription anti-emetic, for use as a complete therapeutic substitute for an IV anti-emetic at the time of chemotherapy treatment, not to exceed a 48 hour dosage regimen

Q0174   Thiethylperazine malcate, 10 mg, oral, FDA approved prescription anti-emetic, for use as a complete therapeutic substitute for an IV anti-emetic at the time of chemotherapy treatment, not to exceed a 48 hour dosage regimen

Q0175   Perphenzaine, 4 mg, oral, FDA approved prescription anti-emetic, for use as a complete therapeutic substitute for an IV anti-emetic at the time of chemotherapy treatment, not to exceed a 48 hour dosage regimen

Q0176   Perphenzaine, 8 mg, oral, FDA approved prescription anti-cmctic, for use as a complete therapeutic substitute for an IV anti-emetic at the time of chemotherapy treatment, not to exceed a 48 hour dosage regimen

Q0177   Hydroxyzine pamoate, 25 mg, oral, FDA approved prescription anti-emetic, for use as a complete therapeutic substitute for an IV anti-emetic at the time of chemotherapy treatment, not to exceed a 48 hour dosage regimen

Q0178   Hydroxyzine pamoate, 50 mg, oral, FDA approved prescription anti-emetic, for use as a complete therapeutic substitute for an IV anti-emetic at the time of chemotherapy treatment, not to exceed a 48 hour dosage regimen

Q0179   Ondansetron HCl, 8 mg, oral, FDA approved prescription anti-emetic, for use as a complete therapeutic substitute for an IV anti-emetic at the time of chemotherapy treatment, not to exceed a 48 hour dosage regimen

Q0180   Dolasetron mesylate, 100 mg, oral, FDA approved prescription anti-emetic, for use as a complete therapeutic substitute for an IV anti-emetic at the time of chemotherapy treatment, not to exceed a 24 hour dosage regimen

Q0181   Unspecified oral dosage form, FDA approved prescription anti-emetic, for use as a complete therapeutic substitute for an IV anti-emetic at the time of chemotherapy treatment, not to exceed a 48 hour dosage regimen

(Q0182)   Code deleted December 31, 2004; use J7343

(Q0183)   Code deleted December 31, 2004; use J7344

(Q0187)   Code deleted December 31, 2005; use J7189

● **Q0480**   Driver for use with pneumatic ventricular assist device, replacement only

● **Q0481**   Microprocessor control unit for use with electric ventricular assist device, replacement only

● **Q0482**   Microprocessor control unit for use with electric/pneumatic combination ventricular assist device, replacement only

● **Q0483**   Monitor/display module for use with electric ventricular assist device, replacement only

● **Q0484**   Monitor/display module for use with electric or electric/pneumatic ventricular assist device, replacement only

● **Q0485**   Monitor control cable for use with electric ventricular assist device, replacement only

● **Q0486**   Monitor control cable for use with electric/pneumatic ventricular assist device, replacement only

● **Q0487**   Leads (pneumatic/electrical) for use with any type electric/pneumatic ventricular assist device, replacement only

● **Q0488**   Power pack base for use with electric ventricular assist device, replacement only

● **Q0489**   Power pack base for use with electric/pneumatic ventricular assist device, replacement only

● **Q0490**   Emergency power source for use with electric ventricular assist device, replacement only

● **Q0491**   Emergency power source for use with electric/pneumatic ventricular assist device, replacement only

● **Q0492**   Emergency power supply cable for use with electric ventricular assist device, replacement only

● **Q0493**   Emergency power supply cable for use with electric/pneumatic ventricular assist device, replacement only

● **Q0494**   Emergency hand pump for use with electric or electric/pneumatic ventricular assist device, replacement only

● **Q0495**   Battery/power pack charger for use with electric or electric/pneumatic ventricular assist device, replacement only

● **Q0496**   Battery for use with electric or electric/pneumatic ventricular assist device, replacement only

● **Q0497**   Battery clips for use with electric or electric/pneumatic ventricular assist device, replacement only

● **Q0498**   Holster for use with electric or electric/pneumatic ventricular assist device, replacement only

● **Q0499**   Belt/vest for use with electric or electric/pneumatic ventricular assist device, replacement only

● **Q0500**   Filters for use with electric or electric/pneumatic ventricular assist device, replacement only

● **Q0501** Shower cover for use with electric or electric/pneumatic ventricular assist device, replacement only

● **Q0502** Mobility cart for pneumatic ventricular assist device, replacement only

● **Q0503** Battery for pneumatic ventricular assist device, replacement only, each

● **Q0504** Power adapter for pneumatic ventricular assist device, replacement only, vehicle type

● **Q0505** Miscellaneous supply or accessory for use with ventricular assist device

● **Q0510** Pharmacy supply fee for initial immunosuppressive drug(s), first month following implant

● **Q0511** Pharmacy supply fee for oral anti-cancer, oral anti-emetic or immunosuppressive drug(s); for the first prescription in a 30-day period

● **Q0512**   for a subsequent prescription in a 30-day period

● **Q0513** Pharmacy dispensing fee for inhalation drug(s); per 30 days

● **Q0514**   per 90 days

● **Q0515** Injection, sermorelin acetate, 1 microgram
MCM: 2049

(Q1001) Code deleted June 30, 2005

(Q1002) Code deleted June 30, 2005

Q1003 New technology intraocular lense category 3 as defined in Federal Register notice

Q1004 New technology intraocular lense category 4 as defined in Federal Register notice

Q1005 New technology intraocular lense category 5 as defined in Federal Register notice

(Q2001) Code deleted December 31, 2005

(Q2002)   Code deleted December 31, 2005; use J9175

(Q2003)   Code deleted December 31, 2005; use J0365

Q2004   Irrigation solution for treatment of bladder calculi, for
example Renacidin, per 500 ml
MCM: 2049

(Q2005)   Code deleted December 31, 2005

(Q2006)   Code deleted December 31, 2005; use J1162

(Q2007)   Code deleted December 31, 2005; use J1430

(Q2008)   Code deleted December 31, 2005; use J1451

Q2009   Injection, fosphenytoin, 50 mg
MCM: 2049

(Q2011)   Code deleted December 31, 2005; use J1640

(Q2012)   Code deleted December 31, 2005; use J2504

(Q2013)   Code deleted December 31, 2005; use J2513

(Q2014)   Code deleted December 31, 2005

Q2017   Injection, teniposide, 50 mg
MCM: 2049

(Q2018)   Code deleted December 31, 2005; use J3355

(Q2019)   Code deleted December 31, 2005; use J0480

(Q2020)   Code deleted December 31, 2005; use J1675

(Q2021)   Code deleted December 31, 2005; use J1945

(Q2022)   Code deleted December 31, 2005; use J7188

(Q3000)   Code deleted December 31, 2005

Q3001   Radioelements for brachytherapy, any type, each
MCM: 15022

(Q3002)   Code deleted December 31, 2005

■ Not valid   ■ Non-covered   Special   ■ Carrier   **331**
for Medicare   by Medicare   coverage   discretion
instructions

(Q3003) Code deleted December 31, 2005

(Q3004) Code deleted December 31, 2005

(Q3005) Code deleted December 31, 2005

(Q3006) Code deleted December 31, 2005

(Q3007) Code deleted December 31, 2005

(Q3008) Code deleted December 31, 2005

(Q3009) Code deleted December 31, 2005

(Q3010) Code deleted December 31, 2005

(Q3011) Code deleted December 31, 2005

(Q3012) Code deleted December 31, 2005

Q3014 Telehealth originating site facility fee

Q3019 ALS vehicle used, emergency transport, no ALS level services furnished

Q3020 ALS vehicle used, non-emergency transport, no ALS level service furnished

Q3025 Injection, interferon beta-1a, 11 mcg for intramuscular use
MCM: 2049

Q3026 Injection, interferon beta-1a, 11 mcg for subcutaneous use

Q3031 Collagen skin test
CIM: 65-9

Q4001 Cast supplies, body cast adult, with or without head, plaster

Q4002 Cast supplies, body cast adult, with or without head, fiberglass

Q4003 Cast supplies, shoulder cast, adult (11 years +), plaster

Q4004 Cast supplies, shoulder cast, adult (11 years +), fiberglass

Q4005 Cast supplies, long arm cast, adult (11 years +), plaster

Q4006 Cast supplies, long arm cast, adult (11 years +), fiberglass

Q4007 Cast supplies, long arm cast, pediatric (0-10 years), plaster

Q4008 Cast supplies, long arm cast, pediatric (0-10 years), fiberglass

Q4009 Cast supplies, short arm cast, adult (11 years +), plaster

Q4010 Cast supplies, short arm cast, adult (11 years +), fiberglass

Q4011 Cast supplies, short arm cast, pediatric (0-10 years), plaster

Q4012 Cast supplies, short arm cast, pediatric (0-10 years), fiberglass

Q4013 Cast supplies, gauntlet cast (includes lower forearm and hand), adult (11 years +), plaster

Q4014 Cast supplies, gauntlet cast (includes lower forearm and hand), adult (11 years +), fiberglass

Q4015 Cast supplies, gauntlet cast (includes lower forearm and hand), pediatric (0-10 years), plaster

Q4016 Cast supplies, gauntlet cast (includes lower forearm and hand), pediatric (0-10 years), fiberglass

Q4017 Cast supplies, long arm splint, adult (11 years +), plaster

Q4018 Cast supplies, long arm splint, adult (11 years +), fiberglass

Q4019 Cast supplies, long arm splint, pediatric (0-10 years), plaster

Q4020 Cast supplies, long arm splint, pediatric (0-10 years), fiberglass

Q4021 Cast supplies, short arm splint, adult (11 years +), plaster

Q4022 Cast supplies, short arm splint, adult (11 years +), fiberglass

Q4023 Cast supplies, short arm splint, pediatric (0-10 years), plaster

Q4024 Cast supplies, short arm splint, pediatric (0-10 years), fiberglass

Q4025 Cast supplies, hip spica (one or both legs), adult (11 years +), plaster

Q4026 Cast supplies, hip spica (one or both legs), adult (11 years +), fiberglass

Q4027 Cast supplies, hip spica (one or both legs), pediatric (0-10 years), plaster

Q4028 Cast supplies, hip spica (one or both legs), pediatric (0-10 years), fiberglass

Q4029 Cast supplies, long leg cast, adult (11 years +), plaster

Q4030 Cast supplies, long leg cast, adult (11 years +), fiberglass

Q4031 Cast supplies, long leg cast, pediatric (0-10 years), plaster

Q4032 Cast supplies, long leg cast, pediatric (0-10 years), fiberglass

Q4033 Cast supplies, long leg cylinder cast, adult (11 years +), plaster

Q4034 Cast supplies, long leg cylinder cast, adult (11 years +), fiberglass

Q4035 Cast supplies, long leg cylinder cast, pediatric (0-10 years), plaster

Q4036 Cast supplies, long leg cylinder cast, pediatric (0-10 years), fiberglass

Q4037 Cast supplies, short leg cast, adult (11 years +), plaster

Q4038 Cast supplies, short leg cast, adult (11 years +), fiberglass

Q4039 Cast supplies, short leg cast, pediatric (0-10 years), plaster

Q4040 Cast supplies, short leg cast, pediatric (0-10 years), fiberglass

Q4041 Cast supplies, long leg splint, adult (11 years +), plaster

Q4042 Cast supplies, long leg splint, adult (11 years +), fiberglass

Q4043 Cast supplies, long leg splint, pediatric (0-10 years), plaster

Q4044 Cast supplies, long leg splint, pediatric (0-10 years), fiberglass

Q4045 Cast supplies, short leg splint, adult (11 years +), plaster

Q4046 Cast supplies, short leg splint, adult (11 years +), fiberglass

Q4047 Cast supplies, short leg splint, pediatric (0-10 years), plaster

Q4048 Cast supplies, short leg splint, pediatric (0-10 years), fiberglass

Q4049 Finger splint, static

Q4050 Cast supplies, for unlisted types and materials of casts

Q4051 Splint supplies, miscellaneous (includes thermoplastics, strapping, fasteners, padding and other supplies)

(Q4054) Code deleted December 31, 2005; use J0882

(Q4055) Code deleted December 31, 2005; use J0886

(Q4075) Code deleted December 31, 2005; use J0133

(Q4076) Code deleted December 31, 2005; use J1265

(Q4077) Code deleted December 31, 2005; use J3285

INJECTION CODES FOR EPO

● **Q4079**   Injection, natalizumab, 1 mg

● **Q4080**   Iloprost, inhalation solution, administered through DME, 20 micrograms

● **Q9945**   Low osmolar contrast material, up to 149 mg/ml iodine concentration, per ml
MCM: 15022

● **Q9946**   Low osmolar contrast material, 150-199 mg/ml iodine concentration, per ml
MCM: 15022

● **Q9947**   Low osmolar contrast material, 200-249 mg/ml iodine concentration, per ml
MCM: 15022

● **Q9948**   Low osmolar contrast material, 250-299 mg/ml iodine concentration, per ml
MCM: 15022

● **Q9949**   Low osmolar contrast material, 300-349 mg/ml iodine concentration, per ml
MCM: 15022

● **Q9950**   Low osmolar contrast material, 350-399 mg/ml iodine concentration, per ml
MCM: 15022

● **Q9951**   Low osmolar contrast material, 400 or greater mg/ml iodine concentration, per ml
MCM: 15022

● **Q9952**   Injection, gadolinium-based magnetic resonance contrast agent, per ml
MCM: 15022

● **Q9953**   Injection, iron-based magnetic resonance contrast agent, per ml
MCM: 15022

● **Q9954**   Oral magnetic resonance contrast agent, per 100 ml
MCM: 15022

● **Q9955**   Injection, perflexane lipid microspheres, per ml

● New code   ▲ Revised code   ( ) Deleted code

● Q9956   Injection, octafluoropropane microspheres, per ml

● Q9957   Injection, perflutren lipid microspheres, per ml

● Q9958   High osmolar contrast material, up to 149 mg/ml iodine concentration, per ml
MCM: 15022

● Q9959   High osmolar contrast material, 150-199 mg/ml iodine concentration, per ml
MCM: 15022

● Q9960   High osmolar contrast material, 200-249 mg/ml iodine concentration, per ml
MCM: 15022

● Q9961   High osmolar contrast material, 250-299 mg/ml iodine concentration, per ml
MCM: 15022

● Q9962   High osmolar contrast material, 300-349 mg/ml iodine concentration, per ml

● Q9963   High osmolar contrast material, 350-399 mg/ml iodine concentration, per ml
MCM: 15022

● Q9964   High osmolar contrast material, 400 or greater mg/ml iodine concentration, per ml
MCM: 15022

● New code ▲ Revised code ( ) Deleted code

DIAGNOSTIC RADIOLOGY SERVICES

Guidelines

In addition to the information presented in the INTRODUCTION, several other items unique to this section are defined or identified here:

1. SPECIAL REPORT: A service, material or supply that is rarely provided, unusual, variable or new may require a special report in determining medical appropriateness for reimbursement purposes. Pertinent information should include an adequate definition or description of the nature, extent, and need for the service, material or supply.

2. MODIFIERS: Listed services may be modified under certain circumstances. When appropriate, the modifying circumstance is identified by adding a modifier to the basic procedure code. CPT and HCPCS National Level II modifiers may be used with CPT and HCPCS National Level II procedure codes. Modifiers commonly used with DIAGNOSTIC RADIOLOGY SERVICES are as follows:

   -CC   Procedure code change (use "CC" when the procedure code submitted was changed either for administrative reasons or because an incorrect code was filed)

   -LT   Left side (used to identify procedures performed on the left side of the body)

   -RT   Right side (used to identify procedures performed on the right side of the body)

   -TC   Technical component. Under certain circumstances, a charge may be made for the technical component alone. Under those circumstances, the technical component charge is identified by adding modifier -TC to the usual procedure number. Technical component charges are institutional charges and are not billed separately by physicians. However, portable x-ray suppliers bill only for the technical component and should use modifier -TC. The charge data from portable x-ray suppliers will then be used to build customary and prevailing profiles.

■ Not valid   ■ Non-covered   Special   ■ Carrier   **339**
  for Medicare   by Medicare   coverage   discretion
                                       instructions

3. CPT CODE CROSS-REFERENCE: There are no equivalent CPT codes for procedures listed in this section.

Diagnostic Radiology Services

R0070   Transportation of portable x-ray equipment and personnel to home or nursing home, per trip to facility or location; one patient seen
MCM: 2070.4, 5244.B

R0075   more than one patient seen, per patient
MCM: 2070.4, 5244.B

R0076   Transportation of portable EKG to facility or location, per patient
CIM: 50-15   MCM: 2070.1, 2070.4

PRIVATE PAYER CODES

Guidelines

HCPCS "S" codes are temporary national codes established by the private payers for private payer use. Prior to using "S" codes on insurance claims to private payers, you should consult with the payer to confirm that the "S" codes are acceptable. "S" codes are not valid for Medicare use.

In addition to the information presented in the INTRODUCTION, several other items unique to this section are defined or identified here.

1. SPECIAL REPORT: A service, material or supply that is rarely provided, unusual, variable or new may require a special report in determining medical appropriateness for reimbursement purposes. Pertinent information should include an adequate definition or description of the nature, extent, and need for the service, material or supply.

2. MODIFIERS: Listed services may be modified under certain circumstances. When appropriate, the modifying circumstance is identified by adding a modifier to the basic procedure code. CPT and HCPCS National Level II modifiers may be used with CPT and HCPCS National Level II procedure codes.

Private Payer Codes

S0012 Butorphanol tartrate, nasal spray, 25 mg

S0014 Tacrine HCl, 10 mg

(S0016) Code deleted March 31, 2005; use S0072

S0017 Injection, aminocaproic acid, 5 g

S0020 Injection, bupivicaine HCl, 30 ml

S0021 Injection, ceftoperazone sodium, 1 g

S0023 Injection, cimetidine HCl, 300 mg

S0028 Injection, fanotidine, 20 mg

S0030   Injection, metronidazole, 500 mg

S0032   Injection, nafcillin sodium, 2 g

S0034   Injection, ofloxacin, 400 mg

S0039   Injection, sulfamethoxazole and trimethoprim, 10 ml

S0040   Injection, ticarcillin disodium and clavulanate potassium, 3.1 g

(S0071)   Code deleted December 31, 2005

(S0072)   Code deleted December 31, 2005

S0073   Injection, aztreonam, 500 mg

S0074   Injection, cefotetan disodium, 500 mg

S0077   Injection, clindamycin phosphate, 300 mg

S0078   Injection, fosphenytoin sodium, 750 mg

S0080   Injection, pentamidine isethionate, 300 mg

S0081   Injection, piperacillin sodium, 500 mg

S0088   Imatinib [Gleevak] 100 mg

S0090   Sildenafil citrate, 25 mg

S0091   Granisetron hydrochloride, 1mg (for circumstances falling under the Medicare statute, use Q0166)

S0092   Injection, hydromorphone hydrochloride, 250 mg (loading dose for infusion pump)

S0093   Injection, morphine sulfate, 500 mg (loading dose for infusion pump)

S0104   Zidovudine, oral, 100 mg

S0106   Bupropion HCl sustained release tablet, 150 mg, per bottle of 60 tablets

(S0107)   Code deleted March 31, 2005; use J2357

---

342   ●   New code   ▲   Revised code   ( )   Deleted code

S0108   Mercaptopurine, oral, 50 mg

(S0114)   Code deleted December 31, 2005

(S0115)   Code deleted December 31, 2004; use CPT

S0116   Bevacizumab, 100 mg

S0117   Tretinoin, topical, 5 grams

S0122   Injection, menotropins, 75 IU

S0126   Injection, follitropin alfa, 75 IU

S0128   Injection, follitropin beta, 75 IU

S0132   Injection, ganirelix acetate, 250 mcg

● **S0133**   Histrelin, implant, 50 mg

S0136   Clozapine, 25 mg

S0137   Didanosine (DDI), 25 mg

S0138   Finasteride, 5 mg

S0139   Minoxidil, 10 mg

S0140   Saquinavir, 200 mg

S0141   Zalcitabine (DDC), 0.375 mg

● **S0142**   Colistimethate sodium, inhalation solution administered through DME, concentrated form, per mg

● **S0143**   Aztreonam, inhalation solution administered through DME, concentrated form, per gram

● **S0145**   Injection, pegylated interferon alfa-2a, 180 mcg per ml

● **S0146**   Injection, pegylated interferon alfa-2b, 10 mcg per 0.5 ml

S0155   Sterile dilutant for epoprostenol, 50 ml

S0156   Exemestane, 25 mg

Not valid for Medicare   Non-covered by Medicare   Special coverage instructions   Carrier discretion

S0157   Becaplermin gel 0.01%, 0.5 gram

(S0158)   Code deleted March 31, 2005; use J1931

(S0159)   Code deleted March 31, 2005; use J0180

S0160   Dextroamphetamine sulfate, 5 mg

S0161   Calcitrol, 0.25 Mg

S0162   Injection, efalizumab, 125 mg

(S0163)   Code deleted December 31, 2004; use CPT

S0164   Injection, pantoprazole sodium, 40 mg

(S0165)   Code deleted December 31, 2004; use CPT

S0170   Anastrozole, oral, 1 mg

S0171   Injection, bumetanide, 0.5 mg

S0172   Chlorambucil, oral, 2 mg

(S0173)   Code deleted December 31, 2005

S0174   Dolasetron mesylate, oral 50 mg (for circumstances falling under the medicare statute, use Q0180)

S0175   Flutamide, oral, 125 mg

S0176   Hydroxyurea, oral, 500 mg

S0177   Levamisole hydrochloride, oral, 50 mg

S0178   Lomustine, oral, 10 mg

S0179   Megestrol acetate, oral, 20 mg

S0181   Ondansetron hydrochloride, oral, 4 mg (for circumstances falling under the medicare statute, use Q0179)

S0182   Procarbazine hydrochloride, oral, 50 mg

S0183   Prochlorperazine maleate, oral, 5 mg (for circumstances falling under the medicare statute, use Q0164 - Q0165)

S0187   Tamoxifen citrate, oral, 10 mg

S0189   Testosterone pellet, 75 mg

S0190   Mifepristone, oral, 200 mg

S0191   Misoprostol, oral, 200 mcg

S0194   Dialysis/stress vitamin supplement, oral, 100 capsules

S0195   Pneumococcal conjugate vaccine, polyvalent, intramuscular, for children from five years to nine years of age who have not previously received the vaccine

S0196   Injectable poly-l-lactic acid, restorative implant, 1 ml, face (deep dermis, subcutaneous layers)

● **S0197**   Prenatal vitamins, 30-day supply

● **S0198**   Injection, pegaptanib sodium, 0.3 mg

S0199   Medically induced abortion by oral ingestion of medication including all associated services and supplies (e.g., patient counseling, office visits, confirmation of pregnancy by HCG, ultrasound to confirm duration of pregnancy, ultrasound to confirm completion of abortion) except drugs

S0201   Partial hospitalization services, less than 24 hours, per diem

S0207   Paramedic intercept, non-hospital-based ALS service (non-voluntary), non-transport

S0208   Paramedic intercept, hospital-based ALS service (non-voluntary), non-transport

S0209   Wheelchair van, mileage, per mile

S0215   Non-emergency transportation; mileage, per mile

S0220   Medical conference by a physician with interdisciplinary team of health professionals or representatives of community agencies to coordinate activities of patient care (patient is present); approximately 30 minutes

---

| | Not valid for Medicare | | Non-covered by Medicare | | Special coverage instructions | | Carrier discretion | **345** |

S0221   Medical conference by a physician with interdisciplinary team of health professionals or representatives of community agencies to coordinate activities of patient care (patient is present); approximately 60 minutes

S0250   Comprehensive geriatric assessment and treatment planning performed by assessment team

S0255   Hospice referral visit (advising patient and family of care options) performed by nurse, social worker, or other designated staff

S0257   Counseling and discussion regarding advance directives or end of life care planning and decisions, with patient and/or surrogate (list separately in addition to code for appropriate evaluation and management service)

S0260   History and physical (outpatient or office) related to surgical procedure (list separately in addition to code for appropriate evaluation and management service)

● S0265   Genetic counseling, under physician supervision, each 15 minutes

S0302   Completed early periodic screening diagnosis and treatment (EPSDT) service (list in addition to code for appropriate evaluation and management service)

S0310   Hospitalist services (list separately in addition to code for appropriate evaluation and management service)

S0315   Disease management program; initial assessment and initiation of the program

S0316   follow-up/reassessment

S0317   Disease management program; per diem

S0320   Telephone calls by a registered nurse to a disease management program member for monitoring purposes; per month

S0340   Lifestyle modification program for management of coronary artery disease, including all supportive services; first quarter/stage

S0341 Lifestyle modification program for management of coronary artery disease, including all supportive services; second or third quarter/stage

S0342 Lifestyle modification program for management of coronary artery disease, including all supportive services; fourth quarter/stage

S0390 Routine foot care; removal and/or trimming of corns, calluses and/or nails and preventive maintenance, per visit

S0395 Impression casting of a foot performed by a practitioner other than the manufacturer of the orthotic

S0400 Global fee for extracorporeal shock wave lithotripsy treatment of kidney stone(s)

S0500 Disposable contact lens, per lens

S0504 Single vision prescription lens (safety, athletic or sunglass), per lens

S0506 Bifocal vision prescription lens (safety, athletic or sunglass), per lens

S0508 Trifocal vision prescription lens (safety, athletic or sunglass), per lens

S0510 Non-prescription lens (safety, athletic or sunglass), per lens

S0512 Daily wear specialty contact lens, per lens

S0514 Color contact lens, per lens

S0516 Safety eyeglass frames

S0518 Sunglasses frames

S0580 Polycarbonate lens (List this code in addition to the basic code for the lens)

S0581 Nonstandard lens (List this code in addition to the basic code for the lens)

S0590 Integral lens service, miscellaneous services reported separately

S0592   Comprehensive contact lens evaluation

● S0595   Dispensing new spectacle lenses for patient supplied frame

S0601   Screening proctoscopy

S0605   Digital rectal examination, annual

S0610   Annual gynecological examination; new patient

S0612   established patient

● S0613   clinical breast examination without pelvic evaluation

S0618   Audiometry for hearing aid evaluation to determine the level and degree of hearing loss

S0620   Routine ophthalmological examination including refraction; new patient

S0621   established patient

S0622   Physical exam for college, new or established patient (list separately in addition to appropriate evaluation and management code)

● S0625   Retinal telescreening by digital imaging of multiple different fund us areas to screen for vision-threatening conditions, including imaging, interpretation and report

S0630   Removal of sutures by a physician other than the physician who originally closed the wound

S0800   Laser in situ keratomileusis (LASIK)

S0810   Photorefractive keratectomy (PRK)

S0812   Phototherapeutic keratectomy (PTK)

S0820   Computerized corneal topography, unilateral

(S0830)   Code deleted March 31, 2004; use CPT

S1001   Deluxe item, patient aware (List in addition to code for basic item)

S1002   Customized item (List in addition to code for basic item)

S1015   IV tubing extension set

S1016   Non-PVC (polyvinyl chloride) intravenous administration set, for use with drugs that are not stable in PVC, e.g., paclitaxel

S1025   Inhaled nitric oxide for the treatment of hypoxic respiratory failure in the neonate; per diem

S1030   Continuous noninvasive glucose monitoring device, purchase (for physician interpretation of data, use CPT code)

S1031   Continuous noninvasive glucose monitoring device, rental, including sensor, sensor replacement, and download to monitor (for physician interpretation of data, use CPT code)

S1040   Cranial remolding orthosis, rigid, with soft interface material, custom fabricated, includes fitting and adjustment(s)

S2053   Transplantation of small intestine and liver allografts

S2054   Transplantation of multivisceral organs

S2055   Harvesting of donor multivisceral organs, with preparation and maintenance of allografts; from cadaver donor

S2060   Lobar lung transplantation

S2061   Donor lobectomy (lung) for transplantation, living donor

S2065   Simultaneous pancreas kidney transplantation

● **S2068**   Breast reconstruction with deep inferior epigastric perforator (diep) flap, including microvascular anastomosis and closure of donor site, unilateral

S2070   Cystourethroscopy, with ureteroscopy and/or pyeloscopy; with endoscopic laser treatment of ureteral calculi (includes ureteral catheterization)

● **S2075**   Laparoscopy, surgical; repair incisional or ventral hernia

● S2076   repair umbilical hernia

● S2077   implantation of mesh or other prosthesis for incisional or ventral hernia repair (list separately in addition to code for incisional or ventral hernia repair)

● S2078   Laparoscopic supracervical hysterectomy (subtotal hysterectomy), with or without removal of tube(s), with or without removal of ovary(s)

● S2079   Laparoscopic esophagomyotomy (heller type)

S2080   Laser-assisted uvulopalatoplasty (laup)

(S2082)   Code deleted December 31, 2005

S2083   Adjustment of gastric band diameter via subcutaneous port by injection or aspiration of saline

(S2085)   Code deleted December 31, 2004; use CPT

(S2090)   Code deleted December 31, 2005

(S2091)   Code deleted December 31, 2005

S2095   Transcatheter occlusion or embolization for tumor destruction, percutaneous, any method, using yttrium-90 microspheres

S2102   Islet cell tissue transplant from pancreas; allogenic

S2103   Adrenal tissue transplant to brain

S2107   Adoptive immunotherapy i.e., development of specific anti-tumor reactivity (e.g. tumor-infiltrating lymphocyte therapy) per course of treatment

S2112   Arthroscopy, knee, surgical for harvesting cartilage (chondrocyte cells)

(S2113)   Code deleted December 31, 2004; use CPT

● S2114   Arthroscopy, shoulder, surgical; tenodesis of biceps

S2115   Osteotomy, periacetabular, with internal fixation

● **S2117**   Arthroereisis, subtalar

S2120   Low density lipoprotein (LDL) apheresis using heparin-induced extracorporeal LDL precipitation

(S2130)   Code deleted December 31, 2004; use CPT

(S2131)   Code deleted December 31, 2004; use CPT

S2135   Neurolysis, by injection, of metatarsal neuroma/ interdigital neuritis, any interspace of the foot

S2140   Cord blood harvesting for transplantation, allogenic

S2142   Cord blood-derived stem cell transplantation, allogenic

S2150   Bone marrow or blood-derived stem cells (peripheral or umbilical), allogeneic or autologous, harvesting, transplantation, and related complications; including: pheresis and cell preparation/storage; marrow ablative therapy; drugs, supplies, hospitalization with outpatient follow-up; medical/surgical, diagnostic, emergency, and rehabilitative services; and the number of days of pre- and post-transplant care in the global definition

S2152   Solid organ(s), complete or segmental, single organ or combination of organs; deceased or living donor(s), procurement, transplantation, and related complications; including: drugs; supplies; hospitalization with outpatient follow-up; medical/surgical, diagnostic, emergency, and rehabilitative services, and the number of days of pre- and post-transplant care in the global definition

S2202   Echosclerotherapy

S2205   Minimally invasive direct coronary artery bypass surgery involving mini-thoracotomy or mini-sternotomy surgery, performed under direct vision; using arterial graft(s), single coronary arterial graft

S2206   using arterial graft(s), two coronary arterial grafts

S2207   using venous graft only, single coronary venous graft

S2208   using single arterial and venous graft(s), single venous graft

---

	Not valid for Medicare		Non-covered by Medicare		Special coverage instructions		Carrier discretion

S2209   using two arterial grafts and single venous graft

(S2211)   Code deleted December 31, 2004; use CPT

S2213   Implantation of gastric electrical stimulation device

S2225   Myringotomy, laser-assisted

S2230   Implantation of magnetic component of semi-implantable hearing device on ossicles in middle ear

S2235   Implantation of auditory brain stem implant

S2250   Uterine artery embolization for uterine fibroids

(S2255)   Code deleted December 31, 2004; use CPT

S2260   Induced abortion, 17 to 24 weeks, any surgical method

S2262   Abortion for maternal indication, 25 weeks or greater

S2265   Abortion for fetal indication, 25-28 weeks

S2266   Abortion for fetal indication, 29-31 weeks

S2267   Abortion for fetal indication, 32 weeks or greater

S2300   Arthroscopy, shoulder, surgical; with thermally-induced capsulorrhaphy

S2340   Chemodenervation of abductor muscle(s) of vocal cord

S2341   Chemodenervation of adductor muscle(s) of vocal cord

S2342   Nasal endoscopy for post-operative debridement following functional endoscopic sinus surgery, nasal and/or sinus cavity(s), unilateral or bilateral

S2348   Decompression procedure, percutaneous, of nucleus pulposus of intervertebral disc, using radiofrequency energy, single or multiple levels, lumbar

S2350   Diskectomy, anterior, with decompression of spinal cord and/or nerve root(s), including osteophytectomy; lumbar, single interspace

S2351 Diskectomy, anterior, with decompression of spinal cord and/or nerve root(s), including osteophytectomy; lumbar, each additional interspace (list separately in addition to code for primary procedure)

S2360 Percutaneous vertebroplasty, one vertebral body, unilateral or bilateral injection; cervical

S2361 Each additional cervical vertebral body (list separately in addition to code for primary procedure)

S2362 Kyphoplasty, one vertebral body, unilateral or bilateral injection

S2363 Kyphoplasty, one vertebral body, unilateral or bilateral injection; each additional vertebral body (list separately in addition to code for primary procedure)

(S2370) Code deleted September 30, 2004

(S2371) Code deleted September 30, 2004

S2400 Repair, congenital diaphragmatic hernia in the fetus using temporary tracheal occlusion, procedure performed in utero

S2401 Repair, urinary tract obstruction in the fetus, procedure performed in utero

S2402 Repair, congenital cystic adenomatoid malformation in the fetus, procedure performed in utero

S2403 Repair, extralobar pulmonary sequestration in the fetus, procedure performed in utero

S2404 Repair, myelomeningocele in the fetus, procedure performed in utero

S2405 Repair of sacrococcygeal teratoma in the fetus, procedure performed in utero

S2409 Repair, congenital malformation of fetus, procedure performed in utero, not otherwise classified

S2411 Fetoscopic laser therapy for treatment of twin-to-twin transfusion syndrome

Not valid for Medicare   Non-covered by Medicare   Special coverage instructions   Carrier discretion

● **S2900** Surgical techniques requiring use of robotic surgical system (list separately in addition to code for primary procedure)

S3000 Diabetic indicator; retinal eye exam, dilated, bilateral

● **S3005** Performance measurement, evaluation of patient self assessment, depression

S3600 Stat laboratory request (situations other than S3601)

S3601 Emergency stat laboratory charge for patient who is homebound or residing in a nursing facility

S3620 Newborn metabolic screening panel, includes test kit, postage and the following tests: hemoglobin; electrophoresis; hydroxyprogesterone; 17-D; phenalanine (PKU); and thyroxine, total

S3625 Maternal serum triple marker screen including alpha-fetoprotein (AFP), estriol, and human chorionic gonadotropin (HCG)

● **S3626** Maternal serum quadruple marker screen including alpha-fetoprotein (AFP), estriol, human chorionic gonadotropin (HCG) and inhibin a

S3630 Eosinophil count, blood, direct

S3645 HIV-1 antibody testing of oral mucosal transudate

S3650 Saliva test, hormone level; during menopause

S3652 to assess preterm labor risk

S3655 Antisperm antibodies test (immunobead)

S3701 Immunoassay for nuclear matrix protein 22 (NMP-22), quantitative

S3708 Gastrointestinal fat absorption study

S3818 Complete gene sequence analysis; BRCA1 gene

S3819 Complete gene sequense analysis; BRCA2 gene

S3820 Complete BRCA1 and BRCA2 gene sequence analysis for susceptibility to breast and ovarian cancer

S3822 Single mutation analysis (in individual with a known BRCA1 or BRCA2 mutation in the family) for susceptibility to breast and ovarian cancer

S3823 Three-mutation BRCA1 and BRCA2 analysis for susceptibility to breast and ovarian cancer in Ashkenazi individuals

S3828 Complete gene sequence analysis; MLH1 gene

S3829 MSH2 gene

S3830 Complete mlh1 and mlh2 gene sequence analysis for hereditary nonpolyposis colorectal cancer (HNPCC) genetic testing

S3831 Single-mutation analysis (in individual with a known mlh1 and mlh2 mutation in the family) for hereditary nonpolyposis colorectal cancer (HNPCC) genetic testing

S3833 Complete APC gene sequence analysis for susceptibility to familial adenomatous polyposis (FAP) and attenuated FAP

S3834 Single-mutation analysis (in individuals with a known APC mutation in the family) for susceptibility to familial adenomatous polyposis (FAP) and attenuated FAP

S3835 Complete gene sequence analysis for cystic fibrosis genetic testing

S3837 Complete gene sequence analysis for hemochromatosis genetic testing

S3840 DNA analysis for germline mutations of the RET proto-oncogene for susceptibility to multiple endocrine neoplasia type 2

S3841 Genetic testing for retinoblastoma

S3842 Genetic testing for von Hippel-Lindau disease

S3843 DNA analysis of the F5 gene for susceptibility to Factor V Leiden thrombophilia

---

Not valid for Medicare   Non-covered by Medicare   Special coverage instructions   Carrier discretion   **355**

S3844   DNA analysis of the connexin 26 gene (GJB2) for susceptibility to congenital, profound deafness

S3845   Genetic testing for alpha-thalassemia

S3846   Genetic testing for hemoglobin E beta-thalassemia

S3847   Genetic testing for Tay-Sachs disease

S3848   Genetic testing for Gaucher disease

S3849   Genetic testing for Niemann-Pick disease

S3850   Genetic testing for sickle cell anemia

S3851   Genetic testing for Canavan disease

S3852   DNA analysis for APOE epsilon 4 allele for susceptibility to Alzheimer's disease

S3853   Genetic testing for myotonic muscular dystrophy

● S3854   Gene expression profiling panel for use in the management of breast cancer treatment

S3890   DNA analysis, fecal, for colorectal cancer screening

S3900   Surface electromyography (EMG)

S3902   Ballistocardiogram

S3904   Masters two step

S4005   Interim labor facility global (labor occurring but not resulting in delivery)

S4011   In vitro fertilization; including but not limited to identification and incubation of mature oocytes, fertilization with sperm, incubation of embryo(s), and subsequent visualization for determination of development

S4013   Complete cycle, gamete intrafallopian transfer (GIFT), case rate

S4014   Complete cycle, zygote intrafallopian transfer (ZIFT), case rate

S4015 Complete in vitro fertilization cycle, case rate not otherwise specified

S4016 Frozen in vitro fertilization cycle, case rate

S4017 Incomplete cycle, treatment canceled prior to stimulation, case rate

S4018 Frozen embryo transfer procedure canceled before transfer, case rate

S4020 In vitro fertilization procedure canceled before aspiration, case rate

S4021 In vitro fertilization procedure canceled after aspiration, case rate

S4022 Assisted oocyte fertilization, case rate

S4023 Donor egg cycle, incomplete, case rate

S4025 Donor services for in vitro fertilization (sperm or embryo), case rate

S4026 Procurement of donor sperm from sperm bank

S4027 Storage of previously frozen embryos

S4028 Microsurgical epididymal sperm aspiration (mesa)

S4030 Sperm procurement and cryopreservation services; initial visit

S4031 Sperm procurement and cryopreservation services; subsequent visit

S4035 Stimulated intrauterine insemination (IU), case rate

S4036 Intravaginal culture (IVC), case rate

S4037 Cryopreserved embryo transfer, case rate

S4040 Monitoring and storage of cryopreserved embryos, per 30 days

S4042 Management of ovulation induction (interpretation of diagnostic tests and studies, non-face-to-face medical management of the patient), per cycle

S4981 Insertion of levonorgestrel-releasing intrauterine system

S4989 Contraceptive intrauterine device (e.g., progestacert IUD), including implants and supplies

S4990 Nicotine patches, legend

S4991 Nicotine patches, non-legend

S4993 Contraceptive pills for birth control

S4995 Smoking cessation gum

S5000 Prescription drug, generic

S5001 Prescription drug, brand name

S5010 5% dextrose and 0.45% normal saline, 1000 ml

S5011 5% dextrose in lactated ringer's, 1000 ml

S5012 5% dextrose with potassium chloride, 1000 ml

S5013 5% dextrose/0..45% normal saline with potassium chloride and magnesium sulfate, 1000 ml

S5014 5% dextrose/0.45% normal saline with potassium chloride and magnesium sulfate, 1500 ml

S5035 Home infusion therapy, routine service of infusion device (e.g., pump maintenance)

S5036 Home infusion therapy, repair of infusion device (e.g., pump repair)

S5100 Day care services, adult; per 15 minutes

S5101 per half day

S5102 per diem

● New code ▲ Revised code ( ) Deleted code

S5105 Day care services, center-based; services not included in program fee, per diem

S5108 Home care training to home care client; per 15 minutes

S5109 per session

S5110 Home care training, family; per 15 minutes

S5111 per session

S5115 Home care training, non-family; per 15 minutes

S5116 per session

S5120 Chore services; per 15 minutes

S5121 per diem

S5125 Attendant care services; per 15 minutes

S5126 per diem

S5130 Homemaker service, NOS; per 15 minutes

S5131 per diem

S5135 Companion care, adult (e.g., IADL/ADL); per 15 minutes

S5136 per diem

S5140 Foster care, adult, per diem

S5141 per month

S5145 Foster care, therapeutic, child; per diem

S5146 per month

S5150 Unskilled respite care, not hospice; per 15 minutes

S5151 per diem

S5160 Emergency response system; installation and testing

S5161   service fee, per month (excludes installation and testing)

S5162   purchase only

S5165   Home modifications; per service

S5170   Home delivered meals, including preparation; per meal

S5175   Laundry service, external, professional; per order

S5180   Home health respiratory therapy, initial evaluation

S5181   Home health respiratory therapy NOS, per diem

S5185   Medication reminder service, non-face-to-face; per month

S5190   Wellness assessment, performed by non-physician

S5199   Personal care item, NOS, each

S5497   Home infusion therapy, catheter care/maintenance, not otherwise classified; includes administrative services, professional pharmacy services, care coordination, and all necessary supplies and equipment (drugs and nursing visits coded separately), per diem

S5498   Home infusion therapy, catheter care/maintenance, simple (single lumen), includes administrative services, professional pharmacy services, care coordination and all necessary supplies and equipment, (drugs and nursing visits coded separately), per diem

S5501   Home infusion therapy, catheter care/maintenance, complex (more than one lumen), includes administrative services, professional pharmacy services, care coordination, and all necessary supplies and equipment (drugs and nursing visits coded separately), per diem

S5502   Home infusion therapy, catheter care/maintenance, implanted access device, includes administrative services, professional pharmacy services, care coordination and all necessary supplies and equipment, (drugs and nursing visits coded separately), per diem (use this code for interim maintenance of vascular access not currently in use)

● New code   ▲ Revised code   ( ) Deleted code

S5517 Home infusion therapy, all supplies necessary for restoration of catheter patency or declotting

S5518 Home infusion therapy, all supplies necessary for catheter repair

S5520 Home infusion therapy, all supplies (including catheter) necessary for a peripherally inserted central venous catheter (PICC) line insertion

S5521 Home infusion therapy, all supplies (including catheter) necessary for a midline catheter insertion

S5522 Home infusion therapy, insertion of peripherally inserted central venous catheter (PICC), nursing services only (no supplies or catheter included)

S5523 Home infusion therapy, insertion of midline central venous catheter, nursing services only (no supplies or catheter included)

S5550 Insulin, rapid onset; 5 units

S5551 Insulin, most rapid onset (lispro or aspart); 5 units

S5552 Insulin, intermediate acting (NPH or lente); 5 units

S5553 Insulin, long acting; 5 units

S5560 Insulin delivery device, reusable pen; 1.5 ml size

S5561 Insulin delivery device, reusable pen; 3 ml size

S5565 Insulin cartridge for use in insulin delivery device other than pump; 150 units

S5566 Insulin cartridge for use in insulin delivery device other than pump; 300 units

S5570 Insulin delivery device, disposable pen (including insulin); 1.5 ml size

S5571 Insulin delivery device, disposable pen (including insulin); 3 ml size

(S8004) Code deleted March 31, 2005; use 78804

S8030   Scleral application of tantalum ring(s) for localization of lesions for proton beam therapy

S8035   Magnetic source imaging

S8037   Magnetic resonance cholangiopancreatography (MRCP)

S8040   Topographic brain mapping

S8042   Magnetic resonance imaging (MRI), low-field

S8049   Intraoperative radiation therapy (single administration)

S8055   Ultrasound guidance for multifetal pregnancy reduction(s), technical component (only to be used when the physician doing the reduction procedure does not perform the ultrasound, guidance is included in the CPT code for multifetal pregnancy reduction - 59866)

S8075   Computer analysis of full-field digital mammogram and further physician review for interpretation, mammography (List separately in addition to code for primary procedure)

S8080   Scintimammography (radioimmunoscintigraphy of the breast), unilateral, including supply of radiopharmaccutical

S8085   Fluorine-18 fluorodeoxyglucose (F-18 FDG) imaging using dual-head coincidence detection system (non-dedicated PET scan)

S8092   Electron beam computed tomography (also known as ultrafast CT, cine CT)

S8093   CT angiography, coronary arteries, with contrast material

(S8095) Code deleted December 31, 2005

S8096   Portable peak flow meter

S8097   Asthma kit (including but not limited to portable peak expiratory flow meter, instructional video, brochure, and/or spacer)

S8100   Holding chamber or spacer for use with an inhaler or nebulizer; without mask

S8101   with mask

S8110   Peak expiratory flow rate (physician services)

S8120   Oxygen contents, gaseous, 1 unit equals 1 cubic foot

S8121   Oxygen contents, liquid, 1 unit equals 1 pound

(S8182) Code deleted December 31, 2004; use CPT

(S8183) Code deleted December 31, 2004; use CPT

S8185   Flutter device

S8186   Swivel adaptor

S8189   Tracheostomy supply, not otherwise classified

S8190   Electronic spirometer (or microspirometer)

S8210   Mucus trap

S8260   Oral orthotic for treatment of sleep apnea, includes fitting, fabrication, and materials

S8262   Mandibular orthopedic repositioning device, each

S8265   Haberman feeder for cleft lip/palate

● S8270 Enuresis alarm, using auditory buzzer and/or vibration device

S8301   Infection control supplies, not otherwise specified

S8415   Supplies for home delivery of infant

S8420   Gradient pressure aid (sleeve and glove combination), custom made

S8421   Gradient pressure aid (sleeve and glove combination), ready made

S8422   Gradient pressure aid (sleeve), custom made, medium weight

S8423   Gradient pressure aid (sleeve), custom made, heavy weight

S8424	Gradient pressure aid (sleeve), ready made
S8425	Gradient pressure aid (glove), custom made, medium weight
S8426	Gradient pressure aid (glove), custom made, heavy weight
S8427	Gradient pressure aid (glove), ready made
S8428	Gradient pressure aid (gauntlet), ready made
S8429	Gradient pressure exterior wrap
S8430	Padding for compression bandage, roll
S8431	Compression bandage, roll
S8450	Splint, prefabricated, digit (specify digit by use of modifier)
S8451	Splint, prefabricated, wrist or ankle
S8452	Splint, prefabricated, elbow
S8460	Camisole, post mastectomy
S8490	Insulin syringes (100 syringes, any size)
● S8940	Equestrian/hippotherapy, per session
S8948	Application of a modality (requiring constant provider attendance) to one or more areas, low-level laser, each 15 minutes
S8950	Complex lymphedema therapy, each 15 min
S8990	Physical or manipulative therapy performed for maintenance rather than restoration
S8999	Resuscitation bag (for use by patient on artificial respiration during power failure or other catastrophic event)
S9001	Home uterine monitor with or without associated nursing services

S9007 Ultrafiltration monitor

S9015 Automated EEG monitoring

S9022 Digital subraction angiography (use in addition to CPT code for the procedure for further identification)

S9024 Paranasal sinus ultrasound

S9025 Omnicardiogram/cardiointegram

S9034 Extracorporeal shockwave lithotripsy for gall stones (if performed with ERCP, use 43265)

S9055 Procuren or other growth factor preparation to promote wound healing

S9056 Coma stimulation per diem

S9061 Home administration of aerosolized drug therapy (e.g., pentamidine); administative services, professional pharmacy services, care coordination, all necesary supplies and equipment (drugs and nursing visits coded separately), per diem

S9075 Smoking cessation treatment

S9083 Global fee urgent care centers

S9088 Services provided in an urgent care center (list in addition to code for service)

S9090 Vertebral axial decompression, per session

S9092 Canolith repositioning, per visit

S9098 Home visit, phototherapy services (e.g., Bili-lite), including equipment rental, nursing services, blood draw, supplies, and other services, per diem

S9109 Congestive heart failure telemonitoring, equipment rental, including telescale, computer system and software, telephone connections, and maintenance, per month

S9117 Back school, per visit

	Not valid for Medicare		Non-covered by Medicare		Special coverage instructions		Carrier discretion

S9122 Home health aide or certified nurse assistant, providing care in the home; per hour

S9123 Nursing care, in the home; by registered nurse, per hour (use for general nursing care only, not to be used when CPT codes 99500-99602 can be used)

S9124 by licensed practical nurse, per hour

S9125 Respite care, in the home, per diem

S9126 Hospice care, in the home, per diem

S9127 Social work visit, in the home, per diem

S9128 Speech therapy, in the home, per diem

S9129 Occupational therapy, in the home, per diem

S9131 Physical therapy; in the home, per diem

S9140 Diabetic management program; follow-up visit to non-MD provider

S9141 follow-up visit to MD provider

S9145 Insulin pump initiation, instruction in initial use of pump (pump not included)

S9150 Evaluation by ocularist

S9208 Home management of pre-term labor, including administrative services, professional pharmacy services, care coordination, and all necessary supplies or equipment (drugs and nursing visits coded separately), per diem (do not use this code with any home infusion per diem code)

S9209 Home management of pre-term premature rupture of membranes (PPROM), including administrative services, professional pharmacy services, care coordination, and all necessary supplies or equipment (drugs and nursing visits coded separately), per diem (do not use this code with any home infusion per diem code)

S9211 Home management of gestational hypertension, includes administrative services, professional pharmacy services, care coordination and all necessary supplies and equipment (drugs and nursing visits coded separately); per diem (do not use this code with any home infusion per diem code)

S9212 Home management of postpartum hypertension, includes administrative services, professional pharmacy services, care coordination, and all necessary supplies and equipment (drugs and nursing visits coded separately), per diem (do not use this code with any home infusion per diem code)

S9213 Home management of preeclampsia, includes administrative services, professional pharmacy services, care coordination, and all necessary supplies and equipment (drugs and nursing services coded separately); per diem (do not use this code with any home infusion per diem code)

S9214 Home management of gestational diabetes, includes administrative services, professional pharmacy services, care coordination, and all necessary supplies and equipment (drugs and nursing visits coded separately); per diem (do not use this code with any home infusion per diem code)

S9325 Home infusion therapy, pain management infusion; administrative services, professional pharmacy services, care coordination, and all necessary supplies and equipment, (drugs and nursing visits coded separately), per diem (do not use this code with S9326, S9327 or S9328)

S9326 Home infusion therapy, continuous (twenty-four hours or more) pain management infusion; administrative services, professional pharmacy services, care coordination and all necessary supplies and equipment (drugs and nursing visits coded separately), per diem

S9327 Home infusion therapy, intermittent (less than twenty-four hours) pain management infusion; administrative services, professional pharmacy services, care coordination, and all necessary supplies and equipment (drugs and nursing visits coded separately), per diem

Not valid for Medicare | Non-covered by Medicare | Special coverage instructions | Carrier discretion

S9328 Home infusion therapy, implanted pump pain management infusion; administrative services, professional pharmacy services, care coordination, and all necessary supplies and equipment (drugs and nursing visits coded separately), per diem

S9329 Home infusion therapy, chemotherapy infusion; administrative services, professional pharmacy services, care coordination, and all necessary supplies and equipment (drugs and nursing visits coded separately), per diem (do not use this code with S9330 or S9331)

S9330 Home infusion therapy, continuous (twenty-four hours or more) chemotherapy infusion; administrative services, professional pharmacy services, care coordination, and all necessary supplies and equipment (drugs and nursing visits coded separately), per diem

S9331 Home infusion therapy, intermittent (less than twenty-four hours) chemotherapy infusion; administrative services, professional pharmacy services, care coordination, and all necessary supplies and equipment (drugs and nursing visits coded separately), per diem

S9335 Home therapy, hemodialysis; administrative services, professional pharmacy services, care coordination, and all necessary supplies and equipment (drugs and nursing services coded separately), per diem

S9336 Home infusion therapy, continuous anticoagulant infusion therapy (e.g., Heparin), administrative services, professional pharmacy services, care coordination and all necessary supplies and equipment (drugs and nursing visits coded separately), per diem

S9338 Home infusion therapy, immunotherapy (e.g., intravenous immunoglobulin, interferon); administrative services, professional pharmacy services, care coordination, and all necessary supplies and equipment (drugs and nursing visits coded separately), per diem

S9339 Home therapy; peritoneal dialysis, administrative services, professional pharmacy services, care coordination and all necessary supplies and equipment (drugs and nursing visits coded separately), per diem

S9340 Home therapy; enteral nutrition; administrative services, professional pharmacy services, care coordination, and all necessary supplies and equipment (enteral formula and nursing visits coded separately), per diem

S9341 Home therapy; enteral nutrition via gravity; administrative services, professional pharmacy services, care coordination, and all necessary supplies and equipment (enteral formula and nursing visits coded separately), per diem

S9342 Home therapy; enteral nutrition via pump; administrative services, professional pharmacy services, care coordination, and all necessary supplies and equipment (enteral formula and nursing visits coded separately), per diem

S9343 Home therapy; enteral nutrition via bolus; administrative services, professional pharmacy services, care coordination, and all necessary supplies and equipment (enteral formula and nursing visits coded separately), per diem

S9345 Home infusion therapy, anti-hemophilic agent infusion therapy (e.g., Factor VIII); administrative services, professional pharmacy services, care coordination, and all necessary supplies and equipment (drugs and nursing visits coded separately), per diem

S9346 Home infusion therapy, alpha-1-proteinase inhibitor (e.g., Prolastin); administrative services, professional pharmacy services, care coordination, and all necessary supplies and equipment (drugs and nursing visits coded separately), per diem

S9347 Home infusion therapy, uninterrupted, long-term, controlled rate intravenous or subcutaneous infusion therapy (e.g. epoprostenol); administrative services, professional pharmacy services, care coordination, and all necessary supplies and equipment (drugs and nursing visits coded separately), per diem

S9348 Home infusion therapy, sympathomimetic/inotropic agent infusion therapy (e.g., Dobutamine); administrative services, professional pharmacy services, care coordination, all necessary supplies and equipment (drugs and nursing visits coded separately), per diem

S9349 Home infusion therapy, tocolytic infusion therapy; administrative services, professional pharmacy services, care coordination, and all necessary supplies and equipment (drugs and nursing visits coded separately), per diem

S9351 Home infusion therapy, continuous anti-emetic infusion therapy; administrative services, professional pharmacy services, care coordination, all necessary supplies and equipment (drugs and nursing visits coded separately), per diem

S9353 Home infusion therapy, continuous insulin infusion therapy; administrative services, professional pharmacy services, care coordination, and all necessary supplies and equipment (drugs and nursing visits coded separately), per diem

S9355 Home infusion therapy, chelation therapy; administrative services, professional pharmacy services, care coordination, and all necessary supplies and equipment (drugs and nursing visits coded separately), per diem

S9357 Home infusion therapy, enzyme replacement intravenous therapy; (e.g., Imiglucerase); administrative services, professional pharmacy services, care coordination, and all necessary supplies and equipment (drugs and nursing visits coded separately), per diem

S9359 Home infusion therapy, anti-tumor necrosis factor intravenous therapy; (e.g., Infliximab); administrative services, professional pharmacy services, care coordination, and all necessary supplies and equipment (drugs and nursing visits coded separately), per diem

S9361 Home infusion therapy, diuretic intravenous therapy; administrative services, professional pharmacy services, care coordination, and all necessary supplies and equipment (drugs and nursing visits coded separately), per diem

S9363 Home infusion therapy, anti-spasmotic intravenous therapy; administrative services, professional pharmacy services, care coordination, and all necessary supplies and equipment (drugs and nursing visits coded separately), per diem

S9364 Home infusion therapy, total parenteral nutrition (TPN); administrative services, professional pharmacy services, care coordination, and all necessary supplies and equipment, including standard TPN formula (lipids, specialty amino acid formulas, drugs other than in standard formula, and nursing visits coded separately) per diem (Do not use with home infusion codes S9365-S9368 using daily volume scales)

S9365 Home infusion therapy, total parenteral nutrition (TPN); one liter per day, administrative services, professional pharmacy services, care coordination, and all necessary supplies and equipment, including standard TPN formula (lipids, specialty amino acid formulas, drugs other than in standard formula, and nursing visits coded separately), per diem

S9366 Home infusion therapy, total parenteral nutrition (TPN); more than one liter but no more than two liters per day, administrative services, professional pharmacy services, care coordination, and all necessary supplies and equipment, including standard TPN formula (lipids, specialty amino acid formulas, drugs other than in standard formula, and nursing visits coded separately), per diem

S9367 Home infusion therapy, total parenteral nutrition (TPN); more than two liters but no more than three liters per day, administrative services, professional pharmacy services, care coordination, and all necessary supplies and equipment, including standard TPN formula (lipids, specialty amino acid formulas, drugs other than in standard formula, and nursing visits coded separately), per diem

S9368 Home infusion therapy, total parenteral nutrition (TPN); more than three liters per day, administrative services, professional pharmacy services, care coordination, and all necessary supplies and equipment, including standard TPN formula (lipids, specialty amino acid formulas, drugs other than in standard formula, and nursing visits coded separately), per diem

S9370 Home therapy, intermittent anti-emetic injection therapy; administrative services, professional pharmacy services, care coordination, and all necessary supplies and equipment (drugs and nursing visits coded separately), per diem

Not valid for Medicare | Non-covered by Medicare | Special coverage instructions | Carrier discretion

S9372 Home therapy; intermittent anticoagulant injection therapy (e.g., heparin); administrative services, professional pharmacy services, care coordination, and all necessary supplies and equipment (drugs and nursing visits coded separately), per diem (do not use this code for flushing of infusion devices with heparin to maintain patency)

S9373 Home infusion therapy, hydration therapy; administrative services, professional pharmacy services, care coordination, and all necessary supplies and equipment (drugs and nursing visits coded separately), per diem (do not use with hydration therapy codes S9374-S9377 using daily volume scales)

S9374 Home infusion therapy, hydration therapy; one liter per day, administrative services, professional pharmacy services, care coordination, and all necessary supplies and equipment (drugs and nursing visits coded separately), per diem

S9375 Home infusion therapy, hydration therapy; more than one liter but no more than two liters per day, administrative services, professional pharmacy services, care coordination, and all necessary supplies and equipment (drugs and nursing visits coded separately), per diem

S9376 Home infusion therapy, hydration therapy; more than two liters but no more than three liters per day, administrative services, professional pharmacy services, care coordination, and all necessary supplies and equipment (drugs and nursing visits coded separately), per diem

S9377 Home infusion therapy, hydration therapy; more than three liters per day, administrative services, professional pharmacy services, care coordination, and all necessary supplies (drugs and nursing visits coded separately), per diem

S9379 Home infusion therapy, infusion therapy, not otherwise classified; administrative services, professional pharmacy services, care coordination, and all necessary supplies and equipment (drugs and nursing visits coded separately), per diem

S9381 Delivery or service to high risk areas requiring escort or extra protection, per visit

S9401 Anticoagulation clinic, inclusive of all services except laboratory tests, per session

S9430 Pharmacy compounding and dispensing services

S9434 Modified solid food supplements for inborn errors of metabolism

S9435 Medical foods for inborn errors of metabolism

S9436 Childbirth preparation/Lamaze classes, non-physician provider, per session

S9437 Childbirth refresher classes, non-physician provider, per session

S9438 Cesarean birth classes, non-physician provider, per session

S9439 VBAC (vaginal birth after cesarean) classes, non-physician provider, per session

S9441 Asthma education, non-physician provider, per session

S9442 Birthing classes, non-physician provider, per session

S9443 Lactation classes, non-physician provider, per session

S9444 Parenting classes, non-physician provider, per session

S9445 Patient education, not otherwise classified, non-physician provider, individual, per session

S9446 Patient education, not otherwise classified, non-physician provider, group, per session

S9447 Infant safety (including CPR) classes, non-physician provider, per session

S9449 Weight management classes, non-physician provider, per session

S9451 Exercise classes, non-physician provider, per session

S9452 Nutrition classes, non-physician provider, per session

S9453 Smoking cessation classes, non-physician provider, per session

S9454 Stress management classes, non-physician provider, per session

S9455 Diabetic management program; group session

S9460 nurse visit

S9465 dietician visit

S9470 Nutritional counseling, dietitian visit

S9472 Cardiac rehabilitation program, non-physician provider, per diem

S9473 Pulmonary rehabilitation program, non-physician provider, per diem

S9474 Enterostomal therapy by a registered nurse certified in enterostomal therapy, per diem

S9475 Ambulatory setting substance abuse treatment or detoxification services, per diem

S9476 Vestibular rehabilitation program, non-physician provider, per diem

S9480 Intensive outpatient psychiatric services, per diem

S9482 Family stabilization services, per 15 minutes

S9484 Crisis intervention mental health services, per hour

S9485 Crisis intervention mental health services, per diem

S9490 Home infusion therapy, corticosteroid infusion; administrative services, professional pharmacy services, care coordination, and all necessary supplies and equipment (drugs and nursing visits coded separately), per diem

S9494 Home infusion therapy, antibiotic, antiviral, or antifungal therapy; administrative services, professional pharmacy services, care coordination, and all necessary supplies and equipment (drugs and nursing visits coded separately), per diem (do not use with home infusion codes for hourly dosing schedules S9497-S9504)

S9497 Home infusion therapy, antibiotic, antiviral, or antifungal therapy; once every 3 hours; administrative services, professional pharmacy services, care coordination, and all necessary supplies and equipment (drugs and nursing visits coded separately), per diem

S9500 Home infusion therapy, antibiotic, antiviral, or antifungal therapy; once every 24 hours; administrative services, professional pharmacy services, care coordination, and all necessary supplies and equipment (drugs and nursing visits coded separately), per diem

S9501 Home infusion therapy, antibiotic, antiviral, or antifungal therapy; once every 12 hours; administrative services, professional pharmacy services, care coordination, and all necessary supplies and equipment (drugs and nursing visits coded separately), per diem

S9502 Home infusion therapy, antibiotic, antiviral, or antifungal therapy; once every 8 hours, administrative services, professional pharmacy services, care coordination, and all necessary supplies and equipment (drugs and nursing visits coded separately), per diem

S9503 Home infusion therapy, antibiotic, antiviral, or antifungal; once every 6 hours; administrative services, professional pharmacy services, care coordination, and all necessary supplies and equipment (drugs and nursing visits coded separately), per diem

S9504 Home infusion therapy, antibiotic, antiviral, or antifungal; once every 4 hours; administrative services, professional pharmacy services, care coordination, and all necessary supplies and equipment (drugs and nursing visits coded separately), per diem

S9529 Routine venipuncture for collection of specimen(s), single home bound, nursing home, or skilled nursing facility patient

S9537 Home therapy, hematopoietic hormone injection therapy (e.g., erythropoietin, G-CSF, GM-CSF); administrative services, professional pharmacy services, care coordination, and all necessary supplies and equipment (drugs and nursing visits coded separately), per diem

S9538 Home transfusion of blood product(s); administrative services, professional pharmacy services, care coordination and all necessary supplies and equipment (blood products, drugs, and nursing visits coded separately), per diem

S9542 Home injectable therapy; not otherwise classified, including administrative services, professional pharmacy services, care coordination, and all necessary supplies and equipment (drugs and nursing visits coded separately), per diem

S9558 Home injectable therapy; growth hormone, including administrative services, professional pharmacy services, care coordination, and all necessary supplies and equipment (drugs and nursing visits coded separately), per diem

S9559 Home injectable therapy; interferon, including administrative services, professional pharmacy services, care coordination, and all necessary supplies and equipment (drugs and nursing visits coded separately), per diem

S9560 Home injectable therapy; hormonal therapy (e.g., leuprolide, goserelin), including administrative services, professional pharmacy services, care coordination, and all necessary supplies and equipment (drugs and nursing visits coded separately), per diem

S9562 Home injectable therapy, palivizumab, including administrative services, professional pharmacy services, care coordination, and all necessary supplies and equipment (drugs and nursing visits coded separately), per diem

S9590 Home therapy, irrigation therapy (e.g. Sterile irrigation of an organ or anatomical cavity); including administrative services, professional pharmacy services, care coordination, and all necessary supplies and equipment (drugs and nursing visits coded separately), per diem

S9810 Home therapy; professional pharmacy services for provision of infusion, specialty drug administration, and/or disease state management, not otherwise classified, per hour (do not use this code with any per diem code)

S9900 Services by authorized Christian Science Practitioner for the process of healing, per diem. Not to be used for rest or study. Excludes in-patient services.

S9970 Health club membership, annual

S9975 Transplant related lodging, meals, and transportation, per diem

S9976 Lodging, per diem, not otherwise classified

S9977 Meals, per diem, not otherwise specified

S9981 Medical records copying fee, administrative

S9982 Medical records copying fee, per page

S9986 Not medically necessary service (patient is aware that service not medically necessary)

S9988 Services provided as part of a phase I clinical trial

S9989 Services provided outside of the United States of America (list in addition to code(s) for services(s))

S9990 Services provided as part of a phase II clinical trial

S9991 Services provided as part of a phase III clinical trial

S9992 Transportation costs to and from trial location and local transportation costs (e.g., fares for taxicab or bus) for clinical trial participant and one caregiver/companion

S9994 Lodging costs (e.g., hotel charges) for clinical trial participant and one caregiver/companion

S9996 Meals for clinical trial participant and one caregiver/companion

S9999 Sales tax

STATE MEDICAID AGENCY CODES

Guidelines

"T" codes were added to HCPCS in 2002. These codes are exclusively for the use of state Medicaid agencies. Prior to using "T" codes on health insurance claims to your state Medicaid processor, you should verify that these codes are acceptable. "T" codes are not valid for Medicare use.

In addition to the information presented in the INTRODUCTION, several other items unique to this section are defined or identified here.

1. SPECIAL REPORT: A service, material or supply that is rarely provided, unusual, variable or new may require a special report in determining medical appropriateness for reimbursement purposes. Pertinent information should include an adequate definition or description of the nature, extent, and need for the service, material or supply.

2. MODIFIERS: Listed services may be modified under certain circumstances. When appropriate, the modifying circumstance is identified by adding a modifier to the basic procedure code. CPT and HCPCS National Level II modifiers may be used with CPT and HCPCS National Level II procedure codes.

State Medicaid Agency Codes

T1000 Private duty/independent nursing service(s), licensed, up to 15 minutes

T1001 Nursing assessment/evaluation

T1002 RN services, up to 15 minutes

T1003 LPN/LVN services, up to 15 minutes

T1004 Services of a qualified nursing aide, up to 15 minutes

T1005 Respite care services, up to 15 minutes

T1006 Alcohol and/or substance abuse services, family/couple counseling

T1007 Alcohol and/or substance abuse services, treatment plan development and/or modification

T1009 Child sitting services for children of the individual receiving alcohol and/or substance abuse services

T1010 Meals for individuals receiving alcohol and/or substance abuse services (when meals are not included in the program)

T1012 Alcohol and/or substance abuse services, skills development

T1013 Sign language or oral interpreter services, per 15 minutes

T1014 Telehealth transmission, per minute, professional services bill separately

T1015 Clinic visit/encounter, all-inclusive

T1016 Case management, each 15 mintues

T1017 Targeted case management, each 15 minutes

T1018 School-based individualized education program (IEP) services, bundled

T1019 Personal care services, per 15 minutes, not for an inpatient or resident of a hospital, nursing facility, ICF/MR or IMD, part of the individualized plan of treatment (code may not be used to identify services provided by home health aide or certified nurse assistant)

T1020 Personal care services, per diem, not for an inpatient or resident of a hospital, nursing facility, ICF/MR or IMD, part of the individualized plan of treatment (code may not be used to identify services provided by home health aide or certified nurse assistant)

T1021 Home health aide or certified nurse assistant, per visit

T1022 Contracted home health agency services, all services provided under contract, per day

T1023 Screening to determine the appropriateness of consideration of an individual for participation in a specified program, project or treatment protocol, per encounter

T1024 Evaluation and treatment by an integrated, specialty team contracted to provide coordinated care to multiple or severely handicapped children, per encounter

T1025 Intensive, extended multidisciplinary services provided in a clinic setting to children with complex medical, physical, medical and psychosocial impairments, per diem

T1026 Intensive, extended multidisciplinary services provided in a clinic setting to children with complex medical, physical, medical and psychosocial impairments, per hour

T1027 Family training and counseling for child development, per 15 mintues

T1028 Assessment of home, physical and family environment, to determine suitability to meet patient's medical needs

T1029 Comprehensive environmental lead investigation, not including laboratory analysis, per dwelling

T1030 Nursing care, in the home, by registered nurse, per diem

T1031 Nursing care, in the home, by licensed practical nurse, per diem

(T1500) Code deleted December 31, 2004; use CPT

T1502 Administration of oral, intramuscular and/or subcutaneous medication by health care agency/professional, per visit

T1999 Miscellaneous therapeutic items and supplies, retail purchases, not otherwise classified. Identify product in "remarks."

T2001 Non-emergency transportation; patient attendant/escort

T2002 Non-emergency tranportation; per diem

T2003 Non-emergency transportation; encounter/trip

T2004   Non-emergency transportation; commercial carrier, multi-pass

T2005   Non-emergency transportation; stretcher van

(T2006)   Code deleted December 31, 2005; use A0998

T2007   Transportation waiting time, air ambulance, and non-emergency vehicle, one-half (1/2) hour increments

T2010   Preadmission screening and resident review (PASRR) Level I Identification Screening, per screen

T2011   Preadmission screening and resident review (PASRR) Level II Evaluation, per evaluation

T2012   Habilitation, educational, waiver; per diem

T2013   Habilitation, educational, waiver; per hour

T2014   Habilitation, prevocational, waiver; per diem

T2015   Habilitation, prevocational, waiver; per hour

T2016   Habilitation, residential, waiver; per diem

T2017   Habilitation, residential, waiver; per hour

T2018   Habilitation, supported employment, waiver; per diem

T2019   Habilitation, supported employment, wiaver; per 15 minutes

T2020   Day habilitation, waiver; per diem

T2021   Day habilitation, waiver; per 15 minutes

T2022   Case management; per month

T2023   Targeted case management; per month

T2024   Service assessment/plan of care development, waiver

T2025   Waiver services; not otherwise specified (NOS)

T2026   Specialized childcare, waiver; per diem

T2027 Specialized childcare, waiver; per 15 minutes

T2028 Specialized supply, not otherwise specified, waiver

T2029 Specialized medical equipment, not otherwise specified, waiver

T2030 Assisted living, waiver; per month

T2031 Assisted living, waiver; per diem

T2032 Residential care, not otherwise specified (NOS), waiver; per month

T2033 Residential care, not otherwise specified (NOS), waiver; per diem

T2034 Crisis intervention waiver; per diem

T2035 Utility services to support medical equipment and assistive technology/devices, waiver

T2036 Therapeutic camping, overnight, waiver; each session

T2037 Therapeutic camping, day, waiver; each session

T2038 Community transition, waiver; per service

T2039 Vehicle modifications, waiver; per service

T2040 Financial management, self-directed, waiver; per 15 minutes

T2041 Supports brokerage, self-directed, waiver; per 15 minutes

T2042 Hospice routine home care; per diem

T2043 Hospice continuous home care; per hour

T2044 Hospice inpatient respite care; per diem

T2045 Hospice general inpatient care; per diem

T2046 Hospice long term care, room and board only; per diem

T2048 Behavioral health; long-term care residential (non-acute care in a residential treatment program where stay is typically longer than 30 days), with room and board, per diem

T2049 Non-emergency transportation; stretcher van, mileage; per mile

T2101 Human breast milk processing, storage and distribution only

T4521 Adult sized disposable incontinence product, brief/diaper, small, each
CIM: 60-9

T4522 Adult sized disposable incontinence product, brief/diaper, medium, each
CIM: 60-9

T4523 Adult sized disposable incontinence product, brief/diaper, large, each
CIM: 60-9

T4524 Adult sized disposable incontinence product, brief/diaper, extra large, each
CIM: 60-9

T4525 Adult sized disposable incontinence product, protective underwear/pull-on, small size, each
CIM: 60-9

T4526 Adult sized disposable incontinence product, protective underwear/pull-on, medium size, each
CIM: 60-9

T4527 Adult sized disposable incontinence product, protective underwear/pull-on, large size, each
CIM: 60-9

T4528 Adult sized disposable incontinence product, protective underwear/pull-on, extra large size, each
CIM: 60-9

T4529 Pediatric sized disposable incontinence product, brief/diaper, small/medium size, each
CIM: 60-9

T4530 Pediatric sized disposable incontinence product, brief/diaper, large size, each
CIM: 60-9

● New code   ▲ Revised code   ( ) Deleted code

T4531 Pediatric sized disposable incontinence product, protective underwear/pull-on, small/medium size, each
CIM: 60-9

T4532 Pediatric sized disposable incontinence product, protective underwear/pull-on, large size, each
CIM: 60-9

T4533 Youth sized disposable incontinence product, brief/diaper, each
CIM: 60-9

T4534 Youth sized disposable incontinence product, protective underwear/pull-on, each
CIM: 60-9

T4535 Disposable liner/shield/guard/pad/undergarment, for incontinence, each
CIM: 60-9

T4536 Incontinence product, protective underwear/pull-on, reusable, any size, each
CIM: 60-9

T4537 Incontinence product, protective underpad, reusable, bed size, each
CIM: 60-9

T4538 Diaper service, reusable diaper, each diaper
CIM: 60-9

T4539 Incontinence product, diaper/brief, reusable, any size, each
CIM: 60-9

T4540 Incontinence product, protective underpad, reusable, chair size, each
CIM: 60-9

T4541 Incontinence product, disposable underpad, large, each

T4542 Incontinence product, disposable underpad, small size, each

T5001 Positioning seat for persons with special orthopedic needs, for use in vehicles

T5999 Supply, not otherwise specified

● New code   ▲ Revised code   ( ) Deleted code

VISION SERVICES

Guidelines

In addition to the information presented in the INTRODUCTION, several other items unique to this section are defined or identified here:

1. SUBSECTION INFORMATION: Some of the listed subheadings or subsections have special needs or instructions unique to that section. Where these are indicated, special "notes" will be presented preceding or following the listings. Those subsections within the VISION SERVICES section that have "notes" are as follows:

Subsection	Code Numbers
Spectacle lenses	V2100-V2499
Contact lenses	V2500-V2599
Low vision aids	V2600-V2615

2. UNLISTED SERVICE OR PROCEDURE: A service or procedure may be provided that is not listed in this edition of HCPCS. When reporting such a service, the appropriate "unlisted procedure" code may be used to indicate the service, identifying it by "special report" as defined below. HCPCS terminology is inconsistent in defining unlisted procedures. The procedure definition may include the term(s) "unlisted", "not otherwise classified", "unspecified", "unclassified", "other" and "miscellaneous". Prior to using these codes, try to determine if a Local Level III code or CPT code is available. The "unlisted procedures" and accompanying codes for VISION SERVICES are as follows:

V2199	Not otherwise classified, single vision lens, bifocal, glass or plastic
V2499	Variable sphericity lens, other type
V2599	Not otherwise classified, contact lens
V2629	Prosthetic eye, other type
V2799	Vision service, miscellaneous

3. SPECIAL REPORT: A service, material or supply that is rarely provided, unusual, variable or new may require a special report in determining medical appropriateness for reimbursement purposes. Pertinent information should include an adequate definition or description of the nature, extent, and need for the service, material or supply.

V CODES

Not valid for Medicare   Non-covered by Medicare   Special coverage instructions   Carrier discretion

4. MODIFIERS: Listed services may be modified under certain circumstances. When appropriate, the modifying circumstance is identified by adding a modifier to the basic procedure code. CPT and HCPCS National Level II modifiers may be used with CPT and HCPCS National Level II procedure codes. Modifiers commonly used with VISION SERVICES are as follows:

-AP Determination of refractive state was not performed in the course of diagnostic ophthalmological examination

-CC Procedure code change (use "CC" when the procedure code submitted was changed either for administrative reasons or because an incorrect code was filed)

-LS FDA-monitored intraocular lens implant

-LT Left side (used to identify procedures performed on the left side of the body)

-PL Progressive addition lenses

-RT Right side (used to identify procedures performed on the right side of the body)

-SF Second opinion ordered by a professional review organization (PRO) per section 9401, P.L. 99-272. (100 percent reimbursement; no Medicare deductible or coinsurance)

-TC Technical component. Under certain circumstances, a charge may be made for the technical component alone. Under those circumstances, the technical component charge is identified by adding modifier -TC to the usual procedure number. Technical component charges are institutional charges and are not billed separately by physicians. However, portable x-ray suppliers bill only for the technical component and should use modifier -TC. The charge data from portable x-ray suppliers will then be used to build customary and prevailing profiles.

-VP Aphakic patient

5. CPT CODE CROSS-REFERENCE: See sections for equivalent CPT code(s) for all listings in this section.

Vision Services

FRAMES

V2020   Frames, purchases
MCM: 2130

V2025   Deluxe frame
MCM: 3045.4

SPECTACLE LENSES

NOTE: If CPT code 92390 or 92395 is reported, recode with the specific lens type listed below. For aphakic temporary spectacle correction, see CPT code 92358.

SINGLE VISION, GLASS OR PLASTIC

V2100   Sphere, single vision; plano to plus or minus 4.00, per lens

V2101   plus or minus 4.12 to plus or minus 7.00d, per lens

V2102   plus or minus 7.12 to plus or minus 20.00d, per lens

V2103   Spherocylinder, single vision, plano to plus or minus 4.00d sphere; .12 to 2.00d cylinder, per lens

V2104   2.12 to 4.00d cylinder, per lens

V2105   4.25 to 6.00d cylinder, per lens

V2106   over 6.00d cylinder, per lens

V2107   Spherocylinder, single vision, plus or minus 4.25d to plus or minus 7.00d sphere; .12 to 2.00d cylinder, per lens

V2108   2.12 To 4.00d cylinder, per lens

V2109   4.25 to 6.00d cylinder, per lens

V2110   over 6.00d cylinder, per lens

V2111   Spherocylinder, single vision, plus or minus 7.25 to plus or minus 12.00d sphere; .25 to 2.25d cylinder, per lens

V2112	2.25d to 4.00d cylinder, per lens
V2113	4.25 to 6.00d cylinder, per lens
V2114	Spherocylinder, single vision, sphere over plus or minus 12.00d per lens
V2115	Lenticular, (myodisc), per lens, single vision
V2118	Aniseikonic lens, single vision
V2121	Lenticular lens, per lens, single MCM: 2130.B
V2199	Not otherwise classified, single vision lens

BIFOCAL, GLASS OR PLASTIC

(Up to and including 28mm seg width, add power up to and including 3.25d)

V2200	Sphere, bifocal, plano to plus or minus 4.00d, per lens
V2201	Sphere, bifocal, plus or minus 4.12 to plus or minus 7.00d, per lens
V2202	Sphere, bifocal, plus or minus 7.12 to plus or minus 20.00d, per lens
V2203	Spherocylinder, bifocal, plano to plus or minus 4.00d sphere; .12 to 2.00d cylinder, per lens
V2204	2.12 to 4.00d cylinder, per lens
V2205	4.25 to 6.00d cylinder, per lens
V2206	over 6.00d cylinder, per lens
V2207	Spherocylinder, bifocal, plus or minus 4.25 to plus or minus 7.00d sphere; .12 to 2.00d cylinder, per lens
V2208	2.12 to 4.00d cylinder, per lens
V2209	4.25 to 6.00d cylinder, per lens
V2210	over 6.00d cylinder, per lens

● New code   ▲ Revised code   ( ) Deleted code

V2211	Spherocylinder, bifocal, plus or minus 7.25 to plus or minus 12.00d sphere; .25 to 2.25d cylinder, per lens
V2212	2.25 to 4.00d cylinder, per lens
V2213	4.25 to 6.00d cylinder, per lens
V2214	Spherocylinder, bifocal, sphere over plus or minus 12.00d, per lens
V2215	Lenticular (myodisc), per lens, bifocal
V2218	Aniseikonic, per lens, bifocal
V2219	Bifocal seg width over 28mm
V2220	Bifocal add over 3.25d
V2221	Lenticular lens, per lens, bifocal MCM: 2130.B
V2299	Specialty bifocal (by report)

TRIFOCAL, GLASS OR PLASTIC

(Up to and including 28mm seg width, add power up to and including 3.25d)

V2300	Sphere, trifocal, plano to plus or minus 4.00d, per lens
V2301	Sphere, trifocal, plus or minus 4.12 to plus or minus 7.00d, per lens
V2302	Sphere, trifocal, plus or minus 7.12 to plus or minus 20.00, per lens
V2303	Spherocylinder, trifocal, plano to plus or minus 4.00d sphere; .12 to 2.00d cylinder, per lens
V2304	2.25 to 4.00d cylinder, per lens
V2305	4.25 to 6.00d cylinder, per lens
V2306	over 6.00d cylinder, per lens

V2307	Spherocylinder, trifocal, plus or minus 4.25 to plus or minus 7.00d sphere; .12 to 2.00d cylinder, per lens
V2308	2.12 to 4.00d cylinder, per lens
V2309	4.25 to 6.00d cylinder, per lens
V2310	over 6.00d cylinder, per lens
V2311	Spherocylinder, trifocal, plus or minus 7.25 to plus or minus 12.00d sphere; .25 to 2.25d cylinder, per lens
V2312	2.25 to 4.00d cylinder, per lens
V2313	4.25 to 6.00d cylinder, per lens
V2314	Spherocylinder, trifocal, sphere over plus or minus 12.00d, per lens
V2315	Lenticular, (myodisc), per lens, trifocal
V2318	Aniseikonic lens, trifocal
V2319	Trifocal seg width over 28mm
V2320	Trifocal add over 3.25d
V2321	Lenticular lens, per lens, trifocal MCM: 2130.B
V2399	Specialty trifocal (by report)

VARIABLE ASPHERICITY

(Welsh 4-drop, hyperaspheric, double drop, etc.)

V2410	Variable asphericity lens; single vision, full field, glass or plastic, per lens
V2430	bifocal, full field, glass or plastic, per lens
V2499	other type

CONTACT LENSES (CPT 92391 OR 92396)

NOTE: If CPT code 92391 or 92396 is reported, recode with specific lens type listed below, per lens.

V2500 Contact lens, PMMA; spherical, per lens

V2501 toric or prism ballast, per lens

V2502 bifocal, per lens

V2503 color vision deficiency, per lens

V2510 Contact lens, gas permeable; spherical, per lens

V2511 toric, prism ballast, per lens

V2512 bifocal, per lens

V2513 extended wear, per lens

V2520 Contact lens hydrophilic; spherical, per lens
CIM: 45-7, 65-1

V2521 toric, or prism ballast, per lens
CIM: 45-7, 65-1

V2522 bifocal, per lens
CIM: 45-7, 65-1

V2523 extended wear, per lens
CIM: 45-7, 65-1

V2530 Contact lens, scleral, gas impermeable, per lens (for contact lens modification, see 92325)

V2531 Contact lens, scleral, gas permeable, per lens (for contact lens modification, see 92325)
CIM: 65-3

V2599 Contact lens, other type

LOW VISION AIDS (CPT 92392)

NOTE: If CPT code 92392 is reported, record with specific systems listed below.

V2600 Hand held low vision aids and other nonspectacle mounted aids

V2610 Single lens spectacle mounted low vision aids

V2615 Telescopic and other compound lens system, including distance vision telescopic, near vision telescopes and compound microscopic lens system

EYE PROSTHESIS

PROSTHETIC EYE (CPT 92330 OR 92393)

V2623 Prosthetic, eye; plastic, custom
MCM: 2133

V2624 Polishing/resurfacing or ocular prosthesis

V2625 Enlargement of ocular prosthesis

V2626 Reduction of ocular prosthesis

V2627 Scleral cover shell
CIM: 65-3

V2628 Fabrication and fitting of ocular conformer

V2629 Prosthetic eye, other type

INTRAOCULAR LENSES

V2630 Anterior chamber intraocular lens
MCM: 2130

V2631 Iris supported intraocular lens
MCM: 2130

V2632 Posterior chamber intraocular lens
MCM: 2130

MISCELLANEOUS

V2700 Balance lens, per lens

V2702 Deluxe lens feature
MCM: 2130.B

V2710 Slab off prism, glass or plastic, per lens

V2715 Prism, per lens

V2718 Press-on lens, fresnell prism, per lens

V2730 Special base curve, glass or plastic, per lens

V2744 Tint, photochromatic, per lens
MCM: 2130.B

V2745 Addition to lens; tint, any color, solid, gradient or equal, excludes photochromatic, any lens material, per lens
MCM: 2130.B

V2750 Anti-reflective coating, per lens
MCM: 2130.B

V2755 U-V lens, per lens
MCM: 2130.B

V2756 Eye glass case

V2760 Scratch resistant coating, per lens

V2761 Mirror coating, any type, solid, gradient or equal, any lens material, per lens
MCM: 2130.B

V2762 Polarization, any lens material, per lens
MCM: 2130.B

V2770 Occluder lens, per lens

V2780 Oversize lens, per lens

V2781 Progressive lens, per lens

V2782 Lens, index 1.54 to 1.65 plastic or 1.60 to 1.79 glass, excluding polycarbonate, per lens
MCM: 2130.B

V2783   Lens, index greater than or equal to 1.66 plastic or greater than or equal to 1.80 glass, excludes polycarbonate, per lens
MCM: 2130.B

V2784   Lens, polycarbonate or equal, any index, per lens
MCM: 2130.B

V2785   Processing, preserving and transporting corneal tissue

V2786   Specialty occupational multifocal lens, per lens
MCM: 2130.B

● **V2788**   Presbyopia correcting function of intraocular lens

V2790   Amniotic membrane for surgical reconstruction, per procedure

V2797   Vision supply, accessory and/or service component of another HCPCS vision code

V2799   Vision service, miscellaneous

HEARING SERVICES

Guidelines

In addition to the information presented in the INTRODUCTION, several other items unique to this section are defined or identified here:

1. PROSTHETIC DEVICES: Prosthetic devices that replace all or part of an internal body organ or the function of a permanently inoperative or malfunctioning internal body organ are covered when furnished on a physician's order. If the medical record and attending physician indicate the condition will be indefinite, the test of permanence is met.

2. SPEECH PATHOLOGY: Services necessary for diagnosing and treating speech disorders that result in communication disabilities, and swallowing disorders, regardless of the presence of a disability, are covered Medicare services if reasonable and necessary. The services must be considered to be an effective treatment for the patient's condition, and the patient's condition must be at a level of severity that requires the service of a qualified speech pathologist.

3. UNLISTED SERVICE OR PROCEDURE: A service or procedure may be provided that is not listed in this edition of HCPCS. When reporting such a service, the appropriate "unlisted procedure" code may be used to indicate the service, identifying it by "special report" as defined below. HCPCS terminology is inconsistent in defining unlisted procedures. The procedure definition may include the term(s) "unlisted", "not otherwise classified", "unspecified", "unclassified", "other" and "miscellaneous". Prior to using these codes, try to determine if a Local Level III code or CPT code is available. The "unlisted procedures" and accompanying codes for HEARING SERVICES are as follows:

   V5299   Hearing service, miscellaneous

4. SPECIAL REPORT: A service, material or supply that is rarely provided, unusual, variable or new may require a special report in determining medical appropriateness for reimbursement purposes. Pertinent information should include an adequate definition or description of the nature, extent, and need for the service, material or supply.

5. MODIFIERS: Listed services may be modified under certain circumstances. When appropriate, the modifying circumstance is identified by adding a modifier to the basic procedure code. CPT and

Not valid   Non-covered   Special   Carrier   **397**
for Medicare   by Medicare   coverage   discretion
                                          instructions

HCPCS National Level II modifiers may be used with CPT and HCPCS National Level II procedure codes. Modifiers commonly used with HEARING SERVICES are as follows:

-CC   Procedure code change (use "CC" when the procedure code submitted was changed either for administrative reasons or because an incorrect code was filed)

-LT   Left side (used to identify procedures performed on the left side of the body)

-RT   Right side (used to identify procedures performed on the right side of the body)

-SF   Second opinion ordered by a professional review organization (PRO) per sectoin 9401, P.L. 99-272 (100 percent reimbursement; no Medicare deductible or coinsurance)

-TC   Technical component. Under certain circumstances, a charge may be made for the technical component alone. Under those circumstances, the technical component charge is identified by adding modifier -TC to the usual procedure number. Technical component charges are institutional charges and are not billed separately by physicians. However, portable x-ray suppliers bill only for the technical component and should use modifier -TC. The charge data from portable x-ray suppliers will then be used to build customary and prevailing profiles.

6.   CPT CODE CROSS-REFERENCE: See sections for equivalent CPT code(s) for all listings in this section.

Hearing Services

V5008   Hearing screening
MCM: 2320

V5010   Assessment for hearing aid

V5011   Fitting/orientation/checking of hearing aid

V5014   Repair/modification of a hearing aid

V5020   Conformity evaluation

V5030   Hearing aid, monaural; body worn, air conduction

V5040   body worn, bone conduction

V5050   in the ear

V5060   behind the ear

V5070   Glasses; air conduction

V5080   bone conduction

V5090   Dispensing fee, unspecified hearing aid

V5095   Semi-implantable middle ear hearing prosthesis

V5100   Hearing aid, bilateral, body worn

V5110   Dispensing fee, bilateral

V5120   Binaural; body

V5130   in the ear

V5140   behind the ear

V5150   glasses

V5160   Dispensing fee, binaural

V5170   Hearing aid, CROS; in the ear

V5180   behind the ear

V5190   glasses

V5200   Dispensing fee, CROS

V5210   Hearing aid, bicros; in the ear

V5220   behind the ear

V5230   glasses

V5240   Dispensing fee, bicros

V5241   Dispensing fee, monaural hearing aid, any type

Not valid   Non-covered   Special   Carrier
for Medicare   by Medicare   coverage   discretion
instructions

V5242 Hearing aid, analog, monaural, cic (completely in the ear canal)

V5243 Hearing aid, analog, monaural, itc (in the canal)

V5244 Hearing aid, digitally programmable analog, monaural, cic

V5245 Hearing aid, digitally programmable, analog, monaural, itc

V5246 Hearing aid, digitally programmable analog, monaural, ite (in the ear)

V5247 Hearing aid, digitally programmable analog, monaural, bte (behind the ear)

V5248 Hearing aid, analog, binaural, cic

V5249 Hearing aid, analog, binaural, itc

V5250 Hearing aid, digitally programmable analog, binaural, cic

V5251 Hearing aid, digitally programmable analog, binaural, itc

V5252 Hearing aid, digitally programmable, binaural, ite

V5253 Hearing aid, digitally programmable, binaural, bte

V5254 Hearing aid, digital, monaural, cic

V5255 Hearing aid, digital, monaural, itc

V5256 Hearing aid, digital, monaural, ite

V5257 Hearing aid, digital, monaural, bte

V5258 Hearing aid, digital, binaural, cic

V5259 Hearing aid, digital, binaural, itc

V5260 Hearing aid, digital, binaural, ite

V5261 Hearing aid, digital, binaural, bte

V5262 Hearing aid, disposable, any type, monaural

V5263 Hearing aid, disposable, any type, binaural

V5264 Ear mold/insert, not disposable, any type

V5265 Ear mold/insert, disposable, any type

V5266 Battery for use in hearing device

V5267 Hearing aid supplies/accessories

V5268 Assistive listening device, telephone amplifier, any type

V5269 Assistive listening device, alerting, any type

V5270 Assistive listening device, television amplifier, any type

V5271 Assistive listening device, television caption decoder

V5272 Assistive listening device, TDD

V5273 Assistive listening device, for use with cochlear implant

V5274 Assistive learning device, not otherwise specified

V5275 Ear impression, each

V5298 Hearing aid, not otherwise classified

V5299 Hearing service, miscellaneous
MCM: 2320

SPEECH-LANGUAGE PATHOLOGY SERVICES

V5336 Repair/modification of augmentative communicative system or device (excludes adaptive hearing aid)

V5362 Speech screening

V5363 Language screening

V5364 Dysphagia screening

Not valid
for Medicare
Non-covered
by Medicare
Special
coverage
instructions
Carrier
discretion
401

● New code   ▲ Revised code   ( ) Deleted code

APPENDIX A: MODIFIERS

HCPCS National Level II Modifiers

The following list is the complete list of HCPCS National Level II modifiers and descriptions.

-A1   Dressing for one wound

-A2   Dressing for two wounds

-A3   Dressing for three wounds

-A4   Dressing for four wounds

-A5   Dressing for five wounds

-A6   Dressing for six wounds

-A7   Dressing for seven wounds

-A8   Dressing for eight wounds

-A9   Dressing for nine or more wounds

-AA   Anesthesia services performed personally by anesthesiologist
MCM: 3350.5

-AD   Medical supervision by a physician; more than four concurrent anesthesia procedures
MCM: 3350.5

-AE   Registered dictician

-AF   Specialty physician

-AG   Primary physician

-AH   Clinical psychologist
MCM: 3350.5

-AJ   Clinical social worker
MCM: 2152, 5113

-AK   Non-participating physician

-AM   Physician, team member service
MCM: 4105.7

-AP   Determination of refractive state was not performed in the course of diagnostic ophthalmological examination

● **-AQ**   Physician providing a service in an unlisted health professional shortage area (HPSA)

-AR   Physician provider services in a physician scarcity area

-AS   Physician assistant, nurse practitioner or clinical nurse specialist services for assistant at surgery

-AT   Acute treatment (this modifier should be used when reporting service 98940, 98941, 98942)

-AU   Item furnished in conjunction with a urological, ostomy, or tracheostomy supply

-AV   Item furnished in conjunction with a prosthetic device, prosthetic or orthotic

-AW   Item furnished in conjunction with a surgical dressing

-AX   Item furnished in conjunction with dialysis services

-BA   Item furnished in conjunction with parenteral enteral nutrition (pen) services

● **-BL**   Special acquisition of blood and blood products

-BO   Orally administered nutrition, not by feeding tube

-BP   The beneficiary has been informed of the purchase and rental options and has elected to purchase the item

-BR   The beneficiary has been informed of the purchase and rental options and has elected to rent the item

-BU   The beneficiary has been informed of the purchase and rental options and after 30 days has not informed the supplier of his/her decision

-CA   Procedure payable only in the inpatient setting when performed emergently on an outpatient who expires prior to admission

-CB   Service ordered by a renal dialysis facility (RDF) physician as part of the ESRD beneficiary's dialysis benefit, is not part of the composite rate, and is separately reimbursable

-CC   Procedure code change (use -CC when the procedure code submitted was changed either for administrative reasons or because an incorrect code was filed)

-CD   AMCC test has been ordered by an ESRD facility or MCP physician that is part of the composite rate and is not separately billable
MCM: 4270.2

-CE   AMCC test has been ordered by an ESRD facility or MCP physician that is a composite rate test but is beyond the normal frequency covered under the rate and is separately reimbursable based on medical necessity
MCM: 4270.2

-CF   AMCC test has been ordered by an ESRD facility or MCP physician that is not part of the composite rate and is separately billable
MCM: 4270.2

-CG   Innovator drug dispensed

● **-CR**   Catastrophe/disaster related

-E1   Upper left, eyelid

-E2   Lower left, eyelid

-E3   Upper right, eyelid

-E4   Lower right, eyelid

-EJ   Subsequent claims for a defined course of therapy, e.g., EPO, sodium hyaluronate, infliximab
MCM: 4273.2

-EM   Emergency reserve supply (for ESRD benefit only)
MCM: 3045.7

-EP   Service provided as part of Medicaid early periodic screening, diagnosis, and treatment (EPSDT) program

-ET   Emergency services

-EY   No physician or other licensed health care provider order for this item or service

-F1   Left hand, second digit

-F2   Left hand, third digit

-F3   Left hand, fourth digit

-F4   Left hand, fifth digit

-F5   Right hand, thumb

-F6   Right hand, second digit

-F7   Right hand, third digit

-F8   Right hand, fourth digit

-F9   Right hand, fifth digit

-FA   Left hand, thumb

● -FB   Item provided without cost to provider, supplier or practitioner (examples, but not limited to: covered under warranty, replaced due to defect, free samples)

-FP   Service provided as part of Medicaid family planning program

-G1   Most recent URR reading of less than 60

-G2   Most recent URR reading of 60 to 64.9

-G3   Most recent URR reading of 65 to 69.9

-G4   Most recent URR reading of 70 to 74.9

-G5   Most recent URR reading of 75 or greater

-G6   ESRD patient for whom less than six dialysis sessions have been provided in a month

-G7   Pregnancy resulted from rape or incest or pregnancy certified by physician as life threatening
           CIM: 35-99   MCM: 2005.1

-G8   Monitored anesthesia care (MAC) for deep complex, complicated, or markedly invasive surgical procedure

-G9   Monitored anesthesia care for patient who has history of severe cardio-pulmonary condition

-GA   Waiver of liability statement on file

-GB   Claim being re-submitted for payment because it is no longer covered under a global payment demonstration

-GC   This service has been performed in part by a resident under the direction of a teaching physician
           MCM: 3350.5, 4116

-GE   This service has been performed by a resident without the presence of a teaching physician under the primary care exception
           MCM: 4116

-GF   Non-physician (eg., nurse practitioner (NP), certified registered nurse anesthetist (CRNA), certified registered nurse (CRN), clinical nurse specialist (CNS), physician assistant (PA)) services in a critical access hospital

-GG   Performance and payment of a screening mammogram and diagnostic mammogram on the same patient, same day

-GH   Diagnostic mammogram converted from screening mammogram on same day

-GJ   "Opt Out" physician or practitioner emergency or urgent service

-GK   Actual item/service ordered by physician, item associated with -GA or -GZ modifier

-GL   Medically unnecessary upgrade provided instead of standard item, no charge, no advance beneficiary notice (ABN)

-GM   Multiple patients on one ambulance trip

-GN   Services delivered under an outpatient speech language pathology plan of care

-GO   Services delivered under an outpatient occupational therapy plan of care

-GP   Services delivered under an outpatient physical therapy plan of care

-GQ   Via asynchronous telecommunications system

● **-GR**   This service was performed in whole or in part by a resident in a department of veterans affairs medical center or clinic, supervised in accordance with VA policy

● **-GS**   Dosage of epo or darbepoietin alfa has been reduced 25% of preceding month's dosage
MCM: 4273.1

-GT   Via interactive audio and video telecommunication systems

-GV   Attending physician not employed or paid under arrangement by the patient's hospice provider
MCM: 4175.5

-GW   Service not related to the hospice patient's terminal condition
MCM: 4175.5

-GY   Item or service statutorily excluded or does not meet the definition of any Medicare benefit

-GZ   Item or service expected to be denied as not reasonable and necessary
MCM: 2000

-H9   Court-ordered

-HA   Child/adolescent program

-HB   Adult program, non geriatric

-HC   Adult program, geriatric

-HD   Pregnant/parenting women's program

-HE   Mental health program

-HF   Substance abuse program

-HG   Opioid addiction treatment program

-HI   Integrated mental health and mental retardation/developmental disabilities program

-HJ   Employee assistance program

-HK   Specialized mental health programs for high-risk populations

-HL   Intern

-HM   Less than bachelor degree level

-HN   Bachelors degree level

-HO   Masters degree level

-HP   Doctoral level

-HQ   Group setting

-HR   Family/couple with client present

-HS   Family/couple without client present

-HT   Multi-disciplinary team

-HU   Funded by child welfare agency

-HV   Funded state addictions agency

-HW   Funded by state mental health agency

-HX   Funded by county/local agency

-HY   Funded by juvenile justice agency

-HZ   Funded by criminal justice agency

● **-J1**   Competitive acquisition program no-pay submission for a prescription number

● **-J2**   Competitive acquisition program, restocking of emergency drugs after emergency administration

● **-J3**   Competitive acquisition program (CAP), drug not available through CAP as written, reimbursed under average sales price methodology

-JW   Drug amount discarded/not administered to any patient

-K0   Lower extremity prosthesis functional level 0: Does not have the ability or potential to ambulate or transfer safely with or without assistance and a prosthesis does not enhance their quality of life or mobility

-K1   Lower extremity prosthesis functional level 1: Has the ability or potential to use a prosthesis for transfers or ambulation on level surfaces at fixed cadence. Typical of the limited and unlimited household ambulator.

-K2   Lower extremity prosthesis functional level 2: Has the ability or potential for ambulation with the ability to traverse low-level environmental barriers such as curbs, stairs or uneven surfaces. Typical of the limited community ambulator.

-K3   Lower extremity prosthesis functional level 3: Has the ability or potential for ambulation with variable cadence. Typical of the community ambulator who has the ability to traverse most environmental barriers and may have vocational, therapeutic or exercise activity that demands prosthetic utilization beyond simple locomotion.

-K4   Lower prosthesis functional level 4: Has the ability or potential for prosthetic ambulation that exceeds the basic ambulation skills, exhibiting high impact, stress or energy levels, typical of the prosthetic demands of the child, active adult, or athlete.

-KA   Add on option/accessory for wheelchair

-KB   Beneficiary requested upgrade for abn, more than 4 modifiers identified on claim

-KC   Replacement of special power wheelchair interface

-KD   Drug or biological infused through DME

-KF   Item designated by FDA as class III device

-KH   DMEPOS item, initial claim, purchase or first month rental

-KI   DMEPOS item, second or third month rental

-KJ   DMEPOS item, parenteral enteral nutrition (PEN) pump or capped rental, months four to fifteen

-KM   Replacement of facial prosthesis including new impression/ moulage

-KN   Replacement of facial prosthesis using previous master model

-KO   Single drug unit dose formulation

-KP First drug of a multiple drug unit dose formulation

-KQ Second or subsequent drug of a multiple drug unit dose formulation

-KR Rental item, billing for partial month

-KS Glucose monitor supply for diabetic beneficiary not treated with insulin

-KX Specific required documentation on file

-KZ New coverage not implemented by managed care

-LC Left circumflex coronary artery

-LD Left anterior descending coronary artery

-LL Lease/rental (use the -LL modifier when DME equipment rental is to be applied against the purchase price)

-LR Laboratory round trip

-LS FDA-monitored intraocular lens implant
CIM: 65-7

-LT Left side (used to identify procedures performed on the left side of the body)

-MS Six-month maintenance and servicing fee for reasonable and necessary parts and labor which are not covered under any manufacturer or supplier warranty

-NR New when rented (use the -NR modifier when DME which was new at the time of rental is subsequently purchased)

-NU New equipment

● **-P1** A normal healthy patient

● **-P2** A patient with mild systemic disease

● **-P3**   A patient with severe systemic disease

● **-P4**   A patient with severe systemic disease that is a constant threat to life

● **-P5**   A moribund patient who is not cxpcctcd to survive without the operation

● **-P6**   A declared brain-dead patient whose organs are being removed for donor purposes

-PL   Progressive addition lenses

-Q2   CMS/ORD demonstration project procedure/service

-Q3   Live kidney donor surgery and related services

-Q4   Service for ordering/referring physician qualifies as a service exemption

-Q5   Service furnished by a substitute physician under a reciprocal billing arrangement
MCM: 3060.6

-Q6   Service furnished by a locum tenens physician
MCM: 3060.7

-Q7   Onc class Λ finding

-Q8   Two class B findings

-Q9   One class B and two class C findings

-QA   FDA investigational device exemption

(-QB)   Code deleted December 31, 2005

-QC   Single channel monitoring

-QD   Recording and storage in solid state memory by a digital recorder

-QE   Prescribed amount of oxygen is less than one liter per minute (LPM)

-QF   Prescribed amount of oxygen exceeds 4 liters per minute (LPM) and portable oxygen is prescribed

-QG   Prescribed amount of oxygen is greater than four liters per minute (LPM)

-QH   Oxygen conserving device is being used with an oxygen delivery system

-QJ   Services/items provided to a prisoner or patient in state or local custody, however the state or local government, as applicable, meets the requirements in 42 cfr 411.4 (B)

-QK   Medical direction of two, three or four concurrent anesthesia procedures involving qualified individuals
MCM: 3350.5

-QL   Patient pronounced dead after ambulance called

-QM   Ambulance service provided under arrangement by a provider of services

-QN   Ambulance service furnished directly by a provider of service

-QP   Documentation is on file showing that the laboratory test(s) was ordered individually or ordered as a CPT-recognized panel other than automated profile codes 80002-80019, G0058, G0059, and G0060.
MCM: 7517.1

(-QQ)   Code deleted December 31, 2005

● **-QR**   Item or service provided in a medicare specified study

-QS   Monitored anesthesia care service
CIM: 15018I

-QT   Recording and storage on tape by an analog tape recorder

(-QU)   Code deleted December 31, 2005

-QV   Item or service provided as routine care in a medical qualifying clinical trial
CIM: 30-1

-QW   CLIA waived test

-QX   CRNA service: with medical direction by a physician

-QY   Medical direction of one Certified Registered Nurse Anesthetist by an anesthesiologist
MCM: 3350.5

-QZ   CRNA service: without medical direction by a physician

-RC   Right coronary artery

-RD   Drug provided to beneficiary, but not administered incident-to

-RP   Replacement and repair (may be used to indicate replacement of DME, orthotic, and prosthetic devices which have been in use for some time. The claim shows the code for the part, followed by the -RP modifier and the charge for the part)

-RR   Rental (use the -RR modifier when DME is to be rented)

-RT   Right side (used to identify procedures performed on the right side of the body)

-SA   Nurse practitioner rendering service in collaboration w   a physician

-SB   Nurse midwife

-SC   Medically necessary service or supply

-SD   Services provided by registered nurse with specialized, highly technical home infusion training

-SE   State and/or federally funded programs/services

-SF   Second opinion ordered by a professional review organization (PRO) per section 9401, P.L. 99-272 (100% reimbursement — no Medicare deductible or coinsurance)

-SG	Ambulatory surgical center (ASC) facility service
-SH	Second concurrently administered infusion therapy
-SJ	Third or more concurrently administered infusion therapy
-SK	Member of high-risk population (use only with codes for immunization)
-SL	State supplied vaccine
-SM	Second surgical opinion
-SN	Third surgical opinion
-SQ	Item ordered by home health
-ST	Related to trauma or injury
-SU	Procedure performed in physician's office (to denote use of facility and equipment)
-SV	Pharmaceuticals delivered to patient's home but not utilized
-SW	Services provided by a certified diabetic educator
-SY	Persons who are in close contact with member of high-risk population (use only with codes for immunization)
-T1	Left foot, second digit
-T2	Left foot, third digit
-T3	Left foot, fourth digit
-T4	Left foot, fifth digit
-T5	Right foot, great toe
-T6	Right foot, second digit

-T7   Right foot, third digit

-T8   Right foot, fourth digit

-T9   Right foot, fifth digit

-TA   Left foot, great toe

-TC   Technical component. Under certain circumstances, a charge may be made for the technical component alone. Under those circumstances the technical component charge is identified by adding modifier -TC to the usual procedure number. Technical component charges are institutional charges and not billed separately by physicians. However, portable x-ray suppliers only bill for technical component and should utilize modifier -TC. The charge data from portable x-ray suppliers will then be used to build customary and prevailing profiles.

-TD   RN

-TE   LPN/LVN

-TF   Intermediate level of care

-TG   Complex/high tech level of care

-TH   Obstetrical treatment/services, prenatal or postpartum

-TJ   Program group, child and/or adolescent

-TK   Extra patient or passenger, non-ambulance
(Note: use modifier "-GM: Multiple patients on one ambulance trip" for ambulance claims)

-TL   Early intervention/individualized family services plan (IFSP)

-TM   Individualized education program (IEP)

-TN   Rural/outside providers customary service area

-TP   Medical transport, unloaded vehicle

-TQ	Basice life support (BLS) transport by a volunteer ambulance provider
-TR	School-based individualized education program (IEP) services provided outside the public school district responsible for the student
-TS	Follow-up service
-TT	Individualized service provided to more than one patient in same setting
-TU	Special payment rate, overtime
-TV	Special payment rates, holidays/weekends
-TW	Back-up equipment
-UE	Used durable medical equipment
-UF	Services provided in the morning
-UG	Services provided in the afternoon
-UH	Services provided in the evening
-UJ	Services provided at night
-UK	Services provided on behalf of the client to someone other than the client (collateral relationship)
-UN	Two patients served
-UP	Three patients served
-UQ	Four patients served
-UR	Five patients served
-US	Six patients served

-VP   Aphakic patient

AMBULANCE SERVICE MODIFIERS

For ambulance service, one-digit modifiers are combined to form a two-digit modifier that identifies the ambulance's place of origin with the first digit, and ambulance's destination with the second digit. They are used in items 12 and 13 on the CMS Form 1491.

One digit modifiers:

-D   Diagnostic or therapeutic site other than -P or -H when these are used as origin codes

-E   Residential, domiciliary, custodial facility (other than an 1819 facility)

-G   Hospital-based dialysis facility (hospital or hospital related)

-H   Hospital

-I   Site of transfer (for example, airport or helicopter pad) between types of ambulance

-J   Non-hospital-based dialysis facility

-N   Skilled nursing facility (SNF) (1819 facility)

-P   Physician's office (includes HMO non-hospital facility, clinic, etc.)

-R   Residence

-S   Scene of accident or acute event

-X   (Destination code only) Intermediate stop at physician's office on the way to the hospital (includes HMO non-hospital facility, clinic, etc.)

PET SCAN MODIFIERS

Use these single-digit alpha characters in combination as two-character modifiers to indicate the results of a current PET scan and a previous test.

-N   Negative

-E   Equivocal

-P   Positive, but not suggestive of extensive ischemia

-S   Positive and suggestive of extensive ischemia (>20 percent of the left ventricle)

APPENDIX B: SUMMARY OF CHANGES

Summary of Official HCPCS Additions, Changes, and Deletions for 2006

-AQ   Physician providing a service in an unlisted health professional shortage area (HPSA)
Code Added

-BL   Special acquisition of blood and blood products
Code Added

-CR   Catastrophe/disaster related
Code Added

-FB   Item provided without cost to provider, supplier or practitioner (examples, but not limited to: covered under warranty, replaced due to defect, free samples)
Code Added

-GR   This service was performed in whole or in part by a resident in a department of veterans affairs medical center or clinic, supervised in accordance with VA policy
Code Added

-GS   Dosage of epo or darbepoietin alfa has been reduced 25% of preceding month's dosage
MCM: 4273.1
Code Added

-J1   Competitive acquisition program no-pay submission for a prescription number
Code Added

-J2   Competitive acquisition program, restocking of emergency drugs after emergency administration
Code Added

-J3   Competitive acquisition program (CAP), drug not available through CAP as written, reimbursed under average sales price methodology
Code Added

-P1   A normal healthy patient
Code Added

-P2   A patient with mild systemic disease
Code Added

-P3   A patient with severe systemic disease
Code Added

-P4   A patient with severe systemic disease that is a constant threat to life
Code Added

-P5   A moribund patient who is not expected to survive without the operation
Code Added

-P6   A declared brain-dead patient whose organs are being removed for donor purposes
Code Added

-QB   **Deleted 2005**

-QQ   **Deleted 2005**

-QR   Item or service provided in a medicare specified study
Code Added

-QU   **Deleted 2005**

A0998   Ambulance response and treatment, no transport
Code Added

A4215   Needle, sterile, any size, each
Description Changed

A4216 Sterile water, saline and/or dextrose (diluent), 10 ml
Description Changed

A4218 Sterile saline or water, metered dose dispenser, 10 ml
Code Added

A4233 Replacement battery, alkaline (other than j cell), for use with medically necessary home blood glucose monitor owned by patient, each
Code Added

A4234 Replacement battery, alkaline, j cell, for use with medically necessary home blood glucose monitor owned by patient, each
Code Added

A4235 Replacement battery, lithium, for use with medically necessary home blood glucose monitor owned by patient, each
Code Added

A4236 Replacement battery, silver oxide, for use with medically necessary home blood glucose monitor owned by patient, each
Code Added

A4254 **Deleted 2005**

A4260 **Deleted 2005 use J7306**

A4363 Ostomy clamp, any type, replacement only, each
Code Added

A4372 Ostomy skin barrier, solid 4x4 or equivalent, standard wear, with built-in convexity, each
Description Changed

A4411 Ostomy skin barrier, solid 4x4 or equivalent, extended wear, with built-in convexity, each
Code Added

A4412 Ostomy pouch, drainable, high output, for use on a barrier with flange (2 piece system), without filter, each
MCM: 2130
Code Added

A4604 Tubing with integrated heating element for use with positive airway pressure device
Code Added

A4630 Replacement batteries, medically necessary, transcutaneous electrical stimulator, owned by patient
Description Changed

A4641 Radiopharmaceutical, diagnostic, not otherwise classified
Description Changed

A4642 Indium in-111 satumomab pendetide, diagnostic, per study dose, up to 6 millicuries
Description Changed

A4643 **Deleted 2005**

A4644 **Deleted 2005**

A4645 **Deleted 2005**

A4646 **Deleted 2005**

A4647 **Deleted 2005**

A4656 **Deleted 2005**

A5119 **Deleted 2005**

A5120 Skin barrier, wipes or swabs, each
MCM: 2130
Code Added

A5509 **Deleted 2005**

A5511 **Deleted 2005**

A5512 For diabetics only, multiple density insert, direct formed, molded to foot after external heat source of 230 degrees fahrenheit or higher, total contact with patient's foot, including arch, base layer minimum of 1/4 inch material of shore a 35 durometer or 3/16 inch material of shore a 40 durometer (or higher), prefabricated, each
Code Added

A5513 For diabetics only, multiple density insert, custom molded from model of patient's foot, total contact with patient's foot, including arch, base layer minimum of 1/4 inch material of shore a 35 durometer or 3/16 inch material of shore a 40 durometer (or higher), includes arch filler and other shaping material, custom fabricated, each
Code Added

A6457 Tubular dressing with or without elastic, any width, per linear yard
Code Added

A6513 Compression burn mask, face and/or neck, plastic or equal, custom fabricated
Code Added

A6530 Gradient compression stocking, below knee, 18-30 mmhg, each
CIM: 60-9
Code Added

A6531 Gradient compression stocking, below knee, 30-40 mmhg, each
MCM: 2079
Code Added

A6532 Gradient compression stocking, below knee, 40-50 mmhg, each
MCM: 2079
Code Added

A6533   Gradient compression stocking, thigh length, 18-30 mmhg, each
CIM: 60-9 MCM: 2133
Code Added

A6534   Gradient compression stocking, thigh length, 30-40 mmhg, each
CIM: 60-9 MCM: 2133
Code Added

A6535   Gradient compression stocking, thigh length, 40-50 mmhg, each
CIM: 60-9 MCM: 2133
Code Added

A6536   Gradient compression stocking, full length/chap style, 18-30 mmhg, each
CIM: 60-9 MCM: 2133
Code Added

A6537   Gradient compression stocking, full length/chap style, 30-40 mmhg, each
CIM: 60-9 MCM: 2133
Code Added

A6538   Gradient compression stocking, full length/chap style, 40-50 mmhg, each
CIM: 60-9 MCM: 2133
Code Added

A6539   Gradient compression stocking, waist length, 18-30 mmhg, each
CIM: 60-9 MCM: 2133
Code Added

A6540   Gradient compression stocking, waist length, 30-40 mmhg, each
CIM: 60-9 MCM: 2133
Code Added

A6541   Gradient compression stocking, waist length, 40-50 mmhg, each
CIM: 60-9 MCM: 2133
Code Added

A6542 Gradient compression stocking, custom made
CIM: 60-9 MCM: 2133
Code Added

A6543 Gradient compression stocking, lymphedema
CIM: 60-9 MCM: 2133
Code Added

A6544 Gradient compression stocking, garter belt
CIM: 60-9 MCM: 2133
Code Added

A6549 Gradient compression stocking, not otherwise specified
CIM: 60-9 MCM: 2133
Code Added

A6550 Wound care set, for negative pressure wound therapy electrical pump, includes all supplies and accessories
Description Changed

A6551 **Deleted 2005**

A7032 Cushion for use on nasal mask interface, replacement only, each
Description Changed

A7033 Pillow for use on nasal cannula type interface, replacement only, pair
Description Changed

A9275 Home glucose disposable monitor, includes test strips
Code Added

A9281 Reaching/grabbing device, any type, any length, each
Code Added

A9282 Wig, any type, each
Code Added

A9500 Technetium TC-99m sestamibi, diagnostic, per study dose, up to 40 millicuries
Description Changed

A9502   Technetium TC-99m tetrofosmin, diagnostic, per study dose, up to 40 millicuries
Description Changed

A9503   Technetium TC-99m medronate, diagnostic, per study dose, up to 30 millicuries
Description Changed

A9504   Technetium TC-99m apcitide, diagnostic, per study dose, up to 20 millicuries
Description Changed

A9505   Thallium TL-201 thallous chloride, diagnostic, per millicurie
Description Changed

A9507   Indium IN-111 capromablue pendetide, diagnostic, per study dose, up to 10 millicuries
Description Changed

A9508   Iodine I-131 ioblueenguane sulfate, diagnostic, per 0.5 millicurie
Description Changed

A9510   Technetium TC-99m disofenin, diagnostic, per study dose, up to 15 millicuries
Description Changed

A9511   **Deleted 2005**

A9512   Technetium TC-99m pertechnetate, diagnostic, per millicurie
Description Changed

A9513   **Deleted 2005**

A9514   **Deleted 2005**

A9515   **Deleted 2005**

A9516   Iodine I-123 sodium iodide capsule(s), diagnostic, per 100 microcuries
Description Changed

A9517   Iodine I-131 sodium iodide capsule(s), therapeutic, per millicurie
Description Changed

A9519   **Deleted 2005**

A9520   **Deleted 2005**

A9521   Technetium TC-99m exametazime, diagnostic, per study dose, up to 25 millicuries
Description Changed

A9522   **Deleted 2005**

A9523   **Deleted 2005**

A9524   Iodine I-131 iodinated serum alblueumin, diagnostic, per 5 microcuries
Description Changed

A9525   **Deleted 2005**

A9526   Nitrogen n-13 ammonia, diagnostic, per study dose, up to 40 millicuries
Description Changed

A9528   Iodine I-131 sodium iodide capsule(s), diagnostic, per millicurie
Description Changed

A9529   Iodine I-131 sodium iodide solution, diagnostic, per millicurie
Description Changed

A9530   Iodine I-131 sodium iodide solution, therapeutic, per millicurie
Description Changed

A9531   Iodine I-131 sodium iodide, diagnostic, per microcurie (up to 100 microcuries)
Description Changed

A9532   Iodine I-125 serum alblueumin, diagnostic, per 5 microcuries
Description Changed

A9533   **Deleted 2005**

A9534   **Deleted 2005**

A9535   Injection, methylene blue, 1 ml
Code Added

A9536   Technetium tc-99m depreotide, diagnostic, per study dose, up to 35 millicuries
Code Added

A9537   Technetium tc-99m mebrofenin, diagnostic, per study dose, up to 15 millicuries
Code Added

A9538   Technetium tc-99m pyrophosphate, diagnostic, per study dose, up to 25 millicuries
Code Added

A9539   Technetium tc-99m pentetate, diagnostic, per study dose, up to 25 millicuries
Code Added

A9540   Technetium tc-99m macroaggregated albumin, diagnostic, per study dose, up to 10 millicuries
Code Added

A9541   Technetium tc-99m sulfur colloid, diagnostic, per study dose, up to 20 millicuries
Code Added

A9542   Indium in-111 ibritumomab tiuxetan, diagnostic, per study dose, up to 5 millicuries
Code Added

A9543   Yttrium y-90 ibritumomab tiuxetan, therapeutic, per treatment dose, up to 40 millicuries
Code Added

A9544   Iodine i-131 tositumomab, diagnostic, per study dose
Code Added

A9545   Iodine i-131 tositumomab, therapeutic, per treatment dose
Code Added

A9546   Cobalt co-57/58, cyanocobalamin, diagnostic, per study dose, up to 1 microcurie
Code Added

A9547   Indium in-111 oxyquinoline, diagnostic, per 0.5 millicurie
Code Added

A9548   Indium in-111 pentetate, diagnostic, per 0.5 millicurie
Code Added

A9549   Technetium tc-99m arcitumomab, diagnostic, per study dose, up to 25 millicuries
Code Added

A9550   Technetium tc-99m sodium gluceptate, diagnostic, per study dose, up to 25 millicurie
Code Added

A9551   Technetium tc-99m succimer, diagnostic, per study dose, up to 10 millicuries
Code Added

A9552   Fluorodeoxyglucose f-18 fdg, diagnostic, per study dose, up to 45 millicuries
Code Added

A9553   Chromium cr-51 sodium chromate, diagnostic, per study dose, up to 250 microcuries
Code Added

A9554   Iodine i-125 sodium iothalamate, diagnostic, per study dose, up to 10 microcuries
Code Added

A9555   Rubidium rb-82, diagnostic, per study dose, up to 60 millicuries
Code Added

A9556   Gallium ga-67 citrate, diagnostic, per millicurie
Code Added

A9557   Technetium tc-99m bicisate, diagnostic, per study dose, up to 25 millicuries
Code Added

A9558   Xenon xe-133 gas, diagnostic, per 10 millicuries
Code Added

A9559   Cobalt co-57 cyanocobalamin, oral, diagnostic, per study dose, up to 1 microcurie
Code Added

A9560   Technetium tc-99m labeled red blood cells, diagnostic, per study dose, up to 30 millicuries
Code Added

A9561   Technetium tc-99m oxidronate, diagnostic, per study dose, up to 30 millicuries
Code Added

A9562   Technetium tc-99m mertiatide, diagnostic, per study dose, up to 15 millicuries
Code Added

A9563   Sodium phosphate p-32, therapeutic, per millicurie
Code Added

A9564   Chromic phosphate p-32 suspension, therapeutic, per millicurie
Code Added

A9565 Indium in-111 pentetreotide, diagnostic, per millicurie
Code Added

A9566 Technetium tc-99m fanolesomab, diagnostic, per study dose, up to 25 millicuries
Code Added

A9567 Technetium tc-99m pentetate, diagnostic, aerosol, per study dose, up to 75 millicuries
Code Added

A9600 Strontium SR-89 chloride, therapeutic, per millicurie
Description Changed

A9605 Samarium SM-153 lexidronamm, therapeutic, per 50 millicuries
Description Changed

A9698 Non-radioactive contrast imaging material, not otherwise classified, per study
MCM: 15022
Code Added

A9699 Radiopharmaceutical, therapeutic, not otherwise classified
Description Changed

B4149 Enteral formula, manufactured bluelcndcrizcd natural foods with intact nutrients, includes proteins, fats, carblueohydrates, vitamins and minerals, may include fiblueer, administered through an enteral feeding tube, 100 calories = 1 unit
Description Changed

B4184 **Deleted 2005**

B4185 Parenteral nutrition solution, per 10 grams lipids
Code Added

B4186 **Deleted 2005**

C1079 **Deleted 2005 use A9546**

C1080   Deleted 2005 use A9544

C1081   Deleted 2005 use A9545

C1082   Deleted 2005 use A9542

C1083   Deleted 2005 use A9543

C1091   Deleted 2005 use A9547

C1092   Deleted 2005 use A9548

C1093   Deleted 2005 use A9566

C1122   Deleted 2005 use A9549

C1200   Deleted 2005

C1201   Deleted 2005 use A9551

C1305   Deleted 2005 use J7340

C1775   Deleted 2005 use A9552

C2634   Brachytherapy source, high activity, iodine-125, greater than 1.01 mci (nist), per source
Description Changed

C2635   Brachytherapy source, high activity, paladium-103, greater than 2.2 mci (nist), per source
Description Changed

C2637   Brachytherapy source, ytterbium-169, per source
Code Added

C9000   Deleted 2005 use A9553

C9007   **Deleted 2005 use J0476**

C9008   **Deleted 2005 use J0475**

C9009   **Deleted 2005 use J0475**

C9013   **Deleted 2005**

C9102   **Deleted 2005 use A9553**

C9103   **Deleted 2005 use A9554**

C9105   **Deleted 2005 use 90371**

C9112   **Deleted 2005 use Q9957**

C9123   **Deleted 2005**

C9200   **Deleted 2005 use J7340**

C9201   **Deleted 2005 use J7342**

C9202   **Deleted 2005 use Q9956**

C9203   **Deleted 2005 use Q9955**

C9205   **Deleted 2005 use J9263**

C9211   **Deleted 2005 use J0215**

C9212   **Deleted 2005 use J0215**

C9218   **Deleted 2005 use J9025**

C9224   Injection, galsulfase, per 5 mg
Code Added

C9225 Injection, fluocinolone acetonide intravitreal implant, per 0.59 mg
Code Added

C9400 **Deleted 2005 use A9505**

C9401 **Deleted 2005 use A9600**

C9402 **Deleted 2005 use A9517**

C9403 **Deleted 2005 use A9528**

C9404 **Deleted 2005 use A9529**

C9405 **Deleted 2005 use A9530**

C9410 **Deleted 2005 use J1190**

C9411 **Deleted 2005 use J2430**

C9413 **Deleted 2005 use J7317**

C9414 **Deleted 2005 use J8560**

C9415 **Deleted 2005 use J9000**

C9417 **Deleted 2005 use J9040**

C9418 **Deleted 2005 use J9060**

C9419 **Deleted 2005 use J9065**

C9420 **Deleted 2005 use J9070**

C9421 **Deleted 2005 use J9093**

C9422   Deleted 2005 use **J9100**

C9423   Deleted 2005 use **J9130**

C9424   Deleted 2005 use **J9150**

C9425   Deleted 2005 use **J9181**

C9426   Deleted 2005 use **J9200**

C9427   Deleted 2005 use **J9208**

C9428   Deleted 2005 use **J9209**

C9429   Deleted 2005 use **J9211**

C9430   Deleted 2005 use **J9218**

C9431   Deleted 2005 use **J9265**

C9432   Deleted 2005 use **J9280**

C9433   Deleted 2005 use **J9340**

C9438   Deleted 2005 use **J7502**

C9704   Deleted 2005 use **0133T**

C9713   Deleted 2005 use **52648**

C9723   Dynamic infrared blood perfusion imaging (DIRI)
Code Added

C9724   Endoscopic full-thickness plication in the gastric cardia
using endoscopic plication system (eps); includes
endoscopy
Code Added

C9725 Placement of endorectal intracavitary applicator for high intensity brachytherapy
Code Added

E0116 Crutch, underarm, other than wood, adjustable or fixed, with pad, tip, handgrip, with or without shock absorber, each
Description Changed

E0169 **Deleted 2005**

E0170 Commode chair with integrated seat lift mechanism, electric, any type
Code Added

E0171 Commode chair with integrated seat lift mechanism, non-electric, any type
Code Added

E0172 Seat lift mechanism placed over or on top of toilet, any type
Code Added

E0485 Oral device/appliance used to reduce upper airway collapsibility, adjustable or non-adjustable, prefabricated, includes fitting and adjustment
Code Added

E0486 Oral device/appliance used to reduce upper airway collapsibility, adjustable or non-adjustable, custom fabricated, includes fitting and adjustment
Code Added

E0637 Combination sit to stand system, any size including pediatric, with seatlift feature, with or without wheels
Description Changed

E0638 Standing frame system, one position (e.g. Upright, supine or prone stander), any size including pediatric, with or without wheels
Description Changed

E0641   Standing frame system, multi-position (e.g. Three-way stander), any size including pediatric, with or without wheels
CIM: 60-9
Code Added

E0642   Standing frame system, mobile (dynamic stander), any size including pediatric
CIM: 60-9
Code Added

E0705   Transfer board or device, any type, each
Code Added

E0752   **Deleted 2005 use L8680**

E0754   **Deleted 2005 use L8681**

E0756   **Deleted 2005**

E0757   **Deleted 2005 use L8682**

E0758   **Deleted 2005 use L8683**

E0759   **Deleted 2005 use L8684**

E0762   Transcutaneous electrical joint stimulation device system, includes all accessories
Code Added

E0764   Functional neuromuscular stimulator, transcutaneous stimulation of muscles of ambulation with computer control, used for walking by spinal cord injured, entire system, after completion of training program
CIM: 35-77
Code Added

E0911   Trapeze bar, heavy duty, for patient weight capacity greater than 250 pounds, attached to bed, with grab bar
CIM: 60-9
Code Added

E0912   Trapeze bar, heavy duty, for patient weight capacity greater than 250 pounds, free standing, complete with grab bar
CIM: 60-9
Code Added

E0935   Continuous passive motion exercise device for use on knee only
Description Changed

E0953   **Deleted 2005 use E2211**

E0954   **Deleted 2005 use E2219**

E0971   Manual wheelchair accessory, anti-tipping device, each
Description Changed

E0972   **Deleted 2005**

E0996   **Deleted 2005 use E2220**

E1000   **Deleted 2005 use E2214**

E1001   **Deleted 2005 use E2224**

E1019   **Deleted 2005**

E1021   **Deleted 2005**

E1025   **Deleted 2005**

E1026   **Deleted 2005**

E1027   **Deleted 2005**

E1038   Transport chair, adult size, patient weight capacity up to and including 300 pounds
Description Changed

E1039 Transport chair, adult size, heavy duty, patient weight capacity greater than 300 pounds
Description Changed

E1210 **Deleted 2005**

E1211 **Deleted 2005**

E1212 **Deleted 2005 use K0010**

E1213 **Deleted 2005 use K0010**

E1239 **Deleted 2005**

E1392 Portable oxygen concentrator, rental
CIM: 60-9
Code Added

E1812 Dynamic knee, extension/flexion device with active resistance control
Code Added

E2207 Wheelchair accessory, crutch and cane holder, each
Code Added

E2208 Wheelchair accessory, cylinder tank carrier, each
Code Added

E2209 Wheelchair accessory, arm trough, each
Code Added

E2210 Wheelchair accessory, bearings, any type, replacement only, each
Code Added

E2211 Manual wheelchair accessory, pneumatic propulsion tire, any size, each
Code Added

E2212   Manual wheelchair accessory, tube for pneumatic propulsion tire, any size, each
Code Added

E2213   Manual wheelchair accessory, insert for pneumatic propulsion tire (removable), any type, any size, each
Code Added

E2214   Manual wheelchair accessory, pneumatic caster tire, any size, each
Code Added

E2215   Manual wheelchair accessory, tube for pneumatic caster tire, any size, each
Code Added

E2216   Manual wheelchair accessory, foam filled propulsion tire, any size, each
Code Added

E2217   Manual wheelchair accessory, foam filled caster tire, any size, each
Code Added

E2218   Manual wheelchair accessory, foam propulsion tire, any size, each
Code Added

E2219   Manual wheelchair accessory, foam caster tire, any size, each
Code Added

E2220   Manual wheelchair accessory, solid (rubber/plastic) propulsion tire, any size, each
Code Added

E2221   Manual wheelchair accessory, solid (rubber/plastic) caster tire (removable), any size, each
Code Added

E2222   Manual wheelchair accessory, solid (rubber/plastic) caster tire with integrated wheel, any size, each
Code Added

E2223   Manual wheelchair accessory, valve, any type, replacement only, each
Code Added

E2224   Manual wheelchair accessory, propulsion wheel excludes tire, any size, each
Code Added

E2225   Manual wheelchair accessory, caster wheel excludes tire, any size, replacement only, each
Code Added

E2226   Manual wheelchair accessory, caster fork, any size, replacement only, each
Code Added

E2371   Power wheelchair accessory, group 27 sealed lead acid battery, (e.g. Gel cell, absorbed glassmat), each
Code Added

E2372   Power wheelchair accessory, group 27 non-sealed lead acid battery, each
Code Added

G0030   **Deleted 2005**

G0031   **Deleted 2005**

G0032   **Deleted 2005**

G0033   **Deleted 2005**

G0034   **Deleted 2005**

G0035   **Deleted 2005**

G0036   Deleted 2005

G0037   Deleted 2005

G0038   Deleted 2005

G0039   Deleted 2005

G0040   Deleted 2005

G0041   Deleted 2005

G0042   Deleted 2005

G0043   Deleted 2005

G0044   Deleted 2005

G0045   Deleted 2005

G0046   Deleted 2005

G0047   Deleted 2005

G0110   Deleted 2005

G0111   Deleted 2005

G0112   Deleted 2005

G0113   Deleted 2005

G0114   Deleted 2005

G0115   Deleted 2005

G0116   Deleted 2005

G0125   Deleted 2005

G0210   Deleted 2005

G0211   Deleted 2005

G0212   Deleted 2005

G0213   Deleted 2005

G0214   Deleted 2005

G0215   Deleted 2005

G0216   Deleted 2005

G0217   Deleted 2005

G0218   Deleted 2005

G0220   Deleted 2005

G0221   Deleted 2005

G0222   Deleted 2005

G0223   Deleted 2005

G0224   Deleted 2005

G0225   Deleted 2005

G0226   Deleted 2005

G0227 Deleted 2005

G0228 Deleted 2005

G0229 Deleted 2005

G0230 Deleted 2005

G0231 Deleted 2005

G0232 Deleted 2005

G0233 Deleted 2005

G0234 Deleted 2005

G0235 Pet imaging, any site, not otherwise specified
CIM: 50-36
Code Added

G0242 Deleted 2005

G0244 Deleted 2005

G0252 Deleted 2005

G0253 Deleted 2005

G0254 Deleted 2005

G0258 Deleted 2005

G0263 Deleted 2005

G0264 Deleted 2005

G0279   Deleted 2005

G0280   Deleted 2005

G0292   Deleted 2005

G0296   Deleted 2005

G0336   Deleted 2005

G0338   Deleted 2005

G0345   Deleted 2005

G0346   Deleted 2005

G0347   Deleted 2005

G0348   Deleted 2005

G0349   Deleted 2005

G0350   Deleted 2005

G0351   Deleted 2005

G0353   Deleted 2005

G0354   Deleted 2005

G0355   Deleted 2005

G0356   Deleted 2005

G0357   Deleted 2005

G0358   Deleted 2005

G0359   Deleted 2005

G0360   Deleted 2005

G0361   Deleted 2005

G0362   Deleted 2005

G0363   Deleted 2005

G0372   Physician service required to establish and document the
         need for a power mobility device (use in addition to
         primary evaluation and management code)
         Code Added

G0375   Smoking and tobacco use cessation counseling visit;
         intermediate, greater than 3 minutes up to 10 minutes
         Code Added

G0376   Smoking and tobacco use cessation counseling visit;
         intensive, greater than 10 minutes
         Code Added

G0378   Hospital observation service, per hour
         Code Added

G0379   Direct admission of patient for hospital observation care
         Code Added

G9033   Amantadine hydrochloride, oral brand, per 100 mg (for
         use in a Medicare-approved demonstration project)
         Code Added

G9041   Sensory integrative techniques to enhance sensory processing and promote adaptive responses to environmental demands, self care/home management training (e.g. Activities of daily living (adl) and compensatory training, meal preparation, safety procedures, and instructions in use of assistive technology devices/adaptive equipment), community/work reintegration training (e.g. shopping, transportation, money management, avocational activities and/or work environment modification analysis, work task analysis), direct one-on-one contact by the provider, each 15 minutes
Code Added

G9042   Sensory integrative techniques to enhance sensory processing and promote adaptive responses to environmental demands, self care/home management training (e.g. Activities of daily living (adl) and compensatory training, meal preparation, safety procedures, and instructions in use of assistive technology devices/adaptive equipment), community/work reintegration training (e.g. shopping, transportation, money management, avocational activities and/or work environment modification analysis, work task analysis), direct one-on-one contact by the provider, each 15 minutes
Code Added

G9043   Sensory integrative techniques to enhance sensory processing and promote adaptive responses to environmental demands, self care/home management training (e.g. Activities of daily living (adl) and compensatory training, meal preparation, safety procedures, and instructions in use of assistive technology devices/adaptive equipment), community/work reintegration training (e.g. shopping, transportation, money management, avocational activities and/or work environment modification analysis, work task analysis), direct one-on-one contact by the provider, each 15 minutes
Code Added

G9044   Sensory integrative techniques to enhance sensory processing and promote adaptive responses to environmental demands, self care/home management training (e.g. Activities of daily living (ADL) and compensatory training, meal preparation, safety procedures, and instructions in use of assistive technology devices/adaptive equipment), community/work reintegration training (e.g. shopping, transportation, money management, avocational activities and/or work environment modification analysis, work task analysis), direct one-on-one contact by the provider, each 15 minutes
Code Added

J0132   Injection, acetylcysteine, 100 mg
Code Added

J0133   Injection, acyclovir, 5 mg
Code Added

J0278   Injection, amikacin sulfate, 100 mg
Code Added

J0365   Injection, aprotonin, 10,000 kiu
MCM: 2049
Code Added

J0480   Injection, basiliximab, 20 mg
MCM: 2049
Code Added

J0795   Injection, corticorelin ovine triflutate, 1 microgram
MCM: 2049
Code Added

J0880   **Deleted 2005**

J0881   Injection, darbepoetin alfa, 1 microgram (non-esrd use)
MCM: 4273.1
Code Added

J0882   Injection, darbepoetin alfa, 1 microgram (for esrd on dialysis)
MCM: 4273.1
Code Added

J0885   Injection, epoetin alfa, (for non-esrd use), 1000 units
MCM: 2049
Code Added

J0886   Injection, epoetin alfa, 1000 units (for esrd on dialysis)
MCM: 4273.1
Code Added

J1162   Injection, digoxin immune fab (ovine), per vial
MCM: 2049
Code Added

J1265   Injection, dopamine hcl, 40 mg
Code Added

J1430   Injection, ethanolamine oleate, 100 mg
MCM: 2049
Code Added

J1451   Injection, fomepizole, 15 mg
MCM: 2049
Code Added

J1563   **Deleted 2005**

J1564   **Deleted 2005**

J1566   Injection, immune globulin, intravenous, lyophilized (e.g. Powder), 500 mg
MCM: 2049
Code Added

J1567   Injection, immune globulin, intravenous, non-lyophilized (e.g. Liquid), 500 mg
MCM: 2049
Code Added

J1640   Injection, hemin, 1 mg
MCM: 2049
Code Added

J1675   Injection, histrelin acetate, 10 micrograms
MCM: 2049
Code Added

J1750   **Deleted 2005**

J1751   Injection, iron dextran 165, 50 mg
Code Added

J1752   Injection, iron dextran 267, 50 mg
Code Added

J1945   Injection, lepirudin, 50 mg
Code Added

J2278   Injection, ziconotide, 1 microgram
Code Added

J2324   **Deleted 2005**

J2325   Injection, nesiritide, 0.1 mg
MCM: 2049
Code Added

J2425   Injection, palifermin, 50 micrograms
Code Added

J2503   Injection, pegaptanib sodium, 0.3 mg
Code Added

J2504   Injection, pegademase bovine, 25 iu
MCM: 2049
Code Added

J2513 Injection, pentastarch, 10% solution, 100 ml
MCM: 2049
Code Added

J2805 Injection, sincalide, 5 micrograms
Code Added

J2850 Injection, secretin, synthetic, human, 1 microgram
Code Added

J3285 Injection, treprostinil, 1 mg
Code Added

J3355 Injection, urofollitropin, 75 iu
MCM: 2049
Code Added

J3471 Injection, hyaluronidase, ovine, preservative free, per 1
usp unit (up to 999 USP units)
Code Added

J3472 Injection, hyaluronidase, ovine, preservative free, per 1000
usp units
Code Added

J7051 **Deleted 2005**

J7188 Injection, von willebrand factor complex, human, iu
CIM: 35.30 MCM: 2049.5
Code Added

J7189 Factor VIIA (antihemophilic factor, recombinant), per 1
microgram
MCM: 2049
Code Added

J7306 Levonorgestrel (contraceptive) implant system, including
implants and supplies
Code Added

J7317 **Deleted 2005**

J7318   Hyaluronan (sodium hyaluronate) or derivative, intra-articular injection, 1 mg
Code Added

J7320   **Deleted 2005**

J7340   Dermal and epidermal, (substitute) tissue of human origin, with or without bioengineered or processed elements, with metabolically active elements, per square centimeter
Description Changed

J7341   Dermal (substitute) tissue of non-human origin, with or without other bioengineered or processed elements, with metabolically active elements, per square centimeter
Code Added

J7342   Dermal (substitute) tissue of human origin, with or without other Bioengineered or processed elements, with metabolically active elements, per square centimeter
Description Changed

J7343   Dermal and epidermal, (substitute) tissue of non-human origin, with or without other bioengineered or processed elements, without metabolically active elements, per square centimeter
Description Changed

J7344   Dermal (substitute) tissue of human origin, with or without other Bioengineered or processed elements, without metabolically active elements, per square centimeter
Description Changed

J7350   Dermal (substitute) tissue of human origin, injectable, with or without other bioengineered or processed elements, But without metabolized active elements, per 10 mg
Description Changed

J7616   **Deleted 2005**

J7617   **Deleted 2005**

J7620   Albuterol, up to 2.5 mg and ipratropium bromide, up to 0.5 mg, non-compounded inhalation solution, administered through DME
MCM: 2100.5
Code Added

J7626   Budesonide inhalation solution, non-compounded, administered through DME, unit dose form, up to 0.5 mg
Description Changed

J7627   Budesonide, powder, compounded for inhalation solution, administered through DME, unit dose form, up to 0.5 mg
Code Added

J7640   Formorterol, inhalation solution administered through DME, unit dose form, 12 micrograms
Code Added

J8498   Anti-emetic drug, rectal/suppository, not otherwise specified
MCM: 2049.5
Code Added

J8515   Cabergoline, oral, 0.25 mg
MCM: 2049.5
Code Added

J8540   Dexamethasone, oral, 0.25 mg
Code Added

J8597   Anti-emetic drug, oral, not otherwise specified
Code Added

J9025   Injection, azacitidine, 1 mg
Code Added

J9027   Injection, clofarabine, 1 mg
Code Added

J9175   Injection, Elliott's b solution, 1 ml
MCM: 2049
Code Added

J9225   Histrelin implant, 50 mg
MCM: 2049
Code Added

J9264   Injection, paclitaxel protein-bound particles, 1 mg
Code Added

K0064   **Deleted 2005 use E2213**

K0066   **Deleted 2005 use E2220**

K0067   **Deleted 2005 use E2211**

K0068   **Deleted 2005 use E2212**

K0074   **Deleted 2005 use E2214**

K0075   **Deleted 2005 use E2219**

K0076   **Deleted 2005 use E2221**

K0078   **Deleted 2005 use E2215**

K0102   **Deleted 2005 use E2207**

K0104   **Deleted 2005 use E2208**

K0106   **Deleted 2005 use E2209**

K0415   **Deleted 2005**

K0416   **Deleted 2005**

K0452   **Deleted 2005 use E2210**

K0600   **Deleted 2005 use E0762**

K0618   Deleted 2005 use L0491

K0619   Deleted 2005 use L0492

K0620   Deleted 2005 use A6457

K0628   Deleted 2005 use A5512

K0629   Deleted 2005 use A5513

K0630   Deleted 2005 use L0621

K0631   Deleted 2005 use L0622

K0632   Deleted 2005 use L0623

K0633   Deleted 2005 use L0624

K0634   Deleted 2005 use L0625

K0635   Deleted 2005 use L0626

K0636   Deleted 2005 use L0627

K0637   Deleted 2005 use L0628

K0638   Deleted 2005 use L0629

K0639   Deleted 2005 use L0630

K0640   Deleted 2005 use L0631

K0641   Deleted 2005 use L0632

K0642   Deleted 2005 use L0633

K0643 Deleted 2005 use L0634

K0644 Deleted 2005 use L0635

K0645 Deleted 2005 use L0636

K0646 Deleted 2005 use L0637

K0647 Deleted 2005 use L0638

K0648 Deleted 2005 use L0639

K0649 Deleted 2005 use L0640

K0669 Wheelchair accessory, wheelchair seat or Back cushion, does not meet specific code criterion or no written coding verification from SADMERC
Description Changed

K0730 Controlled dose inhalation drug delivery system
Code Added

L0491 TLSO, sagittal-coronal control, modular segmented spinal system, two rigid plastic shells, posterior extends from the sacrococcygeal junction and terminates just inferior to the scapular spine, anterior extends from the symphysis pubis to the xiphoid, soft liner, restricts gross trunk motion in the sagittal and coronal planes, lateral strength is provided by overlapping plastic and stabilizing closures, includes straps and closures, prefabricated, includes fitting and adjustment
Code Added

L0492 TLSO, sagittal-coronal control, modular segmented spinal system, three rigid plastic shells, posterior extends from the sacrococcygeal junction and terminates just inferior to the scapular spine, anterior extends from the symphysis pubis to the xiphoid, soft liner, restricts gross trunk motion in the sagittal and coronal planes, lateral strength is provided by overlapping plastic and stabilizing closures, includes straps and closures, prefabricated, includes fitting and adjustment
Code Added

L0621   Sacroiliac orthosis, flexible, provides pelvic-sacral support, reduces motion about the sacroiliac joint, includes straps, closures, may include pendulous abdomen design, prefabricated, includes fitting and adjustment
Code Added

L0622   Sacroiliac orthosis, flexible, provides pelvic-sacral support, reduces motion about the sacroiliac joint, includes straps, closures, may include pendulous abdomen design, custom fabricated
Code Added

L0623   Sacroiliac orthosis, provides pelvic-sacral support, with rigid or semi-rigid panels over the sacrum and abdomen, reduces motion about the sacroiliac joint, includes straps, closures, may include pendulous abdomen design, prefabricated, includes fitting and adjustment
Code Added

L0624   Sacroiliac orthosis, provides pelvic-sacral support, with rigid or semi-rigid panels placed over the sacrum and abdomen, reduces motion about the sacroiliac joint, includes straps, closures, may include pendulous abdomen design, custom fabricated
Code Added

L0625   Lumbar orthosis, flexible, provides lumbar support, posterior extends from L-1 to below L-5 vertebra, produces intracavitary pressure to reduce load on the intervertebral discs, includes straps, closures, may include pendulous abdomen design, shoulder straps, stays, prefabricated, includes fitting and adjustment
Code Added

L0626   Lumbar orthosis, sagittal control, with rigid posterior panel(s), posterior extends from L-1 to below L-5 vertebra, produces intracavitary pressure to reduce load on the intervertebral discs, includes straps, closures, may include padding, stays, shoulder straps, pendulous abdomen design, prefabricated, includes fitting and adjustment
Code Added

L0627 Lumbar orthosis, sagittal control, with rigid anterior and posterior panels, posterior extends from L-1 to below L-5 vertebra, produces intracavitary pressure to reduce load on the intervertebral discs, includes straps, closures, may include padding, shoulder straps, pendulous abdomen design, prefabricated, includes fitting and adjustment
Code Added

L0628 Lumbar-sacral orthosis, flexible, provides lumbo-sacral support, posterior extends from sacrococcygeal junction to T-9 vertebra, produces intracavitary pressure to reduce load on the intervertebral discs, includes straps, closures, may include stays, shoulder straps, pendulous abdomen design, prefabricated, includes fitting and adjustment
Code Added

L0629 Lumbar-sacral orthosis, flexible, provides lumbo-sacral support, posterior extends from sacrococcygeal junction to T-9 vertebra, produces intracavitary pressure to reduce load on the intervertebral discs, includes straps, closures, may include stays, shoulder straps, pendulous abdomen design, custom fabricated
Code Added

L0630 Lumbar-sacral orthosis, sagittal control, with rigid posterior panel(s), posterior extends from sacrococcygeal junction to T-9 vertebra, produces intracavitary pressure to reduce load on the intervertebral discs, includes straps, closures, may include padding, stays, shoulder straps, pendulous abdomen design, prefabricated, includes fitting and adjustment
Code Added

L0631 Lumbar-sacral orthosis, sagittal control, with rigid anterior and posterior panels, posterior extends from sacrococcygeal junction to T-9 vertebra, produces intracavitary pressure to reduce load on the intervertebral discs, includes straps, pendulous abdomen design, prefabricated, includes fitting and adjustment
Code Added

L0632   Lumbar-sacral orthosis, sagittal control, with rigid anterior and posterior panels, posterior extends from sacrococcygeal junction to T-9 vertebra, produces intracavitary pressure to reduce load on the intervertebral discs, includes straps, closures, may include padding, shoulder straps, pendulous abdomen design, custom fabricated
Code Added

L0633   Lumbar-sacral orthosis, sagittal-coronal control, with rigid posterior frame/panel(s), posterior extends from sacrococcygeal junction to T-9 vertebra, lateral strength provided by rigid lateral frame/panels, produces intracavitary pressure to reduce load on intervertebral discs, includes straps, closures, may include padding, stays, shoulder straps, pendulous abdomen design, prefabricated, includes fitting and adjustment
Code Added

L0634   Lumbar-sacral orthosis, sagittal-coronal control, with rigid posterior frame/panel(s), posterior extends from sacrococcygeal junction to T-9 vertebra, lateral strength provided by rigid lateral frame/panel(s), produces intracavitary pressure to reduce load on intervertebral discs, includes straps, closures, may include padding, stays, shoulder straps, pendulous abdomen design, custom fabricated
Code Added

L0635   Lumbar-sacral orthosis, sagittal-coronal control, lumbar flexion, rigid posterior frame/panel(s), lateral articulating design to flex the lumbar spine, posterior extends from sacrococcygeal junction to T-9 vertebra, lateral strength provided by rigid lateral frame/panel(s), produces intracavitary pressure to reduce load on intervertebral discs, includes straps, closures, may include padding, anterior panel, pendulous abdomen design, prefabricated, includes fitting and adjustment
Code Added

L0636 Lumbar sacral orthosis, sagittal-coronal control, lumbar flexion, rigid posterior frame/panels, lateral articulating design to flex the lumbar spine, posterior extends from sacrococcygeal junction to T-9 vertebra, lateral strength provided by rigid lateral frame/panels, produces intracavitary pressure to reduce load on intervertebral discs, includes straps, closures, may include padding, anterior panel, pendulous abdomen design, custom fabricated
Code Added

L0637 Lumbar-sacral orthosis, sagittal-coronal control, with rigid anterior and posterior frame/panels, posterior extends from sacrococcygeal junction to T-9 vertebra, lateral strength provided by rigid lateral frame/panels, produces intracavitary pressure to reduce load on intervertebral discs, includes straps, closures, may include padding, shoulder straps, pendulous abdomen design, prefabricated, includes fitting and adjustment
Code Added

L0638 Lumbar-sacral orthosis, sagittal-coronal control, with rigid anterior and posterior frame/panels, posterior extends from sacrococcygeal junction to T-9 vertebra, lateral strength provided by rigid lateral frame/panels, produces intracavitary pressure to reduce load on intervertebral discs, includes straps, closures, may include padding, shoulder straps, pendulous abdomen design, custom fabricated
Code Added

L0639 Lumbar-sacral orthosis, sagittal-coronal control, rigid shell(s)/panel(s), posterior extends from sacrococcygeal junction to T-9 vertebra, anterior extends from symphysis pubis to xyphoid, produces intracavitary pressure to reduce load on the intervertebral discs, overall strength is provided by overlapping rigid material and stabilizing closures, includes straps, closures, may include soft interface, pendulous abdomen design, prefabricated, includes fitting and adjustment
Code Added

L0640 Lumbar-sacral orthosis, sagittal-coronal control, rigid shell(s)/panel(s), posterior extends from sacrococcygeal junction to T-9 vertebra, anterior extends from symphysis pubis to xyphoid, produces intracavitary pressure to reduce load on the intervertebral discs, overall strength is provided by overlapping rigid material and stabilizing closures, includes straps, closures, may include soft interface, pendulous abdomen design, custom fabricated
Code Added

L0859 Addition to halo procedure, magnetic resonance image compatible systems, rings and pins, any material
Code Added

L0860 **Deleted 2005 use L0859**

L1750 **Deleted 2005 use A4565**

L1832 Knee orthosis, adjustable knee joints (unicentric or polycentric), positional orthosis, rigid support, prefabricated, includes fitting and adjustment
Description Changed

L1843 Knee orthosis, single upright, thigh and calf, with adjustable flexion and extension joint (unicentric or polycentric), medial-lateral and rotation control, with or without varus/valgus adjustment, prefabricated, includes fitting and adjustment
Description Changed

L1844 Knee orthosis, single upright, thigh and calf, with adjustable flexion and extension joint (unicentric or polycentric), medial-lateral and rotation control, with or without varus/valgus adjustment, custom fabricated
Description Changed

L1845 Knee orthosis, double upright, thigh and calf, with adjustable flexion and extension joint (unicentric or polycentric), medial-lateral and rotation control, with or without varus/valgus adjustment, prefabricated, includes fitting and adjustment
Description Changed

L1846   Knee orthosis, double upright, thigh and calf, with adjustable flexion and extension joint (unicentric or polycentric), medial-lateral and rotation control, with or without varus/valgus adjustment, custom fabricated
Description Changed

L2034   Knee ankle foot orthosis, full plastic, single upright, with or without free motion knee, medial lateral rotation control, with or without free motion ankle, custom fabricated
Code Added

L2036   Knee ankle foot orthosis, full plastic, double upright, with or without free motion knee, with or without free motion ankle, custom fabricated
Description Changed

L2037   Knee ankle foot orthosis, full plastic, single upright, with or without free motion knee, with or without free motion ankle, custom fabricated
Description Changed

L2038   Knee ankle foot orthosis, full plastic, with or without free motion knee, multi-axis ankle, custom fabricated
Description Changed

L2039   **Deleted 2005**

L2387   Addition to lower extremity, polycentric knee joint, for custom fabricated knee ankle foot orthosis, each joint
Code Added

L2405   Addition to knee joint, drop lock, each
Description Changed

L3170   Foot, plastic, silicone or equal, heel stabilizer, each
Description Changed

L3215   Orthopedic footwear, ladies shoe, oxford, each
Description Changed

L3216 Orthopedic footwear, ladies shoe, depth inlay, each
Description Changed

L3217 Orthopedic footwear, ladies shoe, hightop, depth inlay, each
Description Changed

L3219 Orthopedic footwear, mens shoe, oxford, each
Description Changed

L3221 Orthopedic footwear, mens shoe, depth inlay, each
Description Changed

L3222 Orthopedic footwear, mens shoe, hightop, depth inlay, each
Description Changed

L3230 Orthopedic footwear, custom shoe, depth inlay, each
Description Changed

L3671 Shoulder orthosis, shoulder cap design, without joints, may include soft interface, straps, custom fabricated, includes fitting and adjustment
Code Added

L3672 Shoulder orthosis, abduction positioning (airplane design), thoracic component and support bar, without joints, may include soft interface, straps, custom fabricated, includes fitting and adjustment
Code Added

L3673 Shoulder orthosis, abduction positioning (airplane design), thoracic component and support bar, includes nontorsion joint/turnbuckle, may include soft interface, straps, custom fabricated, includes fitting and adjustment
Code Added

L3702 Elbow orthosis, without joints, may include soft interface, straps, custom fabricated, includes fitting and adjustment
Code Added

L3763   Elbow wrist hand orthosis, rigid, without joints, may include soft interface, straps, custom fabricated, includes fitting and adjustment
Code Added

L3764   Elbow wrist hand orthosis, includes one or more nontorsion joints, elastic bands, turnbuckles, may include soft interface, straps, custom fabricated, includes fitting and adjustment
Code Added

L3765   Elbow wrist hand finger orthosis, rigid, without joints, may include soft interface, straps, custom fabricated, includes fitting and adjustment
Code Added

L3766   Elbow wrist hand finger orthosis, includes one or more nontorsion joints, elastic bands, turnbuckles, may include soft interface, straps, custom fabricated, includes fitting and adjustment
Code Added

L3905   Wrist hand orthosis, includes one or more nontorsion joints, elastic bands, turnbuckles, may include soft interface, straps, custom fabricated, includes fitting and adjustment
Code Added

L3906   Wrist hand orthosis, without joints, may include soft interface, straps, custom fabricated, includes fitting and adjustment
Description Changed

L3913   Hand finger orthosis, without joints, may include soft interface, straps, custom fabricated, includes fitting and adjustment
Code Added

L3919   Hand orthosis, without joints, may include soft interface, straps, custom fabricated, includes fitting and adjustment
Code Added

L3921   Hand finger orthosis, includes one or more nontorsion joints, elastic bands, turnbuckles, may include soft interface, straps, custom fabricated, includes fitting and adjustment
Code Added

L3923   Hand finger orthosis, without joints, may include soft interface, straps, prefabricated, includes fitting and adjustment
Description Changed

L3933   Finger orthosis, without joints, may include soft interface, custom fabricated, includes fitting and adjustment
Code Added

L3935   Finger orthosis, nontorsion joint, may include soft interface, custom fabricated, includes fitting and adjustment
Code Added

L3961   Shoulder elbow wrist hand orthosis, shoulder cap design, without joints, may include soft interface, straps, custom fabricated, includes fitting and adjustment
Code Added

L3963   **Deleted 2005**

L3967   Shoulder elbow wrist hand orthosis, abduction positioning (airplane design), thoracic component and support bar, without joints, may include soft interface, straps, custom fabricated, includes fitting and adjustment
Code Added

L3971   Shoulder elbow wrist hand orthosis, shoulder cap design, includes one or more nontorsion joints, elastic bands, turnbuckles, may include soft interface, straps, custom fabricated, includes fitting and adjustment
Code Added

L3973 Shoulder elbow wrist hand orthosis, abduction positioning (airplane design), thoracic component and support bar, includes one or more nontorsion joints, elastic bands, turnbuckles, may include soft interface, straps, custom fabricated, includes fitting and adjustment
Code Added

L3975 Shoulder elbow wrist hand finger orthosis, shoulder cap design, without joints, may include soft interface, straps, custom fabricated, includes fitting and adjustment
Code Added

L3976 Shoulder elbow wrist hand finger orthosis, abduction positioning (airplane design), thoracic component and support bar, without joints, may include soft interface, straps, custom fabricated, includes fitting and adjustment
Code Added

L3977 Shoulder elbow wrist hand finger orthosis, shoulder cap design, includes one or more nontorsion joints, elastic bands, turnbuckles, may include soft interface, straps, custom fabricated, includes fitting and adjustment
Code Added

L3978 Shoulder elbow wrist hand finger orthosis, abduction positioning (airplane design), thoracic component and support bar, includes one or more nontorsion joints, elastic bands, turnbuckles, may include soft interface, straps, custom fabricated, includes fitting and adjustment
Code Added

L5703 Ankle, symes, molded to patient model, socket without solid ankle cushion heel (Sach) foot, replacement only
Code Added

L5858 Addition to lower extremity prosthesis, endoskeletal knee shin system, microprocessor control feature, stance phase only, includes electronic sensor(s), any type
Code Added

L5971 All lower extremity prosthesis, solid ankle cushion heel (sach) foot, replacement only
Code Added

L6621   Upper extremity prosthesis addition, flexion/extension
wrist with or without friction, for use with external
powered terminal device
Code Added

L6677   Upper extremity addition, harness, triple control,
simultaneous operation of terminal device and elbow
Code Added

L6883   Replacement socket, below elbow/wrist disarticulation,
molded to patient model, for use with or without external
power
Code Added

L6884   Replacement socket, above elbow disarticulation, molded
to patient model, for use with or without external power
Code Added

L6885   Replacement socket, shoulder disarticulation/interscapular
thoracic, molded to patient model, for use with or without
external power
Code Added

L7400   Addition to upper extremity prosthesis; below elbow/wrist
disarticulation, ultralight material (titanium, carbon fiber
or equal)
Code Added

L7401   Addition to upper extremity prosthesis, above elbow
disarticulation, ultralight material (titanium, carbon fiber
or equal)
Code Added

L7402   Addition to upper extremity prosthesis, shoulder
disarticulation/interscapular thoracic, ultralight material
(titanium, carbon fiber or equal)
Code Added

L7403   Addition to upper extremity prosthesis, below elbow/wrist
disarticulation, acrylic material
Code Added

L7404 Addition to upper extremity prosthesis, above elbow disarticulation, acrylic material
Code Added

L7405 Addition to upper extremity prosthesis, shoulder disarticulation/interscapular thoracic, acrylic material
Code Added

L7600 Prosthetic donning sleeve, any material, each
Code Added

L8100 Deleted 2005 use A6530

L8110 Deleted 2005 use A6531

L8120 Deleted 2005 use A6532

L8130 Deleted 2005 use A6533

L8140 Deleted 2005 use A6534

L8150 Deleted 2005 use A6535

L8160 Deleted 2005 use A6536

L8170 Deleted 2005 use A6537

L8180 Deleted 2005 use A6538

L8190 Deleted 2005 use A6539

L8195 Deleted 2005 use A6540

L8200 Deleted 2005 use A6541

L8210 Deleted 2005 use A6542

L8220   Deleted 2005 use A6543

L8230   Deleted 2005 use A6544

L8239   Deleted 2005 use A6549

L8609   Artificial cornea
Code Added

L8620   Deleted 2005

L8623   Lithium ion battery for use with cochlear implant device speech processor, other than ear level, replacement, each
Code Added

L8624   Lithium ion battery for use with cochlear implant device speech processor, ear level, replacement, each
Code Added

L8680   Implantable neurostimulator electrode, each
CIM: 65-8
Code Added

L8681   Patient programmer (external) for use with implantable programmable neurostimulator pulse generator
CIM: 65-8
Code Added

L8682   Implantable neurostimulator radiofrequency receiver
CIM: 65-8
Code Added

L8683   Radiofrequency transmitter (external) for use with implantable neurostimulator radiofrequency receiver
CIM: 65-8
Code Added

L8684   Radiofrequency transmitter (external) for use with implantable sacral root neurostimulator receiver for bowel and bladder management, replacement
CIM: 65-8
Code Added

L8685   Implantable neurostimulator pulse generator, single array, rechargeable, includes extension
CIM: 65-8
Code Added

L8686   Implantable neurostimulator pulse generator, single array, non-rechargeable, includes extension
CIM: 65-8
Code Added

L8687   Implantable neurostimulator pulse generator, dual array, rechargeable, includes extension
CIM: 65-8
Code Added

L8688   Implantable neurostimulator pulse generator, dual array, non-rechargeable, includes extension
CIM: 65-8
Code Added

L8689   External recharging system for implanted neurostimulator, replacement only
Code Added

Q0136   **Deleted 2005 use J0885**

Q0137   **Deleted 2005 use J0881**

Q0187   **Deleted 2005 use J7189**

Q0480   Driver for use with pneumatic ventricular assist device, replacement only
Code Added

Q0481   Microprocessor control unit for use with electric ventricular assist device, replacement only
Code Added

Q0482   Microprocessor control unit for use with electric/pneumatic combination ventricular assist device, replacement only
Code Added

Q0483 Monitor/display module for use with electric ventricular assist device, replacement only
Code Added

Q0484 Monitor/display module for use with electric or electric/pneumatic ventricular assist device, replacement only
Code Added

Q0485 Monitor control cable for use with electric ventricular assist device, replacement only
Code Added

Q0486 Monitor control cable for use with electric/pneumatic ventricular assist device, replacement only
Code Added

Q0487 Leads (pneumatic/electrical) for use with any type electric/pneumatic ventricular assist device, replacement only
Code Added

Q0488 Power pack base for use with electric ventricular assist device, replacement only
Code Added

Q0489 Power pack base for use with electric/pneumatic ventricular assist device, replacement only
Code Added

Q0490 Emergency power source for use with electric ventricular assist device, replacement only
Code Added

Q0491 Emergency power source for use with electric/pneumatic ventricular assist device, replacement only
Code Added

Q0492 Emergency power supply cable for use with electric ventricular assist device, replacement only
Code Added

Q0493 Emergency power supply cable for use with electric/pneumatic ventricular assist device, replacement only
Code Added

Q0494 Emergency hand pump for use with electric or electric/pneumatic ventricular assist device, replacement only
Code Added

Q0495 Battery/power pack charger for use with electric or electric/pneumatic ventricular assist device, replacement only
Code Added

Q0496 Battery for use with electric or electric/pneumatic ventricular assist device, replacement only
Code Added

Q0497 Battery clips for use with electric or electric/pneumatic ventricular assist device, replacement only
Code Added

Q0498 Holster for use with electric or electric/pneumatic ventricular assist device, replacement only
Code Added

Q0499 Belt/vest for use with electric or electric/pneumatic ventricular assist device, replacement only
Code Added

Q0500 Filters for use with electric or electric/pneumatic ventricular assist device, replacement only
Code Added

Q0501 Shower cover for use with electric or electric/pneumatic ventricular assist device, replacement only
Code Added

Q0502 Mobility cart for pneumatic ventricular assist device, replacement only
Code Added

Q0503 Battery for pneumatic ventricular assist device, replacement only, each
Code Added

Q0504 Power adapter for pneumatic ventricular assist device, replacement only, vehicle type
Code Added

Q0505 Miscellaneous supply or accessory for use with ventricular assist device
Code Added

Q0510 Pharmacy supply fee for initial immunosuppressive drug(s), first month following implant
Code Added

Q0511 Pharmacy supply fee for oral anti-cancer, oral anti-emetic or immunosuppressive drug(s); for the first prescription in a 30-day period
Code Added

Q0512 Pharmacy supply fee for oral anti-cancer, oral anti-emetic or immunosuppressive drug(s); for a subsequent prescription in a 30-day period
Code Added

Q0513 Pharmacy dispensing fee for inhalation drug(s); per 30 days
Code Added

Q0514 Pharmacy dispensing fee for inhalation drug(s); per 90 days
Code Added

Q0515 Injection, sermorelin acetate, 1 microgram
MCM: 2049
Code Added

Q1001 **Deleted 2005**

Q1002 **Deleted 2005**

Q2001   Deleted 2005

Q2002   Deleted 2005 use J9175

Q2003   Deleted 2005 use J0365

Q2005   Deleted 2005

Q2006   Deleted 2005 use J1162

Q2007   Deleted 2005 use J1430

Q2008   Deleted 2005 use J1451

Q2011   Deleted 2005 use J1640

Q2012   Deleted 2005 use J2504

Q2013   Deleted 2005 use J2513

Q2014   Deleted 2005

Q2018   Deleted 2005 use J3355

Q2019   Deleted 2005 use J0480

Q2020   Deleted 2005 use J1675

Q2021   Deleted 2005 use J1945

Q2022   Deleted 2005 use J7188

Q3000   Deleted 2005

Q3002   Deleted 2005

Q3003   Deleted 2005

Q3004   Deleted 2005

Q3005   Deleted 2005

Q3006   Deleted 2005

Q3007   Deleted 2005

Q3008   Deleted 2005

Q3009   Deleted 2005

Q3010   Deleted 2005

Q3011   Deleted 2005

Q3012   Deleted 2005

Q4054   Deleted 2005 use J0882

Q4055   Deleted 2005 use J0886

Q4075   Deleted 2005 use J0133

Q4076   Deleted 2005 use J1265

Q4077   Deleted 2005 use J3285

Q4079   Injection, natalizumab, 1 mg
Code Added

Q4080   Iloprost, inhalation solution, administered through dme, 20 micrograms
Code Added

Q9945 Low osmolar contrast material, up to 149 mg/ml iodine concentration, per ml
Code Added

Q9946 Low osmolar contrast material, 150-199 mg/ml iodine concentration, per ml
MCM: 15022
Code Added

Q9947 Low osmolar contrast material, 200-249 mg/ml iodine concentration, per ml
MCM: 15022
Code Added

Q9948 Low osmolar contrast material, 250-299 mg/ml iodine concentration, per ml
MCM: 15022
Code Added

Q9949 Low osmolar contrast material, 300-349 mg/ml iodine concentration, per ml
MCM: 15022
Code Added

Q9950 Low osmolar contrast material, 350-399 mg/ml iodine concentration, per ml
MCM: 15022
Code Added

Q9951 Low osmolar contrast material, 400 or greater mg/ml iodine concentration, per ml
MCM: 15022
Code Added

Q9952 Injection, gadolinium-based magnetic resonance contrast agent, per ml
MCM: 15022
Code Added

Q9953 Injection, iron-based magnetic resonance contrast agent, per ml
MCM: 15022
Code Added

Q9954 Oral magnetic resonance contrast agent, per 100 ml
MCM: 15022
Code Added

Q9955 Injection, perflexane lipid microspheres, per ml
Code Added

Q9956 Injection, octafluoropropane microspheres, per ml
Code Added

Q9957 Injection, perflutren lipid microspheres, per ml
Code Added

Q9958 High osmolar contrast material, up to 149 mg/ml iodine concentration, per ml
MCM: 15022
Code Added

Q9959 High osmolar contrast material, 150-199 mg/ml iodine concentration, per ml
MCM: 15022
Code Added

Q9960 High osmolar contrast material, 200-249 mg/ml iodine concentration, per ml
MCM: 15022
Code Added

Q9961 High osmolar contrast material, 250-299 mg/ml iodine concentration, per ml
MCM: 15022
Code Added

Q9962 High osmolar contrast material, 300-349 mg/ml iodine concentration, per ml
Code Added

Q9963 High osmolar contrast material, 350-399 mg/ml iodine concentration, per ml
MCM: 15022
Code Added

Q9964 High osmolar contrast material, 400 or greater mg/ml iodine concentration, per
MCM: 15022
Code Added

S0016 **Deleted 2005 use S0072**

S0071 **Deleted 2005**

S0072 **Deleted 2005**

S0107 **Deleted 2005 use J2357**

S0114 **Deleted 2005**

S0133 Histrelin, implant, 50 mg
Code Added

S0142 Colistimethate sodium, inhalation solution administered through DME, concentrated form, per mg
Code Added

S0143 Aztreonam, inhalation solution administered through dme, concentrated form, per gram
Code Added

S0145 Injection, pegylated interferon alfa-2a, 180 mcg per ml
Code Added

S0146 Injection, pegylated interferon alfa-2b, 10 mcg per 0.5 ml
Code Added

S0158 **Deleted 2005 use J1931**

S0159 **Deleted 2005 use J0180**

S0173 **Deleted 2005**

S0197 Prenatal vitamins, 30-day supply
Code Added

S0198   Injection, pegaptanib sodium, 0.3 mg
Code Added

S0265   Genetic counseling, under physician supervision, each 15 minutes
Code Added

S0595   Dispensing new spectacle lenses for patient supplied frame
Code Added

S0613   Annual gynecological examination; clinical breast examination without pelvic evaluation
Code Added

S0625   Retinal telescreening by digital imaging of multiple different fund us areas to screen for vision-threatening conditions, including imaging, interpretation and report
Code Added

S2068   Breast reconstruction with deep inferior epigastric perforator (diep) flap, including microvascular anastomosis and closure of donor site, unilateral
Code Added

S2075   Laparoscopy, surgical; repair incisional or ventral hernia
Code Added

S2076   Laparoscopy, surgical; repair umbilical hernia
Code Added

S2077   Laparoscopy, surgical; implantation of mesh or other prosthesis for incisional or ventral hernia repair (list separately in addition to code for incisional or ventral hernia repair)
Code Added

S2078   Laparoscopic supracervical hysterectomy (subtotal hysterectomy), with or without removal of tube(s), with or without removal of ovary(s)
Code Added

S2079 Laparoscopic esophagomyotomy (heller type)
Code Added

S2082 **Deleted 2005**

S2090 **Deleted 2005**

S2091 **Deleted 2005**

S2114 Arthroscopy, shoulder, surgical; tenodesis of biceps
Code Added

S2117 Arthroereisis, subtalar
Code Added

S2900 Surgical techniques requiring use of robotic surgical
system (list separately in addition to code for primary
procedure)
Code Added

S3005 Performance measurement, evaluation of patient self
assessment, depression
Code Added

S3626 Maternal serum quadruple marker screen including
alpha-fetoprotein (AFP), estriol, human chorionic
gonadotropin (HCG) and inhibin a
Code Added

S3854 Gene expression profiling panel for use in the
management of breast cancer treatment
Code Added

S8004 **Deleted 2005 use 78804**

S8095 **Deleted 2005**

S8270 Enuresis alarm, using auditory buzzer and/or vibration
device
Code Added

S8940   Equestrian/hippotherapy, per session
Code Added

T2006   **Deleted 2005 use A0998**

V2788   Presbyopia correcting function of intraocular lens
Code Added

APPENDIX C:
TABLE OF DRUGS

HCPCS TABLE OF DRUGS

Directions for the Use of the Table:

1. All drugs are listed in strict alphabetical order by generic drug name.

2. HCPCS code numbers for drugs are listed only under the generic drug name. Users should first look for entries under generic names of drugs. When a drug is known only by brand name, look for the brand name and you will be directed to the generic name of the drug (see "generic name").

3. Cancer chemotherapy drugs are preceded by an asterisk (*).

4. In all cases except those preceded by a pound sign (#), the amount stated includes the amount as well as any amount "up to" that which is stated in the column. When a pound sign appears, it designated that the amount of the drug is only the amount listed.

5. A dash (—) appearing in a column signifies that no information is given for that particular variable for the drug listed.

6. Information which is indented and appears beneath the first line for a drug is to be considered a continuation of the line preceding it. All drug entries should be checked for indented lines beneath it as a continuation of that entry.

7. When one drug has more than one entry as a result of different routes of administration or different amounts, the drug name is not repeated. All entries for the same drug are listed beneath that drug.

8. The following abbreviations are used in the "routes of administration" column:

amp   = ampule

DME = durable medical equipment

EPI   = epidural

DRUG
TABLE

g   = gram

IA   = intra-arterial administration

IM   = intramuscular administration

INF   = infusion

INH   = administration by inhaled solution

INJ   = injection

IO   = intraocular

IT   = intrathecal

IU   = international unit

IV   = intravenous administration

mcg   = microgram

mg   = milligram

ml   = milliliter

ORAL= administered orally

OTH   = other routes of administration

PAR   = parenteral

SC   = subcutaneous administration

TABS = tablets

U   = units

VAR   = various routes of administration

DESCRIPTION	DOSE	ROUTE	CODE

A

Abarelix	10 mg		J0128
Abbokinase (see Urokinase)			
Abbokinase, Open Cath (see Urokinase)			
Abciximab	10 mg	IV	J0130
Abelcet (see Amphotericin B Lipid Complex)			
ABLC (see Amphotericin B)			
Acetazolamide sodium	up to 500 mg	IM/IV	J1120
Acetylcysteine, unit dose form	per gram	INH	J7608
Achromycin (see Tetracycline)			
ACTH (see Corticotropin)			
Acthar (see Corticotropin)			
Actimmune (see Interferon gamma 1-B)			
Activase (see Alteplase recombinant)—			
Acyclovir	5 mg	—	Q4075
Adalimumab	20 mg		J0135
Adenocard (see Adenosine)			
Adenoscan (see Adenosine)			
Adenosine	6 mg	IV	J0150
	30 mg	IV	J0152
Adrenalin Chloride (see Adrenalin, epinephrine)			
Adrenalin, epinephrine	up to 1 ml amp	SC/IM	J0170

DESCRIPTION	DOSE	ROUTE	CODE
Adriamycin PFS or RDF (see Doxorubicin HCl)			
Adrucil (see Fluorouracil)			
Agalsidase beta	1 mg		J0180
Aggrastat (see Tirofiban hydrochloride)			
A-hydroCort (see Hydrocortisone sodium phosphate)			
Akineton (see Biperiden)			
Alatrofloxacin mesylate, injection	100 mg	IV	J0200
Albuterol	up to 5 mg	INH	J7621
Albuterol, concentrated form	per mg	INH	J7618
Albuterol, unit dose form	per mg	INH	J7619
Aldesleukin	per single use vial	IM/IV	J9015
Aldomet (see Methyldopate HCl)			
Alefacept	0.5 mg	—	J0215
Alemtuzumab	10 mg	—	J9010
Alferon N (see Interferon alfa-n3)			
Alglucerase	per 10 U	IV	J0205
Alkaban-AQ (see Vinblastine sulfate)			
Alkeran (see Melphalan, oral)			
Alpha 1 - proteinase inhibitor, human	10 mg	IV	J0256
Alprostadil, injection	1.25 mcg	OTH	J0270
Alprostadil, urethral suppository	—	OTH	J0275
Alteplase recombinant	1 mg	IV	J2997

DESCRIPTION	DOSE	ROUTE	CODE
Alupent (see Metaproterenol sulfate or Metaproterenol, compounded)			
Amcort (see Triamcinolone diacetate)			
A-methaPred (see Methylprednisolone sodium succinate)			
Amgen (see Interferon alphacon-1)			
Amifostine	500 mg	IV	J0207
Amikacin sulfate	100 mg		J0278
Aminolevalinic acid HCl	unit dose (354 mg)	OTH	J7308
Aminophylline/ Aminophyllin	up to 250 mg	IV	J0280
Amiodarone HCl	30 mg	IV	J0282
Amitriptyline HCl	up to 20 mg	IM	J1320
Amobarbital	up to 125 mg	IM/IV	J0300
Amphocin (see Amphotericin B)			
Amphotericin B	50 mg	IV	J0285
Amphotericin B, lipid complex	10 mg	IV	J0287-J0289
Ampicillin sodium	up to 500 mg	IM/IV	J0290
Ampicillin sodium/ sulbactam sodium	per 1.5 g	IM/IV	J0295
Amygdalin (see Laetrile, Amygdalin, vitamin B-17)			
Amytal (see Amobarbital)			
Anabolin LA 100 (see Nandrolone decanoate)			
Ancef (see Cefazolin sodium)			

DESCRIPTION	DOSE	ROUTE	CODE

Andrest 90-4 (see
  Testosterone enanthate
  and estradiol valerate)

Andro-Cyp (see
  Testosterone cypionate)

Andro-Cyp 200 (see
  Testosterone cypionate)

Andro LA 200 (see
  Testosterone enanthate)

Andro-Estro 90-4 (see
  Testosterone enanthate
  and estradiol valerate)

Andro/Fem (see
  Testosterone cypionate
  and estradiol cypionate)

Androgyn LA (see
  Testosterone enanthate
  and estradiol valerate)

Androlone-50 (see
  Nandrolone
  phenpropionate)

Androlone-D 100 (see
  Nandrolone decanoate)

Andronaq-50 (see
  Testosterone suspension)

Andronaq-LA (see
  Testosterone cypionate)

Andronate -100 or -200
  (see Testosterone
  cypionate)

Andropository 100 (see
  Testosterone enanthate)

Andryl 200 (see
  Testosterone enanthate)

Anectine (see
  Succinylcholine
  chloride)

DESCRIPTION	DOSE	ROUTE	CODE
Anergan 25 or 50 (see Promethazine HCl)			
Anistreplase	30 U	IV	J0350
Anti-inhibitor	per IU	IV	J7198
Antispas (see Dicyclomine HCl)			
Antithrombin III (human)	per IU	IV	J7197
Anzemet (see Dolasetron mesylate injection)			
A.P.L. (see Chorionic gonadotropin)			
Aprepitant, oral	5 mg	ORAL	J8501
Apresoline (see Hydralazine HCl)			
Aprotinin	10,000 KIU	—	Q2003
AquaMEPHYTON (see Vitamin K)			
Aralen (see Chloroquine HCl)			
Aramine (see Metaraminol)			
Aranesp (see Darbepoetin alfa)			
Arbutamine	1 mg	IV	J0395
Aredia (see Pamidronate disodium)			
Arfonad (see Trimethaphan camsylate)			
Aristocort Forte or Intralesional (see Triamcinolone diacetate)			
Aristospan Intra-Articular or Intralesional (see Triamcinolone hexacetonide)			

DESCRIPTION	DOSE	ROUTE	CODE
Arrestin (see Trimethobenzamide HCl)			
Arsenic trioxide	1 mg	IV	J9017
Asparaginase	10,000 U	IV/IM	J9020
Astramorph PF (see Morphine sulfate)			
Atgam (see Lymphocyte immune globulin)			
Ativan (see Lorazepam)			
Atropine, concentrated form	per mg	INH	J7635
Atropine, unit dose form	per mg	INH	J7636
Atropine sulfate	up to 0.3 mg	IV/IM/SC	J0460
Atrovent (see Ipratropium bromide)			
Aurothioglucose	up to 50 mg	IM	J2910
Autologous cultured chondrocytes, implant	—	—	J7330
Autoplex T (see Hemophilia clotting factors)			
Avonex (see Interferon beta-1a)			
Azacitidine	1 mg		J9025
Azathioprine	50 mg	ORAL	J7500
Azathioprine, parenteral	100 mg	IV	J7501
Azithromycin, dihydrate	1 g	ORAL	Q0144
Azithromycin, injection	500 mg	IV	J0456

B

Baclofen	10 mg	IT	J0475

DESCRIPTION	DOSE	ROUTE	CODE
Baclofen for intrathecal trial	50 mcg	OTH	J0476
Bactocill (see Oxacillin sodium)			
BAL in oil (see Dimercaprol)			
Banflex (see Orphenadrine citrate)			
Basiliximab	20 mg	—	Q2019
BCG (Bacillus Calmette & Guerin) live instillation	per vial	IV	J9031
Beclomethasone inhalation solution, unit dose form	per mg	INH	J7622
Bena-D 10 or 50 (see Diphenhydramine HCl)			
Benadryl (see Diphenhydramine HCl)			
Benahist 10 or 50 (see Diphenhydramine HCl)			
Ben-Allergin-50 (see Diphenhydramine HCl)			
Benefix (see Factor IX, recombinant)			
Benoject-10 or -50 (see Diphenhydramine HCl)			
Bentyl (see Dicyclomine)			
Benztropine mesylate	per 1 mg	IM/IV	J0515
Berubigen (see Vitamin B-12 cyanocobalamin)			
Betalin 12 (see Vitamin B-12 cyanocobalamin)			
Betameth (see Betamethasone sodium phosphate)			

DESCRIPTION	DOSE	ROUTE	CODE
Betamethasone acetate & Betamethasone sodium phosphate	per 3 mg	IM	J0702
Betamethasone inhalation solution, unit dose form	per mg	INH	J7624
Betamethasone sodium phosphate	per 4 mg	IM/IV	J0704
Betaseron (see Interferon beta-1b)			
Bethanechol chloride	up to 5 mg	SC	J0520
Bevacizumab	10 mg		J9035
Bicillin C-R, and Bicillin C-R 900/300 (see Penicillin G procaine & Penicillin G benzathine)			
Bicillin L-A (see Penicillin G benzathine)			
BiCNU (see Carmustine)			
Biperiden lactate	per 5 mg	IM/IV	J0190
Bitolterol mesylate, concentrated form	per mg	INH	J7628
Bitolterol mesylate, unit dose form	per mg	INH	J7629
Bivalirudin	1 mg	—	J0583
Blenoxane (see Bleomycin sulfate)			
Bleomycin sulfate	15 U	IM/IV/SC	J9040
Bortezomib	0.1 mg		J9041
Botulinum toxin type A	per unit	IM	J0585
Botulinum toxin type B	per 100 U	IM	J0587
Brethine (see Terbutaline sulfate or Terbutaline, compounded)			
Bricanyl subcutaneous (see Terbutaline sulfate)			

DESCRIPTION	DOSE	ROUTE	CODE
Brompheniramine maleate	per 10 mg	IM/SC/IV	J0945
Bronkephrine (see Ethylnorepinephrine HCl)			
Bronkosol (see Isoetharine HCl)			
Budesonide inhalation solution, concentrated form	0.25 mg	INH	J7633
Budesonide inhalation solution, unit dose form	0.25 mg	INH	J7626
Buprenorphine HCl	0.1 mg	—	J0592
Busulfan	2 mg	ORAL	J8510
Butorphanol tartrate	2 mg		J0595

C

Cabergoline	0.5 mg	ORAL	Q2001
Cafcit (see Caffeine citrate)			
Caffeine citrate	5 mg	IV	J0706
Cainc-1 or -2 (see Lidocaine HCl)			
Calcijex (see Calcitriol)			
Calcimar (see Calcitonin-salmon)			
Calcitonin-salmon	up to 400 U	SC/IM	J0630
Calcitriol	0.1 mcg	IM	J0636
Calcium disodium versenate (see Edetate calcium disodium)			
Calcium gluconate	per 10 ml	IV	J0610
Calcium glycerophosphate and calcium lactate	per 10 ml	IM/SC	J0620

DESCRIPTION	DOSE	ROUTE	CODE
Calphosan (see Calcium glycerophosphate and calcium lactate)			
Camptosar (see Irinotecan)			
Capecitabine	150 mg	ORAL	J8520
	500 mg	ORAL	J8521
Carbocaine (see Mepivacaine)			
Carbocaine with Neo-Cobefrin (see Mepivacaine)			
Carboplatin	50 mg	IV	J9045
Carmustine	100 mg	IV	J9050
Carnitor (see Levocarnitine)			
Carticel (see Autologous cultured chondrocytes)			
Caspofungin acetate	5 mg	IV	J0637
Cefadyl (see Cephapirin sodium)			
Cefazolin sodium	up to 500 mg	IV/IM	J0690
Cefepime hydrochloride	500 mg	IV	J0692
Cefizox (see Ceftizoxime sodium)			
Cefotaxime sodium	per 1 gram	IV/IM	J0698
Cefoxitin sodium	1 g	IV/IM	J0694
Ceftazidime	per 500 mg	IV/IM	J0713
Ceftizoxime sodium	per 500 mg	IV/IM	J0715
Ceftriaxone sodium	per 250 mg	IV/IM	J0696
Cefuroxime sodium, sterile	per 750 mg	IM/IV	J0697
Celestone phosphate (see Betamethasone sodium phosphate)			

DESCRIPTION	DOSE	ROUTE	CODE
Celestone soluspan (see Betamethasone acetate and betamethasone sodium phosphate)			
CellCept (see Mycophenolate mofetil)			
Cel-U-Jec (see Betamethasone sodium phosphate)			
Cenacort Forte (see Triamcinolone diacetate)			
Cenacort A-40 (see Triamcinolone acetonide)			
Cephalothin sodium	up to 1 g	IM/IV	J1890
Cephapirin sodium	up to 1 g	IV/IM	J0710
Ceredase (see Alglucerase)			
Cerezyme (see Imiglucerase)			
Cerubidine (see Daunorubicin HCl)			
Cetuximab	10 mg		J9055
Chealamide (see Endrate ethylenediamine-tetra-acetic acid)			
Chloramphenicol sodium succinate	up to 1 g	IV	J0720
Chlordiazepoxide HCl	up to 100 mg	IM/IV	J1990
Chloromycetin sodium succinate (see Chloramphenicol sodium succinate)			
Chloroprocaine HCl	per 30 ml	VAR	J2400
Chloroquine HCl	up to 250 mg	IM	J0390
Chlorothiazide sodium	per 500 mg	IV	J1205
Chlorpromazine HCl	up to 50 mg	IM/IV	J3230

DESCRIPTION	DOSE	ROUTE	CODE
Chlorpromazine HCl, oral	10 mg	ORAL	Q0171
	25 mg	ORAL	Q0172
Chorex-5 or -10 (see Chorionic gonadotropin)			
Chorignon (see Chorionic gonadotropin)			
Chorionic gonadotropin	per 1,000 USP U	IM	J0725
Choron 10 (see Chorionic gonadotropin)			
Cidofovir	375 mg	IV	J0740
Cilastatin sodium/ imipenem	per 250 mg	IV/IM	J0743
Cipro IV (see Ciprofloxacin)			
Ciprofloxacin	200 mg	IV	J0744
Cisplatin, powder or soln.	per 10 mg	IV	J9060
Cisplatin	50 mg	IV	J9062
Cladribine	per 1 mg	IV	J9065
Claforan (see Cefotaxime sodium)			
Clonidine hydrochloride	1 mg	EPI	J0735
Cobex (see Vitamin B-12 cyanocobalamin)			
Codeine phosphate	per 30 mg	IM/IV/SC	J0745
Codimal-A (see Brompheniramine maleate)			
Cogentin (see Benztropine mesylate)			
Colchicine	per 1 mg	IV	J0760
Colistimethate sodium	up to 150 mg	IM/IV	J0770
Coly-Mycin M (see Colistimethate sodium)			
Compa-Z (see Prochlorperazine)			

DESCRIPTION	DOSE	ROUTE	CODE
Compazine (see Prochlorperazine)			
Cophene-B (see Brompheniramine maleate)			
Copper contraceptive, intrauterine	—	OTH	J7300
Cordarone (see Amiodarone HCl)			
Corgonject-5 (see Chorionic gonadotropin)			
Corticorelin ovine triflutate	per dose	—	Q2005
Corticotropin	up to 40 U	IV/IM/SC	J0800
Cortrosyn (see Cosyntropin)			
Cosmegen (see Dactinomycin)			
Cosyntropin	per 0.25 mg	IM/IV	J0835
Cotranzine (see Prochlorperazine)			
Cromolyn sodium, unit dose form	per 10 mg	INH	J7631
Crysticillin 300 A.S. or 600 A.S. (see Penicillin G procaine)			
Cyclophosphamide	100 mg	IV	J9070
	200 mg	IV	J9080
	500 mg	IV	J9090
	1.0 g	IV	J9091
	2.0 g	IV	J9092
Cyclophosphamide, lyophilized	100 mg	IV	J9093
	200 mg	IV	J9094
	500 mg	IV	J9095
	1.0 g	IV	J9096
	2.0 g	IV	J9097

DESCRIPTION	DOSE	ROUTE	CODE
Cyclophosphamide, oral	25 mg	ORAL	J8530
Cyclosporine, oral	25 mg	ORAL	J7515
	100 mg	ORAL	J7502
Cyclosporine, parenteral	250 mg	IV	J7516
Cytarabine	100 mg	SC/IV	J9100
	500 mg	SC/IV	J9110
Cytarabine, liposome	10 mg	—	J9098
Cytomegalovirus immune globulin intravenous (human)	per vial	IV	J0850
Cytostar-U (see Cytarabine)			
Cytovene (see Ganciclovir sodium)			
Cytoxan (see Cyclophosphamide; cyclophosphamide, lyophilized; and cyclophosphamide, oral)			

D

D-5-W, infusion	1,000 cc	IV	J7070
Dacarbazine	100 mg	IV	J9130
	200 mg	IV	J9140
Daclizumab, parenteral	25 mg	IV	J7513
Dactinomycin	0.5 mg	IV	J9120
Dalalone (see Dexamethasone sodium phosphate)			
Dalalone-LA (see Dexamethasone acetate)			
Dalteparin sodium	per 2,500 IU	SC	J1645
Daptomycin	1 mg		J0878

DESCRIPTION	DOSE	ROUTE	CODE
Darbepoetin alfa	1 mcg	—	Q4054
	5 mcg	—	J0880
	1000 units	—	Q0137
Daunorubicin citrate, liposomal formulation	10 mg	IV	J9151
Daunorubicin	10 mg	IV	J9150
Daunoxome (see Daunorubicin citrate)			
DDAVP (see Desmopressin acetate)			
Decadron (see Dexamethasone sodium phosphate)			
Decadron-LA (see Dexamethasone acetate)			
Decadron Phosphate (see Dexamethasone sodium phosphate)			
Deca-Durabolin (see Nandrolone decanoate)			
Decaject (see Dexamethasone sodium phosphate)			
Decaject-LA (see Dexamethasone acetate)			
Decolone-50 or -100 (see Nandrolone decanoate)			
De-Comberol (see Testosterone cypionate and estradiol cypionate)			
Deferoxamine mesylate	500 mg	IM/SC/IV	J0895
Dehist (see Brompheniramine maleate)			

DESCRIPTION	DOSE	ROUTE	CODE
Deladumone or Deladumone OB (see Testosterone enanthate and estradiol valerate)			
Delatest (see Testosterone enanthate)			
Delatestadiol (see Testosterone enanthate and estradiol valerate)			
Delatestryl (see Testosterone enanthate)			
Delestrogen (see Estradiol valerate)			
Delta-Cortef (see Prednisolone, oral)			
Demadex (see Torsemide)			
Demerol HCl (see Meperidine HCl)			
Denileukin diftitox	300 mcg	—	J9160
DepAndro 100 or 200 (see Testosterone cypionate)			
DepAndrogyn (see Testosterone cypionate and estradiol cypionate)			
DepGynogen (see Depo-estradiol cypionate)			
DepMedalone 40 or 80 (see Methylprednisolone acetate)			
Depo-estradiol cypionate	up to 5 mg	IM	J1000
Depogen (see Depo-estradiol cypionate)			
Depoject (see Methylprednisolone acetate)			

DESCRIPTION	DOSE	ROUTE	CODE
Depo-Medrol (see Methylprednisolone acetate)			
Depopred 40 or 80 (see Methylprednisolone acetate)			
Depo-Provera (see Medroxyprogesterone acetate)			
Depotest (see Testosterone cypionate)			
Depo-Testadiol (see Testosterone cypionate and estradiol cypionate)			
Depotestogen (see Testosterone cypionate and estradiol cypionate)			
Depo-Testosterone (see Testosterone cypionate)			
Desferal Mesylate (see Deferoxamine mesylate)			
Desmopressin acetate	1 mcg	IV/SC	J2597
Dexacen-4 (see Dexamethasone sodium phosphate)			
Dexacen LA-8 (see Dexamethasone acetate)			
Dexamethasone, concentrated form	per mg	INH	J7637
Dexamethasone, unit form	per mg	INH	J7638
Dexamethasone acetate	1 mg	IM	J1094
Dexamethosone sodium phosphate	1 mg	IM/IV/OTH	J1100
Dexasone (see Dexamethasone sodium phosphate)			

DESCRIPTION	DOSE	ROUTE	CODE
Dexasone LA (see Dexamethasone acetate)			
Dexferrum (see Iron dextran)			
Dexone (see Dexamethasone sodium phosphate)			
Dexone LA (see Dexamethasone acetate)			
Dexrazoxane hydrochloride	250 mg	IV	J1190
Dextran 40	500 ml	IV	J7100
Dextran 75	500 ml	IV	J7110
Dextrose 5%/normal saline	500 ml = 1 U	IV	J7042
Dextrose/water (5%)	500 ml = 1 U	IV	J7060
D.H.E. 45 (see Dihydroergotamine)			
Diamox (see Acetazolamide sodium)			
Diazepam	up to 5 mg	IM/IV	J3360
Diazoxide	up to 300 mg	IV	J1730
Dibent (see Dicyclomine HCl)			
Dicylomine HCl	up to 20 mg	IM	J0500
Didronel (see Etidronate disodium)			
Diethylstilbestrol diphosphate	250 mg	IV	J9165
Diflucan (see Fluconazole)			
Digoxin	up to 0.5 mg	IM/IV	J1160
Digoxin immune fab (ovine)	per vial	—	Q2006
Dihydrex (see Diphenhydramine HCl)			
Dihydroergotamine mesylate	per 1 mg	IM/IV	J1110

DESCRIPTION	DOSE	ROUTE	CODE
Dilantin (see Phenytoin sodium)			
Dilaudid (see Hydromorphone HCl)			
Dilocaine (see Lidocaine HCl)			
Dilomine (see Dicyclomine HCl)			
Dilor (see Dyphylline)			
Dimenhydrinate	up to 50 mg	IM/IV	J1240
Dimercaprol	per 100 mg	IM	J0470
Dimethyl sulfoxide (see DMSO, Dimethyl-sulfoxide)			
Dinate (see Dimenhydrinate)			
Dioval or Dioval 40 or Dioval XX (see Estradiol valerate)			
Diphenacen-50 (see Diphenhydramine HCl)			
Diphenhydramine HCl, injection	up to 50 mg	IV/IM	J1200
Diphenhydramine HCl, oral	50 mg	ORAL	Q0163
Dipyridamole	per 10 mg	IV	J1245
Disotate (see Endrate ethylenediamine-tetra-acetic acid)			
Di-Spaz (see Dicyclomine HCl)			
Ditate-DS (see Testosterone enanthate and estradiol valerate)			
Diuril sodium (see Chlorothiazide sodium)			

DESCRIPTION	DOSE	ROUTE	CODE
D-Med 80 (see Methylprednisolone acetate)			
DMSO, Dimethyl sulfoxide	50%, 50 ml	OTH	J1212
Dobutamine HCl	per 250 mg	IV	J1250
Dobutrex (see Dobutamine HCl)			
Docetaxel	20 mg	IV	J9170
Dolasetron mesylate, injection	10 mg	IV	J1260
Dolasetron mesylate, tablets	100 mg	ORAL	Q0180
Dolophine HCl (see Methadone HCl)			
Dommanate (see Dimenhydrinate)			
Dopamine HCl	40 mg	—	Q4076
Dornase alpha, inhalation solution, unit dose form	per mg	INH	J7639
Doxercalciferol	1 mcg	IV	J1270
Doxil (see Doxorubicin HCl, lipid)			
Doxorubicin HCl	10 mg	IV	J9000
Doxorubicin HCl, all lipid	10 mg	IV	J9001
Dramamine (see Dimenhydrinate)			
Dramanate (see Dimenhydrinate)			
Dramilin (see Dimenhydrinate)			
Dramocen (see Dimenhydrinate)			
Dramoject (see Dimenhydrinate)			

DESCRIPTION	DOSE	ROUTE	CODE
Dronabinol, oral	2.5 mg	ORAL	Q0167
	5 mg	ORAL	Q0168
Droperidol	up to 5 mg	IM/IV	J1790
Droperidol and fentanyl citrate	up to 2 ml amp	IM/IV	J1810
Drug(s) administered through metered dose inhaler	—	INH	J3535
DTIC-Dome (see Dacarbazine)			
Dua-Gen LA (see Testosterone enanthate and estradiol valerate cypionate)			
Duoval PA (see Testosterone enanthate and estradiol valerate)			
Durabolin (see Nandrolone phenpropionate)			
Duraclon (see Clonidine HCl)			
Dura-Estrin (see Depo-estradiol cypionate)			
Duracillin A.S. (see Penicillin G procaine)			
Duragen-10, -20, or -40 (see Estradiol valerate)			
Duralone-40 or -80 (see Methylprednisolone acetate)			
Duralutin (see Hydroxyprogesterone caproate)			
Duramorph (see Morphine sulfate)			

DESCRIPTION	DOSE	ROUTE	CODE
Duratest-100 or -200 (see Testosterone cypionate)			
Duratestrin (see Testosterone cypionate and estradiol cypionate)			
Durathate 200 (see Testosterone enanthate)			
Dymenate (see Dimenhydrinate)			
Dyphylline	up to 500 mg	IM	J1180

E

Edetate calcium disodium	up to 1,000 mg	IV/SC/IM	J0600
Edetate disodium	per 150 mg	IV	J3520
Elavil (see Amitriptyline HCl)			
Ellence (see Epirubicin HCl)			
Elliots b solution	per ml	OTH	Q2002
Elspar (see Asparaginase)			
Emete-Con (see Benzquinamide)			
Eminase (see Anisteplase)			
Enbrel (see Etanercept)			
Endrate ethylenediamine-tetra-acetic acid (see Edetate disodium)			
Enovil (see Amitriptyline HCl)			
Enoxaparin sodium	10 mg	SC	J1650
Epinephrine, adrenalin	up to 1 ml amp	SC/IM	J0170
Epirubicin HCl	2 mg	—	J9178
Epoetin alfa	1,000 units	—	Q4055

DESCRIPTION	DOSE	ROUTE	CODE
Epoprostenol	0.5 mg	IV	J1325
Eptifibatide, injection	5 mg	IM/IV	J1327
Ergonovine maleate	up to 0.2 mg	IM/IV	J1330
Ertapenem sodium	500 mg	—	J1335
Erythromycin lactobionate	500 mg	IV	J1364
Estra-D (see Depo-estradiol cypionate)			
Estra-L 20 or 40 (see Estradiol valerate)			
Estra-Testrin (see Testosterone enanthate and estradiol valerate)			
Estradiol cypionate (see Depo-estradiol cypionate)			
Estradiol LA, or Estradiol LA-20, or Estradiol LA-40 (see Estradiol valerate)			
Estradiol valerate	up to 10 mg	IM	J1380
	up to 20 mg	IM	J1390
	up to 40 mg	IM	J0970
Estro-Cyp (see Depo-estradiol cypionate)			
Estrogen, conjugated	per 25 mg	IV/IM	J1410
Estroject LA (see Depo-estradiol cypionate)			
Estrone	per 1 mg	IM	J1435
Estrone 5 (see Estrone)			
Estrone aqueous (see Estrone)			
Estronol (see Estrone)			

DESCRIPTION	DOSE	ROUTE	CODE
Estronol-LA (see Depo-estradiol cypionate)			
Etanercept, injection	25 mg	IM/IV	J1438
Ethanolamine	100 mg	—	Q2007
Ethyol (see Amifostine)			
Etidronate disodium	per 300 mg	IV	J1436
Etopophos (see Etoposide)			
Etoposide	10 mg	IV	J9181
	100 mg	IV	J9182
Etoposide, oral	50 mg	ORAL	J8560
Everone (see Testosterone enanthate)			

F

Factor VIIa (coagulation factor, recombinant)	per mg	IV	Q0187
Factor VIII (anti-hemophilic factor, human)	per IU	IV	J7190
Factor VIII (anti-hemophilic factor, porcine)	per IU	IV	J7191
Factor VIII (anti-hemophilic factor, recombinant)	per IU	IV	J7192
Factor IX (anti-hemophilic factor, purified, non-recombinant)	per IU	IV	Q0160
Factor IX (anti-hemophilic factor, recombinant)	per IU	IV	Q0161
Factor IX, complex	per IU	IV	J7194
Factors, other hemophilia clotting	per IU	IV	J7196

DESCRIPTION	DOSE	ROUTE	CODE
Factrel (see Gonadorelin HCl)			
Feiba VH Immuno (see Factors, other hemophilia clotting)			
Fentanyl citrate	0.1 mg	IM/IV	J3010
Ferrlecit (see Sodium ferricgluconate complex in sucrose injection)			
Filgrastim (G-CSF)	300 mcg	SC/IV	J1440
	480 mcg	SC/IV	J1441
Flexoject (sce Orphenadrine citrate)			
Flexon (see Orphenadrine citrate)			
Flolan (see Epoprostenol)			
Floxuridine	500 mg	IV	J9200
Fluconazole	200 mg	IV	J1450
Fludara (see Fludarabine phosphate)			
Fludarabine phosphate	50 mg	IV	J9185
Flunisolide inhalation solution, unit dose form	per mg	INH	J7641
Fluorouracil	500 mg	IV	J9190
Folex, or Folex PFS (see Methotrexate sodium)			
Follutein (see Chorionic gonadotropin)			
Fomepizole	1.5 mg	—	Q2008
Fomivirsen sodium	1.65 mg	IO	J1452
Fondaparinux sodium	0.5 mg	—	J1652
Formoterol	12 mcg	INH	J7640
Fortaz (see Ceftazidime)			
Foscarnet sodium	per 1,000 mg	IV	J1455

DESCRIPTION	DOSE	ROUTE	CODE
Foscavir (see Foscarnet sodium)			
Fosphenytoin	50 mg	—	Q2009
FUDR (see Floxuridine)			
Fulvestrant	25 mg	—	J9395
Fungizone intravenous (see Amphotericin B)			
Furomide M.D. (see Furosemide)			
Furosemide	up to 20 mg	IM/IV	J1940

G

Gallium nitrate	1 mg		J1457
Gamastan (see Gamma globulin and immune globulin)			
Gamma globulin	1 cc	IM	J1460
	2 cc	IM	J1470
	3 cc	IM	J1480
	4 cc	IM	J1490
	5 cc	IM	J1500
	6 cc	IM	J1510
	7 cc	IM	J1520
	8 cc	IM	J1530
	9 cc	IM	J1540
	10 cc	IM	J1550
	over 10 cc	IM	J1560
Gammar (see Gamma globulin and immune globulin)			
Gammar-IV (see Immune globulin intravenous (human))			
Gamulin RH (see Rho(D) immune globulin)			

DESCRIPTION	DOSE	ROUTE	CODE
Ganciclovir, implant	4.5 mg	OTH	J7310
Ganciclovir sodium	500 mg	IV	J1570
Garamycin, gentamicin	up to 80 mg	IM/IV	J1580
Gatifloxacin	10 mg	IV	J1590
Gefitinib	250 mg		J8565
Gemcitabine HCl	200 mg	IV	J9201
Gemsar (see Gemcitabine HCl)			
Gemtuzumab ozogamicin	5 mg	IV	J9300
Gentamicin sulfate (see Garamycin, gentamicin)			
Gentran (see Dextran 40)			
Gentran 75 (see Dextran 75)			
Gesterol 50 (see Progestcrone)			
Glatiramer acetate	20 mg	—	J1595
Glucagon HCl	per 1 mg	SC/IM/IV	J1610
Glukor (see Chorionic gonadotropin)			
Glycopyrrolate, concentrated form	per 1 mg	INH	J7642
Glycopyrrolate, unit dose form	per 1 mg	INH	J7643
Gold sodium thiomalate	up to 50 mg	IM	J1600
Gonadorelin HCl	per 100 mcg	SC/IV	J1620
Gonic (see Chorionic gonadotropin)			
Goserelin acetate implant	per 3.6 mg	SC	J9202
Granisetron HCl, injection	100 mcg	IV	J1626
Granisetron HCl, oral	1 mg	ORAL	Q0166
Gynogen LA-10, -20, or -40 (see Estradiol valerate)			

DESCRIPTION	DOSE	ROUTE	CODE

H

Haldol (see Haloperidol)

Haloperidol	up to 5 mg	IM/IV	J1630
Haloperidol decanoate	per 50 mg	IM	J1631

Hectoral (see Doxercalciferol)

Hemin	per 1 mg	—	Q2011

Hemofil M (see Factor VIII)

Hemophilia clotting factors (e.g., anti-inhibitors)	per IU	IV	J7198
Hemophilia clotting factors, NOC	per IU	IV	J7199
Hepatitis B vaccine	—	—	Q3021-Q3023

Hep-Lock or Hep-Lock U/P (see Heparin sodium (heparin lock flush))

Heparin sodium	1,000 U	IV/SC	J1644
Heparin sodium (heparin lock flush)	10 U	IV	J1642

Herceptin (see Trastuzumab)

Hexadrol Phosphate (see Dexamethasone sodium phosphate)

Histaject (see Brompheniramine maleate)

Histerone 50 or 100 (see Testosterone suspension)

Histrelin acetate	10 mg	—	Q2020

DESCRIPTION	DOSE	ROUTE	CODE
Hyalgan (see Sodium hyaluronate)			
Hyaluronidase	up to 150 U	SC/IV	J3470
Hyaluronidase, ovine			J3471, J3472
Hyate:C (see Factor VIII (anti-hemophilic factor (porcine)))			
Hybolin improved (see Nandrolone phenpropionate)			
Hybolin decanoate (see Nandrolone decanoate)			
Hycamtin (see Topotecan)			
Hydralazine HCl	up to 20 mg	IV/IM	J0360
Hydrate (see Dimenhydrinate)			
Hydrocortisone acetate	up to 25 mg	IV/IM/SC	J1700
Hydrocortisone sodium phosphate	up to 50 mg	IV/IM/SC	J1710
Hydrocortisone succinate sodium	up to 100 mg	IV/IM/SC	J1720
Hydrocortone acetate (see Hyrocortisone acetate)			
Hydrocortone Phosphate (see Hydrocortisone sodium phosphate)			
Hydromorphone HCl	up to 4 mg	SC/IM/IV	J1170
Hydroxyzine HCl	up to 25 mg	IM	J3410
Hydroxyzine pamoate	25 mg	ORAL	Q0177
	50 mg	ORAL	Q0178
Hylan G-F 20	16 mg	OTH	J7320
Hyoscyamine sulfate	up to 0.25 mg	SC/IM/IV	J1980
Hyperstat IV (see Diazoxide)			

DESCRIPTION	DOSE	ROUTE	CODE
Hyper-Tet (see Tetanus immune globulin, human)			
HypRho-D (see Rho(D) immune globulin)			
Hyrexin-50 (see Diphenhydramine HCl)			
Hyzine-50 (see Hydroxyzine HCl)			

I

Ibutilide fumarate	1 mg	IV	J1742
Idamycin (see Idarubicin HCl)			
Idarubicin HCl	5 mg	IV	J9211
Ifex (see Ifosfamide)			
Ifosfamide	per 1 g	IV	J9208
Ilotycin (see Erythromycin gluceptate)			
Imatinib	100 mg		S0088
Imferon (see Iron dextran)			
Imiglucerase	per U	IV	J1785
Imitrex (see Sumatriptan succinate)			
Immune globulin	500 mg	IV	J1561
Immune globulin, anti-thymocyte globulin	250 mg	IV	J7504
Immune globulin, intravenous	1 g	IV	J1563
	10 mg	IV	J1564
Immunosuppressive drug, not otherwise classified	—	—	J7599
Imuran (see Azathioprine)			
Inapsine (see Droperidol)			

DESCRIPTION	DOSE	ROUTE	CODE
Inderal (see Propranolol HCl)			
Infed (see Iron dextran)			
Infergen (see Interferon alfa-1)			
Infliximab, injection	10 mg	IM/IV	J1745
Innohep (see Tinzarparin)			
Innovar (see Droperidol with fentanyl citrate)			
Insulin	5 U	SC	J1815
Insulin lispro	50 U	SC	J1817
Intal (see Cromolyn sodium)			
Integrilin, injection (see Eptifibatide)			
Interferon			
alphacon-1, recombinant	1 mcg	SC	J9212
alfa-2A, recombinant	3 million U	SC/IM	J9213
alfa-2B, recombinant	1 million U	SC/IM	J9214
alfa-N3, (human leukocyte derived)	250,000 IU	IM	J9215
beta-1A	33 mcg	IM	J1825
	11 mcg	IM	Q3025
	11 mcg	SC	Q3026
beta-1B	0.25 mg	SC	J1830
gamma-1B	3 million U	SC	J9216
Intrauterine copper contraceptive (see Copper contraceptive, intrauterine)			
Ipratropium bromide, unit dose form	per mg	INH	J7644
Irinotecan	20 mg	IV	J9206
Iron dextran	50 mg	IV/IM	J1750

DESCRIPTION	DOSE	ROUTE	CODE
Iron sucrose	1 mg	IV	J1756
Irrigation solution for Tx of bladder calculi	per 50 ml	OTH	Q2004
Isocaine HCl (see Mepivacaine)			
Isoetharine HCl, concentrated form	per mg	INH	J7648
Isoetharine HCl, unit dose form	per mg	INH	J7649
Isoproterenol HCl, concentrated form	per mg	INH	J7658
Isoproterenol HCl, unit dose form	per mg	INH	J7659
Isuprel (see Isoproterenol HCl)			
Itraconazole	50 mg	IV	J1835

J

Jenamicin (see Garamycin, gentamicin)

K

Kabikinase (see Streptokinase)

Kaleinate (see Calcium gluconate)

Kanamycin sulfate	up to 75 mg	IM/IV	J1850
	up to 500 mg	IM/IV	J1840

Kantrex (see Kanamycin sulfate)

Keflin (see Cephalothin sodium)

DESCRIPTION	DOSE	ROUTE	CODE
Kefurox (see Cefuroxime sodium)			
Kefzol (see Cefazolin sodium)			
Kenaject-40 (see Triamcinolone acetonide)			
Kenalog-10 or -40 (see Triamcinolone acetonide)			
Kestrone 5 (see Estrone)			
Ketorolac tromethamine	per 15 mg	IM/IV	J1885
Key-Pred 25 or 50 (see Prednisolone acetate)			
Key-Pred-SP (see Prednisolone sodium phosphate)			
K-Flex (see Orphenadrine citrate)			
Klebcil (see Kanamycin sulfate)			
Koate-HP (see Factor VIII)			
Kogenate (see Factor VIII)			
Konakion (see Vitamin K, phytonadione, etc.)			
Konyne-80 (see Factor IX, complex)			
Kutapressin	up to 2 ml	SC/IM	J1910
Kytril (see Granisetron HCl)			

L

L.A.E. 20 (see Estradiol valerate)

DESCRIPTION	DOSE	ROUTE	CODE
Laetrile, amygdalin, vitamin B-17	—	—	J3570
Lanoxin (see Digoxin)			
Largon (see Propiomazine HCl)			
Laronidase	0.1 mg		J1931
Lasix (see Furosemide)			
L-Caine (see Lidocaine HCl)			
Lepirudin	50 mg	—	Q2021
Leucovorin calcium	per 50 mg	IM/IV	J0640
Leukine (see Sargramostim (GM-CSF))			
Leuprolide acetate	per 1 mg	IM	J9218
Leuprolide acetate, implant	65 mg	—	J9219
Leuprolide acetate (for depot suspension)	3.75 mg	IM	J1950
	7.5 mg	IM	J9217
Leustatin (see Cladribine)			
Levabuterol HCl, concentrated form	0.5 mg	INH	J7618
Levabuterol HCl, unit dose form	0.5 mg	INH	J7619
Levaquin I.U. (see Levofloxacin)			
Levocarnitine	per 1 g	IV	J1955
Levo-Dromoran (see Levorphanol tartrate)			
Levofloxacin	250 mg	IV	J1956
Levonorgestrel releasing intrauterine contraceptive	52 mg	OTH	J7302
Levorphanol tartrate	up to 2 mg	SC/IV	J1960
Levsin (see Hyoscyamine sulfate)			

DESCRIPTION	DOSE	ROUTE	CODE
Levulan Kerastick (see Aminolevulinic acid HCl)			
Librium (see Chlordiazepoxide HCl)			
Lidocaine HCl	10 mg	IV	J2001
Lidoject-1 or -2 (see Lidocaine HCl)			
Lincocin (see Lincomycin HCl)			
Lincomycin HCl	up to 300 mg	IV	J2010
Linezolid	200 mg	IV	J2020
Liquaemin sodium (see Heparin sodium)			
Lioresal (see Baclofen)			
LMD (10%) (see Dextran 40)			
Lorazepam	2 mg	IM/IV	J2060
Lovenox (see Enoxaparin sodium)			
Lufyllin (see Dyphylline)			
Luminal sodium (see Phenobarbital sodium)			
Lunelle (see Medroxyprogesterone acetate/estradiol cypionate)			
Lupron (see Leuprolide acetate)			
Lymphocyte immune globulin, anti-thymocyte globulin, equine	250 mg	IV	J7504
Lymphocyte immune globulin, anti-thymocyte globulin, rabbit	25 mg	IV	J7511

DESCRIPTION	DOSE	ROUTE	CODE
Lyophilized (see Cyclophosphamide, lyophilized)			

M

Magnesium sulfate	500 mg	—	J3475
Mannitol	25% in 50 ml	IV	J2150
Marmine (see Dimenhydrinate)			
Maxipime (see Cefepime hydrochloride)			
Mechlorethamine HCl (nitrogen mustard), HN2	10 mg	IV	J9230
Medralone 40 or 80 (see Methylprednisolone acetate)			
Medrol (see Methylprednisolone)			
Medroxyprogesterone acetate	50 mg	IM	J1051
	150 mg	IM	J1055
Medroxyprogesterone acetate/estradiol cypionate	5 mg/25 mg	IM	J1056
Mefoxin (see Cefoxitin sodium)			
Melphalan HCl	50 mg	IV	J9245
Melphalan, oral	2 mg	ORAL	J8600
Menoject LA (see Testosterone cypionate and estradiol cypionate)			
Mepergan injection (see Meperidine and promethazine HCl)			

DESCRIPTION	DOSE	ROUTE	CODE
Meperidine HCl	per 100 mg	IM/IV/SC	J2175
Meperidine and promethazine HCl	up to 50 mg	IM/IV	J2180
Mepivacaine HCl	per 10 ml	VAR	J0670
Mcropcnem	100 mg	—	J2185
Mesna	200 mg	IV	J9209
Mesnex (see Mesna)			
Metaprel (see Metaproterenol sulfate)			
Metaproterenol sulfate, concentrated form	per 10 mg	INH	J7668
Metaproterenol sulfate, unit dose form	per 10 mg	INH	J7669
Metaraminol bitartrate	per 10 mg	IV/IM/SC	J0380
Metastron (see Strontium-89 chloride)			
Methacholine chloride	1 mg		J7674
Methadone HCl	up to 10 mg	IM/SC	J1230
Methergine (see Methylergonovine maleate)			
Methocarbamol	up to 10 ml	IV/IM	J2800
Methotrexate, oral	2.5 mg	ORAL	J8610
Methotrexate sodium	5 mg	IV/IM/IT/IA	J9250
	50 mg	IV/IM/IT/IA	J9260
Methotrexate LPF (see Methotrexate sodium)			
Methyldopate HCl	up to 250 mg	IV	J0210
Methylene blue	1 ml		A9535
Methylergonovine maleate	up to 0.2 mg	IM/IV	J2210
Methylprednisolone, oral	per 4 mg	ORAL	J7509
Methylprednisolone acetate	20 mg	IM	J1020
	40 mg	IM	J1030
	80 mg	IM	J1040

DESCRIPTION	DOSE	ROUTE	CODE
Methylprednisone sodium succinate	up to 40 mg	IM/IV	J2920
	up to 125 mg	IM/IV	J2930
Metoclopramide HCl	up to 10 mg	IV	J2765
Miacalcin (see Calcitonin-salmon)			
Midazolam HCl	per 1 mg	IM/IV	J2250
Milrinone lactate	5 mg	IV	J2260
Mirena (see Levonorgestrel releasing intrauterine contraceptive)			
Mithracin (see Plicamycin)			
Mitomycin	5 mg	IV	J9280
	20 mg	IV	J9290
	40 mg	IV	J9291
Mitoxantrone HCl	per 5 mg	IV	J9293
Monocid (see Cefonicid sodium)			
Monoclate-P (see Factor VIII)			
Monoclonal antibodies, parenteral	5 mg	IV	J7505
Mononine (see Factor IX, purified, non-recombinant)			
Morphine sulfate	up to 10 mg	IM/IV/SC	J2270
	100 mg	IM/IV/SC	J2271
Morphine sulfate, preservative free	per 10 mg	SC/IM/IV	J2275
Moxifloxacin	100 mg	—	J2280
M-Prednisol-40 or -80 (see Methylprednisolone acetate)			

DESCRIPTION	DOSE	ROUTE	CODE
Mucomyst (see Acetylcysteine or Acetylcysteine, compounded)			
Mucosol (see Acetylcysteine)			
Muromonab-CD3	5 mg	IV	J7505
Muse (see Alprostadil)			
Mustargen (see Mechlorethamine HCl)			
Mutamycin (see Mitomycin)			
Mycophenolate mofetil	250 mg	ORAL	J7517
Mycophenolic acid	180 mg		J7518
Myleran (see Busulfan)			
Mylotarg (see Gemtuzumab ozogamicin)			
Myobloc (see Botulinum toxin type B)			
Myochrysine (see Gold sodium thiomalate)			
Myolin (see Orphenadrine citrate)			

N

Nalbuphine HCl	per 10 mg	IM/IV/SC	J2300
Naloxone HCl	per 1 mg	IM/IV/SC	J2310
Nandrobolic LA (see Nandrolone decanoate)			
Nandrolone decanoate	up to 50 mg	IM	J2320
	up to 100 mg	IM	J2321
	up to 200 mg	IM	J2322
Narcan (see Naloxone HCl)			

DESCRIPTION	DOSE	ROUTE	CODE
Naropin (see Ropivacaine HCl)			
Nasahist B (see Brompheniramine maleate)			
Nasal vaccine inhalation	—	INH	J3530
Natalizumab	1 mg		Q4079
Navane (see Thiothixene)			
Navelbine (see Vinorelbine tartrate)			
ND Stat (see Brompheniramine maleate)			
Nebcin (see Tobramycin sulfate)			
NebuPent (see Pentamidine isethionate)			
Nembutal sodium solution (see Pentobarbital sodium)			
Neocyten (see Orphenadrine citrate)			
Neo-Durabolic (see Nandrolone decanoate)			
Neoquess (see Dicyclomine HCl)			
Neosar (see Cyclophosphamide)			
Neostigmine methylsulfate	up to 0.5 mg	IM/IV/SC	J2710
Neo-Synephrine (see Phenylephrine HCl)			
Nervocaine 1% or 2% (see Lidocaine HCl)			
Nesacaine or Nesacaine-MPF (see Chloroprocaine HCl)			

DESCRIPTION	DOSE	ROUTE	CODE
Nesiritide	0.5 mg	—	J2324
Neumega (see Oprelvekin)			
Neupogen (see Filgrastim (G-CSF))			
Neutrexin (see Trimetrexate glucuronate)			
Nipent (see Pentostatin)			
Nordryl (see Diphenhydramine HCl)			
Norflex (see Orphenadrine citrate)			
Norzine (see Thiethylperazine maleate)			
Not otherwise classified drugs	—	—	J3490
Not otherwise classified drugs, other than INH administered through DME	—	—	J7799
Not otherwise classified drugs, INH administered through DME	—	—	J7699
Not otherwise classified drugs, anti-neoplastic	—	—	J9999
Not otherwise classified drugs, chemothera-peutic	—	ORAL	J8999
Not otherwise classified drugs, immunosup-pressive	—	—	J7599
Not otherwise classified drugs, non-chemothera-peutic	—	ORAL	J8499
Novantrone (see Mitoxantrone HCl)			

DESCRIPTION	DOSE	ROUTE	CODE
Novo Seven (see Factor VIIa)			
NPH (see Insulin)			
Nubain (see Nalbuphine HCl)			
Nulicaine (see Lidocaine HCl)			
Numorphan or Numorphan H.P. (see Oxymorphone HCl)			

O

Octreotide acetate, injection	1 mg	IM/IV	J2352
Oculinum (see Botulinum toxin type A)			
O-Flex (see Orphenadrine citrate)			
Omalizumab	5 mg		J2357
Omnipen-N (see Ampicillin)			
Oncaspar (see Pegaspargase)			
Oncovin (see Vincristine sulfate)			
Ondansetron HCl	1 mg	IV	J2405
Ondansetron HCl, oral	8 mg	ORAL	Q0179
Oprelvekin	5 mg	SC	J2355
Oraminic II (see Brompheniramine maleate)			
Ormazine (see Chlorpromazine HCl)			
Orphenadrine citrate	up to 60 mg	IV/IM	J2360

DESCRIPTION	DOSE	ROUTE	CODE
Orphenate (see Orphenadrine citrate)			
Or-Tyl (see Dicyclomine)			
Oxacillin sodium	up to 250 mg	IM/IV	J2700
Oxaliplatin	0.5 mg	—	J9263
Oxymorphone HCl	up to 1 mg	IV/SC/IM	J2410
Oxytetracycline HCl	up to 50 mg	IM	J2460
Oxytocin	up to 10 U	IV/IM	J2590

P

Paclitaxel	30 mg	IV	J9265
Paclitaxel protein-bound particles	1 mg		J9264
Palifermin	50 mcg		J2425
Palonosetron Hcl	25 mcg		J2469
Pamidronate disodium	per 30 mg	IV	J2430
Papaverine HCl	up to 60 mg	IV/IM	J2440
Paragard T 380 A (see Copper contraceptive, intrauterine)			
Paraplatin (see Carboplatin)			
Paricalcitol, injection	1 mcg	IV/IM	J2501
Pegademase bovine	25 IU	—	Q2012
Pegaptinib	0.3 mg		J2503
Pegaspargase	single dose vial	IM/IV	J9266
Pegfilgrastim	6 mg	—	J2505
Pemetrexed	10 mg		J9305
Penicillin G benzathine	up to 600,000 U	IM	J0560
	up to 1,200,000 U	IM	J0570
	up to 2,400,000 U	IM	J0580

DESCRIPTION	DOSE	ROUTE	CODE
Penicillin G benzathine & penicillin G procaine	up to 600,000 U	IM	J0530
	up to 1,200,000 U	IM	J0540
	up to 2,400,000 U	IM	J0550
Penicillin G potassium	up to 600,000 U	IM/IV	J2540
Penicillin G procaine, aqueous	up to 600,000 U	IM/IV	J2510
Pentamidine isethionate	per 300 mg	INH	J2545
Pentastarch, 10%	per 100 ml	—	Q2013
Pentazocine HCl	up to 30 mg	IM/SC/IV	J3070
Pentobarbital sodium	per 50 mg	IM/IV/OTH	J2515
Pentostatin	per 10 mg	IV	J9268
Permapen (see Penicillin G benzathine)			
Perphenazine, injection	up to 5 mg	IM/IV	J3310
Perphenazine, tablets	4 mg	ORAL	Q0175
	8 mg	ORAL	Q0176
Persantine IV (see Dipyridamole)			
Pfizerpen (see Penicillin G potassium)			
Pfizerpen AS (see Penicillin G procaine)			
Phenazine 25 or 50 (see Promethazine HCl)			
Phenergan (see Promethazine HCl)			
Phenobarbital sodium	up to 120 mg	IM/IV	J2560
Phentolamine mesylate	up to 5 mg	IM/IV	J2760
Phenylephrine HCl	up to 1 ml	SC/IM/IV	J2370
Phenytoin sodium	per 50 mg	IM/IV	J1165
Photofrin (see Porfimer sodium)			
Phytonadione (Vitamin K)	per 1 mg	IM/SC/IV	J3430

DESCRIPTION	DOSE	ROUTE	CODE
Piperacillin/Tazobactam sodium, injection	1.125 g	IV	J2543
Pitocin (see Oxytocin)			
Plantinol AQ, see Cisplatin			
Plas + SD (see Plasma, pooled multiple donor)			
Plasma, cryoprecipitate reduced	each U	—	P9044
Plasma, pooled multiple donor, frozen	each U	IV	P9023
Platinol or Platinol AQ (see Cisplatin)			
Plicamycin	2,500 mcg	IV	J9270
Polocaine (see Mepivacaine)			
Polycillin-N (see Ampicillin)			
Porfimer sodium	75 mg	IV	J9600
Potassium chloride	per 2 mEq	IV	J3480
Pralidoxime chloride	up to 1 g	IV/IM/SC	J2730
Predalone-50 (see Prednisolone acetate)			
Predcor-25 or -50 (see Prednisolone acetate)			
Predicort-50 (see Prednisolone acetate)			
Prednisone	per 5 mg	ORAL	J7506
Prednisolone, oral	per 5 mg	ORAL	J7510
Prednisolone acetate	up to 1 ml	IM	J2650
Predoject-50 (see Prednisolone acetate)			
Pregnyl (see Chorionic gonadotropin)			
Premarin intravenous (see Estrogen, conjugated)			

DESCRIPTION	DOSE	ROUTE	CODE
Prescription, chemotherapeutic, NOS	—	ORAL	J8999
Prescription, nonchemotherapeutic, NOS	—	ORAL	J8499
Primacor (see Milrinone lactate)			
Primaxin IM or IV (see Cilastatin sodium, imipenem)			
Priscoline HCl (see Tolazoline HCl)			
Pro-Depo (see Hydroxyprogesterone caproate)			
Procainamide HCl	up to 1 g	IM/IV	J2690
Prochlorperazine	up to 10 mg	IM/IV	J0780
Prochlorperazine maleate, oral	5 mg	ORAL	Q0164
	10 mg	ORAL	Q0165
Profasi HP (see Chorionic gonadotropin)			
Profilnine Heat-Treated (see Factor IX)			
Progestaject (see Progesterone)			
Progesterone	per 50 mg	—	J2675
Prograf (see Tacrolimus, oral or parenteral)			
Prokine (see Sargramostim (GM-CSF))			
Prolastin (see Alpha 1 -proteinase inhibitor, human)			
Proleukin (see Aldesleukin)			

DESCRIPTION	DOSE	ROUTE	CODE
Prolixin decanoate (see Fluphenazine decanoate)			
Promazine HCl	up to 25 mg	IM	J2950
Promethazine HCl, injection	up to 50 mg	IM/IV	J2550
Promethazine HCl, oral	12.5 mg	ORAL	Q0169
	25 mg	ORAL	Q0170
Pronestyl (see Procainamide HCl)			
Proplex T or SX-T (see Factor IX)			
Propranolol HCl	up to 1 mg	IV	J1800
Prorex-25 or -50 (see Promethazine HCl)			
Prostaphlin (see Procainamide HCl)			
Prostigmin (see Neostigmine methylsulfate)			
Protamine sulfate	per 10 mg	IV	J2720
Protirelin	per 250 mcg	IV	J2725
Prothazine (see Promethazine HCl)			
Protopam chloride (see Pralidoxime chloride)			
Proventil (see Albuterol sulfate, compounded)			
Prozine-50 (see Promazine HCl)			
Pulminicort respules (see Budesonide)			
Pyridoxine HCl	100 mg	—	J3415

DESCRIPTION	DOSE	ROUTE	CODE

Q

Quelicin (see
  Succinylcholine
  chloride)

| Quinupristin/dalfopristin | 500 mg (150/350) | IV | J2770 |

R

| Ranitidine HCl, injection | 25 mg | IV/IM | J2780 |

Rapamune (see Sirolimus)

| Rasburicase | 0.5 mg | — | J2783 |

Recombinant (see Factor
  VIII)

Redisol (see Vitamin B-12
  cyanocobalamin)

Regitine (see Phentolamine
  mesylate)

Reglan (see
  Metoclopramide HCl)

Regular (see Insulin)

Relefact TRH (see
  Protirelin)

Remicade (see Infliximab,
  injection)

Reo Pro (see Abciximab)

Rep-Pred 40 or 80 (see
  Methylprednisolone
  acetate)

RespiGam (see Respiratory
  syncytial virus)

| Respiratory syncytial virus immuneglobulin | 50 mg | IV | J1565 |

Retavase (see Reteplase)

DESCRIPTION	DOSE	ROUTE	CODE
Reteplase	18.8 mg	IV	J2993
Retrovir (see Zidovudine)			
Rheomacrodex (see Dextran 40)			
Rhesonativ (see Rho(D) immune globulin, human)			
Rheumatrex Dose Pack (see Methotrexate, oral)			
Rho(D) immune globulin, human	1 dose pkg, 300 mcg	IM	J2790
	1 dose pkg, 50 mcg	IM	J2798
Rho(D) immune globulin, human, solvent detergent	100 IU	IV	J2792
RhoGAM (see Rho(D) immune globulin, human)			
Ringer's lactate infusion	up to 1,000 cc	IV	J7120
Risperidone	0.5 mg		J2794
Rituxan (see Rituximab)			
Rituximab	100 mg	IU	J9310
Robaxin (see Methocarbamol)			
Rocephin (see Ceftriaxone sodium)			
Roferon-A (see Interferon alfa-2A, recombinant)			
Ropivacaine HCl	1 mg	——	J2795
Rubex (see Doxorubicin HCl)			
Rubramin PC (see Vitamin B-12 cyanocobalamin)			

DESCRIPTION	DOSE	ROUTE	CODE

S

Saline solution, 5% dextrose	500 ml	IV	J7042
Saline solution, normal infusion	250 cc	IV	J7050
	1,000 cc	IV	J7030
Saline solution, sterile	500 ml = 1 U	IV/OTH	J7040
	up to 5 cc	IV/OTH	J7051
Sandimmune (see Cyclosporine)			
Sandoglobulin (see Immune globulin intravenous (human))			
Sandostatin Lar Depot (see Octreotide)			
Sargramostim (GM-CSF)	50 mcg	IV	J2820
Secobarbital sodium	up to 250 mg	IM/IV	J2860
Seconal (see Secobarbital sodium)			
Selestoject (see Betamethasone sodium phosphate)			
Sermorelin acetate	0.5 mg	—	Q2014
Sinusol-B (see Brompheniramine maleate)			
Sirolimus	1 mg	ORAL	J7520
Sodium chloride 0.9%	per 2 ml	IV	J2912
Sodium ferricgluconate in sucrose	12.5 mg	—	J2916
Sodium hyaluronate	5 mg	OTH	J7316
Solganal (see Aurothioglucose)			

DESCRIPTION	DOSE	ROUTE	CODE
Solu-Cortef (see Hydrocortisone sodium phosphate (J1710))			
Solu-Medrol (see Methylprednisolone sodium succinate)			
Solurex (see Dexamethasone sodium phosphate)			
Solurex LA (see Dexamethasone acetate)			
Somatrem	1 mg	—	J2940
Somatropin	1 mg	—	J2941
Sparine (see Promazine HCl)			
Spasmoject (see Dicyclomine HCl)			
Spectinomycin HCl	up to 2 g	IM	J3320
Sporanox (see Itraconazole)			
Staphcillin (see Methicillin sodium)			
Stilphostrol (see Diethylstilbestrol diphosphate)			
Streptase (see Streptokinase)			
Streptokinase	per 250,000 IU	IV	J2995
Streptomycin	up to 1 g	IM	J3000
Streptomycin sulfate (see Streptomycin)			
Streptozocin	1 g	IV	J9320
Strontium-89 chloride	per 10 ml	IV	J3005
Sublimaze (see Fentanyl citrate)			

DESCRIPTION	DOSE	ROUTE	CODE
Succinylcholine chloride	up to 20 mg	IV/IM	J0330
Sumatriptan succinate	6 mg	SC	J3030
Supartz (see Sodium hyaluronate)			
Surostrin (see Succinycholine chloride)			
Sus-Phrine (see Adrenalin, epinephrine)			
Synercid (see Quinupristan/ dalfopristin)			
Synkavite (see Vitamin K, phytonadione, etc.)			
Syntocionon (see Oxytocin)			
Synvisc (see Hylan G-F 20)			
Sytobex (see Vitamin B-12 cyanocobalamin)			

T

Tacrolimus, oral	per 1 mg	ORAL	J7507
Tacrolimus, parenteral	5 mg	—	J7525
Talwin (see Pentazocine HCl)			
Taractan (see Chlorprothixene)			
Taxol (see Paclitaxel)			
Taxotere (see Docetaxel)			
Tazidime (see Ceftazidime)			
TEEV (see Testosterone enanthate and Estradiol valerate)			
Temozolmide	5 mg	ORAL	J8700
Tenecteplase	50 mg	—	J3100

DESCRIPTION	DOSE	ROUTE	CODE
Teniposide	50 mg	—	Q2017
Tequin (see Gatifloxin)			
Terbutaline sulfate	up to 1 mg	SC/IV	J3105
Terbutaline sulfate, concentrated form	per 1 mg	INH	J7680
Terbutaline sulfate, unit dose form	per 1 mg	INH	J7681
Teriparatide	10 mcg	—	J3110
Terramycin IM (see Oxytetracycline HCl)			
Testa-C (see Testosterone cypionate)			
Testadiate (see Testosterone enanthate and Estradiol valerate)			
Testadiate-Depo (see Testosterone cypionate)			
Testaject-LA (see Testosterone cypionate)			
Testaqua (see Testosterone suspension)			
Test-Estro Cypionates or Test-Estro-C (see Testosterone cypionate and Estradiol cypionate)			
Testex (see Testosterone propionate)			
Testoject-50 (see Testosterone suspension)			
Testoject-LA (see Testosterone cypionate)			
Testone LA 100 or 200 (see Testosterone enanthate)			
Testosterone aqueous (see Testosterone suspension)			

DESCRIPTION	DOSE	ROUTE	CODE
Testosterone cypionate	up to 100 mg	IM	J1070
	1 cc, 200 mg	IM	J1080
Testosterone cypionate & Estradiol cypionate	up to 1 ml	IM	J1060
Testosterone enanthate	up to 100 mg	IM	J3120
	up to 200 mg	IM	J3130
Testosterone enanthate & Estradiol valerate	up to 1 cc	IM	J0900
Testosterone propionate	up to 100 mg	IM	J3150
Testosterone suspension	up to 50 mg	IM	J3140
Testradiol 90/4 (see Testosterone enanthate)			
Testrin PA (see Testosterone enanthate)			
Tetanus immune globulin, human	up to 250 U	IM	J1670
Tetracycline	up to 250 mg	IM/IV	J0120
Thallous chloride Tl 201	per mci	—	A9505
Theelin Aqueous (see Estrone)			
Theophylline	per 40 mg	IV	J2810
TheraCys (see BCG live)			
Thiamine HCl	100 mg	—	J3411
Thiethylperazine maleate, injection	up to 10 mg	IM	J3280
Thiethylperazine maleate, oral	10 mg	ORAL	Q0174
Thiotepa	15 mg	IV	J9340
Thorazine (see Chlorpromazine HCl)			
Thymoglobulin (see Immune globulin, anti-thymocyte)			
Thypinone (see Protirelin)			

DESCRIPTION	DOSE	ROUTE	CODE
Thyrogen (see Thyrotropin alfa)			
Thyrotropin alfa, injection	0.9 mg	IM/SC	J3240
Tice BCG (see BCG live)			
Ticon (see Trimethobenzamide HCl)			
Tigan (see Trimethobenzamide HCl)			
Tiject-20 (see Trimethobenzamide HCl)			
Tinzarparin	1,000 IU	SC	J1655
Tirofiban hydrochloride	12.5 mg	IM/IV	J3245
	0.25 mg		J3246
TNKase (see Tenecteplase)			
Tobi (see Tobramycin, inhalation solution)			
Tobramycin, inhalation solution	300 mg	INH	J7682
Tobramycin sulfate	up to 80 mg	IM/IV	J3260
Tofranil (see Imipramine HCl)			
Tolazoline HCl	up to 25 mg	IV	J2670
Topotecan	4 mg	IV	J9350
Toradol (see Ketorolac tromethamine)			
Torecan (see Thiethylperazine maleate)			
Tornalate (see Bitolterol mesylate)			
Torsemide	10 mg/ml	IV	J3265

DESCRIPTION	DOSE	ROUTE	CODE
Totacillin-N (see Ampicillin)			
Trastuzumab	10 mg	IV	J9355
Treprostinil	1 mg		Q4077
Tri-Kort (see Triamcinolone acetonide)			
Triam-A (see Triamcinolone acetonide)			
Triamcinolone, concentrated form	per 1 mg	INH	J7683
Triamcinolone, unit dose form	per 1 mg	INH	J7684
Triamcinolone acetonide	per 10 mg	IM	J3301
Triamcinolone diacetate	per 5 mg	IM	J3302
Triamcinolone hexacetonide	per 5 mg	VAR	J3303
Triflupromazine HCl	up to 20 mg	IM/IV	J3400
Trilafon (see Perphenazine)			
Trilog (see Triamcinolone acetonide)			
Trilone (see Triamcinolone diacetate)			
Trimethobenzamide HCl, injection	up to 200 mg	IM	J3250
Trimethobenzamide HCl, oral	250 mg	ORAL	Q0173
Trimetrexate glucoronate	per 25 mg	IV	J3305
Triptorelin pamoate	3.75 mg	—	J3315
Trisenox (see Arsenic trioxide)			
Trobicin (see Spectinomycin HCl)			

DESCRIPTION	DOSE	ROUTE	CODE
Trovan (see Alatrofloxacin mesylate)			
Tysabri, see Natalizumab			

U

Ultrazine-10 (see Prochlorperazine)			
Unasyn (see Ampicillin sodium/sulbactam sodium)			
Unclassified drugs (see also Not elsewhere classified)	—	—	J3490
Unspecified oral antiemetic	—	—	Q0181
Urea	up to 40 g	IV	J3350
Ureaphil (see Urea)			
Urecholine (see Bethanechol chloride)			
Urofollitropin	75 IU	—	Q2018
Urokinase	5,000 IU vial	IV	J3364
	250,000 IU vial	IV	J3365

V

V-Gan 25 or 50 (see Promethazine HCl)			
Valergen 10, 20, or 40 (see Estradiol valerate)			
Valertest No. 1 or No. 2 (see Testosterone enanthate and Estradiol valerate)			
Valium (see Diazepam)			
Valrubicin, intravesical	200 mg	OTH	J9357

DESCRIPTION	DOSE	ROUTE	CODE
Valstar (see Valrubicin)			
Vancocin (see Vancomycin HCl)			
Vancoled (see Vancomycin HCl)			
Vancomycin HCl	up to 500 mg	IV/IM	J3370
Vasoxyl (see Methoxamine HCl)			
Velban (see Vinblastine sulfate)			
Velsar (see Vinblastine sulfate)			
Venofer (see Iron sucrose)			
Ventolin (see Albuterol sulfate)			
VePesid (see Etoposide and Etoposide, oral)			
Versed (see Midazolam HCl)			
Verteporfin	15 mg	IV	J3395
	0.1 mg		J3396
Vesprin (see Triflupromazine HCl)			
Viadur (see Leuprolide acetate implant)			
Vinblastine sulfate	1 mg	IV	J9360
Vincasar PFS (see Vincristine sulfate)			
Vincristine sulfate	1 mg	IV	J9370
	2 mg	IV	J9375
	5 mg	IV	J9380
Vinorelbine tartrate	per 10 mg	IV	J9390
Vistaject-25 (see Hydroxyzine HCl)			

DESCRIPTION	DOSE	ROUTE	CODE
Vistaril (see Hydroxyzine HCl)			
Vistide (see Cidofovir)			
Visudyne (sec Verteporfin)			
Vitamin B-12 cyanocobalamin	up to 1,000 mcg	IM/SC	J3420
Vitamin K, phytonadione, menadione, menadiol sodium diphosphate	per 1 mg	IM/SC/IV	J3430
Von Willebrand factor complex, human	per IU	IV	Q2022
Voriconazole	10 mg		J3465

W

Wehamine (see
Dimenhydrinate)

Wehdryl (see
Diphenhydramine HCl)

Wellcovorin (see
Leucovorin calcium)

Win Rho SD (see Rho(D)
immuneglobulin, human,
solvent detergent)

Wyamine sulfate (see
Mephentermine sulfate)

Wycillin (see Penicillin G
procaine)

Wydase (see
Hyaluronidase)

X

Xeloda (see Capecitabine)

Xopenex (see Albuterol)

DESCRIPTION	DOSE	ROUTE	CODE
Xylocaine HCl (see Lidocaine HCl)			

Z

Zanosar (see Streptozocin)			
Zantac (see Ranitidine HCl)			
Zemplar (see Paricalcitol)			
Zenapax (see Daclizumab)			
Zetran (see Diazepam)			
Ziconotide	1 mcg		J2278
Zidovudine	10 mg	IV	J3485
Zinacef (see Cefuroxime sodium)			
Ziprasidone mesylate	10 mg	—	J3486
Zithromax (see Azithromycin dihydrate)			
Zithromax I.V. (see Azithromycin, injection)			
Zofran (see Ondansetron HCl)			
Zoladex (see Goserelin acetate implant)			
Zoledronic acid	—	—	J3487
Zolicef (see Cefazolin sodium)			
Zosyn (see Piperacillin)			
Zyvox (see Linezoid)			

APPENDIX D: MEDICARE REFERENCES

COVERAGE INSTRUCTION MANUAL (CIM) REFERENCES

The following Medicare references refer to policy issues identified in the main body of the HCPCS code section. Coverage Instruction Manual references are identified with the term CIM: followed by the reference number(s).

30-1 ROUTINE COSTS IN CLINICAL TRIALS

Effective for items and services furnished on or after September 19, 2000, Medicare covers the routine costs of qualifying clinical trials, as such costs are defined below, as well as reasonable and necessary items and services used to diagnose and treat complications arising from participation in all clinical trials. All other Medicare rules apply.

Routine costs of a clinical trial include all items and services that are otherwise generally available to Medicare beneficiaries (i.e., there exists a benefit category, it is not statutorily excluded, and there is not a national noncoverage decision) that are provided in either the experimental or the control arms of a clinical trial except:

- The investigational item or service, itself;
- Items and services provided solely to satisfy data collection and analysis needs and that are not used in the direct clinical management of the patient (e.g., monthly CT scans for a condition usually requiring only a single scan); and
- Items and services customarily provided by the research sponsors free of charge for any enrollee in the trial.

Routine costs in clinical trials include:

- Items or services that are typically provided absent a clinical trial (e.g., conventional care);
- Items or services required solely for the provision of the investigational item or service (e.g., administration of a noncovered chemotherapeutic agent), the clinically appropriate monitoring of the effects of the item or service, or the prevention of complications; and
- Items or services needed for reasonable and necessary care arising from the provision of an investigational item or service--in particular, for the diagnosis or treatment of complications.

This policy does not withdraw Medicare coverage for items and services that may be covered according to local medical review policies or the regulations on category B investigational device exemptions (IDE) found in 42 CFR 405.201-405.215, 411.15, and 411.406. For information about LMRPs, refer to www.lmrp.net, a searchable database of Medicare contractors' local policies.

For noncovered items and services, including items and services for which Medicare payment is statutorily prohibited, Medicare only covers the treatment of complications arising from the delivery of the noncovered item or service and unrelated reasonable and necessary care. (Refer to MCM §§2300.1 and MIM 3101.) However, if the item or service is not covered by virtue of a national noncoverage policy in the Coverage Issues Manual and is the focus of a qualifying clinical trial, the routine costs of the clinical trial (as defined above) will be covered by Medicare but the noncovered item or service, itself, will not.

A. Requirements for Medicare Coverage of Routine Costs.—Any clinical trial receiving Medicare coverage of routine costs must meet the following three requirements:

1. The subject or purpose of the trial must be the evaluation of an item or service that falls within a Medicare benefit category (e.g., physicians' service, durable medical equipment, diagnostic test) and is not statutorily excluded from coverage (e.g., cosmetic surgery, hearing aids).
2. The trial must not be designed exclusively to test toxicity or disease pathophysiology. It must have therapeutic intent.
3. Trials of therapeutic interventions must enroll patients with diagnosed disease rather than healthy volunteers. Trials of diagnostic interventions may enroll healthy patients in order to have a proper control group.

The three requirements above are insufficient by themselves to qualify a clinical trial for Medicare coverage of routine costs. Clinical trials also should have the following desirable characteristics; however, some trials, as described below, are presumed to meet these characteristics and are automatically qualified to receive Medicare coverage:

1. The principal purpose of the trial is to test whether the intervention potentially improves the participants' health outcomes;
2. The trial is well-supported by available scientific and medical information or it is intended to clarify or establish the health outcomes of interventions already in common clinical use;
3. The trial does not unjustifiably duplicate existing studies;
4. The trial design is appropriate to answer the research question being asked in the trial;
5. The trial is sponsored by a credible organization or individual capable of executing the proposed trial successfully;
6. The trial is in compliance with Federal regulations relating to the protection of human subjects; and
7. All aspects of the trial are conducted according to the appropriate standards of scientific integrity.

B. Qualification Process for Clinical Trials.—Using the authority found in §1142 of the Act (cross-referenced in §1862(a)(1)(E) of the Act), the Agency for Healthcare Research and Quality (AHRQ) will convene a multi-agency Federal panel (the "panel") composed of representatives of the Department of Health and Human Services research agencies (National Institutes of Health (NIH), Centers for Disease Control and Prevention (CDC), the Food and Drug Administration (FDA), AHRQ, and the Office of Human Research Protection), and the research arms of the Department of Defense (DOD) and the Department of Veterans Affairs (VA) to develop qualifying criteria that will indicate a strong probability that a trial exhibits the desirable characteristics listed above. These criteria will be easily verifiable, and where possible, dichotomous. Trials that meet these qualifying criteria will receive Medicare coverage of their associated routine costs. This panel is not reviewing or approving individual trials. The multi-agency panel will meet periodically to review and evaluate the program and recommend any necessary refinements to HCFA.

Clinical trials that meet the qualifying criteria will receive Medicare coverage of routine costs after the trial's lead principal investigator certifies that the trial meets the criteria. This process will require the principal investigator to enroll the trial in a Medicare clinical trials registry, currently under development.

Some clinical trials are automatically qualified to receive Medicare coverage of their routine costs because they have been deemed by AHRQ, in consultation with the other agencies represented on the multi-agency panel to be highly likely to have the above-listed seven desirable characteristics of clinical trials. The principal investigators of these automatically qualified trials do not need to certify that the trials meet the qualifying criteria, but must enroll the trials in the Medicare clinical trials registry for administrative purposes, once the registry is established.

Effective September 19, 2000, clinical trials that are deemed to be automatically qualified are:

1. Trials funded by NIH, CDC, AHRQ, HCFA, DOD, and VA;
2. Trials supported by centers or cooperative groups that are funded by the NIH, CDC, AHRQ, HCFA, DOD and VA;
3. Trials conducted under an investigational new drug application (IND) reviewed by the FDA; and
4. Drug trials that are exempt from having an IND under 21 CFR 312.2(b)(1) will be deemed automatically qualified until the qualifying criteria are developed and the certification process is in place. At that time the principal investigators of these trials must certify that the trials meet the qualifying criteria in order to maintain Medicare coverage of routine costs. This certification process will only affect the future status of the trial and will not be used to retroactively change the earlier deemed status.

Medicare will cover the routine costs of qualifying trials that either have been deemed to be automatically qualified or have certified that they meet the qualifying criteria unless the CMS Chief Clinical Officer subsequently finds that a clinical trial does not meet the qualifying criteria jeopardizes the safety or welfare of Medicare beneficiaries.

Should HCFA find that a trial's principal investigator misrepresented that the trial met the necessary qualifying criteria in order to gain Medicare coverage of routine costs, Medicare coverage of the routine costs would be denied under §1862(a)(1)(E) of the Act. In the case of such a denial, the Medicare beneficiaries enrolled in the trial would not be held liable (i.e., would be held harmless from collection) for the costs consistent with the provisions of §§1879, 1842(l), or 1834(j)(4) of the Act, as applicable. Where appropriate, the billing providers would be held liable for the costs and fraud investigations of the billing providers and the trial's principal investigator may be pursued.

Medicare regulations require Medicare+Choice (M+C) organizations to follow CMS national coverage decisions. This NCD raises special issues that require some modification of most M+C organizations' rules governing provision of items and services in and out of network. The items and services covered under this NCD are inextricably linked to the clinical trials with which they are associated and cannot be covered outside of the context of those clinical trials. M+C organizations therefore must cover these services regardless of whether they are available through in-network providers. M+C organizations may have reporting requirements when enrollees participate in clinical trials, in order to track and coordinate their members' care, but cannot require prior authorization or approval.

35-1 COLONIC IRRIGATION—NOT COVERED

Colonic irrigation is a procedure to wash out or lavage material on the walls of the bowel to an unlimited distance without inducing defecation. This procedure is distinguished from all types of enemas which are primarily used to induce defecation.

There are no conditions for which colonic irrigation is medically indicated and no evidence of therapeutic value. Accordingly, colonic irrigation cannot be considered reasonable and necessary within the meaning of section 1862(a)(1) of the law.

35-10 HYPERBARIC OXYGEN THERAPY

For purposes of coverage under Medicare, hyperbaric oxygen (HBO) therapy is a modality in which the entire body is exposed to oxygen under increased atmospheric pressure.

A. Covered Conditions.—Program reimbursement for HBO therapy will be limited to that which is administered in a chamber (including the one man unit) and is limited to the following conditions:

1. Acute carbon monoxide intoxication, (ICD-9 -CM diagnosis 986).
2. Decompression illness, (ICD-9-CM diagnosis 993.2, 993.3).
3. Gas embolism, (ICD-9-CM diagnosis 958.0, 999.1).
4. Gas gangrene, (ICD-9-CM diagnosis 0400).
5. Acute traumatic peripheral ischemia. HBO therapy is an adjunctive treatment to be used in combination with accepted standard therapeutic measures when loss of function, limb, or life is threatened. (ICD-9-CM diagnosis 902.53, 903.01, 903.1, 904.0, 904.41.)
6. Crush injuries and suturing of severed limbs. As in the previous conditions, HBO therapy would be an adjunctive treatment when loss of function, limb, or life is threatened. (ICD-9-CM diagnosis 927.00-927.03, 927.09-927.11, 927.20-927.21, 927.8-927.9, 928.00-928.01, 928.10-928.11, 928.20-928.21, 928.3, 928.8-928.9, 929.0, 929.9, 996.90-996.99.)
7. Progressive necrotizing infections (necrotizing fasciitis), (ICD-9-CM diagnosis 728.86).
8. Acute peripheral arterial insufficiency, (ICD-9-CM diagnosis 444.21, 444.22, 444.81).
9. Preparation and preservation of compromised skin grafts (not for primary management of wounds), (ICD-9CM diagnosis 996.52; excludes artificial skin graft).
10. Chronic refractory osteomyelitis, unresponsive to conventional medical and surgical management, (ICD-9-CM diagnosis 730.10-730.19).
11. Osteoradionecrosis as an adjunct to conventional treatment, (ICD-9-CM diagnosis 526.89).
12. Soft tissue radionecrosis as an adjunct to conventional treatment, (ICD-9-CM diagnosis 990).
13. Cyanide poisoning, (ICD-9-CM diagnosis 987.7, 989.0).
14. Actinomycosis, only as an adjunct to conventional therapy when the disease process is refractory to antibiotics and surgical treatment, (ICD-9-CM diagnosis 039.0-039.4, 039.8, 039.9).

15. Diabetic wounds of the lower extremities in patients who meet the following three criteria:

    a. Patient has type I or type II diabetes and has a lower extremity wound that is due to diabetes;
    b. Patient has a wound classified as Wagner grade III or higher; and
    c. Patient has failed an adequate course of standard wound therapy.

The use of HBO therapy is covered as adjunctive therapy only after there are no measurable signs of healing for at least 30-days of treatment with standard wound therapy and must be used in addition to standard wound care. Standard wound care in patients with diabetic wounds includes: assessment of a patient's vascular status and correction of any vascular problems in the affected limb if possible, optimization of nutritional status, optimization of glucose control, debridement by any means to remove devitalized tissue, maintenance of a clean, moist bed of granulation tissue with appropriate moist dressings, appropriate off-loading, and necessary treatment to resolve any infection that might be present. Failure to respond to standard wound care occurs when there are no measurable signs of healing for at least 30 consecutive days. Wounds must be evaluated at least every 30 days during administration of HBO therapy. Continued treatment with HBO therapy is not covered if measurable signs of healing have not been demonstrated within any 30-day period of treatment.

B. Noncovered Conditions.—All other indications not specified under §35-10 (A) are not covered under the Medicare program. No program payment may be made for any conditions other than those listed in §35-10(A).

No program payment may be made for HBO in the treatment of the following conditions:

    1. Cutaneous, decubitus, and stasis ulcers.
    2. Chronic peripheral vascular insufficiency.
    3. Anaerobic septicemia and infection other than clostridial.
    4. Skin burns (thermal).
    5. Senility.
    6. Myocardial infarction.
    7. Cardiogenic shock.
    8. Sickle cell anemia.
    9. Acute thermal and chemical pulmonary damage, i.e., smoke inhalation with pulmonary insufficiency.
    10. Acute or chronic cerebral vascular insufficiency.
    11. Hepatic necrosis.
    12. Aerobic septicemia.
    13. Nonvascular causes of chronic brain syndrome (Pick's disease, Alzheimer's disease, Korsakoff's disease).
    14. Tetanus.
    15. Systemic aerobic infection.
    16. Organ transplantation.
    17. Organ storage.
    18. Pulmonary emphysema.
    19. Exceptional blood loss anemia.
    20. Multiple Sclerosis.
    21. Arthritic Diseases.
    22. Acute cerebral edema.

C. Topical Application of Oxygen.—This method of administering oxygen does not meet the definition of HBO therapy as stated above. Also, its clinical efficacy has not been established. Therefore, no Medicare reimbursement may be made for the topical application of oxygen. (Cross reference: §35-31.)

35-13 PROLOTHERAPY, JOINT SCLEROTHERAPY, AND LIGAMENTOUS INJECTIONS WITH SCLEROSING AGENTS—NOT COVERED

The medical effectiveness of the above therapies has not been verified by scientifically controlled studies. Accordingly, reimbursement for these modalities should be denied on the ground that they are not reasonable and necessary as required by §1862(a)(1) of the law.

35-20 TREATMENT OF MOTOR FUNCTION DISORDERS WITH ELECTRIC NERVE STIMULATION—NOT COVERED

While electric nerve stimulation has been employed to control chronic intractable pain for some time, its use in the treatment of motor function disorders, such as multiple sclerosis, is a recent innovation, and the medical effectiveness of such therapy has not been verified by scientifically controlled studies. Therefore, where electric nerve stimulation is employed to treat motor function disorders, no reimbursement may be made for the stimulator or for the services related to its implantation since this treatment cannot be considered reasonable and necessary.

See §§35-27 and 65-8.

NOTE: For Medicare coverage of deep brain stimulation for essential tremor and Parkinson's disease, see §65-19.

35-27 BIOFEEDBACK THERAPY

Biofeedback therapy provides visual, auditory or other evidence of the status of certain body functions so that a person can exert voluntary control over the functions, and thereby alleviate an abnormal bodily condition. Biofeedback therapy often uses electrical devices to transform bodily signals indicative of such functions as heart rate, blood pressure, skin temperature, salivation, peripheral vasomotor activity, and gross muscle tone into a tone or light, the loudness or brightness of which shows the extent of activity in the function being measured.

Biofeedback therapy differs from electromyography, which is a diagnostic procedure used to record and study the electrical properties of skeletal muscle. An electromyography device may be used to provide feedback with certain types of biofeedback.

Biofeedback therapy is covered under Medicare only when it is reasonable and necessary for the individual patient for muscle re-education of specific muscle groups or for treating pathological muscle abnormalities of spasticity, incapacitating muscle spasm, or weakness, and more conventional treatments (heat, cold, massage, exercise, support) have not been successful. This therapy is not covered for treatment of ordinary muscle tension states or for psychosomatic conditions.

See HCFA-Pub. 14-3, §§2200ff, 2215, and 4161; HCFA-Pub. 13-3, §§3133.3, 3148, and 3149; HCFA-Pub. 10, §§242 and 242.5 for special physical therapy requirements. See also §35-20 and 65-8.)

35-27.1 BIOFEEDBACK THERAPY FOR THE TREATMENT OF URINARY INCONTINENCE

Biofeedback therapy for the treatment of urinary incontinence (Effective for services performed on or after July 1, 2001.) This policy applies to biofeedback therapy rendered by a practitioner in an office or other facility setting.

Biofeedback is covered for the treatment of stress and/or urge incontinence in cognitively intact patients who have failed a documented trial of pelvic muscle exercise (PME)training. Biofeedback is not a treatment, per se, but a tool to help patients learn how to perform PME. Biofeedback-assisted PME incorporates the use of an electronic or mechanical device to relay visual and/or auditory evidence of pelvic floor muscle tone, in order to improve awareness of pelvic floor musculature and to assist patients in the performance of PME.

A failed trial of PME training is defined as no clinically significant improvement in urinary incontinence after completing 4 weeks of an ordered plan of pelvic muscle exercises to increase periurethral muscle strength.

Contractors may decide whether or not to cover biofeedback as an initial treatment modality.

Home use of biofeedback therapy is not covered.

35-30 BLOOD PLATELET TRANSFUSIONS

Effective for services performed on or after August 1, 1978, blood platelet transplants are safe and effective for the correction of thrombocytopenia and other blood defects. It is covered under Medicare when treatment is reasonable and necessary for the individual patient.

35-30.1 STEM CELL TRANSPLANTATION

Stem cell transplantation is a process in which stem cells are harvested from either a patient's or donor's bone marrow or peripheral blood for intravenous infusion. The transplant can be used to effect hematopoietic reconstitution following severely myelotoxic doses of chemotherapy (HDCT) and/or radiotherapy used to treat various malignancies. Allogeneic stem cell transplant may also be used to restore function in recipients having an inherited or acquired deficiency or defect.

A. Allogeneic Stem Cell Transplantation.—Allogeneic stem cell transplantation (ICD-9-CM procedure codes 41.02, 41.03, 41.05, and 41.08) is a procedure in which a portion of a healthy donor's stem cell or bone marrow is obtained and prepared for intravenous infusion.

   1. Covered Conditions.—The following uses of allogeneic bone marrow transplantation are covered under Medicare:

- Effective for services performed on or after August 1, 1978, for the treatment of leukemia, leukemia in remission (ICD-9-CM codes 204.00 through 208.91), or aplastic anemia (ICD-9-CM codes 284.0 through 284.9) when it is reasonable and necessary; and
- Effective for services performed on or after June 3, 1985, for the treatment of severe combined immunodeficiency disease (SCID) (ICD-9-CM code 279.2), and for the treatment of Wiskott - Aldrich syndrome (ICD-9-CM 279.12).

   2. Noncovered Conditions.—Effective May 24, 1996, allogeneic stem cell transplantation is not covered as treatment for multiple myeloma (ICD-9-CM codes 203.0 and 238.6).

B. Autologous Stem Cell Transplantation (Effective for Services Performed on or After 04/28/89).—Autologous stem cell transplantation (ICD-9-CM procedure codes 41.01, 41.04, 41.07, and 41.09) is a technique for restoring stem cells using the patient's own previously stored cells.

   1. Covered Conditions.—Autologous stem cell transplantation (ICD-9-CM codes 41.01, 41.04, 41.07, 41.09, CPT-4 code 38241) is considered reasonable and necessary under §1862(a)(1)(A) of the Act for the following conditions and is covered under Medicare for patients with:

- Acute leukemia in remission (ICD-9-CM codes 204.01, lymphoid; 205.01, myeloid; 206.01, monocytic; 207.01, acute erythremia and erythroleukemia; and 208.01 unspecified cell type) who have a high probability of relapse and who have no human leucocyte antigens (HLA)-matched;
- Resistant non-Hodgkin's lymphomas (ICD-9-CM codes 200.00-200.08, 200.10-200.18, 200.20-200.28, 200.80-200.88, 202.00-202.08, 202.80-202.88, and 202.90-202.98) or those presenting with poor prognostic features following an initial response;
- Recurrent or refractory neuroblastoma (see ICD-9-CM Neoplasm by site, malignant); or
- Advanced Hodgkin's disease (ICD-9-CM codes 201.00-201.98) who have failed conventional therapy and have no HLA-matched donor;

Effective October 1, 2000, single AuSCT is only covered for Durie-Salmon Stage II or III patients that fit the following requirement:

   a. Newly diagnosed or responsive multiple myeloma. This includes those patients with previously untreated disease, those with at least a partial response to prior chemotherapy (defined as a 50 percent decrease either in measurable paraprotein [serum and/or urine] or in bone marrow infiltration, sustained for at least 1 month), and those in responsive relapse; and
   b. Adequate cardiac, renal, pulmonary, and hepatic function.

NOTE: Tandem transplantation for multiple myeloma remains non-covered.

   2. Noncovered Conditions.—Insufficient data exist to establish definite conclusions regarding the efficacy of autologous stem cell transplantation for the following conditions:

- Acute leukemia not in remission (ICD-9-CM codes 204.00, 205.00, 206.00, 207.00 and 208.00);
- Chronic granulocytic leukemia (ICD-9-CM codes 205.10 and 205.11);
- Solid tumors (other than neuroblastoma) (ICD-9-CM codes 140.0-199.1);
- Up to October 1, 2000, multiple myeloma;

35-34 FABRIC WRAPPING OF ABDOMINAL ANEURYSMS—NOT COVERED

Fabric wrapping of abdominal aneurysms is not a covered Medicare procedure. This is a treatment for abdominal aneurysms which involves wrapping aneurysms with cellophane or fascia lata. This procedure has not been shown to prevent eventual rupture. In extremely rare instances, external wall reinforcement may be indicated when the current accepted treatment (excision of the aneurysm and reconstruction with synthetic materials) is not a viable alternative, but external wall reinforcement is not fabric wrapping. Accordingly, fabric wrapping of abdominal aneurysms is not considered reasonable and necessary within the meaning of §1862(a)(1) of the Act.

35-46 ASSESSING PATIENT'S SUITABILITY FOR ELECTRICAL NERVE STIMULATION THERAPY

Electrical nerve stimulation is an accepted modality for assessing a patient's suitability for ongoing treatment with a transcutaneous or an implanted nerve stimulator. Accordingly, program payment may be made for the following techniques when used to determine the potential therapeutic usefulness of an electrical nerve stimulator:

A. Transcutaneous Electrical Nerve Stimulation (TENS).--This technique involves attachment of a transcutaneous nerve stimulator to the surface of the skin over the peripheral nerve to be stimulated. It is used by the patient on a trial basis and its effectiveness in modulating pain is monitored by the physician, or physical therapist. Generally, the physician or physical therapist is able to determine whether the patient is likely to derive a significant therapeutic benefit from continuous use of a transcutaneous stimulator within a trial period of 1 month; in a few cases this determination may take longer to make. Document the medical necessity for such services which are furnished beyond the first month. (See §45-25 for an explanation of coverage of medically necessary supplies for the effective use of TENS.)

If TENS significantly alleviates pain, it may be considered as primary treatment; if it produces no relief or greater discomfort than the original pain electrical nerve stimulation therapy is ruled out. However, where TENS produces incomplete relief, further evaluation with percutaneous electrical nerve stimulation may be considered to determine whether an implanted peripheral nerve stimulator would provide significant relief from pain. (See §35-46B.)

Usually, the physician or physical therapist providing the services will furnish the equipment necessary for assessment. Where the physician or physical therapist advises the patient to rent the TENS from a supplier during the trial period rather than supplying it himself/herself, program payment may be made for rental of the TENS as well as for the services of the physician or physical therapist who is evaluating its use. However, the combined program payment which is made for the physician's or physical therapist's services and the rental of the stimulator from a supplier should not exceed the amount which would be payable for the total service, including the stimulator, furnished by the physician or physical therapist alone.

B. Percutaneous Electrical Nerve Stimulation (PENS).--This diagnostic procedure which involves stimulation of peripheral nerves by a needle electrode inserted through the skin is performed only in a physician's office, clinic, or hospital outpatient department. Therefore, it is covered only when performed by a physician or incident to physician's service. If pain is effectively controlled by percutaneous stimulation, implantation of electrodes is warranted.

As in the case of TENS (described in subsection A), generally the physician should be able to determine whether the patient is likely to derive a significant therapeutic benefit from continuing use of an implanted nerve stimulator within a trial period of 1 month. In a few cases, this determination may take longer to make. The medical necessity for such diagnostic services which are furnished beyond the first month must be documented.

NOTE: Electrical nerve stimulators do not prevent pain but only alleviate pain as it occurs. A patient can be taught how to employ the stimulator, and once this is done, can use it safely and effectively without direct physician supervision. Consequently, it is inappropriate for a patient to visit his/her physician, physical therapist, or an outpatient clinic on a continuing basis for treatment of pain with electrical nerve stimulation. Once it is determined that electrical nerve stimulation should be continued as therapy and the patient has been trained to use the stimulator, it is expected that a stimulator will be implanted or the patient will employ the TENS on a continual basis in his/her home. Electrical nerve stimulation treatments furnished by a physician in his/her office, by a physical therapist or outpatient clinic are excluded from coverage by §1862(a)(1) of the Act. (See §65-8 for an explanation of coverage of the therapeutic use of implanted peripheral nerve stimulators under the prosthetic devices benefit. See §60-20 for an explanation of coverage of the therapeutic use of TENS under the durable medical equipment benefit.)

35-47 BREAST RECONSTRUCTION FOLLOWING MASTECTOMY (Effective for services performed on and after May 15, 1980.)

During recent years, there has been a considerable change in the treatment of diseases of the breast such as fibrocystic disease and cancer. While extirpation of the disease remains of primary importance, the quality of life following initial treatment is increasingly recognized as of great concern. The increased use of breast reconstruction procedures is due to several factors:

- A change in epidemiology of breast cancer, including an apparent increase in incidence;
- Improved surgical skills and techniques;
- The continuing development of better prostheses; and
- Increasing awareness by physicians of the importance of postsurgical psychological adjustment.

Reconstruction of the affected and the contralateral unaffected breast following a medically necessary mastectomy is considered a relatively safe and effective noncosmetic procedure. Accordingly, program payment may be made for breast reconstruction surgery following removal of a breast for any medical reason.

Program payment may not be made for breast reconstruction for cosmetic reasons. (Cosmetic surgery is excluded from coverage under §1862(a)(l0) of the Social Security Act.)

35-48 OSTEOGENIC STIMULATION

Electrical stimulation to augment bone repair can be attained either invasively or noninvasively. Invasive devices provide electrical stimulation directly at the fracture site either through percutaneously placed cathodes or by implantation of a coiled cathode wire into the fracture site. The power pack for the latter device is implanted into soft tissue near the fracture site and subcutaneously connected to the cathode, creating a self-contained system with no external components. The power supply for the former device is externally placed and the leads connected to the inserted cathodes. With the noninvasive device, opposing pads, wired to an external power supply, are placed over the cast. An electromagnetic field is created between the pads at the fracture site.

1. Noninvasive Stimulator.—The noninvasive stimulator device is covered only for the following indications:

   - Nonunion of long bone fractures;
   - Failed fusion, where a minimum of nine months has elapsed since the last surgery;
   - Congenital pseudarthroses; and
   - As an adjunct to spinal fusion surgery for patients at high risk of pseudarthrosis due to previously failed spinal fusion at the same site or for those undergoing multiple level fusion. A multiple level fusion involves 3 or more vertebrae (e.g., L3-L5, L4-S1, etc).

2. Invasive (Implantable) Stimulator.—The invasive stimulator device is covered only for the following indications:

   - Nonunion of long bone fractures; and
   - As an adjunct to spinal fusion surgery for patients at high risk of pseudarthrosis due to previously failed spinal fusion at the same site or for those undergoing multiple level fusion.

A multiple level fusion involves 3 or more vertebrae (e.g., L3-L5, L4-S1, etc).

Effective for services performed on or after September 15, 1980, nonunion of long bone fractures, for both noninvasive and invasive devices, is considered to exist only after 6 or more months have elapsed without healing of the fracture.

Effective for services performed on or after April 1, 2000, nonunion of long bone fractures, for both noninvasive and invasive devices, is considered to exist only when serial radiographs have confirmed that fracture healing has ceased for three or more months prior to starting treatment with the electrical osteogenic stimulator. Serial radiographs must include a minimum of two sets of radiographs, each including multiple views of the fracture site, separated by a minimum of 90 days.

B. Ultrasonic Osteogenic Stimulators.—An ultrasonic osteogenic stimulator is a non-invasive device that emits low intensity, pulsed ultrasound. The ultrasound signal is applied to the skin surface at the fracture location via ultrasound, conductive gel in order to stimulate fracture healing.

Effective for services performed on or after January 1, 2001, ultrasonic osteogenic stimulators are covered as medically reasonable and necessary for the treatment of non-union fractures. In demonstrating nonunion of fractures, we would expect:

1. A minimum of two sets of radiographs obtained prior to starting treatment with the osteogenic stimulator, separated by a minimum of 90 days. Each radiograph must include multiple views of the fracture site accompanied with a written interpretation by a physician stating that there has been no clinically significant evidence of fracture healing between the two sets of radiographs.
2. Indications that the patient failed at least one surgical intervention for the treatment of the fracture.

Non-unions of the skull, vertebrae, and those that are tumor-related are excluded from coverage. The ultrasonic osteogenic stimulator may not be used concurrently with other non-invasive osteogenic devices. The national non-coverage policy related to ultrasonic osteogenic stimulators for fresh fractures and delayed unions remains in place. This policy relates only to non-union as defined above.

35-49 HYPERTHERMIA FOR TREATMENT OF CANCER (Effective for services performed on or after December 31, 1984.)

Local hyperthermia for treatment of cancer consists of the use of heat to make tumors more susceptible to cancer therapy measures.

Local hyperthermia is covered under Medicare when used in connection with radiation therapy for the treatment of primary or metastatic cutaneous or subcutaneous superficial malignancies It is not covered when used alone or in connection with chemotherapy.

35-50 COCHLEOSTOMY WITH NEUROVASCULAR TRANSPLANT FOR MENIERE'S DISEASE—NOT COVERED

Ménière's disease (or syndrome) is a common cause of paroxysmal vertigo. Ménière's syndrome is usually treated medically. When medical treatment fails, surgical treatment may be required.

While there are two recognized surgical procedures used in treating Ménière's disease (decompression of the endolymphatic hydrops and labyrinthectomy), there is no scientific evidence supporting the safety and effectiveness of cochleostomy with neurovascular transplant in treatment of Ménière's syndrome. Accordingly, Medicare does not cover cochleostomy with neurovascular transplant for treatment of Ménière's disease.

35-51 HEMODIALYSIS FOR TREATMENT OF SCHIZOPHRENIA—NOT COVERED

Scientific evidence supporting use of hemodialysis as a safe and effective means of treatment for schizophrenia is inconclusive at this time. Accordingly, Medicare does not cover hemodialysis for treatment of schizophrenia.

35-52 LASER PROCEDURES

Medicare recognizes the use of lasers for many medical indications. Procedures performed with lasers are sometimes used in place of more conventional techniques. In the absence of a specific noncoverage instruction, and where a laser has been approved for marketing by the Food and Drug Administration, contractor discretion may be used to determine whether a procedure performed with a laser is reasonable and necessary and, therefore, covered.

The determination of coverage for a procedure performed using a laser is made on the basis that the use of lasers to alter, revise, or destroy tissue is a surgical procedure. Therefore, coverage of laser procedures is restricted to practitioners with training in the surgical management of the disease or condition being treated.

35-53 ADULT LIVER TRANSPLANTATION

A. General.—Effective July 15, 1996, adult liver transplantation when performed on beneficiaries with end stage liver disease other than hepatitis B or malignancies is covered under Medicare when performed in a facility which is approved by CMS as meeting institutional coverage criteria.

Effective December 10, 1999, adult liver transplantation when performed on beneficiaries with end stage liver disease other than malignancies is covered under Medicare when performed in a facility which is approved by CMS as meeting institutional coverage criteria.

Effective September 1, 2001, Medicare covers adult liver transplantation for hepatocellular carcinoma when the following conditions are met:

1. The patient is not a candidate for subtotal liver resection;
2. The patient's tumor(s) is less than or equal to 5 cm in diameter;
3. There is no macrovascular involvement;
4. There is no identifiable extrahepatic spread of tumor to surrounding lymph nodes, lungs, abdominal organs or bone; and
5. The transplant is furnished in a facility which is approved by CMS as meeting institutional coverage criteria for liver transplants (See 65 FR 15006).

Adult liver transplantation for other malignancies remains excluded from coverage.

Coverage of adult liver transplantation is effective as of the date of the facility's approval, but for applications received before July 13, 1991, can be effective as early as March 8, 1990. (See *Federal Register* 56 FR 15006 dated April 12, 1991.)

B. Follow-up Care.—Follow-up care or retransplantation (ICD-9-M 996.82, Complications of Transplanted Organ, Liver0 required as a result of a covered liver transplant is covered, provided such services are otherwise reasonable and necessary. Follow-up care is also covered for patients who have been discharged from a hospital after receiving noncovered liver transplant. Coverage for follow-up care is for items and services that are reasonable and necessary as determined by Medicare guidelines. (See *Intermediary Manual*, §3101.14 and *Carriers Manual*, §2300.1.)

C. Immunosuppressive Drugs.--See *Intermediary Manual*, §3600.8 and *Carriers Manual*; §§2050.5, 4471, and 5249.

35-53.1 PEDIATRIC LIVER TRANSPLANTATION

Effective for services performed on or after February 9, 1984, liver transplantation is covered for children (under age 18) with extrahepatic biliary atresia or any other form of end stage liver disease, except that coverage is not provided for children with a malignancy extending beyond the margins of the liver or those with persistent viremia.

Effective for services performed on or after April 12, 1991, liver transplantation is covered for Medicare beneficiaries when performed in a pediatric hospital that performs pediatric liver transplants if the hospital submits an application which CMS approves documenting that:

- The hospital's pediatric liver transplant program is operated jointly by the hospital and another facility that has been found by CMS to meet the institutional coverage criteria in the *Federal Register* notice of April 12, 1991;

- The unified program shares the same transplant surgeons and quality assurance program (including oversight committee, patient protocol, and patient selection criteria); and
- The hospital is able to provide the specialized facilities, services, and personnel that are required by pediatric liver transplant patients.

35-54 REFRACTIVE KERATOPLASTY—NOT COVERED

Refractive keratoplasty is surgery to reshape the cornea of the eye to correct vision problems such as myopia (nearsightedness) and hyperopia (farsightedness). Refractive keratoplasty procedures include keratomileusis, in which the front of the cornea is removed, frozen, reshaped, and stitched back on the eye to correct either near or farsightedness; keratophakia, in which a reshaped donor cornea is inserted in the eye to correct farsightedness; and radial keratotomy, in which spoke-like slits are cut in the cornea to weaken and flatten the normally curved central portion to correct nearsightedness.

The correction of common refractive errors by eyeglasses, contact lenses or other prosthetic devices is specifically excluded from coverage. The use of radial keratotomy and/or keratoplasty for the purpose of refractive error compensation is considered a substitute or alternative to eye glasses or contact lenses, which are specifically excluded by §1862 (a)(7) of the Act (except in certain cases in connection with cataract surgery). In addition, many in the medical community consider such procedures cosmetic surgery, which is excluded by section §1862(a)(10) of the Act. Therefore, radial keratotomy and keratoplasty to treat refractive defects are not covered.

Keratoplasty that treats specific lesions of the cornea, such as phototherapeutic keratectomy that removes scar tissue from the visual field, deals with an abnormality of the eye and is not cosmetic surgery. Such cases may be covered under §1862(a)(1)(A) of the Act.

The use of lasers to treat ophthalmic disease constitutes ophthalmologic surgery. Coverage is restricted to practitioners who have completed an approved training program in ophthalmologic surgery.

35-55 TRANSVENOUS (CATHETER) PULMONARY EMBOLECTOMY—NOT COVERED

Transvenous (catheter) pulmonary embolectomy is a procedure for removing pulmonary emboli by passing a catheter through the femoral vein. It is not covered under Medicare because it is still experimental.

35-56 FLUIDIZED THERAPY DRY HEAT FOR CERTAIN MUSCULOSKELETAL DISORDERS

Fluidized therapy is a high intensity heat modality consisting of a dry whirlpool of finely divided solid particles suspended in a heated air stream, the mixture having the properties of a liquid. Use of fluidized therapy dry heat is covered as an acceptable alternative to other heat therapy modalities in the treatment of acute or subacute traumatic or nontraumatic musculoskeletal disorders of the extremities.

35-57 ELECTROENCEPHALOGRAPHIC MONITORING DURING SURGICAL PROCEDURES INVOLVING THE CEREBRAL VASCULATURE

Electroencephalographic (EEG) monitoring is a safe and reliable technique for the assessment of gross cerebral blood flow during general anesthesia and is covered under Medicare. Very characteristic changes in the EEG occur when cerebral perfusion is inadequate for cerebral function. EEG monitoring as an indirect measure of cerebral perfusion requires the expertise of an electroencephalographer, a neurologist trained in EEG, or an advanced EEG technician for its proper interpretation.

The EEG monitoring may be covered routinely in carotid endarterectomies and in other neurological procedures where cerebral perfusion could be reduced. Such other procedures might include aneurysm surgery where hypotensive anesthesia is used or other cerebral vascular procedures where cerebral blood flow may be interrupted.

35-57.1 ELECTROENCEPHALOGRAPHIC (EEG) MONITORING DURING OPEN-HEART SURGERY—NOT COVERED

The value of EEG monitoring during open heart surgery and in the immediate post-operative period is debatable because there are little published data based on well designed studies regarding its clinical effectiveness. The procedure is not frequently used and does not enjoy widespread acceptance of benefit.

Accordingly, Medicare does not cover EEG monitoring during open heart surgery and during the immediate post-operative period.

35-58 THORACIC DUCT DRAINAGE (TDD) IN RENAL TRANSPLANTS

Thoracic duct drainage (TDD) is an immunosuppressive technique used in renal transplantation. This procedure, which removes lymph from kidney transplant recipients as a means of achieving suppression of the immune mechanism, is currently being used both pre-transplant and post-transplant in conjunction with more conventional immunotherapy. TDD is performed on an inpatient basis, and the inpatient stay is covered for patients admitted for treatment in advance of a kidney transplant as well as for those receiving it post-transplant.

TDD is a covered technique when furnished to a kidney transplant recipient or an individual approved to receive kidney transplantation in a hospital approved to perform kidney transplantation.

35-59 ENDOSCOPY

Endoscopy is a technique in which a long flexible tube-like instrument is inserted into the body orally or rectally, permitting visual inspection of the gastrointestinal tract. Although primarily a diagnostic tool, endoscopy includes certain therapeutic procedures such as removal of polyps, and endoscopic papillotomy, by which stones are removed from the bile duct.

Endoscopic procedures are covered when reasonable and necessary for the individual patient.

35-64 CHELATION THERAPY FOR TREATMENT OF ATHEROSCLEROSIS

Chelation therapy is the application of chelation techniques for the therapeutic or preventive effects of removing unwanted metal ions from the body. The application of chelation therapy using ethylenediamine-tetra-acetic acid (EDTA) for the treatment and prevention of atherosclerosis is controversial. There is no widely accepted rationale to explain the beneficial effects attributed to this therapy. Its safety is questioned and its clinical effectiveness has never been established by well designed, controlled clinical trials. It is not widely accepted and practiced by American physicians. EDTA chelation therapy for atherosclerosis is considered experimental. For these reasons, EDTA chelation therapy for the treatment or prevention of atherosclerosis is not covered.

Some practitioners refer to this therapy as chemoendarterectomy and may also show a diagnosis other than atherosclerosis, such as arteriosclerosis or calcinosis. Claims employing such variant terms should also be denied under this section.

Cross-reference: §45-20

35-65 GASTRIC FREEZING

Gastric freezing for chronic peptic ulcer disease is a non-surgical treatment which was popular about 20 years ago but now is seldom done. It has been abandoned due to a high complication rate, only temporary improvement experienced by patients, and lack of effectiveness when tested by double-blind, controlled clinical trials. Since the procedure is now considered obsolete, it is not covered.

35-74 EXTERNAL COUNTERPULSATION (ECP) FOR SEVERE ANGINA—COVERED

External counterpulsation (ECP), commonly referred to as enhanced external counterpulsation, is a non-invasive outpatient treatment for coronary artery disease refractory to medical and/or surgical therapy. Although ECP devices are cleared by the Food and Drug Administration (FDA) for use in treating a variety of cardiac conditions, including stable or unstable angina pectoris, acute myocardial infarction and cardiogenic shock, the use of this device to treat cardiac conditions other than stable angina pectoris is not covered, since only that use has developed sufficient evidence to demonstrate its medical effectiveness. Non-coverage of hydraulic versions of these types of devices remains in force.

Coverage is provided for the use of ECP for patients who have been diagnosed with disabling angina (Class III or Class IV, Canadian Cardiovascular Society Classification or equivalent classification) who, in the opinion of a cardiologist or cardiothoracic surgeon, are not readily amenable to surgical intervention, such as PTCA or cardiac bypass because: (1) their condition is inoperable, or at high risk of operative complications or post-operative failure; (2) their coronary anatomy is not readily amenable to such procedures; or (3) they have co-morbid states which create excessive risk.

A full course of therapy usually consists of 35 one-hour treatments, which may be offered once or twice daily, usually 5 days per week. The patient is placed on a treatment table where their lower trunk and lower extremities are wrapped in a series of three compressive air cuffs which inflate and deflate in synchronization with the patient's cardiac cycle.

35-77 NEUROMUSCULAR ELECTRICAL STIMULATION (NMES)

Neuromuscular electrical stimulation (NMES) involves the use of a device that transmits an electrical impulse to activate muscle groups by way of electrodes. There are two broad categories of NMES. One type of device stimulates the muscle when the patient is in a resting state to treat muscle atrophy. The second type is used to enhance functional activity of neurologically impaired patients.

Treatment of Muscle Atrophy
Coverage of NMES to treat muscle atrophy is limited to the treatment of patients with disuse atrophy where the nerve supply to the muscle is intact, including brain, spinal cord and peripheral nerves and other non-neurological reasons for disuse atrophy. Examples include casting or splinting of a limb, contracture due to scarring of soft tissue as in burn lesions, and hip orthotic training begins). (See CIM 45-25 for an explanation of coverage of medically necessary supplies for the effective use of NMES).

Use for Walking in Patients with Spinal Cord Injury (SCI)
The type of NMES that is used to enhance the ability to walk of SCI patients is commonly referred to as functional electrical stimulation (FES). These devices are surface units that use electrical impulses to activate paralyzed or weak muscles in precise sequence. Coverage for the use of NMES/FES is limited to SCI patients, for walking, who have completed a training program, which consists of at least 32 physical therapy sessions with the device over a period of 3 months. The trial period of physical therapy will enable the physician treating the patient for his or her spinal cord injury to properly evaluate the person's ability to use these devices frequently and for the long term. Physical therapy sessions are only covered in the inpatient hospital, outpatient hospital, comprehensive outpatient rehabilitation facilities, and outpatient rehabilitation facilities. The physical therapy necessary to perform this training must be directly performed by the physical therapist as part of a one-on-one training program; this service cannot be done unattended.

The goal of physical therapy must be to train SCI patients on the use of NMES/FES devices to achieve walking, not to reverse or retard muscle atrophy.

Coverage for NMES/FES for walking will be limited to SCI patients with all of the following characteristics:

1) persons with intact lower motor units (L1 and below) (both muscle and peripheral nerve);
2) persons with muscle and joint stability for weight bearing at upper and lower extremities that can demonstrate balance and control to maintain an upright support posture independently;
3) persons that demonstrate brisk muscle contraction to NMES and have sensory perception of electrical stimulation sufficient for muscle contraction;
4) persons that possess high motivation, commitment and cognitive ability to use such devices for walking;
5) persons that can transfer independently and can demonstrate independent standing tolerance for at least 3 minutes;
6) persons that can demonstrate hand and finger function to manipulate controls;
7) persons with at least 6-month post recovery spinal cord injury and restorative surgery;
8) persons without hip and knee degenerative disease and no history of long bone fracture secondary to osteoporosis; and
9) persons who have demonstrated a willingness to use the device long-term.

NMES/FES for walking will not be covered in SCI patients with any of the following:

1) persons with cardiac pacemakers;
2) severe scoliosis or severe osteoporosis;
3) skin disease or cancer at area of stimulation;
4) irreversible contracture; or
5) autonomic dysreflexia.

The only settings where therapists with the sufficient skills to provide these services are employed, are inpatient hospitals, outpatient hospitals, comprehensive outpatient rehabilitation facilities and outpatient rehabilitation facilities. The physical therapy necessary to perform this training must be part of a one-on-one training program.

Additional therapy after the purchase of the DME would be limited by our general policies on coverage of skilled physical therapy.

All other uses of NMES remain non-covered.

(*Also reference Medicare Carriers' Manual, Part 3, Claims-§2210 and Medicare Intermediary Manual, Part 3, Claims-§3653 - See - Maintenance Program 271.1*)

35-82 PANCREAS TRANSPLANTS

Pancreas transplantation is performed to induce an insulin independent, euglycemic state in diabetic patients. The procedure is generally limited to those patients with severe secondary complications of diabetes, including kidney failure. However, pancreas transplantation is sometimes performed on patients with labile diabetes and hypoglycemic unawareness.

Medicare has had a policy of not covering pancreas transplantation for many years as the safety and effectiveness of the procedure had not been demonstrated. The Office of Health Technology Assessment performed an assessment on pancreas-kidney transplantation in 1994. They found reasonable graft survival outcomes for patients receiving either simultaneous pancreas-kidney transplantation and pancreas after kidney transplantation.

Effective July 1, 1999, Medicare will cover whole organ pancreas transplantation (ICD-9-CM code 52.80, or 52.82, CPT code 48554) only when it is performed simultaneous with or after a kidney transplant (ICD-9-CM code 55.69, CPT code 50360, or 50365). If the pancreas transplant occurs after the kidney transplant, immunosuppressive therapy will begin with the date of discharge from the inpatient stay for the pancreas transplant.

35-93 LUNG VOLUME REDUCTION SURGERY (REDUCTION PNEUMOPLASTY, ALSO CALLED LUNG SHAVING OR LUNG CONTOURING) UNILATERAL OR BILATERAL BY OPEN OR THORACOSCOPIC APPROACH FOR TREATMENT OF EMPHYSEMA OR CHRONIC OBSTRUCTIVE PULMONARY DISEASE—NOT GENERALLY COVERED

Lung volume reduction surgery (LVRS) or reduction pneumoplasty, also referred to as lung shaving or lung contouring, is performed on patients with emphysema and chronic obstructive pulmonary disease (COPD) in order to allow the underlying compressed lung to expand, and thus, establish improved respiratory function. The goal of this procedure is to offer a better quality of life for patients with emphysema and COPD. In addition, LVRS may be offered as a "bridge to transplant" for patients who otherwise may not have been considered candidates for lung transplantation.

Unilateral or bilateral LVRS by open or thoracoscopic approach is not generally covered, because there is insufficient medical evidence available to base a determination that this procedure is generally safe and effective. Therefore, LVRS generally cannot be considered reasonable and necessary under §1862(a)(1)(A) of the Act in most cases.

When this policy was first established in December 1995, HCFA committed Medicare to reviewing the scientific literature as it was published in order to modify coverage policy as clinical data were developed. HCFA has reviewed data that suggest the need for a randomized clinical trial regarding the safety and effectiveness of LVRS. On April 24, 1996, the Health Care Financing Administration (HCFA) and the National Heart, Lung and Blood Institute (NHLBI) of the National Institutes of Health announced their intention to collaborate on a multi-center, randomized clinical study evaluating the effectiveness of LVRS. On December 20, 1996, HCFA and NHLBI announced the clinical centers and the data coordinating center that will be participating in the study. HCFA has determined that LVRS is reasonable and necessary when it is provided under the conditions detailed by the protocol of the HCFA/NHLBI clinical study. Therefore, Medicare will cover LVRS in those limited circumstances when it is provided to a Medicare beneficiary under the protocols established for the study. Coverage will be provided where the care is furnished in facilities that are approved as meeting the criteria established by HCFA and NHLBI for this study.

35-98 ELECTRICAL STIMULATION FOR THE TREATMENT OF WOUNDS

Electrical stimulation (ES) has been used or studied for many different applications, one of which is accelerating wound healing. The types of ES used for healing chronic venous and arterial wound and pressure ulcers are direct current (DC), alternating current (AC), pulsed current (PC), pulsed electromagnetic induction (PEMI), and spinal cord stimulation (SCS). An example of AC is transcutaneous electrical stimulation (TENS). The PEMI includes Pulsed Electromagnetic Field (PEMF) and Pulsed Electromagnetic Energy (PEE) using pulsed radio frequency energy, both of which are nonthermal i.e., they do not produce heat. Some ES use generators to create energy in the means such as coils, rather than by leads or surface electrodes.

There is insufficient evidence to determine any clinically significant differences in healing rates. Therefore, ES cannot be covered by Medicare because its effectiveness has not been adequately demonstrated.

35-99 ABORTION

Abortions are not covered Medicare procedures except:

1. If the pregnancy is the result of an act of rape or incest; or
2. In the case where a woman suffers from a physical disorder, physical injury, or physical illness, including a life-endangering physical condition caused by or arising from the pregnancy itself, that would, as certified by a physician, place the woman in danger of death unless an abortion is performed.

This restricted coverage applies to CPT codes 59840, 59841, 59850, 59851, 59852, 59855, 59856, 59857, and 59866.

35-100 PHOTODYNAMIC THERAPY

Photodynamic therapy is a medical procedure which involves the infusion of a photosensitive (light-activated) drug with a very specific absorption peak. This drug is chemically designed to have a unique affinity for the diseased tissue intended for treatment. Once introduced to the body, the drug accumulates and is retained in diseased tissue to a greater degree than in normal tissue. Infusion is followed by the targeted irradiation of this tissue with a non-thermal laser, calibrated to emit light at a wavelength that corresponds to the drug's absorption peak. The drug then becomes active and locally treats the diseased tissue.

Ocular photodynamic therapy (OPT)

OPT is used in the treatment of ophthalmologic diseases. OPT is only covered when used in conjunction with verteporfin (see §45-30 PHOTOSENSITIVE DRUGS).

A. Classic Subfoveal Choroidal Neovascular (CNV) Lesions.—OPT is covered with a diagnosis of neovascular age-related macular degeneration (AMD) with predominately classic subfoveal choroidal neovascular (CNV) lesions (where the area of classic CNV occupies = 50% of the area of the entire lesion) at the initial visit as determined by a fluorescein angiogram. Subsequent follow-up visits will require a fluorescein angiogram prior to treatment. There are no requirements regarding visual acuity, lesion size, and number of re-treatments.
B. Occult Subfoveal Choroidal Neovascular (CNV) Lesions.—OPT is noncovered for patients with a diagnosis of age-related macular degeneration (AMD) with occult and no classic CNV lesions.
C. Other Conditions.—Use of OPT with verteporfin for other types of AMD (e.g., patients with minimally classic CNV lesions, atrophic, or dry AMD) is noncovered. OPT with verteporfin for other ocular indications such as pathologic myopia or presumed ocular histoplasmosis syndrome, is eligible for coverage through individual contractor discretion.

35-102 ELECTRICAL STIMULATION FOR THE TREATMENT OF WOUNDS (Effective for services on and after April 1, 2003)

Electrical stimulation (ES) has been used or studied for many different applications, one of which is accelerating wound healing. Electrical stimulation for the treatment of wounds is the application of electrical current through electrodes placed directly on the skin in close proximity to the wound. Electrical stimulation for the treatment of wounds will only be covered for chronic Stage III or Stage IV pressure ulcers, arterial ulcers, diabetic ulcers and venous stasis ulcers. All other uses of electrical stimulation for the treatment of wounds are noncovered. Chronic ulcers are defined as ulcers that have not healed within 30 days of occurrence. Electrical stimulation will not be covered as an initial treatment modality.

The use of electrical stimulation for the treatment of wounds is considered an adjunctive therapy. Electrical stimulation will be covered only after appropriate standard wound therapy has been tried for at least 30-days and there are no measurable signs of healing. This 30-day period can begin while the wound is acute. Measurable signs of improved healing include a decrease in wound size, either surface area or volume, decrease in amount of exudates and decrease in amount of necrotic tissue. Standard wound care includes: optimization of nutritional status; debridement by any means to remove devitalized tissue; maintenance of a clean, moist bed of granulation tissue with appropriate moist dressings; and necessary treatment to resolve any infection that may be present. Standard wound care based on the specific type of wound includes: frequent repositioning of a patient with pressure ulcers (usually every 2 hours); off-loading of pressure and good glucose control for diabetic ulcers; establishment of adequate circulation for arterial ulcers; and the use of a compression system for patients with venous ulcers.

Continued treatment with electrical stimulation is not covered if measurable signs of healing have not been demonstrated within any 30-day period of treatment. Electrical stimulation must be discontinued when the wound demonstrates 100 per-cent epithelialzed wound bed.

Any form of electromagnetic therapy for the treatment of chronic wounds will not be covered. This service can only be covered when performed by a physician, physical therapist, or incident to a physician service. Evaluation of the wound is an integral part of wound therapy. When a physician, physical therapist, or a clinician incident to a physician, performs electrical stimulation, that practitioner must evaluate the wound and contact the treating physician if the wound worsens. If electrical stimulation is being used, wounds must be evaluated at least monthly by the treating physician.

Unsupervised use of electrical stimulation for wound therapy will not be covered, as this use has not been found to be medically reasonable and necessary.

45-4 VITAMIN B12 INJECTIONS TO STRENGTHEN TENDONS, LIGAMENTS, ETC., OF THE FOOT—NOT COVERED

Vitamin B12 injections to strengthen tendons, ligaments, etc., of the foot are not covered under Medicare because (1) there is no evidence that vitamin B12 injections are effective for the purpose of strengthening weakened tendons and ligaments, and (2) this is nonsurgical treatment under the subluxation exclusion. Accordingly, vitamin B12 injections are not considered reasonable and necessary within the meaning of §1862(a)(1) of the Act.

See Intermediary Manual, §§3101.3 and 3158 and Carriers Manual, §§2050.5 and 2323.

45-7 HYDROPHILIC CONTACT LENS FOR CORNEAL BANDAGE

Some hydrophilic contact lenses are used as moist corneal bandages for the treatment of acute or chronic corneal pathology, such as bullous keratopathy, dry eyes, corneal ulcers and erosion, keratitis, corneal edema, descemetocele, corneal ectasis, Mooren's ulcer, anterior corneal dystrophy, neurotrophic keratoconjunctivitis, and for other therapeutic reasons.

Payment may be made under §1861(s)(2) of the Act for a hydrophilic contact lens approved by the Food and Drug Administration (FDA) and used as a supply incident to a physician's service. Payment for the lens is included in the payment for the physician's service to which the lens is incident. Contractors are authorized to accept an FDA letter of approval or other FDA published material as evidence of FDA approval. (See §65-1 for coverage of a hydrophilic contact lens as a prosthetic device.)

See Intermediary Manual, §3112.4 and Carriers Manual, §§2050.1 and 15010.

45-10 LAETRILE AND RELATED SUBSTANCES—NOT COVERED

Laetrile (and the other drugs called by the various terms mentioned below) have been used primarily in the treatment or control of cancer. Although the terms "Laetrile," "laetrile," "amygdaline," "Sarcarcinase," "vitamin B-17," and "nitriloside" have been used interchangeably, the chemical identity of the substances to which these terms refer has varied.

The FDA has determined that neither Laetrile nor any other drug called by the various terms mentioned above, nor any other product which might be characterized as a "nitriloside" is generally recognized (by experts qualified by scientific training and experience to evaluate the safety and effectiveness of drugs) to be safe and effective for any therapeutic use. Therefore, use of this drug cannot be considered to be reasonable and necessary within the meaning of §1862(a)(1) of the Act and program payment may not be made for its use or any services furnished in connection with its administration.

A hospital stay only for the purpose of having laetrile (or any other drug called by the terms mentioned above) administered is not covered. Also, program payment may not be made for laetrile (or other drug noted above) when it is used during the course of an otherwise covered hospital stay, since the FDA has found such drugs to not be safe and effective for any therapeutic purpose.

45-16 CERTAIN DRUGS DISTRIBUTED BY THE NATIONAL CANCER INSTITUTE (Effective for services furnished on or after October 1, 1980.)

Under its Cancer Therapy Evaluation, the Division of Cancer Treatment of the National Cancer Institute (NCI), in cooperation with the Food and Drug Administration, approves and distributes certain drugs for use in treating terminally ill cancer patients. One group of these drugs, designated as Group C drugs, unlike other drugs distributed by the NCI, are not limited to use in clinical trials for the purpose of testing their efficacy. Drugs are classified as Group C drugs only if there is sufficient evidence demonstrating their efficacy within a tumor type and that they can be safely administered.

A physician is eligible to receive Group C drugs from the Division of Cancer Treatment only if the following requirements are met:

- A physician must be registered with the NCI as an investigator by having completed an FD-Form 1573;
- A written request for the drug, indicating the disease to be treated, must be submitted to the NCI;
- The use of the drug must be limited to indications outlined in the NCI's guidelines; and
- All adverse reactions must be reported to the Investigational Drug Branch of the Division of Cancer Treatment.

In view of these NCI controls on distribution and use of Group C drugs, intermediaries may assume, in the absence of evidence to the contrary, that a Group C drug and the related hospital stay are covered if all other applicable coverage requirements are satisfied.

If there is reason to question coverage in a particular case, the matter should be resolved with the assistance of the local PSRO, or if there is none, the assistance of your medical consultants.

Information regarding those drugs which are classified as Group C drugs may be obtained from:

Office of the Chief, Investigational Drug Branch
Division of Cancer Treatment, CTEP, Landow Building
Room 4C09, National Cancer Institute
Bethesda, Maryland 20205

45-20 ETHYLENEDIAMINE-TETRA-ACETIC (EDTA) CHELATION THERAPY FOR TREATMENT OF ATHEROSCLEROSIS

The use of EDTA as a chelating agent to treat atherosclerosis, arteriosclerosis, calcinosis, or similar generalized condition not listed by the FDA as an approved use is not covered. Any such use of EDTA is considered experimental.

See §35-64 for an explanation of this conclusion.

45-22 LYMPHOCYTE IMMUNE GLOBULIN, ANTI-THYMOCYTE GLOBULIN (EQUINE)

The lymphocyte immune globulin preparations are biologic drugs not previously approved or licensed for use in the management of renal allograft rejection. A number of other lymphocyte immune globulin products of equine, lapine, and murine origin are currently under investigation for their potential usefulness in controlling allograft rejections in human transplantation. These biologic drugs are viewed as adjunctive to traditional immunosuppressive products such as steroids and anti-metabolic drugs. At present, lymphocyte immune globulin preparations are not recommended to replace conventional immunosuppressive drugs, but to supplement them and to be used as alternatives to elevated or accelerated dosing with conventional immunosuppressive agents.

The FDA has approved one lymphocyte immune globulin preparation for marketing, lymphocyte immune globulin, anti-thymocyte globulin (equine). This drug is indicated for the management of allograft rejection episodes in renal transplantation. It is covered under Medicare when used for this purpose. Other forms of lymphocyte globulin preparation which the FDA approves for this indication in the future may be covered under Medicare.

45-23 DIMETHYL SULFOXIDE (DMSO)

DMSO is an industrial solvent produced as a chemical byproduct of paper production from wood pulp. The Food and Drug Administration has determined that the only purpose for which DMSO is safe and effective for humans is in the treatment of the bladder condition, interstitial cystitis.

Therefore, the use of DMSO for all other indications is not considered to be reasonable and necessary. Payment may be made for its use only when reasonable and necessary for a patient in the treatment of interstitial cystitis.

45-24 ANTI-INHIBITOR COAGULANT COMPLEX (AICC)

Anti-inhibitor coagulant complex, AICC, is a drug used to treat hemophilia in patients with factor VIII inhibitor antibodies. AICC has been shown to be safe and effective and has Medicare coverage when furnished to patients with hemophilia A and inhibitor antibodies to factor VIII who have major bleeding episodes and who fail to respond to other, less expensive therapies.

45-25 SUPPLIES USED IN THE DELIVERY OF TRANSCUTANEOUS ELECTRICAL NERVE STIMULATION (TENS) AND NEURO-MUSCULAR ELECTRICAL STIMULATION (NMES)—(Effective for services rendered (i.e., items rented or purchased) on or after July 14, 1988.)

Transcutaneous Electrical Nerve Stimulation (TENS) and/or Neuromuscular Electrical Stimulation (NMES) can ordinarily be delivered to patients through the use of conventional electrodes, adhesive tapes and lead wires. There may be times, however, where it might be medically necessary for certain patients receiving TENS or NMES treatment to use, as an alternative to conventional electrodes, adhesive tapes and lead wires, a form-fitting conductive garment (i.e., a garment with conductive fibers which are separated from the patients' skin by layers of fabric).

A form-fitting conductive garment (and medically necessary related supplies) may be covered under the program only when:

1. It has received permission or approval for marketing by the Food and Drug Administration;
2. It has been prescribed by a physician for use in delivering covered TENS or NMES treatment; and
3. One of the medical indications outlined below is met:

   - The patient cannot manage without the conductive garment because there is such a large area or so many sites to be stimulated and the stimulation would have to be delivered so frequently that it is not feasible to use conventional electrodes, adhesive tapes and lead wires;
   - The patient cannot manage without the conductive garment for the treatment of chronic intractable pain because the areas or sites to be stimulated are inaccessible with the use of conventional electrodes, adhesive tapes and lead wires;
   - The patient has a documented medical condition such as skin problems that preclude the application of conventional electrodes, adhesive tapes and lead wires;
   - The patient requires electrical stimulation beneath a cast either to treat disuse atrophy, where the nerve supply to the muscle is intact, or to treat chronic intractable pain; or
   - The patient has a medical need for rehabilitation strengthening (pursuant to a written plan of rehabilitation) following an injury where the nerve supply to the muscle is intact.

A conductive garment is not covered for use with a TENS device during the trial period specified in §35-46 unless:

4. The patient has a documented skin problem prior to the start of the trial period; and
5. The carrier's medical consultants are satisfied that use of such an item is medically necessary for the patient.

(See conditions for coverage of the use of TENS in the diagnosis and treatment of chronic intractable pain in §§35-46 and 60-20 and the use of NMES in the treatment of disuse atrophy in §35-77.)

45-30 PHOTOSENSITIVE DRUGS

Photosensitive drugs are the light-sensitive agents used in photodynamic therapy. Once introduced into the body, these drugs selectively identify and adhere to diseased tissue. The drugs remain inactive until they are exposed to a specific wavelength of light, by means of a laser, that corresponds to their absorption peak. The activation of a photosensitive drug results in a photochemical reaction which treats the diseased tissue without affecting surrounding normal tissue.

Verteporfin

Verteporfin, a benzoporphyrin derivative, is an intravenous lipophilic photosensitive drug with an absorption peak of 690 nm. This drug was first approved by the Food and Drug Administration (FDA) on April 12, 2000, and subsequently, approved for inclusion in the United States Pharmacopoeia on July 18, 2000, meeting Medicare's definition of a drug as defined under §1861(t)(1) of the Social Security Act. Effective July 1, 2001, Verteporfin is only covered when used in conjunction with ocular photodynamic therapy (see §35-100 PHOTODYNAMIC THERAPY) when furnished intravenously incident to a physician's service. For patients with age-related macular degeneration, Verteporfin is only covered with a diagnosis of neovascular age-related macular degeneration (ICD-9-CM 362.52) with predominately classic subfoveal choroidal neovascular (CNV) lesions (where the area of classic CNV occupies = 50% of the area of the entire lesion) at the initial visit as determined by a fluorescein angiogram (CPT code 92235). Subsequent follow-up visits will require a fluorescein angiogram prior to treatment. OPT with verteporfin is covered for the above indication and will remain noncovered for all other indications related to AMD (see CIM § CIM § 35-100). OPT with Verteporfin for use in non-AMD conditions is eligible for coverage through individual contractor discretion.

50-1 CARDIAC PACEMAKER EVALUATION SERVICES (Effective for services rendered on or after October 1, 1984.)

Medicare covers a variety of services for the post-implant follow-up and evaluation of implanted cardiac pacemakers. The following guidelines are designed to assist contractors in identifying and processing claims for such services.

NOTE: These new guidelines are limited to lithium battery-powered pacemakers, because mercury-zinc battery-powered pacemakers are no longer being manufactured and virtually all have been replaced by lithium units. Contractors still receiving claims for monitoring such units should continue to apply the guidelines published in 1980 to those units until they are replaced.

There are two general types of pacemakers in current use--single-chamber pacemakers, which sense and pace the ventricles of the heart, and dual-chamber pacemakers which sense and pace both the atria and the ventricles. These differences require different monitoring patterns over the expected life of the units involved. One fact of which contractors should be aware is that many dual-chamber units may be programmed to pace only the ventricles; this may be done either at the time the pacemaker is implanted or at some time afterward. In such cases, a dual-chamber unit, when programmed or reprogrammed for ventricular pacing, should be treated as a single-chamber pacemaker in applying screening guidelines.

The decision as to how often any patient's pacemaker should be monitored is the responsibility of the patient's physician who is best able to take into account the condition and circumstances of the individual patient. These may vary over time, requiring modifications of the frequency with which the patient should be monitored. In cases where monitoring is done by some entity other than the patient's physician, such as a commercial monitoring service or hospital outpatient department, the physician's prescription for monitoring is required and should be periodically renewed (at least annually) to assure that the frequency of monitoring is proper for the patient. Where a patient is monitored both during clinic visits and transtelephonically, the contractor should be sure to include frequency data on both types of monitoring in evaluating the reasonableness of the frequency of monitoring services received by the patient.

Since there are over 200 pacemaker models in service at any given point, and a variety of patient conditions that give rise to the need for pacemakers, the question of the appropriate frequency of monitoring is a complex one. Nevertheless, it is possible to develop guidelines within which the vast majority of pacemaker monitoring will fall and contractors should do this, using their own data and experience, as well as the frequency guidelines which follow, in order to limit extensive claims development to those cases requiring special attention.

Guidelines for Transtelephonic Monitoring of Cardiac Pacemakers

A. General.—Transtelephonic monitoring of pacemakers is coming into increasingly widespread use, with the services being furnished by commercial suppliers, hospital outpatient departments and physicians' offices.

Telephone monitoring of cardiac pacemakers as described below is medically efficacious in identifying early signs of possible pacemaker failure, thus reducing the number of sudden pacemaker failures requiring emergency replacement. All systems which monitor the pacemaker rate (bpm) in both the free-running and/or magnetic mode are effective in detecting subclinical pacemaker failure due to battery depletion. More sophisticated systems are also capable of detecting internal electronic problems within the pulse generator itself and other potential problems. In the case of dual chamber pacemakers in particular, such monitoring may detect failure of synchronization of the atria and ventricles, and the need for adjustment and reprogramming of the device.

NOTE: The transmitting device furnished to the patient is simply one component of the diagnostic system, and is not covered as durable medical equipment. Those engaged in transtelephonic pacemaker monitoring should reflect the costs of the transmitters in setting their charges for monitoring.

B. Definition of Transtelephonic Monitoring.—In order for transtelephonic monitoring services to be covered, the services must consist of the following elements:

1. A minimum 30-second readable strip of the pacemaker in the free-running mode;
2. Unless contraindicated, a minimum 30-second readable strip of the pacemaker in the magnetic mode; and
3. A minimum 30 seconds of readable ECG strip.

C. Frequency Guidelines for Transtelephonic Monitoring.—The guidelines below constitute a system which contractors should use, in conjunction with their knowledge of local medical practices, to screen claims for transtelephonic monitoring prior to payment. It is important to note that they are not recommendations with respect to a minimum frequency for such monitoring, but rather a maximum frequency (within which payment may be made without further claims development). As with previous guidelines, more frequent monitoring may be covered in cases where contractors are satisfied that such monitoring are medically necessary; e.g., based on the condition of the patient, or with respect to pacemakers exhibiting unexpected defects or premature failure. Contractors should seek written justification for more frequent monitoring from the patient's physician and/or any monitoring service involved.

These guidelines are divided into two broad categories—Guideline I, which will apply to the majority of pacemakers now in use, and Guideline II, which will apply only to pacemaker systems (pacemaker and leads) for which sufficient long-term clinical information exists to assure that they meet the standards of the Inter-Society Commission for Heart Disease Resources (ICHD) for longevity and end-of-life decay. (The ICHD standards are: (1) 90 percent cumulative survival at 5 years following implant; and (2) an end-of-life decay of less than a 50 percent drop of output voltage and less than 20 percent deviation of magnet rate, or a drop of 5 beats per minute or less, over a period of 3 months or more.) Contractors should consult with their medical advisers and other appropriate individuals and organizations (such as the North American Society of Pacing and Electrophysiology, which publishes product reliability information) should questions arise over whether a pacemaker system meets the ICHD standards.

The two groups of guidelines are then further broken down into two general categories--single chamber and dual-chamber pacemakers. Contractors should be aware that the frequency with which a patient is monitored may be changed from time to time for a number of reasons, such as a change in the patient's overall condition, a reprogramming of the patient's pacemaker, the development of better information on the pacemaker's longevity or failure mode, etc. Consequently, changes in the proper set of guidelines may be required. Contractors should inform physicians and monitoring services to alert contractors to any changes in the patient's monitoring prescription that might necessitate changes in the screening guidelines applied to that patient. (Of particular importance is the reprogramming of a dual-chamber pacemaker to a single-chamber mode of operation. Such reprogramming would shift the patient from the appropriate dual-chamber guideline to the appropriate single-chamber guideline.)

Guideline I
1. Single-chamber pacemakers:
   1st month—every 2 weeks.
   2nd through 36th month—every 8 weeks.
   37th month to failure—every 4 weeks.

2. Dual-chamber pacemaker:
   1st month—every 2 weeks.
   2nd through 6th month—every 4 weeks.
   7th through 36th month—every 8 weeks.
   37th month to failure—every 4 weeks.

Guideline II
1. Single-chamber pacemakers:
   1st month—every 2 weeks.
   2nd through 48th month—every 12 weeks.
   49th through 72nd month—every 8 weeks.
   Thereafter—every 4 weeks.

2. Dual-chamber pacemaker:
   1st month—every 2 weeks.
   2nd through 30th month—every 12 weeks.
   31st through 48th month—every 8 weeks.
   Thereafter—every 4 weeks.

D. Pacemaker Clinic Services
   1. General.—Pacemaker monitoring is also covered when done by pacemaker clinics. Clinic visits may be done in conjunction with transtelephonic monitoring or as a separate service; however, the services rendered by a pacemaker clinic are more extensive than those currently possible by telephone. They include, for example, physical examination of patients and reprogramming of pacemakers. Thus, the use of one of these types of monitoring does not preclude concurrent use of the other.
   2. Frequency Guidelines—As with transtelephonic pacemaker monitoring, the frequency of clinic visits is the decision of the patient's physician, taking into account, among other things, the medical condition of the patient. However, contractors can develop monitoring guidelines that will prove useful in screening claims. The following are recommendations for monitoring guidelines on lithium-battery pacemakers:
      a. For single-chamber pacemakers - twice in the first 6 months following implant, then once every 12 months.
      b. For dual-chamber pacemakers - twice in the first 6 months, then once every 6 months.

50-4 GRAVLEE JET WASHER

The Gravlee Jet Washer is a sterile, disposable, diagnostic device for detecting endometrial cancer. The use of this device is indicated where the patient exhibits clinical symptoms or signs suggestive of endometrial disease, such as irregular or heavy vaginal bleeding.

Program payment cannot be made for the washer or the related diagnostic services when furnished in connection with the examination of an asymptomatic patient. Payment for routine physical checkups is precluded under the statute.

(See §1862(a)(7) of the Act.) (See Intermediary Manual, §3157 and Carriers Manual, §2320.)

50-10 VABRA ASPIRATOR

The VABRA aspirator is a sterile, disposable, vacuum aspirator which is used to collect uterine tissue for study to detect endometrial carcinoma. The use of this device is indicated where the patient exhibits clinical symptoms or signs suggestive of endometrial disease, such as irregular or heavy vaginal bleeding.

Program payment cannot be made for the aspirator or the related diagnostic services when furnished in connection with the examination of an asymptomatic patient. Payment for routine physical checkups is precluded under the statute (§1862(a)(7) of the Act).

Cross-reference: Intermediary Manual, §3157; Carriers Manual §2320; §50-4

50-15 ELECTROCARDIOGRAPHIC SERVICES

Reimbursement may be made under Part B for electrocardiographic (EKG) services rendered by a physician or incident to his/her services or by an approved laboratory or an approved supplier of portable X-ray services. Since there is no coverage for EKG services of any type rendered on a screening basis or as part of a routine examination, the claim must indicate the signs and symptoms or other clinical reason necessitating the services.

A separate charge by an attending or consulting physician for EKG interpretation is allowed only when it is the normal practice to make such charge in addition to the regular office visit charge. No payment is made for EKG interpretations by individuals other than physicians.

On a claim involving EKG services furnished by a laboratory or a portable X-ray supplier, identify the physician ordering the service and, when the charge includes both the taking of the tracing and its interpretation, include the identity of the physician making the interpretation. No separate bill for the services of a physician is paid unless it is clear that he/she was the patient's attending physician or was acting as a consulting physician. The taking of an EKG in an emergency, i.e., when the patient is or may be experiencing what is commonly referred to as a heart attack, is covered as a laboratory service or a diagnostic service by a portable X-ray supplier only when the evidence shows that a physician was in attendance at the time the service was performed or immediately thereafter.

Where EKG services are rendered in the patient's home and the laboratory's or portable X-ray supplier's charge is higher than that imposed for the same service when performed in the laboratory or portable X-ray supplier's office, the medical need for home service should be documented. In the absence of such justification, reimbursement for the service if otherwise medically necessary should be based on the reasonable charge applicable when performed in the laboratory or X-ray supplier's office.

The documentation required in the various situations mentioned above must be furnished not only when the laboratory or portable X-ray supplier bills the patient or carrier for its service, but also when such a facility bills the attending physician who, in turn, bills the patient or carrier for the EKG services. (In addition to the evidence required to document the claim, the laboratory or portable X-ray supplier must maintain in its records the referring physician's written order and the identity of the employee taking the tracing.)

Long Term EKG Monitoring, also referred to as long-term EKG recording, Holter recording, or dynamic electrocardiography, is a diagnostic procedure which provides a continuous record of the electrocardiographic activity of a patient's heart while he is engaged in his daily activities.

The basic components of the long-term EKG monitoring systems are a sensing element, the design of which may provide either for the recording of electrocardiographic information on magnetic tape or for detecting significant variations in rate or rhythm as they occur, and a component for either graphically recording the electrocardiographic data or for visual or computer assisted analysis of the information recorded on magnetic tape. The long-term EKG permits the examination in the ambulant or potentially ambulant patient of as many as 70,000 heartbeats in a 12-hour recording while the standard EKG which is obtained in the recumbent position, yields information on only 50 to 60 cardiac cycles and provides only a limited data base on which diagnostic judgments may be made.

Many patients with cardiac arrhythmias are unaware of the presence of an irregularity in heart rhythm. Due to the transient nature of many arrhythmias and the short intervals in which the rhythm of the heart is observed by conventional standard EKG techniques, the offending arrhythmias can go undetected. With the extended examination provided by the long-term EKG, the physician is able not only to detect but also to classify various types of rhythm disturbances and waveform abnormalities and note the frequency of their occurrence. The knowledge of the reaction of the heart to daily activities with respect to rhythm, rate, conduction disturbances, and changes are of great assistance in directing proper therapy and this modality is valuable in both inpatient and outpatient diagnosis and therapy. Long-term monitoring of ambulant or potentially ambulant inpatients provides significant potential for reducing the length of stay for post-coronary infarct patients in the intensive care setting and may result in earlier discharge from the hospital with greater assurance of safety to the patients. The indications for the use of this technique, noted below, are similar for both inpatients and outpatients.

The long-term EKG has proven effective in detecting transient episodes of cardiac dysrhythmia and in permitting the correlation of these episodes with cardiovascular symptomatology. It is also useful for patients who have symptoms of obscure etiology suggestive of cardiac arrhythmia. Examples of such symptoms include palpitations, chest pain, dizziness, light-headedness, near syncope, syncope, transient ischemic episodes, dyspnea, and shortness of breath.

This technique would also be appropriate at the time of institution of any arrhythmic drug therapy and may be performed during the course of therapy to evaluate response. It is also appropriate for evaluating a change of dosage and may be indicated shortly before and after the discontinuation of anti-arrhythmic medication. The therapeutic response to a drug whose duration of action and peak of effectiveness is defined in hours cannot be properly assessed by examining 30-40 cycles on a standard EKG rhythm strip. The knowledge that all patients placed on anti-arrhythmic medication do not respond to therapy and the known toxicity of anti-arrhythmic agents clearly indicate that proper assessment should be made on an individual basis to determine whether medication should be continued and at what dosage level.

The long-term EKG is also valuable in the assessment of patients with coronary artery disease. It enables the documentation of etiology of such symptoms as chest pain and shortness of breath. Since the standard EKG is often normal during the intervals between the episodes of precordial pain, it is essential to obtain EKG information while the symptoms are occurring. The long-term EKG has enabled the correlation of chest symptoms with the objective evidence of ST-segment abnormalities. It is appropriate for patients who are recovering from an acute myocardial infarction or coronary insufficiency before and after discharge from the hospital, since it is impossible to predict which of these patients is subject to ventricular arrhythmias on the basis of the presence or absence of rhythm disturbances during the period of initial coronary care. The long-term EKG enables the physician to identify patients who are at a higher risk of dying suddenly in the period following an acute myocardial infarction. It may also be reasonable and necessary where the high-risk patient with known cardiovascular disease advances to a substantially higher level of activity which might trigger increased or new types of arrhythmias necessitating treatment. Such a high-risk case would be one in which there is documentation that acute phase arrhythmias have not totally disappeared during the period of convalescence.

In view of recent developments in cardiac pacemaker monitoring techniques (see CIA 50-1), the use of the long-term EKG for routine assessment of pacemaker function can no longer be justified. Its use for the patient with an internal pacemaker would be covered only when he has symptoms suggestive of arrhythmia not revealed by the standard EKG or rhythm strip.

These guidelines are intended as a general outline of the circumstances under which the use of this diagnostic procedure would be warranted. Each patient receiving a long-term EKG should be evaluated completely, prior to performance of this diagnostic study. A complete history and physical examination should be obtained and the indications for use of the long-term EKG should be reviewed by the referring physician.

The performance of a long-term EKG does not necessarily require the prior performance of a standard EKG. Nor does the demonstration of a normal standard EKG preclude the need for a long-term EKG. Finally, the demonstration of an abnormal standard EKG does not obviate the need for a long-term EKG if there is suspicion that the dysrhythmia is transient in nature.

A period of recording of up to 24 hours would normally be adequate to detect most transient arrhythmias and provide essential diagnostic information. The medical necessity for longer periods of monitoring must be documented.

Medical documentation for adjudicating claims for the use of the long-term EKG should be similar to other EKG services, X-ray services, and laboratory procedures. Generally, a statement of the diagnostic impression of the referring physician with an indication of the patient's relevant signs and symptoms should be sufficient for purposes of making a determination regarding the reasonableness and medical necessity for the use of this procedure. However, the intermediaries or carriers should require whatever additional documentation their medical consultants deem necessary to properly adjudicate the individual claim where the information submitted is not adequate.

It should be noted that the recording device furnished to the patient is simply one component of the diagnostic system and a separate charge for it will not be recognized under the durable medical equipment benefit.

Patient-Activated EKG Recorders, distributed under a variety of brand names, permit the patient to record an EKG upon manifestation of symptoms, or in response to a physician's order (e.g., immediately following strong exertion).Most such devices also permit the patient to simultaneously voice-record in order to describe symptoms and/or activity. In addition, some of these devices permit transtelephonic transmission of the recording to a physician's office, clinic, hospital, etc., having a decoder/recorder for review and analysis, thus eliminating the need to physically transport the tape. Some of these devices also permit a "time sampling" mode of operation. However, the "time sampling" mode is not covered—only the patient-activated mode of operation, when used for the indications described below, is covered at this time.

Services in connection with patient-activated EKG recorders are covered when used as an alternative to the long-term EKG monitoring (described above) for similar indications--detecting and characterizing symptomatic arrhythmias, regulation of anti-arrhythmic drug therapy, etc. Like long-term EKG monitoring, use of these devices is covered for evaluating patients with symptoms of obscure etiology suggestive of cardiac arrhythmia such as palpitations, chest pain, dizziness, lightheadedness, near syncope, syncope, transient ischemic episodes, dyspnea and shortness of breath.

As with long-term EKG monitors, patient-activated EKG recorders may be useful for both inpatient and outpatient diagnosis and therapy. While useful for assessing some post-coronary infarct patients in the hospital setting, these devices should not, however, be covered for outpatient monitoring of recently discharged post-infarct patients.

Computer Analyzed Electrocardiograms.—Computer interpretation of EKG's is recognized as a valid and effective technique which will improve the quality and availability of cardiology services. Reimbursement may be made for such computer service when furnished in the setting and under the circumstances required for coverage of other electrocardiographic services. Where either a laboratory's or a portable x-ray supplier's charge for EKG services includes the physician review and certification of the printout as well as the computer interpretation, the certifying physician must be identified on the HCFA-1490 before the entire charge can be considered a reimbursable charge. Where the laboratory's (or portable x-ray supplier's) reviewing physician is not identified, the carrier should conclude that no professional component is involved and make its charge determination accordingly. If the supplying laboratory (or portable x-ray supplier when supplied by such a facility) does not include professional review and certification of the hard copy, a charge by the patient's physician may be recognized for the service. In any case the charge for the physician component should be substantially less than that for physician interpretation of the conventional EKG tracing in view of markedly reduced demand on the physician's time where computer interpretation is involved.

Considering the unit cost reduction expected of this innovation, the total charge for the complete EKG service (taking of tracing and interpretation) when computer interpretation is employed should never exceed that considered reasonable for the service when physician interpretation is involved.

Transtelephonic Electrocardiographic Transmissions (Formerly Referred to as EKG Telephone Reporter Systems).—Effective for services furnished on and after March 1, 1980, coverage is extended to include the use of transtelephonic electrocardiographic (EKG) transmissions as a diagnostic service for the indications described below, when performed with equipment meeting the standards described below, subject to the limitations and conditions specified below. Coverage is further limited to the amounts payable with respect to the physician's service in interpreting the results of such transmissions, including charges for rental of the equipment. The device used by the beneficiary is part of a total diagnostic system and is not considered durable medical equipment.

1. Covered Uses.—The use of transtelephonic EKGs is covered for the following uses:

   a. To detect, characterize, and document symptomatic transient arrhythmias;
   b. To overcome problems in regulating antiarrhythmic drug dosage;
   c. To carry out early posthospital monitoring of patients discharged after myocardial infarction; (only if 24-hour coverage is provided, see 4. below).

Since cardiology is a rapidly changing field, some uses other than those specified above may be covered if, in the judgment of the contractor's medical consultants, such a use was justifiable in the particular case. The enumerated uses above represent uses for which a firm coverage determination has been made, and for which contractors may make payment without extensive claims development or review.

2. Specifications for Devices—The devices used by the patient are highly portable (usually pocket-sized) and detect and convert the normal EKG signal so that it can be transmitted via ordinary telephone apparatus to a receiving station. At the receiving end, the signal is decoded and transcribed into a conventional EKG. There are numerous devices available which transmit EKG readings in this fashion. For purposes of Medicare coverage, however, the transmitting devices must meet at least the following criteria:
   a. They must be capable of transmitting EKG Leads, I, II, or III;
   b. These lead transmissions must be sufficiently comparable to readings obtained by a conventional EKG to permit proper interpretation of abnormal cardiac rhythms.
3. Potential for Abuse - Need for Screening Guidelines.--While the use of these devices may often compare favorably with more costly alternatives, this is the case only where the information they contribute is actively utilized by a knowledgeable practitioner as part of overall medical management of the patient. Consequently, it is vital that contractors be aware of the potential

for abuse of these devices, and adopt necessary screening and physician education policies to detect and halt potentially abusive situations. For example, use of these devices to diagnose and treat suspected arrhythmias as a routine substitute for more conventional methods of diagnosis, such as a careful history, physical examination, and standard EKG and rhythm strip would not be appropriate. Moreover, contractors should require written justification for use of such devices in excess of 30 consecutive days in cases involving detection of transient arrhythmias.

Contractors may find it useful to review claims for these devices with a view toward detecting patterns of practice which may be useful in developing schedules which may be adopted for screening such claims in the future.

4. Twenty-four Hour Coverage.—No payment may be made for the use of these devices to carry out early posthospital monitoring of patients discharged after myocardial infarction unless provision is made for 24 hour coverage in the manner described below.

Twenty-four hour coverage means that there must be, at the monitoring site (or sites) an experienced EKG technician receiving calls; tape recording devices do not meet this requirement. Further, such technicians should have immediate access to a physician, and have been instructed in when and how to contact available facilities to assist the patient in case of emergencies.

Cross-reference: HCFA-Pub. 13-3, §§3101.5, 3110, 3112.3, HCFA-Pub. 14-3, §§2070, 2255, 2050.1

50-20 DIAGNOSTIC PAP SMEARS (Effective for services performed on and after May 15, 1978)

A diagnostic pap smear and related medically necessary services are covered under Medicare Part B when ordered by a physician under one of the following conditions:

- Previous cancer of the cervix, uterus, or vagina that has been or is presently being treated;
- Previous abnormal pap smear;
- Any abnormal findings of the vagina, cervix, uterus, ovaries, or adnexa;
- Any significant complaint by the patient referable to the female reproductive system; or
- Any signs or symptoms that might in the physician's judgment reasonably be related to a gynecologic disorder.

In respect to the last bullet, the contractor's medical staff must determine whether in a particular case a previous malignancy at another site is an indication for a diagnostic pap smear or whether the test must be considered a screening pap smear as described in §50-20.1.

Use the following CPT codes for indicating diagnostic pap smears:

- 88150 Cytopathology, smears, cervical or vaginal (e.g., Papanicolaou), up to three smears; screening by technician under physician supervision; or
- 88151 Cytopathology, smears, cervical or vaginal (e.g., Papanicolaou), up to three smears; requiring interpretation by physician.

50-20.1 SCREENING PAP SMEARS AND PELVIC EXAMINATIONS FOR EARLY DETECTION OF CERVICAL OR VAGINAL CANCER (For screening pap smears, effective for services performed on or after July 1, 1990. For pelvic examinations including clinical breast examination, effective for services furnished on or after January 1, 1998.)

A screening pap smear (use HCPCS code P3000 Screening Papanicolaou smear, cervical or vaginal, up to three smears; by technician under physician supervision or P3001 Screening Papanicolaou smear, cervical or vaginal, up to three smears requiring interpretation by physician). (Use HCPCS codes G0123 Screening Cytopathology, cervical or vaginal (any reporting system), collected in preservative fluid, automated thin layer preparation, screening by cytotechnologist under physician supervision or G0124 Screening Cytopathology, cervical or vaginal (any reporting system) collected in preservative fluid, automated thin layer preparation, requiring interpretation by physician) and related medically necessary services provided to a woman for the early detection of cervical cancer (including collection of the sample of cells and a physician's interpretation of the test results) and pelvic examination (including clinical breast examination) (use HCPCS code G0101 cervical or vaginal cancer screening; pelvic and clinical breast examination) are covered under Medicare Part B when ordered by a physician (or authorized practitioner) under one of the following conditions:

- She has not had such a test during the preceding 3 years or is a woman of childbearing age (§1861(nn) of the Act).
- There is evidence (on the basis of her medical history or other findings) that she is at high risk of developing cervical cancer and her physician (or authorized practitioner) recommends that she have the test performed more frequently than every 3 years.
- High risk factors for cervical and vaginal cancer are:
- Early onset of sexual activity (under 16 years of age)
- Multiple sexual partners (five or more in a lifetime)
- History of sexually transmitted disease (including HIV infection)
- Fewer than three negative or any pap smears within the previous 7 years; and
- DES (diethylstilbestrol) - exposed daughters of women who took DES during pregnancy.
- NOTE: Claims for pap smears must indicate the beneficiary's low or high risk status by including the appropriate ICD-9-CM on the line item (Item 24E of the HCFA-1500).
- V76.2, special screening for malignant neoplasms of the cervix, indicates low risk; and
- V15.89, other specified personal history presenting hazards to health, indicates high risk.

If pap smear or pelvic exam claims do not point to one of these diagnosis codes, the claim will reject in the Common Working File. Claims can contain up to four diagnosis codes, but the one pointed to on the line item must be either V76.2 or V15.89.

Definitions:
A woman as described in §1861(nn) of the Act is a woman who is of childbearing age and has had a pap smear test during any of the preceding 3 years that indicated the presence of cervical or vaginal cancer or other abnormality, or is at high risk of developing cervical or vaginal cancer.

A woman of childbearing age is one who is premenopausal and has been determined by a physician or other qualified practitioner to be of childbearing age, based upon the medical history or other findings.

"Other qualified practitioner", as defined in 42 CFR 410.56(a) includes a certified nurse midwife (as defined in §1861(gg) of the Act), or a physician assistant, nurse practitioner, or clinical nurse specialist (as defined in §1861(aa) of the Act) who is authorized under State law to perform the examination.

Screening Pelvic Examination:
Section 4102 of the Balanced Budget Act of 1997 provides for coverage of screening pelvic examinations (including a clinical breast examination) for all female beneficiaries, effective January 1, 1998, subject to certain frequency and other limitations. A screening pelvic examination (including a clinical breast examination) should include at least seven of the following 11 elements:

- Inspection and palpation of breasts for masses or lumps, tenderness, symmetry, or nipple discharge.
- Digital rectal examination including sphincter tone, presence of hemorrhoids, and rectal masses. Pelvic examination (with or without specimen collection for smears and cultures) including:
- External genitalia (for example, general appearance, hair distribution, or lesions).
- Urethral meatus (for example, size, location, lesions, or prolapse).
- Urethra (for example, masses, tenderness, or scarring).
- Bladder (for example, fullness, masses, or tenderness).
- Vagina (for example, general appearance, estrogen effect, discharge lesions, pelvic support, cystocele, or rectocele).
- Cervix (for example, general appearance, lesions, or discharge).
- Uterus (for example, size, contour, position, mobility, tenderness, consistency, descent, or support).
- Adnexa/parametria (for example, masses, tenderness, organomegaly, or nodularity).
- Anus and perineum.

This description is from *Documentation Guidelines for Evaluation and Management Services*, published in May 1997 and was developed by the Health Care Financing Administration and the American Medical Association.

50-21 MAMMOGRAMS (Effective for mammograms performed on or after May 15, 1978.)

A radiological mammogram is a covered diagnostic test under the following conditions:

- A patient has distinct signs and symptoms for which a mammogram is indicated;
- A patient has a history of breast cancer; or
- A patient is asymptomatic but, on the basis of the patient's history and other factors the physician considers significant, the physician's judgment is that a mammogram is appropriate.

Use of mammograms in routine screening of (1) asymptomatic women aged 50 and over, and (2) asymptomatic women aged 40 or over whose mothers or sisters have had the disease, is considered medically appropriate, but would not be covered for Medicare purposes.

Cross-reference: Carriers Manual, §2070, Intermediary Manual, §3101.5.

50-24 HAIR ANALYSIS—NOT COVERED

Hair analysis to detect mineral traces as an aid in diagnosing human disease is not a covered service under Medicare.

The correlation of hair analysis to the chemical state of the whole body is not possible at this time, and therefore this diagnostic procedure cannot be considered to be reasonable and necessary under §1862(a)(1) of the law.

50-26 DENTAL EXAMINATION PRIOR TO KIDNEY TRANSPLANTATION

Despite the "dental services exclusion" in §1862(a)(12) of the Act (see Intermediary Manual,§3162; Carriers Manual, §2336), an oral or dental examination performed on an inpatient basis as part of a comprehensive workup prior to renal transplant surgery is a covered service. This is because the purpose of the examination is not for the care of the teeth or structures directly supporting the teeth. Rather, the examination is for the identification, prior to a complex surgical procedure, of existing medical problems where the increased possibility of infection would not only reduce the chances for successful surgery but would also expose the patient to additional risks in undergoing such surgery.

Such a dental or oral examination would be covered under Part A of the program if performed by a dentist on the hospital's staff, or under Part B if performed by a physician. (When performing a dental or oral examination, a dentist is not recognized as a physician under §1861(r) of the law.)(See Carriers Manual §2020.3.)

50-34 OBSOLETE OR UNRELIABLE DIAGNOSTIC TESTS

A. Diagnostic Tests (Effective for services performed on or after May 15, 1980).—Do not routinely pay for the following diagnostic tests because they are obsolete and have been replaced by more advanced procedures. The listed tests may be paid for only if the medical need for the procedure is satisfactorily justified by the physician who performs it. When the services are subject to PRO review, the PRO is responsible for determining that satisfactory medical justification exists. When the services are not subject to PRO review, the intermediary or carrier is responsible for determining that satisfactory medical justification exists. This includes:

- Amylase, blood isoenzymes, electrophoretic,
- Chromium, blood,
- Guanase, blood,
- Zinc sulphate turbidity, blood,
- Skin test, cat scratch fever,
- Skin test, lymphopathia venereum,
- Circulation time, one test,
- Cephalin flocculation,
- Congo red, blood,
- Hormones, adrenocorticotropin quantitative animal tests,
- Hormones, adrenocorticotropin quantitative bioassay,
- Thymol turbidity, blood,
- Skin test, actinomycosis,
- Skin test, brucellosis,
- Skin test, psittacosis,
- Skin test, trichinosis,

- Calcium, feces, 24-hour quantitative,
- Starch, feces, screening,
- Chymotrypsin, duodenal contents,
- Gastric analysis, pepsin,
- Gastric analysis, tubeless,
- Calcium saturation clotting time,
- Capillary fragility test (Rumpel-Leede),
- Colloidal gold,
- Bendien's test for cancer and tuberculosis,
- Bolen's test for cancer,
- Rehfuss test for gastric acidity, and
- Serum seromucoid assay for cancer and other diseases.

B. Cardiovascular Tests (Effective for services performed on or after January 1, 1997).--Do not pay for the following phonocardiography and vectorcardiography diagnostic tests because they have been determined to be outmoded and of little clinical value. They include:

- CPT code 93201, Phonocardiogram with or without ECG lead; with supervision during recording with interpretation and report (when equipment is supplied by the physician),

50-36 POSITRON EMISSION TOMOGRAPHY (PET) SCANS

I. General Description
Positron emission tomography (PET) is a noninvasive diagnostic imaging procedure that assesses the level of metabolic activity and perfusion in various organ systems of the [human] body. A positron camera (tomograph) is used to produce cross-sectional tomographic images, which are obtained from positron emitting radioactive tracer substances (radiopharmaceuticals) such as 2-[F-18] Fluoro-D-Glucose (FDG), that are administered intravenously to the patient.

The following indications may be covered for PET under certain circumstances. Details of Medicare PET coverage are discussed later in this section. Unless otherwise indicated, the clinical conditions below are covered when PET utilizes FDG as a tracer.

NOTE: This manual section lists all Medicare-covered uses of PET scans. A particular use of PET scans is not covered unless this manual specifically provides that such use is covered. Although this section lists some non-covered uses of PET scans, it does not constitute an exhaustive list of all non-covered uses.

Clinical Condition	Effective Date	Coverage
Solitary Pulmonary Nodules (SPNs)	January 1, 1998	Characterization
Lung Cancer (Non Small Cell)	January 1, 1998	Initial staging
Lung Cancer (Non Small Cell)	July 1, 2001	Diagnosis, staging and restaging
Esophageal Cancer	July 1, 2001	Diagnosis, staging and restaging
Colorectal Cancer	July 1, 1999	Determining location of tumors if rising CEA level suggests recurrence
Colorectal Cancer	July 1, 2001	Diagnosis, staging and restaging

Lymphoma	July 1, 1999	Staging and restaging only when used as an alternative to Gallium scan
Lymphoma	July 1, 2001	Diagnosis, staging and restaging
Melanoma	July 1, 1999	Evaluating recurrence prior to surgery as an alternative to a Gallium scan
Melanoma	July 1, 2001	Diagnosis, staging and restaging; Noncovered for evaluating regional nodes
Breast Cancer	October 1, 2002	As an adjunct to standard imaging modalities for staging patients with distant metastasis or restaging patients with locoregional recurrence or metastasis; as an adjunct to standard imaging modalities for monitoring tumor response to treatment for women with locally advanced and metastatic breast cancer when a change in therapy is anticipated
Head and Neck Cancers (excluding CNS and thyroid	July 1, 2001	Diagnosis, staging and restaging
Thyroid Cancer	October 1, 2003	Restaging of recurrent or residual thyroid cancers of follicular cell origin that have been previously treated by thyroidectomy and radioiodine ablation and have a serum thyroglobulin >10ng/ml and negative I-131 whole body scan performed
Myocardial Viability	July 1, 2001 toSeptember 30, 2002	Covered only following inconclusive SPECT
Myocardial Viability	October 1, 2002	Primary or initial diagnosis, or following an inconclusive SPECT prior to revascularization. SPECT may not be used following an inconclusive PET scan

Refractory Seizures	July 1, 2001	Covered for pre-surgical evaluation only
Perfusion of the heart using Rubidium 82* tracer	March 14, 1995	Covered for noninvasive imaging of the perfusion of the heart
Perfusion of the heart using ammonia N-13* tracer	October 1, 2003	Covered for noninvasive imaging of the perfusion of the heart

*Not FDG-PET.

II. General Conditions of Coverage for FDG PET
   A. Allowable FDG PET Systems
      1. Definitions: For purposes of this section:
         a. "Any FDA approved" means all systems approved or cleared for marketing by the FDA to image radionuclides in the body.
         b. "FDA approved" means that the system indicated has been approved or cleared for marketing by the FDA to image radionuclides in the body.
         c. "Certain coincidence systems" refers to the systems that have all the following features:

- Crystal at least 5/8-inch thick;
- Techniques to minimize or correct for scatter and/or randoms; and
- Digital detectors and iterative reconstruction.

Scans performed with gamma camera PET systems with crystals thinner than 5/8-inch will not be covered by Medicare. In addition, scans performed with systems with crystals greater than or equal to 5/8-inch in thickness, but that do not meet the other listed design characteristics are not covered by Medicare.

      2. Allowable PET systems by covered clinical indication:

Allowable Type of FDG PET System

Covered Clinical Condition	Before 7/1/2001	7/1/ 2001 -12/31/2001	On or after 1/1/2002
Characterization of single pulmonary nodules	Effective 1/1/1998, any FDA approved	Any FDA approved	FDA approved: Full ring Partial ring Certain coincidence systems
Initial staging of lung cancer (non small cell)	Effective 1/1/1998, any FDA approved	Any FDA approved	FDA approved: Full ring Partial ring Certain coincidence systems
Determining location of colorectal tumors if rising CEA level suggests recurrence	Effective 7/1/1999, any FDA approved	Any FDA approved	FDA approved: Full ring Partial ring Certain coincidence systems

Staging or restaging of lymphoma only when used as an alternative to a gallium scan	Effective 7/1/1999, any FDA approved	Any FDA approved	FDA approved: Full ring Partial ring Certain coincidence systems
Evaluating recurrence of melanoma prior to surgery as an alternative to a gallium scan	Effective 7/1/1999, any FDA approved.	Any FDA approved	FDA approved: Full ring Partial ring Certain coincidence systems
Diagnosis, staging, and restaging of colorectal cancer	Not covered by Medicare	Full ring	FDA approved: Full ring Partial ring
Diagnosis, staging, and restaging of esophageal cancer	Not covered by Medicare	Full ring	FDA approved: Full ring Partial ring
Diagnosis, staging, and restaging of head and neck cancers (excluding CNS and thyroid)	Not covered by Medicare	Full ring	FDA approved: Full ring Partial ring

Diagnosis, staging, and restaging of lung cancer (non small cell)	Not covered by Medicare	Full ring	FDA approved: Full ring Partial ring
Diagnosis, staging, and restaging of lymphoma	Not covered by Medicare	Full ring	FDA approved: Full ring Partial ring
Diagnosis, staging, and restaging of melanoma (noncovered for evaluating regional nodes)	Not covered by Medicare	Full ring	FDA approved: Full ring Partial ring

Determination of myocardial viability only following an inconclusive SPECT	Not covered by Medicare	Full ring	FDA approved: Full ring Partial ring
Presurgical evaluation of refractory seizures	Not covered by Medicare	Full ring	FDA approved: Full ring
Breast Cancer	Not covered	Not covered	Effective October 1, 2002, full and partial ring

Thyroid Cancer	Not covered	Not covered	Effective October 1, 2003, full and partial ring
Myocardial Viability Primary or initial diagnosis prior to revascularization	Not covered	Not covered	Effective October 1, 2002, full and partial ring

B. Regardless of any other terms or conditions, all uses of FDG PET scans, in order to be covered by the Medicare program, must meet the following general conditions prior to June 30, 2001:

1. Submission of claims for payment must include any information Medicare requires to assure that the PET scans performed were: (a) medically necessary, (b) did not unnecessarily duplicate other covered diagnostic tests, and (c) did not involve investigational drugs or procedures using investigational drugs, as determined by the Food and Drug Administration (FDA).
2. The PET scan entity submitting claims for payment must keep such patient records as Medicare requires on file for each patient for whom a PET scan claim is made.

C. Regardless of any other terms or conditions, all uses of FDG PET scans, in order to be covered by the Medicare program, must meet the following general conditions as of July 1, 2001:

1. The provider of the PET scan should maintain on file the doctor's referral and documentation that the procedure involved only FDA approved drugs and devices, as is normal business practice.
2. The ordering physician is responsible for documenting the medical necessity of the study and that it meets the conditions specified in the instructions. The physician should have documentation in the beneficiary's medical record to support the referral to the PET scan provider.

IV. Covered Indications for PET Scans and Limitations/Requirements for Usage

For all uses of PET relating to malignancies the following conditions apply:

1. Diagnosis: PET is covered only in clinical situations in which the PET results may assist in avoiding an invasive diagnostic procedure, or in which the PET results may assist in determining the optimal anatomical location to perform an invasive diagnostic procedure. In general, for most solid tumors, a tissue diagnosis is made prior to the performance of PET scanning. PET scans following a tissue diagnosis are performed for the purpose of staging, not diagnosis. Therefore, the use of PET in the diagnosis of lymphoma, esophageal, and colorectal cancers as well as in melanoma should be rare.

    PET is not covered for other diagnostic uses, and is not covered for screening (testing of patients without specific signs and symptoms of disease).

2. Staging and or Restaging: PET is covered in clinical situations in which 1) (a) the stage of the cancer remains in doubt after completion of a standard diagnostic workup, including conventional imaging (computed tomography, magnetic resonance imaging, or ultrasound) or (b) the use of PET would also be considered reasonable and necessary if it could potentially replace one or more conventional imaging studies when it is expected that conventional study information is insufficient for the clinical management of the patient and 2) clinical management of the patient would differ depending on the stage of the cancer identified. PET will be covered for restaging after the completion of treatment for the purpose of detecting residual disease, for detecting suspected recurrence or to determine the extent of a known recurrence. Use of PET would also be considered reasonable and necessary if it could potentially replace one or more conventional imaging studies when it is expected that conventional study information is insufficient for the clinical management of the patient.

3. Monitoring: Use of PET to monitor tumor response during the planned course of therapy (i.e., when no change in therapy is being contemplated) is not covered except for breast cancer. Restaging only occurs after a course of treatment is completed, and this is covered, subject to the conditions above.

NOTE: In the absence of national frequency limitations, contractors, should, if necessary, develop frequency requirements on any or all of the indications covered on and after July 1, 2001.

IV. Coverage of PET for Perfusion of the Heart

A. Rubidium 82
Effective for services performed on or after March 14, 1995, PET scans performed at rest or with pharmacological stress used for noninvasive imaging of the perfusion of the heart for the diagnosis and management of patients with known or suspected coronary artery disease using the FDA-approved radiopharmaceutical Rubidium 82 (Rb 82) are covered, provided the requirements below are met.

Requirements:

- The PET scan, whether at rest alone, or rest with stress, is performed in place of, but not in addition to, a single photon emission computed tomography (SPECT); or
- The PET scan, whether at rest alone or rest with stress, is used following a SPECT that was found to be inconclusive. In these cases, the PET scan must have been considered necessary in order to determine what medical or surgical intervention is required to treat the patient. (For purposes of this requirement, an inconclusive test is a test(s) whose results are equivocal, technically uninterpretable, or discordant with a patient's other clinical data and must be documented in the beneficiary's file.)
- For any PET scan for which Medicare payment is claimed for dates of services prior to July 1, 2001, the claimant must submit additional specified information on the claim form (including proper codes and/or modifiers), to indicate the results of the PET scan. The claimant must also include information on whether the PET scan was done after an inconclusive noninvasive cardiac test. The information submitted with respect to the previous noninvasive cardiac test must specify the type of test done prior to the PET scan and whether it was inconclusive or unsatisfactory. These explanations are in the form of special G codes used for billing PET scans using Rb 82. Beginning July 1, 2001, claims should be submitted with the appropriate codes.

B. Ammonia N-13
Effective for services performed on or after October 1, 2003, PET scans performed at rest or with pharmacological stress used for noninvasive imaging of the perfusion of the heart for the diagnosis and management of patients with known or suspected coronary artery disease using the FDA-approved radiopharmaceutical ammonia N-13 are covered, provided the requirements below are met.

Requirements:

- The PET scan, whether at rest alone, or rest with stress, is performed in place of, but not in addition to, a single photon emission computed tomography (SPECT); or
- The PET scan, whether at rest alone or rest with stress, is used following a SPECT that was found to be inconclusive. In these cases, the PET scan must have been considered necessary in order to determine what medical or surgical intervention is required to treat the patient. (For purposes of this requirement, an inconclusive test is a test whose results are equivocal, technically uninterpretable, or discordant with a patient's other clinical data and must be documented in the beneficiary's file.)

V. Coverage of FDG PET for Lung Cancer
The coverage for FDG PET for lung cancer, effective January 1, 1998, has been expanded. Beginning July 1, 2001, usage of FDG PET for lung cancer has been expanded to include diagnosis, staging, and restaging (see section III) of the disease.

A. Effective for services performed on or after January 1, 1998, Medicare covers regional FDG PET chest scans, on any FDA approved scanner, for the characterization of single pulmonary nodules (SPNs). The primary purpose of such characterization should be to determine the likelihood of malignancy in order to plan future management and treatment for the patient.

Beginning July 1, 2001, documentation should be maintained in the beneficiary's medical file at the referring physician's office to support the medical necessity of the procedure, as is normal business practice.

Requirements:

- There must be evidence of primary tumor. Claims for regional PET chest scans for characterizing SPNs should include evidence of the initial detection of a primary lung tumor, usually by computed tomography (CT). This should include, but is not restricted to, a report on the results of such CT or other detection method, indicating an indeterminate or possibly malignant lesion, not exceeding four centimeters (cm) in diameter.
- PET scan claims must include the results of concurrent thoracic CT (as noted above), which is necessary for anatomic information, in order to ensure that the PET scan is properly coordinated with other diagnostic modalities.
- In cases of serial evaluation of SPNs using both CT and regional PET chest scanning, such PET scans will not be covered if repeated within 90 days following a negative PET scan.

NOTE: A tissue sampling procedure (TSP) is not routinely covered in the case of a negative PET scan for characterization of SPNs, since the patient is presumed not to have a malignant lesion, based upon the PET scan results. When there has been a negative PET, the provider must submit additional information with the claim to support the necessity of a TSP, for review by the Medicare contractor.

B. Effective for services performed from January 1, 1998 through June 30, 2001, Medicare approved coverage of FDG PET for initial staging of non-small-cell lung carcinoma (NSCLC).

Limitations: This service is covered only when the primary cancerous lung tumor has been pathologically confirmed; claims for PET must include a statement or other evidence of the detection of such primary lung tumor. The evidence should include, but is not restricted to, a surgical pathology report, which documents the presence of an NSCLC. Whole body PET scan results and results of concurrent computed tomography (CT) and follow-up lymph node biopsy must be properly coordinated with other diagnostic modalities. Claims must include both:

- The results of concurrent thoracic CT, necessary for anatomic information, and
- The results of any lymph node biopsy performed to finalize whether the patient will be a surgical candidate. The ordering physician is responsible for providing this biopsy result to the PET facility.

NOTE: Where the patient is considered a surgical candidate, (given the presumed absence of metastatic NSCLC unless medical review supports a determination of medical necessity of a biopsy) a lymph node biopsy will not be covered in the case of a negative CT and negative PET. A lymph node biopsy will be covered in all other cases, i.e., positive CT + positive PET; negative CT + positive PET; positive CT + negative PET.

C. Beginning July 1, 2001, Medicare covers FDG PET for diagnosis, staging, and restaging of NSCLC. Documentation should be maintained in the beneficiary's medical file to support the medical necessity of the procedure, as is normal business practice.

Requirements: PET is covered in either/or both of the following circumstances:

- Diagnosis - PET is covered only in clinical situations in which the PET results may assist in avoiding an invasive diagnostic procedure, or in which the PET results may assist in determining the optimal anatomical location to perform an invasive diagnostic procedure. In general, for most solid tumors, a tissue diagnosis is made prior to the performance of PET scanning. PET scans following a tissue diagnosis are performed for the purpose of staging, not diagnosis. Therefore, the use of PET in the diagnosis of lymphoma, esophageal, and colorectal cancers as well as in melanoma should be rare.
- Staging and/or Restaging - PET is covered in clinical situations in which 1) (a) the stage of the cancer remains in doubt after completion of a standard diagnostic workup, including conventional imaging (computed tomography, magnetic resonance imaging, or ultrasound) or (b) the use of PET would also be considered reasonable and necessary if it could potentially replace one or more conventional imaging studies when it is expected that conventional study information is insufficient for the clinical management of the patient and 2) clinical management of the patient would differ depending on the stage of the cancer identified. PET will be covered for restaging after the completion of treatment for the purpose of detecting residual disease, for detecting suspected recurrence or to determine the extent of a known recurrence. Use of PET would also be considered reasonable and necessary if it could potentially replace one or more conventional imaging studies when it is expected that conventional study information is insufficient for the clinical management of the patient.

Documentation should be maintained in the beneficiary's medical record at the referring physician's office to support the medical necessity of the procedure, as is normal business practice.

VI. Coverage of FDG PET for Esophageal Cancer

A. Beginning July 1, 2001, Medicare covers FDG PET for the diagnosis, staging, and restaging of esophageal cancer. Medical evidence is present to support the use of FDG PET in Presurgical staging of esophageal cancer.

Requirements: PET is covered in either/or both of the following circumstances:

- Diagnosis - PET is covered only in clinical situations in which the PET results may assist in avoiding an invasive diagnostic procedure, or in which the PET results may assist in determining the optimal anatomical location to perform an invasive diagnostic procedure. In general, for most solid tumors, a tissue diagnosis is made prior to the performance of PET scanning. PET scans following a tissue diagnosis are performed for the purpose of staging, not diagnosis. Therefore, the use of PET in the diagnosis of lymphoma, esophageal and colorectal cancers as well as in melanoma should be rare.
- Staging and/or Restaging - PET is covered in clinical situations in which 1)(a) the stage of the cancer remains in doubt after completion of a standard diagnostic workup, including conventional imaging (computed tomography, magnetic resonance imaging, or ultrasound) or (b) the use of PET would also be considered reasonable and necessary if it could potentially replace one or more conventional imaging studies when it is expected that conventional study information is insufficient for the clinical management of the patient, and 2) clinical management of the patient would differ depending on the stage of the cancer identified. PET will be covered for restaging after the completion of treatment for the purpose of detecting residual disease, for detecting suspected recurrence, or to determine the extent of a known recurrence. Use of PET would also be considered reasonable and necessary if it could potentially replace one or more conventional imaging studies when it is expected that conventional study information is insufficient for the clinical management of the patient.

Documentation should be maintained in the beneficiary's medical record at the referring physician's office to support the medical necessity of the procedure, as is normal business practice.

VII. Coverage of FDG PET for Colorectal Cancer

Medicare coverage of FDG PET for colorectal cancer where there is a rising level of carcinoembryonic antigen (CEA) was effective July 1, 1999 through June 30, 2001. Beginning July 1, 2001, usage of FDG PET for colorectal cancer has been expanded to include diagnosis, staging, and restaging of the disease (see part III).

A. Effective July 1, 1999, Medicare covers FDG PET for patients with recurrent colorectal carcinomas, which are suggested by rising levels of the biochemical tumor marker CEA.

1. Frequency Limitations: Whole body PET scans for assessment of recurrence of colorectal cancer cannot be ordered more frequently than once every 12 months unless medical necessity documentation supports a separate re-elevation of CEA within this period.

2. Limitations: Because this service is covered only in those cases in which there has been a recurrence of colorectal tumor, claims for PET should include a statement or other evidence of previous colorectal tumor, through June 30, 2001.

B. Beginning July 1, 2001, Medicare coverage has been expanded for colorectal carcinomas for diagnosis, staging and re-staging. New medical evidence supports the use of FDG PET as a useful tool in determining the presence of hepatic/extrahepatic metastases in the primary staging of colorectal carcinoma, prior to selecting a treatment regimen. Use of FDG PET is also supported in evaluating recurrent colorectal cancer beyond the limited presentation of a rising CEA level where the patient presents clinical signs or symptoms of recurrence.

Requirements: PET is covered in either/both of the following circumstances:
Diagnosis - PET is covered only in clinical situations in which the PET results may assist in avoiding an invasive diagnostic procedure, or in which the PET results may assist in determining the optimal anatomical location to perform an invasive diagnostic procedure. In general, for most solid tumors, a tissue diagnosis is made prior to the performance of PET scanning. PET scans following a tissue diagnosis are performed for the purpose of staging, not diagnosis. Therefore, the use of PET in the diagnosis of lymphoma, esophageal, and colorectal cancers as well as in melanoma should be rare.

- Staging and/or Restaging - PET is covered in clinical situations in which 1) (a) the stage of the cancer remains in doubt after completion of a standard diagnostic workup, including conventional imaging (computed tomography, magnetic resonance imaging, or ultrasound) or (b) the use of PET would also be considered reasonable and necessary if it could potentially replace one or more conventional imaging studies when it is expected that conventional study information is insufficient for the clinical management of the patient and 2) clinical management of the patient would differ depending on the stage of the cancer identified. PET will be covered for restaging after the completion of treatment for the purpose of detecting residual disease, for detecting suspected recurrence, or to determine the extent of a known recurrence. Use of PET would also be considered reasonable and necessary if it could potentially replace one or more conventional imaging studies when it is expected that conventional study information is insufficient for the clinical management of the patient.

Documentation that these conditions are met should be maintained by the referring physician in the beneficiary's medical record, as is normal business practice.

VIII. Coverage of FDG PET for Lymphoma

Medicare coverage of FDG PET to stage and re-stage lymphoma as alternative to a Gallium scan, was effective July 1, 1999. Beginning July 1, 2001, usage of FDG PET for lymphoma has been expanded to include diagnosis, staging and restaging (see section III) of the disease.

A. Effective July 1, 1999, FDG PET is covered for the staging and restaging of lymphoma.

Requirements:

- PET is covered only for staging or follow-up restaging of lymphoma. Claims must include a statement or other evidence of previous diagnosis of lymphoma when used as an alternative to a Gallium scan
- To ensure that the PET scan is properly coordinated with other diagnostic modalities, claims must include the results of concurrent computed tomography (CT) and/or other diagnostic modalities when they are necessary for additional anatomic information.
- In order to ensure that the PET scan is covered only as an alternative to a Gallium scan, no PET scan may be covered in cases where it is done within 50 days of a Gallium scan done by the same facility where the patient has remained during the 50-day period. Gallium scans done by another facility less than 50 days prior to the PET scan will not be counted against this screen. The purpose of this screen is to assure that PET scans are covered only when done as an alternative to a Gallium scan within the same facility. We are aware that, in order to assure proper patient care, the treating physician may conclude that previously performed Gallium scans are either inconclusive or not sufficiently reliable.

Frequency Limitation for Restaging: PET scans will be allowed for restaging no sooner than 50 days following the last staging PET scan or Gallium scan, unless sufficient evidence is presented to convince the Medicare contractor that the restaging at an earlier date is medically necessary. Since PET scans for restaging are generally done following cycles of chemotherapy, and since such cycles usually take at least 8 weeks, we believe this screen will adequately prevent medically unnecessary scans while allowing some adjustments for unusual cases. In all cases, the determination of the medical necessity for a PET scan for re-staging lymphoma is the responsibility of the local Medicare contractor.

Beginning July 1, 2001, documentation should be maintained in the beneficiary's medical record at the referring physician's office to support the medical necessity of the procedure, as is normal business practice.

B. Effective for services performed on or after July 1, 2001, the Medicare program has broadened coverage of FDG PET for the diagnosis, staging and restaging of lymphoma.

Requirements: PET is covered in either/both of the following circumstances:

- Diagnosis - PET is covered only in clinical situations in which the PET results may assist in avoiding an invasive diagnostic procedure, or in which the PET results may assist in determining the optimal anatomical location to perform an invasive diagnostic procedure. In general, for most solid tumors, a tissue diagnosis is made prior to the performance of PET scanning. PET scans following a tissue diagnosis are performed for the purpose of staging, not diagnosis. Therefore, the use of PET in the diagnosis of lymphoma, esophageal, and colorectal cancers as well as in melanoma should be rare.

- Staging and/or Restaging - PET is covered in clinical situations in which 1) (a) the stage of the cancer remains in doubt after completion of a standard diagnostic workup, including conventional imaging (computed tomography, magnetic resonance imaging, or ultrasound) or (b) the use of PET would also be considered reasonable and necessary if it could potentially replace one or more conventional imaging studies when it is expected that conventional study information is insufficient for the clinical management of the patient, and 2) clinical management of the patient would differ depending on the stage of the cancer identified. PET will be covered for restaging after the completion of treatment for the purpose of detecting residual disease, for detecting suspected recurrence, or to determine the extent of a known recurrence. Use of PET would also be considered reasonable and necessary if it could potentially replace one or more conventional imaging studies when it is expected that conventional study information is insufficient for the clinical management of the patient.

Documentation that these conditions are met should be maintained by the referring physician in the beneficiary's medical record, as is normal business practice.

IX. Coverage of FDG PET for Melanoma

Medicare covered the evaluation of recurrent melanoma prior to surgery when used as an alternative to a Gallium scan, effective July 1, 1999. For services furnished on or after July 1, 2001 FDG PET is covered for the diagnosis, staging, and restaging of malignant melanoma (see part III). FDG PET is not covered for the use of evaluating regional nodes in melanoma patients.

A. Effective for services furnished July 1, 1999 through June 30, 2001, in the case of patients with recurrent melanoma prior to surgery, FDG PET (when used as an alternative to a Gallium scan) is covered for tumor evaluation.

Frequency Limitations: Whole body PET scans cannot be ordered more frequently than once every 12 months, unless medical necessity documentation, maintained in the beneficiaries medical record, supports the specific need for anatomic localization of possible recurrent tumor within this period.

Limitations: The FDG PET scan is covered only as an alternative to a Gallium scan. PET scans can not be covered in cases where it is done within 50 days of a Gallium scan done by the same PET facility where the patient has remained under the care of the same facility during the 50-day period. Gallium scans done by another facility less than 50 days prior to the PET scan will not be counted against this screen. The purpose of this screen is to assure that PET scans are covered only when done as an alternative to a Gallium scan within the same facility. We are aware that, in order to assure proper patient care, the treating physician may conclude that previously performed Gallium scans are either inconclusive or not sufficiently reliable to make the determination covered by this provision. Therefore, we will apply this 50-day rule only to PET scans done by the same facility that performed the Gallium scan.

Beginning July 1, 2001, documentation should be maintained in the beneficiary's medical file at the referring physician's office to support the medical necessity of the procedure, as is normal business practice.

B. Effective for services performed on or after July 1, 2001 FDG PET scan coverage for the diagnosis, staging and restaging of melanoma (not the evaluation regional nodes) has been broadened.

Limitations: PET scans are not covered for the evaluation of regional nodes.

Requirements: PET is covered in either/both of the following circumstances:

Diagnosis - PET is covered only in clinical situations in which the PET results may assist in avoiding an invasive diagnostic procedure, or in which the PET results may assist in determining the optimal anatomical location to perform an invasive diagnostic procedure. In general, for most solid tumors, a tissue diagnosis is made prior to the performance of PET scanning. PET scans following a tissue diagnosis are performed for the purpose of staging, not diagnosis. Therefore, the use of PET in the diagnosis of lymphoma, esophageal, and colorectal cancers as well as in melanoma should be rare.

- Staging and/or Restaging - PET is covered in clinical situations in which 1) (a) the stage of the cancer remains in doubt after completion of a standard diagnostic workup, including conventional imaging (computed tomography, magnetic resonance imaging, or ultrasound) or (b) the use of PET would also be considered reasonable and necessary if it could potentially replace one or more conventional imaging studies when it is expected that conventional study information is insufficient for the clinical management of the patient, and

2) clinical management of the patient would differ depending on the stage of the cancer identified. PET will be covered for restaging after the completion of treatment for the purpose of detecting residual disease, for detecting suspected recurrence, or to determine the extent of a known recurrence. Use of PET would also be considered reasonable and necessary if it could potentially replace one or more conventional imaging studies when it is expected that conventional study information is insufficient for the clinical management of the patient.

Documentation that these conditions are met should be maintained by the referring physician in the beneficiary's medical file, as is normal business practice.

X. Coverage of FDG PET for Head and Neck Cancers

Effective for services performed on or after July 1, 2001, Medicare will provide coverage for cancer of the head and neck, excluding the central nervous system (CNS) and thyroid. The head and neck cancers encompass a diverse set of malignancies of which the majority is squamous cell carcinomas. Patients may present with metastases to cervical lymph nodes but conventional forms of diagnostic imaging fail to identify the primary tumor. Patients that present with cancer of the head and neck are left with two options either to have a neck dissection or to have radiation of both sides of the neck with random biopsies. PET scanning attempts to reveal the site of primary tumor to prevent the adverse effects of random biopsies or unneeded radiation.

Limitations: PET scans for head and neck cancers are not covered for CNS or thyroid cancers (prior to October 1, 2003). Refer to section XIV for coverage for thyroid cancer effective October 1, 2003.

Requirements: PET is covered in either/or both of the following circumstances:

- Diagnosis - PET is covered only in clinical situations in which the PET results may assist in avoiding an invasive diagnostic procedure, or in which the PET results may assist in determining the optimal anatomical location to perform an invasive diagnostic procedure. In general, for most solid tumors, a tissue diagnosis is made prior to the performance of PET scanning. PET scans following a tissue diagnosis are performed for the purpose of staging, not diagnosis. Therefore, the use of PET in the diagnosis of lymphoma, esophageal, and colorectal cancers as well as in melanoma should be rare.
- Staging and/or Restaging - PET is covered in clinical situations in which 1) (a) the stage of the cancer remains in doubt after completion of a standard diagnostic workup, including conventional imaging (computed tomography, magnetic resonance imaging, or ultrasound) or (b) the use of PET would also be considered reasonable and necessary if it could potentially replace one or more conventional imaging studies when it is expected that conventional study information is insufficient for the clinical management of the patient, and 2) clinical management of the patient would differ depending on the stage of the cancer identified. PET will be covered for restaging after the completion of treatment for the purpose of detecting residual disease, for detecting suspected recurrence, or to determine the extent of a known recurrence. Use of PET would also be considered reasonable and necessary if it could potentially replace one or more conventional imaging studies when it is expected that conventional study information is insufficient for the clinical management of the patient.

Documentation that these conditions are met should be maintained by the referring physician in the beneficiary's medical record, as is normal business practice.

XI. Coverage of FDG PET for Myocardial Viability

The identification of patients with partial loss of heart muscle movement or hibernating myocardium is important in selecting candidates with compromised ventricular function to determine appropriateness for revascularization. Diagnostic tests such as FDG PET distinguish between dysfunctional but viable myocardial tissue and scar tissue in order to affect management decisions in patients with ischemic cardiomyopathy and left ventricular dysfunction.

FDG PET is covered for the determination of myocardial viability following an inconclusive SPECT from July 1, 2001 through September 30, 2002. Only full ring PET scanners are covered from July 1, 2001 through December 31, 2001. However, as of January 1, 2002, full and partial ring scanners are covered.

Beginning October 1, 2002, Medicare covers FDG PET for the determination of myocardial viability as a primary or initial diagnostic study prior to revascularization, or following an inconclusive SPECT. Studies performed by full and partial ring scanners are covered.

Limitations: In the event that a patient has received a single photon computed tomography test (SPECT) with inconclusive results, a PET scan may be covered. However, if a patient received a FDG PET study with inconclusive results, a follow up SPECT is not covered.

Documentation that these conditions are met should be maintained by the referring physician in the beneficiary's medical record, as is normal business practice.

(See §50-58 of the CIM for SPECT coverage.)

XII. Coverage of FDG PET for Refractory Seizures

Beginning July 1, 2001, Medicare will cover FDG-PET for pre-surgical evaluation for the purpose of localization of a focus of refractory seizure activity.

Limitations: Covered only for pre-surgical evaluation.

Documentation that these conditions are met should be maintained by the referring physician in the beneficiary's medical record, as is normal business practice.

XIII. Breast Cancer

Beginning October 1, 2002, Medicare covers FDG PET as an adjunct to other imaging modalities for staging patients with distant metastasis, or restaging patients with locoregional recurrence or metastasis. Monitoring treatment of a breast cancer tumor when a change in therapy is contemplated is also covered as an adjunct to other imaging modalities.

Limitations: Effective October 1, 2002, Medicare continues to have a national non-coverage determination for initial diagnosis of breast cancer and staging of axillary lymph nodes. Medicare coverage for staging patients with distant metastasis or restaging patients with locoregional recurrence or metastasis; and for monitoring tumor response to treatment for women with locally advanced and metastatic breast cancer when a change in therapy is anticipated, is only covered as an adjunct to other imaging modalities.

Documentation that these conditions are met should be maintained by the referring physician in the beneficiary's medical record, as is normal business practice.

XIV. Thyroid Cancer

1. Effective for services furnished on or after October 1, 2003, Medicare covers the use of FDG PET for thyroid cancer only for restaging of recurrent or residual thyroid cancers of follicular cell origin that have been previously treated by thyroidectomy and radioiodine ablation and have a serum thyroglobulin >10ng/ml and negative I-131 whole body scan performed.

2. All other uses of FDG PET in the diagnosis and treatment of thyroid cancer remain noncovered.

XV. Soft Tissue Sarcoma - NOT COVERED

Following a thorough review of the scientific literature, including a technology assessment on the topic, Medicare maintains its national noncoverage determination for all uses of FDG PET for soft tissue sarcoma.

XVI. Dementia and Neurogenerative Diseases - NOT COVERED

Following a thorough review of the scientific literature, including a technology assessment on the topic and consideration by the Medicare Coverage Advisory Committee, Medicare maintains its national noncoverage determination for all uses of FDG-PET for the diagnosis and management of dementia or other neurogenerative diseases

50-42 AMBULATORY BLOOD PRESSURE MONITORING

Ambulatory blood pressure monitoring (ABPM) involves the use of a non-invasive device which is used to measure blood pressure in 24-hour cycles. These 24-hour measurements are stored in the device and are later interpreted by the physician. ABPM must be performed for at least 24 hours to meet coverage criteria.

ABPM is only covered for those patients with suspected white coat hypertension. Suspected white coat hypertension is defined as 1) office blood pressure >140/90 mm Hg on at least three separate clinic/office visits with two separate measurements made at each visit; 2) at least two documented blood pressure measurements taken outside the office which are <140/90 mm Hg; and 3) no evidence of end-organ damage. The information obtained by ABPM is necessary in order to determine the appropriate management of the patient. ABPM is not covered for any other uses. In the rare circumstance that ABPM needs to be performed more than once in a patient, the qualifying criteria described above must be met for each subsequent ABPM test.

For those patients that undergo ABPM and have an ambulatory blood pressure of <135/85 with no evidence of end-organ damage, it is likely that their cardiovascular risk is similar to that of normotensives. They should be followed over time. Patients for which ABPM demonstrates a blood pressure of >135/85 may be at increased cardiovascular risk, and a physician may wish to consider antihypertensive therapy.

50-44 BONE (MINERAL) DENSITY STUDIES—Effective for services rendered on or after March 4, 1983.

Bone (mineral) density studies are used to evaluate diseases of bone and/or the responses of bone diseases to treatment. The studies assess bone mass or density associated with such diseases as osteoporosis, osteomalacia, and renal osteodystrophy. Various single or combined methods of measurement may be required to: (a) diagnose bone disease, (b) monitor the course of bone changes with disease progression, or (c) monitor the course of bone changes with therapy. Bone density is usually studied by using photodensitometry, single or dual photon absorptiometry, or bone biopsy.

The following bone (mineral) density studies are covered under medicare:

A. Single Photon Absorptiometry.—A non-invasive radiological technique that measures absorption of a monochromatic photon beam by bone material. The device is placed directly on the patient, uses a low dose of radionuclide, and measures the mass absorption efficiency of the energy used. It provides a quantitative measurement of the bone mineral of cortical and trabecular bone, and is used in assessing an individual's treatment response at appropriate intervals.

Single photon absorptiometry is covered under Medicare when used in assessing changes in bone density of patients with osteodystrophy or osteoporosis when performed on the same individual at intervals of 6 to 12 months.

B. Bone Biopsy.—A physiologic test which is a surgical, invasive procedure. A small sample of bone (usually from the ilium) is removed, generally by a biopsy needle. The biopsy sample is then examined histologically, and provides a qualitative measurement of the bone mineral of trabecular bone. This procedure is used in ascertaining a differential diagnosis of bone disorders and is used primarily to differentiate osteomalacia from osteoporosis.

Bone biopsy is covered under Medicare when used for the qualitative evaluation of bone no more than four times per patient, unless there is special justification given. When used more than four times on a patient, bone biopsy leaves a defect in the pelvis and may produce some patient discomfort.

C. Photodensitometry.—(radiographic absorptiometry).—A noninvasive radiological procedure that attempts to assess bone mass by measuring the optical density of extremity radiographs with a photodensitometer, usually with a reference to a standard density wedge placed on the film at the time of exposure. This procedure provides a quantitative measurement of the bone mineral of cortical bone, and is used for monitoring gross bone change.

The following bone (mineral) density study is not covered under medicare:

Dual Photon Absorptiometry.—A noninvasive radiological technique that measures absorption of a dichromatic beam by bone material. This procedure is not covered under Medicare because it is still considered to be in the investigational stage.

Displacement cardiography, including cardiokymography and photokymography, is a noninvasive diagnostic test used in evaluating coronary artery disease.

A. Cardiokymography.—(Effective For Services Rendered On Or After October 12, 1988).

Cardiokymography is a covered service only when it is used as an adjunct to electrocardiographic stress testing in evaluating coronary artery disease and only when the following clinical indications are present:

- For male patients, atypical angina pectoris or nonischemic chest pain; or
- For female patients, angina, either typical or atypical.

B. Photokymography.—NOT COVERED

Photokymography remains excluded from coverage.

50-50   DISPLACEMENT CARDIOGRAPHY

Displacement cardiography, including cardiokymography and photokymography, is a noninvasive diagnostic test used in evaluating coronary artery disease.

A. Cardiokymography.—(Effective For Services Rendered On Or After October 12, 1988).

Cardiokymography is a covered service only when it is used as an adjunct to electrocardiographic stress testing in evaluating coronary artery disease and only when the following clinical indications are present:

- For male patients, atypical angina pectoris or nonischemic chest pain; or
- For female patients, angina, either typical or atypical.

B. Photokymography.—NOT COVERED

Photokymography remains excluded from coverage.

50-55 PROSTATE CANCER SCREENING TESTS—COVERED (Effective for services furnished on or after January 1, 2000)

A. General.—Section 4103 of the Balanced Budget Act of 1997 provides for coverage of certain prostate cancer screening tests subject to certain coverage, frequency, and payment limitations. Effective for services furnished on or after January 1, 2000. Medicare will cover prostate cancer screening tests/procedures for the early detection of prostate cancer. Coverage of prostate cancer screening tests includes the following procedures furnished to an individual for the early detection of prostate cancer:

- Screening digital rectal examination; and
- Screening prostate specific antigen blood test.

B. Screening Digital Rectal Examinations. Screening digital rectal examinations (HCPCS code G0102) are covered at a frequency of once every 12 months for men who have attained age 50 (at least 11 months have passed following the month in which the last Medicare-covered screening digital rectal examination was performed). Screening digital rectal examination means a clinical examination of an individual's prostate for nodules or other abnormalities of the prostate. This screening must be performed by a doctor of medicine or osteopathy (as defined in §1861(r)(1) of the Act), or by a physician assistant, nurse practitioner, clinical nurse specialist, or certified nurse midwife (as defined in §1861(aa) and §1861(gg) of the Act) who is authorized under State law to perform the examination, fully knowledgeable about the beneficiary's medical condition, and would be responsible for using the results of any examination performed in the overall management of the beneficiary's specific medical problem.

C. Screening Prostate Specific Antigen Tests. Screening prostate specific antigen tests (code G0103) are covered at a frequency of once every 12 months for men who have attained age 50 (at least 11 months have passed following the month in which the last Medicare-covered screening prostate specific antigen test was performed). Screening prostate specific antigen tests (PSA) means a test to detect the marker for adenocarcinoma of prostate. PSA is a reliable immunocytochemical marker for primary and metastatic adenocarcinoma of prostate. This screening must be ordered by the beneficiary's physician or by the beneficiary's physician assistant, nurse practitioner, clinical nurse specialist, or certified nurse midwife (the term "attending physician" is defined in §1861(r)(1) of the Act to mean a doctor of medicine or osteopathy and the terms "physician assistant, nurse practitioner, clinical nurse specialist, or certified nurse midwife" are defined in §1861(aa) and §1861(gg) of the Act) who is fully knowledgeable about the beneficiary's medical condition, and who would be responsible for using the results of any examination (test) performed in the overall management of the beneficiary's specific medical problem.

50-57.1 CURRENT PERCEPTION THRESHOLD/SENSORY NERVE CONDUCTION THRESHOLD TEST (sNCT) NONCOVERED

The Current Perception Threshold/Sensory Nerve Conduction Threshold (sNCT) test is a diagnostic test used to diagnose sensory neuropathies. The device is a noninvasive test that uses transcutaneous electrical stimuli to evoke a sensation. There is insufficient scientific or clinical evidence to consider this device reasonable and necessary within the meaning of Section 1862(a)(1)(A) of the law and will not be covered by Medicare.

55-1 WATER PURIFICATION AND SOFTENING SYSTEMS USED IN CONJUNCTION WITH HOME DIALYSIS

A. Water Purification Systems.—Water used for home dialysis should be chemically free of heavy trace metals and/or organic contaminants which could be hazardous to the patient. It should also be as free of bacteria as possible but need not be biologically sterile. Since the characteristics of natural water supplies in most areas of the country are such that some type of water purification system is needed, such a system used in conjunction with a home dialysis (either peritoneal or hemodialysis) unit is covered under Medicare.

There are two types of water purification systems which will satisfy these requirements:

- Deionization—The removal of organic substances, mineral salts of magnesium and calcium (causing hardness), compounds of fluoride and chloride from tap water using the process of filtration and ion exchange; or
- Reverse Osmosis—The process used to remove impurities from tap water utilizing pressure to force water through a porous membrane.

Use of both a deionization unit and reverse osmosis unit in series, theoretically to provide the advantages of both systems, has been determined medically unnecessary since either system can provide water which is both chemically and bacteriologically pure enough for acceptable use in home dialysis. In addition, spare deionization tanks are not covered since they are essentially a precautionary supply rather than a current requirement for treatment of the patient.

Activated carbon filters used as a component of water purification systems to remove unsafe concentrations of chlorine and chloramines are covered when prescribed by a physician.

B. Water Softening System.—Except as indicated below, a water softening system used in conjunction with home dialysis is excluded from coverage under Medicare as not being reasonable and necessary within the meaning of §1862(a)(1) of the law. Such a system, in conjunction with a home dialysis unit, does not adequately remove the hazardous heavy metal contaminants (such as arsenic) which may be present in trace amounts.

A water softening system may be covered when used to pretreat water to be purified by a reverse osmosis (RO) unit for home dialysis where:

- The manufacturer of the RO unit has set standards for the quality of water entering the RO (e.g., the water to be purified by the RO must be of a certain quality if the unit is to perform as intended);
- The patient's water is demonstrated to be of a lesser quality than required; and
- The softener is used only to soften water entering the RO unit, and thus, used only for dialysis. (The softener need not actually be built into the RO unit, but must be an integral part of the dialysis system.)

C. Developing Need When a Water Softening System is Replaced with a Water Purification Unit in an Existing Home Dialysis System.—The medical necessity of water purification units must be carefully developed when they replace water softening systems in existing home dialysis systems. A purification system may be ordered under these circumstances for a number of reasons. For example, changes in the medical community's opinions regarding the quality of water necessary for safe dialysis may lead the physician to decide the quality of water previously used should be improved, or the water quality itself may have deteriorated. Patients may have dialyzed using only an existing water softener previous to Medicare ESRD coverage because of inability to pay for a purification system. On the other hand, in some cases, the installation of a purification system is not medically necessary. Thus, when such a case comes to your attention, ask the physician to furnish the reason for the changes. Supporting documentation, such as the supplier's recommendations or water analysis, may be required. All such cases should be reviewed by your medical consultants.

Cross-reference: Intermediary Manual, §§3113, 3643 (item 1c); Carriers Manual, §§2100, 2100.2 2130, 2105 (item 1c); Hospital Manual, §235.

60-3 WHITE CANE FOR USE BY A BLIND PERSON—NOT COVERED

A white cane for use by a blind person is more an identifying and self-help device rather than an item which makes a meaningful contribution in the treatment of an illness or injury.

60-4 HOME USE OF OXYGEN

A. General.—Medicare coverage of home oxygen and oxygen equipment under the durable medical equipment (DME) benefit (see §1861(s)(6)of the Act) is considered reasonable and necessary only for patients with significant hypoxemia who meet the medical documentation, laboratory evidence, and health conditions specified in subsections B, C, and D. This section also includes special coverage criteria for portable oxygen systems. Finally, a statement on the absence of coverage of the professional services of a respiratory therapist under the DME benefit is included in subsection F.

B. Medical documentation.—Initial claims for oxygen services must include a completed Form HCFA-484 (Certificate of Medical Necessity: Oxygen)to establish whether coverage criteria are met and to ensure that the oxygen services provided are consistent with the physician's prescription or other medical documentation. The treating physician's prescription or other medical documentation must indicate that other forms of treatment (e.g., medical and physical therapy directed at secretions, bronchospasm and infection) have been tried, have not been sufficiently successful, and oxygen therapy is still required. While there is no substitute for oxygen therapy, each patient must receive optimum therapy before long-term home oxygen therapy is ordered. Use Form HCFA-484 for recertifications. (See Medicare Carriers Manual §3312 for completion of Form HCFA-484.)

The medical and prescription information in section B of Form HCFA-484 can be completed only by the treating physician, the physician's employee, or another clinician (e.g., nurse, respiratory therapist, etc.) as long as that person is not the DME supplier. Although hospital discharge coordinators and medical social workers may assist in arranging for physician-prescribed home oxygen, they do not have the authority to prescribe the services. Suppliers may not enter this information. While this section may be completed by nonphysician clinician or a physician employee, it must be reviewed and the form HCFA-484 signed by the attending physician.

A physician's certification of medical necessity for oxygen equipment must include the results of specific testing before coverage can be determined.

Claims for oxygen must also be supported by medical documentation in the patient's record. Separate documentation is used with electronic billing. (See Medicare Carriers Manual, Part 3, §4105.5.) This documentation may be in the form of a prescription written by the patient's attending physician who has recently examined the patient (normally within a month of the start of therapy) and must specify:

- A diagnosis of the disease requiring home use of oxygen;
- The oxygen flow rate; and

An estimate of the frequency, duration of use (e.g., 2 liters per minute, 10 minutes per hour, 12 hours per day), and duration of need (e.g., 6 months or lifetime).

NOTE: A prescription for "Oxygen PRN" or "Oxygen as needed" does not meet this last requirement. Neither provides any basis for determining if the amount of oxygen is reasonable and necessary for the patient.

A member of the carrier's medical staff should review all claims with oxygen flow rates of more than 4 liters per minute before payment can be made.

The attending physician specifies the type of oxygen delivery system to be used (i.e., gas, liquid, or concentrator) by signing the completed form HCFA-484. In addition the supplier or physician may use the space in section C for written confirmation of additional details of the physician's order. The additional order information contained in section C may include the means of oxygen delivery (mask, nasal, cannula, etc.), the specifics of varying flow rates, and/or the noncontinuous use of oxygen as appropriate. The physician confirms this order information with their signature in section D.

New medical documentation written by the patient's attending physician must be submitted to the carrier in support of revised oxygen requirements when there has been a change in the patient's condition and need for oxygen therapy.

Carriers are required to conduct periodic, continuing medical necessity reviews on patients whose conditions warrant these reviews and on patients with indefinite or extended periods of necessity as described in Medicare Carriers Manual, Part 3, §4105.5. When indicated, carriers may also request documentation of the results of a repeat arterial blood gas or oximetry study.

NOTE: Section 4152 of OBRA 1990 requires earlier recertification and retesting of oxygen patients who begin coverage with an arterial blood gas result at or above a partial pressure of 55 or an arterial oxygen saturation percentage at or above 89. (See Medicare Carriers Manual §4105.5 for certification and retesting schedules.)

C. Laboratory Evidence.—Initial claims for oxygen therapy must also include the results of a blood gas study that has been ordered and evaluated by the attending physician. This is usually in the form of a measurement of the partial pressure of oxygen (PO2) in arterial blood. (See Medicare Carriers Manual, Part 3, §2070.1 for instructions on clinical laboratory tests.) A measurement of arterial oxygen saturation obtained by ear or pulse oximetry, however, is also acceptable when ordered and evaluated by the attending physician and performed under his or her supervision or when performed by a qualified provider or supplier of laboratory services. When the arterial blood gas and the oximetry studies are both used to document the need for home oxygen therapy and the results are conflicting, the arterial blood gas study is the preferred source of documenting medical need. A DME supplier is not considered a qualified provider or supplier of laboratory services for purposes of these guidelines. This prohibition does not extend to the results of blood gas test conducted by a hospital certified to do such tests. The conditions under which the laboratory tests are performed must be specified in writing and submitted with the initial claim, i.e., at rest, during exercise, or during sleep.

The preferred sources of laboratory evidence are existing physician and/or hospital records that reflect the patient's medical condition. Since it is expected that virtually all patients who qualify for home oxygen coverage for the first time under these guidelines have recently been discharged from a hospital where they submitted to arterial blood gas tests, the carrier needs to request that such test results be submitted in support of their initial claims for home oxygen. If more than one arterial blood gas test is performed during the patient's hospital stay, the test result obtained closest to, but no earlier than 2 days prior to the hospital discharge date is required as evidence of the need for home oxygen therapy.

For those patients whose initial oxygen prescription did not originate during a hospital stay, blood gas studies should be done while the patient is in the chronic stable state, i.e., not during a period of an acute illness or an exacerbation of their underlying disease."
Carriers may accept a attending physician's statement of recent hospital test results for a particular patient, when appropriate, in lieu of copies of actual hospital records.

A repeat arterial blood gas study is appropriate when evidence indicates that an oxygen recipient has undergone a major change in their condition relevant to home use of oxygen. If the carrier has reason to believe that there has been a major change in the patient's physical condition, it may ask for documentation of the results of another blood gas or oximetry study.

D. Health Conditions.—Coverage is available for patients with significant hypoxemia in the chronic stable state if: (1) the attending physician has determined that the patient has a health condition outlined in subsection D.1, (2) the patient meets the blood gas evidence requirements specified in subsection D.3, and (3) the patient has appropriately tried other alternative treatment measures without complete success. (See subsection B.)

   1. Conditions for Which Oxygen Therapy May Be Covered.—

- A severe lung disease, such as chronic obstructive pulmonary disease, diffuse interstitial lung disease, whether of known or unknown etiology; cystic fibrosis bronchiectasis; widespread pulmonary neoplasm; or
- Hypoxia-related symptoms or findings that might be expected to improve with oxygen therapy. Examples of these symptoms and findings are pulmonary hypertension, recurring congestive heart failure due to chronic cor pulmonale, erythrocytosis, impairment of the cognitive process, nocturnal restlessness, and morning headache.

2. Conditions for Which Oxygen Therapy Is Not Covered.—

- Angina pectoris in the absence of hypoxemia. This condition is generally not the result of a low oxygen level in the blood, and there are other preferred treatments;
- Breathlessness without cor pulmonale or evidence of hypoxemia. Although intermittent oxygen use is sometimes prescribed to relieve this condition, it is potentially harmful and psychologically addicting;
- Severe peripheral vascular disease resulting in clinically evident desaturation in one or more extremities. There is no evidence that increased PO2 improves the oxygenation of tissues with impaired circulation; or
- Terminal illnesses that do not affect the lungs.

3. Covered Blood Gas Values.—If the patient has a condition specified in subsection D.1, the carrier must review the medical documentation and laboratory evidence that has been submitted for a particular patient (see subsections B and C) and determine if coverage is available under one of the three group categories outlined below.

   a. Group I.—Except as modified in subsection d, coverage is provided for patients with significant hypoxemia evidenced by any of the following:

   (1) An arterial PO2 at or below 55 mm Hg, or an arterial oxygen saturation at or below 88 percent, taken at rest, breathing room air.
   (2) An arterial PO2 at or below 55 mm Hg, or an arterial oxygen saturation at or below 88 percent, taken during sleep for a patient who demonstrates an arterial PO2 at or above 56 mm Hg, or an arterial oxygen saturation at or above 89 percent, while awake; or a greater than normal fall in oxygen level during sleep (a decrease in arterial PO2 more than 10 mm Hg, or decrease in arterial oxygen saturation more than 5 percent) associated with symptoms or signs reasonably attributable to hypoxemia (e.g., impairment of cognitive processes and nocturnal restlessness or insomnia). In either of these cases, coverage is provided only for use of oxygen during sleep, and then only one type of unit will be covered. Portable oxygen, therefore, would not be covered in this situation.
   (3) An arterial PO2 at or below 55 mm Hg or an arterial oxygen saturation at or below 88 percent, taken during exercise for a patient who demonstrates an arterial PO2 at or above 56 mm Hg, or an arterial oxygen saturation at or above 89 percent, during the day while at rest. In this case, supplemental oxygen is provided for during exercise if there is evidence the use of oxygen improves the hypoxemia that was demonstrated during exercise when the patient was breathing room air.

   b. Group II.—Except as modified in subsection d, coverage is available for patients whose arterial PO2 is 56-59 mm Hg or whose arterial blood oxygen saturation is 89 percent, if there is evidence of:

   (1) Dependent edema suggesting congestive heart failure;
   (2) Pulmonary hypertension or cor pulmonale, determined by measurement of pulmonary artery pressure, gated blood pool scan, echocardiogram, or "P" pulmonale on EKG (P wave greater than 3 mm in standard leads II, III, or AVFL; or
   (3) Erythrocythemia with a hematocrit greater than 56 percent.

   c. Group III.—Except as modified in subsection d, carriers must apply a rebuttable presumption that a home program of oxygen use is not medically necessary for patients with arterial PO2 levels at or above 60 mm Hg, or arterial blood oxygen saturation at or above 90 percent. In order for claims in this category to be reimbursed, the carrier's reviewing physician needs to review any documentation submitted in rebuttal of this presumption and grant specific approval of the claims. HCFA expects few claims to be approved for coverage in this category.
   d. Variable Factors That May Affect Blood Gas Values.—In reviewing the arterial PO2 levels and the arterial oxygen saturation percentages specified in subsections D. 3. a, b and c, the carrier's medical staff must take into account variations in oxygen measurements that may result from such factors as the patient's age, the altitude level, or the patient's decreased oxygen carrying capacity.

E. Portable Oxygen Systems.—A patient meeting the requirements specified below may qualify for coverage of a portable oxygen system either (1) by itself or (2) to use in addition to a stationary oxygen system. A portable oxygen system is covered for a particular patient if:

- The claim meets the requirements specified in subsections A-D, as appropriate; and
- The medical documentation indicates that the patient is mobile in the home and would benefit from the use of a portable oxygen system in the home. Portable oxygen systems are not covered for patients who qualify for oxygen solely based on blood gas studies obtained during sleep.

F. Respiratory Therapists.—Respiratory therapists' services are not covered under the provisions for coverage of oxygen services under the Part B durable medical equipment benefit as outlined above. This benefit provides for coverage of home use of oxygen and oxygen equipment, but does not include a professional component in the delivery of such services.

(See §60-9; Intermediary Manual, Part 3, §3113ff; and Medicare Carriers Manual, Part 3, §2100ff.)

60-5 POWER-OPERATED VEHICLES THAT MAY BE USED AS WHEELCHAIRS

Power-operated vehicles that may be appropriately used as wheelchairs are covered under the durable medical equipment provision.

These vehicles have been appropriately used in the home setting for vocational rehabilitation and to improve the ability of chronically disabled persons to cope with normal domestic, vocational and social activities. They may be covered if a wheelchair is medically necessary and the patient is unable to operate a wheelchair manually.

A specialist in physical medicine, orthopedic surgery, neurology, or rheumatology must provide an evaluation of the patient's medical and physical condition and a prescription for the vehicle to assure that the patient requires the vehicle and is capable of using it safely. When an intermediary determines that such a specialist is not reasonably accessible, e.g., more than 1 day's round trip from the beneficiary's home, or the patient's condition precludes such travel, a prescription from the beneficiary's physician is acceptable.

The intermediary's medical staff reviews all claims for a power-operated vehicle, including the specialists' or other physicians' prescriptions and evaluations of the patient's medical and physical conditions, to insure that all coverage requirements are met. (See §60-9 and Intermediary Manual, Part 3, §3629.)

60-6 SPECIALLY SIZED WHEELCHAIRS

Payment may be made for a specially sized wheelchair even though it is more expensive than a standard wheelchair. For example, a narrow wheelchair may be required because of the narrow doorways of a patient's home or because of a patient's slender build. Such difference in the size of the wheelchair from the standard model is not considered a deluxe feature.

A physician's certification or prescription that a special size is needed is not required where you can determine from the information in file or other sources that a specially sized wheelchair (rather than a standard one) is needed to accommodate the wheelchair to the place of use or the physical size of the patient.

To determine the reasonable charge in these cases, use the criteria set out in Carriers Manual, §§5022, 5022.1, 5200, and 5205, as necessary.

Cross-reference: Intermediary Manual, §§3113.2C, 3642.1, 3643 (item 3); Carriers Manual, §§2100.2c, 2105, 4105.2, 5107; Hospital Manual, §§235.2c, 420.1 (item 13).

60-7 SELF-CONTAINED PACEMAKER MONITORS

Self-contained pacemaker monitors are accepted devices for monitoring cardiac pacemakers. Accordingly, program payment may be made for the rental or purchase of either of the following pacemaker monitors when it is prescribed by a physician for a patient with a cardiac pacemaker:

A. Digital Electronic Pacemaker Monitor.—This device provides the patient with an instantaneous digital readout of his pacemaker pulse rate. Use of this device does not involve professional services until there has been a change of five pulses (or more) per minute above or below the initial rate of the pacemaker; when such change occurs, the patient contacts his physician.

B. Audible/Visible Signal Pacemaker Monitor.—This device produces an audible and visible signal which indicates the pacemaker rate. Use of this device does not involve professional services until a change occurs in these signals; at such time, the patient contacts his physician.

NOTE: The design of the self-contained pacemaker monitor makes it possible for the patient to monitor his pacemaker periodically and minimizes the need for regular visits to the outpatient department of the provider.

Therefore, documentation of the medical necessity for pacemaker evaluation in the outpatient department of the provider should be obtained where such evaluation is employed in addition to the self-contained pacemaker monitor used by the patient in his home.

Cross-reference: §50-1

60-8 SEAT LIFT

Reimbursement may be made for the rental or purchase of a medically necessary seat lift when prescribed by a physician for a patient with severe arthritis of the hip or knee and patients with muscular dystrophy or other neuromuscular diseases when it has been determined the patient can benefit therapeutically from use of the device. In establishing medical necessity for the seat lift, the evidence must show that the item is included in the physician's course of treatment, that it is likely to effect improvement, or arrest or retard deterioration in the patient's condition, and that the severity of the condition is such that the alternative would be chair or bed confinement.

Coverage of seat lifts is limited to those types which operate smoothly, can be controlled by the patient, and effectively assist a patient in standing up and sitting down without other assistance. Excluded from coverage is the type of lift which operates by a spring release mechanism with a sudden, catapult-like motion and jolts the patient from a seated to a standing position. Limit the payment for units which incorporate a recliner feature along with the seat lift to the amount payable for a seat lift without this feature.

Cross reference: Carriers Manual, § 5107

60-9 DURABLE MEDICAL EQUIPMENT REFERENCE LIST

The durable medical equipment (DME) list which follows is designed to facilitate your processing of DME claims. This section is designed to be used as a quick reference tool for determining the coverage status of certain pieces of DME and especially for those items which are commonly referred to by both brand and generic names. The information contained herein is applicable (where appropriate) to all DME coverage determinations discussed in the DME portion of this manual. The list is organized into two columns. The first column lists alphabetically various generic categories of equipment on which national coverage decisions have been made by HCFA; and the second column notes the coverage status of each equipment category.

In the case of equipment categories that have been determined by HCFA to be covered under the DME benefit, the list outlines the conditions of coverage that must be met if payment is to be allowed for the rental or purchase of the DME by a particular patient, or cross-refers to another section of the manual where the applicable coverage criteria are described in more detail. With respect to equipment categories that cannot be covered as DME, the list includes a brief explanation of why the equipment is not covered. This DME list will be updated periodically to reflect any additional national coverage decisions that HCFA may make with regard to other categories of equipment.

When you receive a claim for an item of equipment which does not appear to fall logically into any of the generic categories listed, you have the authority and responsibility for deciding whether those items are covered under the DME benefit. These decisions must be made by each contractor based on the advice of its medical consultants, taking into account:

- The general DME coverage instructions in the Carriers Manual, §2100ff and Intermediary Manual, §3113ff (see below for brief summary);
- Whether the item has been approved for marketing by the Food and Drug Administration (FDA) (see Carriers Manual, §2303.1 and Intermediary Manual, §3151.1) and is otherwise generally considered to be safe and effective for the purpose intended; and
- Whether the item is reasonable and necessary for the individual patient.
- As provided in the Carriers Manual, § 2100.1, and Intermediary Manual, §3113.1, the term DME is defined as equipment which
- Can withstand repeated use; i.e., could normally be rented, and used by successive patients;
- Is primarily and customarily used to serve a medical purpose;
- Generally is not useful to a person in the absence of illness or injury; and
- Is appropriate for use in a patient's home.

Durable Medical Equipment Reference List:

Item	Coverage Status
Air Cleaners	deny--environmental control equipment; not primarily medical in nature (§1861(n) of the Act)
Air Conditioners	deny--environmental control equipment; not primarily medical in nature (§1861(n) of the Act)
Air-Fluidized Bed	(See §60-19.)
Alternating Pressure Pads, and Mattresses and Lambs Wool Pads	covered if patient has, or is highly susceptible to, decubitus ulcers and patient's physician has specified that he will be supervising its use in connection with his course of treatment.
Audible/Visible Signal Pacemaker Monitor	(See Self-Contained Pacemaker Monitor.)
Augmentative Communication Device	(See Speech Generating Devices, §60-23.)
Bathtub Lifts	deny--convenience item; not primarily medical in nature (§1861(n) of the Act)
Bathtub Seats	deny--comfort or convenience item; hygienic equipment; not primarily medical in nature (§1861(n) of the Act)

Bead Bed	(See §60-19.)
Bed Baths (home type)	deny--hygienic equipment; not primarily medical in nature (§1861(n) of the Act)
Bed Lifter (bed elevator)	deny--not primarily medical in nature (§1861(n) of the Act.
Bedboards	deny--not primarily medical in nature (§1861(n) of the Act)

Bed Pans (autoclavable hospital type)	covered if patient is bed confined
Bed Side Rails	(See Hospital Beds, §60-18.)
Beds-Lounge (power or manual)	deny--not a hospital bed; comfort or convenience item; not primarily medical in nature (§1861(n) of the Act)
Beds--Oscillating	deny--institutional equipment; inappropriate for home use
Bidet Toilet Seat	(See Toilet Seats.)
Blood Glucose Analyzer Reflectance Colorimeter	deny--unsuitable for home use (See §60-11.)
Blood Glucose Monitor	covered if patient meets certain conditions (See §60-11.)
Braille Teaching Texts	deny--educational equipment; not primarily medical in nature (§1861(n) of the Act)
Canes	covered if patient's condition impairs ambulation (See §60-3.)
Carafes	deny--convenience item; not primarily medical in nature (§1861(n) of the Act)
Catheters	deny--nonreusable disposable supply (§1861(n) of the Act)

Commodes	covered if patient is confined to bed or room. NOTE: The term "room confined" means that the patient's condition is such that leaving the room is medically contraindicated. The accessibility of bathroom facilities generally would not be a factor in this determination. However, confinement of a patient to his home in a case where there are no toilet facilities in the home may be equated to room confinement. Moreover, payment may also be made if a patient's medical condition confines him to a floor of his home and there is no bathroom located on that floor (See hospital beds in §60-18 for definition of "bed confinement".)

Communicator	(See §60-23, Speech Generating Devices)

Continuous Passive Motion	Continuous passive motion devices are devices covered for patients who have received a total knee replacement. To qualify for coverage, use of the device must commence within 2 days following surgery. In addition, coverage is limited to that portion of the three week period following surgery during which the device is used in the patient's home. There is insufficient evidence to justify coverage of these devices for longer periods of time or for other applications.
Continuous Positive Airway Pressure (CPAP)	(See §60-17.)
Crutches	covered if patient's condition impairs Ambulation
Cushion Lift Power Seat	(See Seat Lifts.)
Dehumidifiers (room or central heating system type)	deny--environmental control equipment; not primarily medical in nature (§1861(n) of the Act
Diathermy Machines (standard pulses wave types)	deny--inappropriate for home use (See and §35-41.)

Digital Electronic Pacemaker Monitor	(See Self-Contained Pacemaker Monitor.)
Disposable Sheets and Bags	deny--nonreusable disposable supplies (§1861(n) of the Act)
Elastic Stockings	deny--nonreusable supply; not rental-type items (§1861(n) of the Act)
Electric Air Cleaners	deny--(See Air Cleaners.) (§1861(n) of the Act)
Electric Hospital Beds	(See Hospital Beds §60-18.)
Electrical Stimulation for Wounds	deny--inappropriate for home use
Electrostatic Machines	deny--(See Air Cleaners and Air Conditioners.) (§1861(n) of the Act)
Elevators	deny--convenience item; not primarily medical in nature (§1861(n) of the Act)
Emesis Basins	deny--convenience item; not primarily medical in nature (§1861(n) of the Act)
Esophageal Dilator	deny--physician instrument; inappropriate for patient use
Exercise Equipment	deny--not primarily medical in nature (§1861(n) of the Act)
Fabric Supports	deny--nonreusable supplies; not rental-type it (§1861(n) of the Act)

Face Masks (oxygen)	covered if oxygen is covered (See § 60-4.)
Face Masks (surgical)	deny--nonreusable disposable items (§1861(n) of the Act)
Flowmeter	(See Medical Oxygen Regulators)
Fluidic Breathing Assister	(See IPPB Machines.)
Fomentation Device	(See Heating Pads.)
Gel Flotation Pads and Mattresses	(See Alternating Pressure Pads and Mattresses.)
Grab Bars	deny--self-help device; not primarily medical in nature (§1861(n) of the Act)
Heat and Massage Foam Cushion Pad	deny--not primarily medical in nature; personal comfort item (§§ 1861(n) and 1862(a)(6) of the Act)
Heating and Cooling Plants	deny--environmental control equipment; not primarily medical in nature(§1861(n) of the Act)

Heating Pads	covered if the contractor's medical staff determines patient's medical condition is one for which the application of heat in the form of a heating pad is therapeutically effective.
Heat Lamps	covered if the contractor's medical staff determines patient's medical condition is one for which the application of heat in the form of a heat lamp is therapeutically effective.
Hospital Beds	(See § 60-18.)
Hot Packs	(See Heating Pads.)
Humidifiers (oxygen)	(See Oxygen Humidifiers.)
Humidifiers (room or central heating system types)	deny--environmental control equipment; not medical in nature (§1861(n) of the Act)
Hydraulic Lift	(See Patient Lifts.)
Incontinent Pads	deny--nonreusable supply; hygienic item (§ 1861(n) of the Act.)
Infusion Pumps	For external and implantable pumps, see §60-14. If the pump is used with an enteral or parenteral malnutritional therapy system, see §§65-10 - 65.10.2 0.2 for special coverage rules.
Injectors (hypodermic jet devices for injection of insulin	deny-- noncovered self-administered drug supply, §1861(s)(2)(A) of the Act)

IPPB Machines	covered if patient's ability to breathe is severely impaired

Iron Lungs	(See Ventilators.)
Irrigating Kit	deny--nonreusable supply; hygienic equipment (§1861(n) of the Act)
Lambs Wool Pads	covered under same conditions as alternating pressure pads and mattresses
Leotards	deny--(See Pressure Leotards.) (§1861(n)of the Act)
Lymphedema Pumps	covered (See §60-16.)(segmental and non-segmental therapy types)
Massage Devices	deny--personal comfort items; not primarily medical in nature (§§1861(n) and 1862(a)(6) of the Act)
Mattress	covered only where hospital bed is medically necessary (Separate Charge for replacement mattresses should not be allowed where hospital bed with mattress is rented.) (See §60-18.)
Medical Oxygen Regulators	covered if patient's ability to breathe is severely impaired (See §60-4.)
Mobile Geriatric Chair	(See Rolling Chairs.)
Motorized Wheelchairs	(See Wheelchairs (power operated).)
Muscle Stimulators	Covered for certain conditions (See §35-77.)
Nebulizers	covered if patient's ability to breathe is severely impaired
Oscillating Beds	deny--institutional equipment--inappropriate for home use
Overbed Tables	deny--convenience item; not primarily medical in nature (§1861(n) of the Act)
Oxygen	covered if the oxygen has been prescribed for use in connection with medically necessary durable medical equipment (See §60-4.)

Oxygen Humidifiers	covered if a medical humidifier has been prescribed for use in connection with medically necessary durable medical equipment for purposes of moisturizing oxygen (See §60-4.)
Oxygen Regulators (Medical)	(See Medical Oxygen Regulators.)

Oxygen Tents	(See § 60-4.)
Paraffin Bath Units (Portable)	(See Portable Paraffin Bath Units.)
Paraffin Bath Units (Standard)	deny--institutional equipment; inappropriate for home use
Parallel Bars	deny--support exercise equipment; primarily for institutional use; in the home setting other devices (e.g., a walker) satisfy the patient's need
Patient Lifts	covered if contractor's medical staff determines patient's condition is such that periodic movement is necessary to effect improvement or to arrest or retard deterioration in his condition.
Percussors	covered for mobilizing respiratory tract secretions in patients with chronic obstructive lung disease, chronic bronchitis, or emphysema, when patient or operator of powered percussor has received appropriate training by a physician or therapist, and no one competent to administer manual therapy is available.
Portable Oxygen Systems	1. Regulated (adjustable --covered under conditions specified in flow rate)§60-4. Refer all claims to medical staff for this determination. 2. Preset (flow rate --deny--emergency, first-aid, or not adjustable) precautionary equipment; essentially not therapeutic in nature
Portable Paraffin Bath Units	covered when the patient has undergone a successful trial period of paraffin therapy ordered by a physician and the patient's condition is expected to be relieved by long term use of this modality.
Portable Room Heaters	deny--environmental control equipment; not primarily medical in nature (§1861(n) of the Act)
Portable Whirlpool Pumps	deny--not primarily medical in nature; personal comfort items (§§1861(n) and 1862(a)(6) of the Act)
Postural Drainage Boards	covered if patient has a chronic pulmonary condition
Preset Portable Oxygen Units	deny--emergency, first-aid, or precautionary equipment; essentially not therapeutic in nature

Pressure Leotards	deny—nonreusable supply, not rental-type item (§1861(n) of the Act)
Pulse Tachometer	deny—not reasonable or necessary for monitoring pulse of homebound patient with or without a cardiac pacemaker
Quad-Canes	(See Walkers.)
Raised Toilet Seats	deny—convenience item; hygienic equipment; not primarily medical in nature (§1861(n) of the Act)
Reflectance Colorimeters	(See Blood Glucose Analyzers.)
Respirators	(See Ventilators.)
Rolling Chairs	covered if the contractor's medical staff determines that the patient's condition is such that there is a medical need for this item and it has been prescribed by the patient's physician in lieu of a wheelchair. Coverage is limited to those rollabout chairs having casters of at least 5 inches in diameter and specifically designed to meet the needs of ill, injured or otherwise impaired individuals. Coverage is denied for the wide range of chairs with smaller casters as are found in general use in homes, offices, and institutions for many purposes not related to the care or treatment of ill or injured persons. This type is not primarily medical in nature. (§1861(n) of the Act)
Safety Roller	(See §60-15.)
Sauna Baths	deny—not primarily medical in nature; personal comfort items (§§1861(n) and 1862(a)(6) of the Act)
Seat Lift	covered under the conditions specified in §60-8. Refer all to medical staff for this determination.
Self-Contained Pacemaker Monitor	covered when prescribed by a physician for a patient with a cardiac pacemaker (See §§50-1C and 60-7.)
Sitz Bath	covered if the contractor's medical staff determines patient has an infection or injury of the perineal area and the item has been prescribed by the patient's physician as a part of his planned regimen of treatment in the patient's home.

Spare Tanks of Oxygen	deny--convenience or precautionary supply
Speech Teaching Machine	deny--education equipment; not primarily medical in nature (§1861(n) of the Act)

Stairway Elevators	deny--(See Elevators.) (§1861(n) of the Act)
Standing Table	deny--convenience item; not primarily medical in nature (§1861(n) of the Act)

Steam Packs	these packs are covered under the same condition as a heating pad (See Heating Pads.)
Suction Machine	covered if the contractor's medical staff determines that the machine specified in the claim is medically required and appropriate for home use without technical or professional supervision.
Support Hose	deny (See Fabric Supports.) (§1861(n) of the Act)
Surgical Leggings	deny--nonreusable supply; not rental-type item (§1861(n) of the Act)
Telephone Alert Systems	deny--these are emergency communications systems and do not serve a diagnostic or therapeutic purpose

Telephone Arms	deny--convenience item; not medical in nature (§1861(n) of the Act)
Toilet Seats	deny--not medical equipment (§1861(n)of the Act)
Traction Equipment	covered if patient has orthopedic impairment requiring traction equipment which prevents ambulation during the period of use (Consider covering devices usable during ambulation; e.g., cervical traction collar, under the brace provision)
Trapeze Bars	covered if patient is bed confined and the patient needs a trapeze bar to sit up because of respiratory condition, to change body position for other medical reasons, or to get in and out of bed.
Treadmill Exerciser	deny--exercise equipment; not primarily medical in nature(§1861(n) of the Act)

Ultraviolet Cabinet	covered for selected patients with generalized intractable psoriasis. Using appropriate consultation, the contractor should determine whether medical and other factors justify treatment at home rather than at alternative sites, e.g., outpatient department of a hospital.
Urinals (autoclavable hospital type)	covered if patient is bed confined
Vaporizers	covered if patient has a respiratory illness

Ventilators	covered for treatment of neuromuscular diseases, thoracic restrictive diseases, and chronic respiratory failure consequent to chronic obstructive pulmonary disease. Includes both positive and negative pressure types.
Walkers	covered if patient's condition impairs ambulation (See also §60-15.)
Water and Pressure Pads and Mattresses	(See Alternating Pressure Pads and Mattresses.)
Wheelchairs	covered if patient's condition is such that without the use of a wheelchair he would otherwise be bed or chair confined. An individual may qualify for a wheelchair and still be considered bed confined.

Wheelchairs (power operated) and wheelchairs with other special features	covered if patient's condition is such and that a wheelchair is medically necessary and the patient is unable to operate the wheelchair manually. Any claim involving a power wheelchair or a wheelchair with other special features should be referred for medical consultation since payment for the special features is limited to those which are medically required because of the patient's condition. (See §60-5 for power operated and §60-6 for specially sized wheelchairs.) NOTE: A power-operated vehicle that may appropriately be used as a wheelchair can be covered. (See §60-5 for coverage details.)

Whirlpool Bath Equipment	covered if patient is homebound and has a (standard) condition for which the whirlpool bath can be expected to provide substantial therapeutic benefit justifying its cost. Where patient is not homebound but has such a condition, payment is restricted to the cost of providing the services elsewhere; e.g., an outpatient department of a participating hospital, if that alternative is less costly. In all cases, refer claim to medical staff for a determination.
Whirlpool Pumps	deny--(See Portable Whirlpool Pumps.) (§1861(n) of the Act)
White Cane	deny--(See §60-3.)

60-11 HOME BLOOD GLUCOSE MONITORS

There are several different types of blood glucose monitors that use reflectance meters to determine blood glucose levels. Medicare coverage of these devices varies, both with respect to the type of device and the medical condition of the patient for whom the device is prescribed.

Reflectance colorimeter devices used for measuring blood glucose levels in clinical settings are not covered as durable medical equipment for use in the home because their need for frequent professional re-calibration makes them unsuitable for home use. However, some types of blood glucose monitors which use a reflectance meter specifically designed for home use by diabetic patients may be covered as durable medical equipment, subject to the conditions and limitations described below.

Blood glucose monitors are meter devices that read color changes produced on specially treated reagent strips by glucose concentrations in the patient's blood. The patient, using a disposable sterile lancet, draws a drop of blood, places it on a reagent strip and, following instructions which may vary with the device used, inserts it into the device to obtain a reading. Lancets, reagent strips, and other supplies necessary for the proper functioning of the device are also covered for patients for whom the device is indicated. Home blood glucose monitors enable certain patients to better control their blood glucose levels by frequently checking and appropriately contacting their attending physician for advice and treatment. Studies indicate that the patient's ability to carefully follow proper procedures is critical to obtaining satisfactory results with these devices. In addition, the cost of the devices, with their supplies, limits economical use to patients who must make frequent checks of their blood glucose levels. Accordingly, coverage of home blood glucose monitors is limited to patients meeting the following conditions:

- The patient has been diagnosed as having diabetes;
- The patient's physician states that the patient is capable of being trained to use the particular device prescribed in an appropriate manner. In some cases, the patient may not be able to perform this function, but a responsible individual can be trained to use the equipment and monitor the patient to assure that the intended effect is achieved. This is permissible if the record is properly documented by the patient's physician; and
- The device is designed for home rather than clinical use.

There is also a blood glucose monitoring system designed especially for use by those with visual impairments. The monitors used in such systems are identical in terms of reliability and sensitivity to the standard blood glucose monitors described above. They differ by having such features as voice synthesizers, automatic timers, and specially designed arrangements of supplies and materials to enable the visually impaired to use the equipment without assistance.

These special blood glucose monitoring systems are covered under Medicare if the following conditions are met:

- The patient and device meet the three conditions listed above for coverage of standard home blood glucose monitors; and
- The patient's physician certifies that he or she has a visual impairment severe enough to require use of this special monitoring system.

The additional features and equipment of these special systems justify a higher reimbursement amount than allowed for standard blood glucose monitors. Separately identify claims for such devices and establish a separate reimbursement amount for them. For those carriers using HCPCS, the procedure code and definition is: E0609--Blood Glucose Monitor--with special features (e.g., voice synthesizers, automatic timer).

60-14 INFUSION PUMPS

The following indications for treatment using infusion pumps are covered under medicare:

A. External Infusion Pumps.—

1. Iron Poisoning (Effective for Services Performed On or After 9/26/84).—When used in the administration of deferoxamine for the treatment of acute iron poisoning and iron overload, only external infusion pumps are covered.
2. Thromboembolic Disease (Effective for Services Performed On or After 9/26/84).—When used in the administration of heparin for the treatment of thromboembolic disease and/or pulmonary embolism, only external infusion pumps used in an institutional setting are covered.
3. Chemotherapy for Liver Cancer (Effective for Services Performed On or After 1/29/85).—The external chemotherapy infusion pump is covered when used in the treatment of primary hepatocellular carcinoma or colorectal cancer where this disease is unresectable or where the patient refuses surgical excision of the tumor.
4. Morphine for Intractable Cancer Pain (Effective for Services Performed On or After 4/22/85).—Morphine infusion via an external infusion pump is covered when used in the treatment of intractable pain caused by cancer (in either an inpatient or outpatient setting, including a hospice).
5. Continuous subcutaneous insulin infusion pumps (CSII) (Effective for Services Performed On or After 4/1/2000).—

An external infusion pump and related drugs/supplies are covered as medically necessary in the home setting in the following situation:

Treatment of Diabetes

In order to be covered, patients must meet criterion A or B:

(A) The patient has completed a comprehensive diabetes education program, and has been on a program of multiple daily injections of insulin (i.e. at least 3 injections per day), with frequent self-adjustments of insulin dose for at least 6 months prior to initiation of the insulin pump, and has documented frequency of glucose self-testing an average of at least 4 times per day during the 2 months prior to initiation of the insulin pump, and meets one or more of the following criteria while on the multiple daily injection regimen:

(1) Glycosylated hemoglobin level (HbAlc) > 7.0 percent
(2) History of recurring hypoglycemia
(3) Wide fluctuations in blood glucose before mealtime
(4) Dawn phenomenon with fasting blood sugars frequently Exceeding 200 mg/dl
(5) History of severe glycemic excursions

(B) The patient with diabetes has been on a pump prior to enrollment in Medicare and has documented frequency of glucose self-testing an average of at least 4 times per day during the month prior to Medicare enrollment.

Diabetes needs to be documented by a fasting C-peptide level that is less than or equal to 110 percent of the lower limit of normal of the laboratory's measurement method. (Effective for Services Performed on or after January 1, 2002.)

Continued coverage of the insulin pump would require that the patient has been seen and evaluated the treating physician at least every 3 months.

The pump must be ordered by and follow-up care of the patient must be managed by a physician who manages multiple patients with CSII and who works closely with a team including nurses, diabetes educators, and dietitians who are knowledgeable in the use of CSII.

6. Other uses of external infusion pumps are covered if the contractor's medical staff verifies the appropriateness of the therapy and of the prescribed pump for the individual patient.

NOTE: Payment may also be made for drugs necessary for the effective use of an external infusion pump as long as the drug being used with the pump is itself reasonable and necessary for the patient's treatment.

B. Implantable Infusion Pumps.—

1. Chemotherapy for Liver Cancer (Effective for Services Performed On or After 9/26/84).—The implantable infusion pump is covered for intra-arterial infusion of 5-FUdR for the treatment of liver cancer for patients with primary hepatocellular carcinoma or Duke's Class D colorectal cancer, in whom the metastases are limited to the liver, and where (1) the disease is unresectable or (2) where the patient refuses surgical excision of the tumor.
2. Anti-Spasmodic Drugs for Severe Spasticity.—An implantable infusion pump is covered when used to administer anti-spasmodic drugs intrathecally (e.g., baclofen) to treat chronic intractable spasticity in patients who have proven unresponsive to less invasive medical therapy as determined by the following criteria:

   • As indicated by at least a 6-week trial, the patient cannot be maintained on noninvasive methods of spasm control, such as oral anti-spasmodic drugs, either because these methods fail to control adequately the spasticity or produce intolerable side effects, and
   • Prior to pump implantation, the patient must have responded favorably to a trial intrathecal dose of the anti-spasmodic drug.

3. Opioid Drugs for Treatment of Chronic Intractable Pain.—An implantable infusion pump is covered when used to administer opioid drugs (e.g., morphine) intrathecally or epidurally for treatment of severe chronic intractable pain of malignant or nonmalignant origin in patients who have a life expectancy of at least 3 months and who have proven unresponsive to less invasive medical therapy as determined by the following criteria:

   • The patient's history must indicate that he/she would not respond adequately to non-invasive methods of pain control, such as systemic opioids (including attempts to eliminate physical and behavioral abnormalities which may cause an exaggerated reaction to pain); and
   • A preliminary trial of intraspinal opioid drug administration must be undertaken with a temporary intrathecal/epidural catheter to substantiate adequately acceptable pain relief and degree of side effects (including effects on the activities of daily living) and patient acceptance.

4. Coverage of Other Uses of Implanted Infusion Pumps .—Determinations may be made on coverage of other uses of implanted infusion pumps if the contractor's medical staff verifies that:

The drug is reasonable and necessary for the treatment of the individual patient;

   • It is medically necessary that the drug be administered by an implanted infusion pump; and
   • The FDA approved labeling for the pump must specify that the drug being administered and the purpose for which it is administered is an indicated use for the pump.

5. Implantation of Infusion Pump Is Contraindicated.—The implantation of an infusion pump is contraindicated in the following patients:

   • Patients with a known allergy or hypersensitivity to the drug being used (e.g., oral baclofen, morphine, etc.);
   • Patients who have an infection;
   • Patients whose body size is insufficient to support the weight and bulk of the device; and
   • Patients with other implanted programmable devices since crosstalk between devices may inadvertently change the prescription.

NOTE: Payment may also be made for drugs necessary for the effective use of an implantable infusion pump as long as the drug being used with the pump is itself reasonable and necessary for the patient's treatment.

The following indications for treatment using infusion pumps are not covered under medicare:

A. External Infusion Pumps.—

 1. Vancomycin (Effective for Services Beginning On or After September 1, 1996).—Medicare coverage of vancomycin as a durable medical equipment infusion pump benefit is not covered. There is insufficient evidence to support the necessity of using an external infusion pump, instead of a disposable elastomeric pump or the gravity drip method, to administer vancomycin in a safe and appropriate manner.

B. Implantable Infusion Pump.—

 1. Thromboembolic Disease (Effective for Services Performed On or After 9/26/84).—According to the Public Health Service, there is insufficient published clinical data to support the safety and effectiveness of the heparin implantable pump. Therefore, the use of an implantable infusion pump for infusion of heparin in the treatment of recurrent thromboembolic disease is not covered.
 2. Diabetes—Implanted infusion pumps for the infusion of insulin to treat diabetes is not covered. The data do not demonstrate that the pump provides effective administration of insulin.

60-15 SAFETY ROLLER (Effective for Claims Adjudicated On or After 6/3/85)

"Safety roller" is the generic name applied to devices for patients who cannot use standard wheeled walkers. They may be appropriate, and therefore covered, for some patients who are obese, have severe neurological disorders, or restricted use of one hand, which makes it impossible to use a wheeled walker that does not have the sophisticated braking system found on safety rollers.

In order to assure that payment is not made for a safety roller when a less expensive standard wheeled walker would satisfy the patient's medical needs, carriers refer safety roller claims to their medical consultants. The medical consultant determines whether some or all of the features provided in a safety roller are necessary, and therefore covered and reimbursable. If it is determined that the patient could use a standard wheeled walker, the charge for the safety roller is reduced to the charge of a standard wheeled walker.

Some obese patients who could use a standard wheeled walker if their weight did not exceed the walker's strength and stability limits can have it reinforced and its wheel base expanded. Such modifications are routine mechanical adjustments and justify a moderate surcharge. In these cases the carrier reduces the charge for the safety roller to the charge for the standard wheeled walker plus the surcharge for modifications.

In the case of patients with medical documentation showing severe neurological disorders or restricted use of one hand which makes it impossible for them to use a wheeled walker that does not have a sophisticated braking system, a reasonable charge for the safety roller may be determined without relating it to the reasonable charge for a standard wheeled walker. (Such reasonable charge should be developed in accordance with the instructions in Medicare Carriers Manual §§5010 and 5205.)

Cross reference: Carriers Manual §§2100ff., §60-9.

60-16 PNEUMATIC COMPRESSION DEVICES

Pneumatic compression devices consist of an inflatable garment for the arm or leg and an electrical pneumatic pump that fills the garment with compressed air. The garment is intermittently inflated and deflated with cycle times and pressures that vary between devices. Pneumatic devices are covered for the treatment of lymphedema or for the treatment of chronic venous insufficiency with venous stasis ulcers.

Lymphedema
Lymphedema is the swelling of subcutaneous tissues due to the accumulation of excessive lymph fluid. The accumulation of lymph fluid results from impairment to the normal clearing function of the lymphatic system and/or from an excessive production of lymph. Lymphedema is divided into two broad classes according to etiology. Primary lymphedema is a relatively uncommon, chronic condition which may be due to such causes as Milroy's Disease or congenital anomalies. Secondary

lymphedema, which is much more common, results from the destruction of or damage to formerly functioning lymphatic channels, such as surgical removal of lymph nodes or post radiation fibrosis, among other causes.

Pneumatic compression devices are covered in the home setting for the treatment of lymphedema if the patient has undergone a four-week trial of conservative therapy and the treating physician determines that there has been no significant improvement or if significant symptoms remain after the trial. The trial of conservative therapy must include use of an appropriate compression bandage system or compression garment, exercise, and elevation of the limb. The garment may be prefabricated or custom-fabricated but must provide adequate graduated compression.

Chronic Venous Insufficiency with Venous Stasis Ulcers
Chronic venous insufficiency (CVI) of the lower extremities is a condition caused by abnormalities of the venous wall and valves, leading to obstruction or reflux of blood flow in the veins. Signs of CVI include hyperpigmentation, stasis dermatitis, chronic edema, and venous ulcers.

Pneumatic compression devices are covered in the home setting for the treatment of CVI of the lower extremities only if the patient has one or more venous stasis ulcer(s) which have failed to heal after a 6 month trial of conservative therapy directed by the treating physician. The trial of conservative therapy must include a compression bandage system or compression garment, appropriate dressings for the wound, exercise, and elevation of the limb.

General Coverage Criteria
Pneumatic compression devices are covered only when prescribed by a physician and when they are used with appropriate physician oversight, i.e., physician evaluation of the patient's condition to determine medical necessity of the device, assuring suitable instruction in the operation of the machine, a treatment plan defining the pressure to be used and the frequency and duration of use, and ongoing monitoring of use and response to treatment.

The determination by the physician of the medical necessity of a pneumatic compression device must include (1) the patient's diagnosis and prognosis; (2) symptoms and objective findings, including measurements which establish the severity of the condition; (3) the reason the device is required, including the treatments which have been tried and failed; and (4) the clinical response to an initial treatment with the device. The clinical response includes the change in pre-treatment measurements, ability to tolerate the treatment session and parameters, and ability of the patient (or caregiver) to apply the device for continued use in the home.

The only time that a segmented, calibrated gradient pneumatic compression device (HCPCS code E0652) would be covered is when the individual has unique characteristics that prevent them from receiving satisfactory pneumatic compression treatment using a nonsegmented device in conjunction with a segmented appliance or a segmented compression device without manual control of pressure in each chamber.

Cross reference: §60-9.

60-17 CONTINUOUS POSITIVE AIRWAY PRESSURE (CPAP)

CPAP is a non-invasive technique for providing single levels of air pressure from a flow generator, via a nose mask, through the nares. The purpose is to prevent the collapse of the oropharyngeal walls and the obstruction of airflow during sleep, which occurs in obstructive sleep apnea (OSA).

Effective for services furnished between and including January 12, 1987 and March 31, 2002:

The diagnosis of OSA requires documentation of at least 30 episodes of apnea, each lasting a minimum of 10 seconds, during 6-7 hours of recorded sleep. The use of CPAP is covered under Medicare when used in adult patients with moderate or severe OSA for whom surgery is a likely alternative to CPAP.

Initial claims must be supported by medical documentation (separate documentation where electronic billing is used), such as a prescription written by the patient's attending physician, that specifies:

- a diagnosis of moderate or severe obstructive sleep apnea, and
- surgery is a likely alternative.

The claim must also certify that the documentation supporting a diagnosis of OSA (described above) is available.

Effective for services furnished on or after April 1, 2002:

The use of CPAP devices are covered under Medicare when ordered and prescribed by the licensed treating physician to be used in adult patients with OSA if either of the following criteria using the Apnea-Hypopnea Index (AHI) are met:

- AHI = 15 events per hour, or
- AHI = 5 and = 14 events per hour with documented symptoms of excessive daytime sleepiness, impaired cognition, mood disorders or insomnia, or documented hypertension, ischemic heart disease or history of stroke.

The AHI is equal to the average number of episodes of apnea and hypopnea per hour and must be based on a minimum of 2 hours of sleep recorded by polysomnography using actual recorded hours of sleep (i.e., the AHI may not be extrapolated or projected).

Apnea is defined as a cessation of airflow for at least 10 seconds. Hypopnea is defined as an abnormal respiratory event lasting at least 10 seconds with at least a 30% reduction in thoracoabdominal movement or airflow as compared to baseline, and with at least a 4% oxygen desaturation.

The polysomnography must be performed in a facility - based sleep study laboratory, and not in the home or in a mobile facility.

Initial claims for CPAP devices must be supported by information contained in the medical record indicating that the patient meets Medicare's stated coverage criteria.

Cross reference: §60-9.

60-18 HOSPITAL BEDS

A. General Requirements for Coverage of Hospital Beds.—A physician's prescription, and such additional documentation as the contractors' medical staffs may consider necessary, including medical records and physicians' reports, must establish the medical necessity for a hospital bed due to one of the following reasons:

- The patient's condition requires positioning of the body; e.g., to alleviate pain, promote good body alignment, prevent contractures, avoid respiratory infections, in ways not feasible in an ordinary bed; or
- The patient's condition requires special attachments that cannot be fixed and used on an ordinary bed.

B. Physician's Prescription.—The physician's prescription, which must accompany the initial claim, and supplementing documentation when required, must establish that a hospital bed is medically necessary. If the stated reason for the need for a hospital bed is the patient's condition requires positioning, the prescription or other documentation must describe the medical condition, e.g., cardiac disease, chronic obstructive pulmonary disease, quadriplegia or paraplegia, and also the severity and frequency of the symptoms of the condition, that necessitates a hospital bed for positioning.

If the stated reason for requiring a hospital bed is the patient's condition requires special attachments, the prescription must describe the patient's condition and specify the attachments that require a hospital bed.

C. Variable Height Feature.—In well documented cases, the contractors' medical staffs may determine that a variable height feature of a hospital bed, approved for coverage under subsection A above, is medically necessary and, therefore, covered, for one of the following conditions:

- Severe arthritis and other injuries to lower extremities; e.g., fractured hip. The condition requires the variable height feature to assist the patient to ambulate by enabling the patient to place his or her feet on the floor while sitting on the edge of the bed;
- Severe cardiac conditions. For those cardiac patients who are able to leave bed, but who must avoid the strain of "jumping" up or down;

- Spinal cord injuries, including quadriplegic and paraplegic patients, multiple limb amputee and stroke patients. For those patients who are able to transfer from bed to a wheelchair, with or without help; or
- Other severely debilitating diseases and conditions, if the variable height feature is required to assist the patient to ambulate.

D. Electric Powered Hospital Bed Adjustments.—Electric powered adjustments to lower and raise head and foot may be covered when the contractor's medical staff determines that the patient's condition requires frequent change in body position and/or there may be an immediate need for a change in body position (i.e., no delay can be tolerated) and the patient can operate the controls and cause the adjustments. Exceptions may be made to this last requirement in cases of spinal cord injury and brain damaged patients.

E. Side Rails.—If the patient's condition requires bed side rails, they can be covered when an integral part of, or an accessory to, a hospital bed.

Cross reference: Carriers Manual, §5015.4

60-19 AIR-FLUIDIZED BED (Effective for services rendered on or after: 07/30/90)

An air-fluidized bed uses warm air under pressure to set small ceramic beads in motion which simulate the movement of fluid. When the patient is placed in the bed, his body weight is evenly distributed over a large surface area which creates a sensation of "floating." Medicare payment for home use of the air-fluidized bed for treatment of pressure sores can be made if such use is reasonable and necessary for the individual patient.

A decision that use of an air-fluidized bed is reasonable and necessary requires that:

- The patient has a stage 3 (full thickness tissue loss) or stage 4 (deep tissue destruction) pressure sore;
- The patient is bedridden or chair bound as a result of severely limited mobility;
- In the absence of an air-fluidized bed, the patient would require institutionalization;
- The air-fluidized bed is ordered in writing by the patient's attending physician based upon a comprehensive assessment and evaluation of the patient after completion of a course of conservative treatment designed to optimize conditions that promote wound healing. This course of treatment must have been at least one month in duration without progression toward wound healing. This month of prerequisite conservative treatment may include some period in an institution as long as there is documentation available to verify that the necessary conservative treatment has been rendered.
- Use of wet-to-dry dressings for wound debridement, begun during the period of conservative treatment and which continue beyond 30 days, will not preclude coverage of air-fluidized bed. Should additional debridement again become necessary, while a patient is using an air-fluidized bed (after the first 30-day course of conservative treatment) that will not cause the air-fluidized bed to become non-covered. In all instances documentation verifying the continued need for the bed must be available.
- Conservative treatment must include:

    -Frequent repositioning of the patient with particular attention to relief of pressure over bony prominences (usually every 2 hours);
    -Use of a specialized support surface (Group II) designed to reduce pressure and shear forces on healing ulcers and to prevent new ulcer formation;
    -Necessary treatment to resolve any wound infection;
    -Optimization of nutrition status to promote wound healing;
    -Debridement by any means (including wet to dry dressings-which does not require an occlusive covering) to remove devitalized tissue from the wound bed;
    -Maintenance of a clean, moist bed of granulation tissue with appropriate moist dressings protected by an occlusive covering, while the wound heals.

- A trained adult caregiver is available to assist the patient with activities of daily living, fluid balance, dry skin care, repositioning, recognition and management of altered mental status, dietary needs, prescribed treatments, and management and support of the air-fluidized bed system and its problems such as leakage;
- A physician directs the home treatment regimen, and reevaluates and recertifies the need for the air-fluidized bed on a monthly basis; and
- All other alternative equipment has been considered and ruled out.

Home use of the air-fluidized bed is not covered under any of the following circumstances:

- The patient has coexisting pulmonary disease (the lack of firm back support makes coughing ineffective and dry air inhalation thickens pulmonary secretions);
- The patient requires treatment with wet soaks or moist wound dressings that are not protected with an impervious covering such as plastic wrap or other occlusive material; an air-fluidized bed;
- The caregiver is unwilling or unable to provide the type of care required by the patient on an air-fluidized bed;
- Structural support is inadequate to support the weight of the air-fluidized bed system (it generally weighs 1600 pounds or more);
- Electrical system is insufficient for the anticipated increase in energy consumption; or
- Other known contraindications exist.

Coverage of an air-fluidized bed is limited to the equipment itself. Payment for this covered item may only be made if the written order from the attending physician is furnished to the supplier prior to the delivery of the equipment. Payment is not included for the caregiver or for architectural adjustments such as electrical or structural improvement.

Cross reference: Carriers Manual, §5102.2.

60-21 INTRAPULMONARY PERCUSSIVE VENTILATOR (IPV)—NOT COVERED

IPV is a mechanized form of chest physical therapy. Instead of a therapist clapping or slapping the patient's chest wall, the IPV delivers mini-bursts (more than 200 per minute) of respiratory gasses to the lungs via a mouthpiece. Its intended purpose is to mobilize endobronchial secretions and diffuse patchy atelectasis. The patient controls variables such as inspiratory time, peak pressure and delivery rates.

Studies do not demonstrate any advantage of IPV over that achieved with good pulmonary care in the hospital environment and there are no studies in the home setting. There are no data to support the effectiveness of the device. Therefore, IPV in the home setting is not covered.

60-23 SPEECH GENERATING DEVICES

Effective January 1, 2001, augmentative and alternative communication devices or communicators, which are hereafter referred to as "speech generating devices" are now considered to fall within the DME benefit category established by §1861(n) of the Social Security Act. They may be covered if the contractor's medical staff determines that the patient suffers from a severe speech impairment and that the medical condition warrants the use of a device based on the following definitions.

Definition of Speech Generating Devices
Speech generating devices are defined as speech aids that provide an individual who has a severe speech impairment with the ability to meet his functional speaking needs. Speech generating are characterized by:

- Being a dedicated speech device, used solely by the individual who has a severe speech impairment;
- May have digitized speech output, using pre-recorded messages, less than or equal to 8 minutes recording time;
- May have digitized speech output, using pre-recorded messages, greater than 8 minutes recording time;
- May have synthesized speech output, which requires message formulation by spelling and device access by physical contact with the device-direct selection techniques;
- May have synthesized speech output, which permits multiple methods of message formulation and multiple methods of device access; or
- May be software that allows a laptop computer, desktop computer or personal digital assistant (PDA) to function as a speech generating device.

Devices that would not meet the definition of speech generating devices and therefore, do not fall within the scope of §1861(n) are characterized by:

- Devices that are not dedicated speech devices, but are devices that are capable of running software for purposes other than for speech generation, e.g., devices that can also run a word processing package, an accounting program, or perform other non-medical function.
- Laptop computers, desktop computers, or PDAs, which may be programmed to perform the same function as a speech generating device, are non-covered since they are not primarily medical in nature and do not meet the definition of DME. For this reason, they cannot be considered speech generating devices for Medicare coverage purposes.
- A device that is useful to someone without severe speech impairment is not considered a speech generating device for Medicare coverage purposes.

60-24 NON-IMPLANTABLE PELVIC FLOOR ELECTRICAL STIMULATOR

Non-implantable pelvic floor electrical stimulators provide neuromuscular electrical stimulation through the pelvic floor with the intent of strengthening and exercising pelvic floor musculature. Stimulation is generally delivered by vaginal or anal probes connected to an external pulse generator.

The methods of pelvic floor electrical stimulation vary in location, stimulus frequency (Hz), stimulus intensity or amplitude (mA), pulse duration (duty cycle), treatments per day, number of treatment days per week, length of time for each treatment session, overall time period for device use and between clinic and home settings. In general, the stimulus frequency and other parameters are chosen based on the patient's clinical diagnosis.

Pelvic floor electrical stimulation with a non-implantable stimulator is covered for the treatment of stress and/or urge urinary incontinence in cognitively intact patients who have failed a documented trial of pelvic muscle exercise (PME) training.

A failed trial of PME training is defined as no clinically significant improvement in urinary continence after completing 4 weeks of an ordered plan of pelvic muscle exercises designed to increase periurethral muscle strength.

60-25 NONCONTACT NORMOTHERMIC WOUND THERAPY (NNWT)

NNWT is a device reported to promote wound healing by warming a wound to a predetermined temperature. The device consists of a noncontact wound cover into which a flexible, battery powered, infrared heating card is inserted. There is insufficient scientific or clinical evidence to consider this device as reasonable and necessary for the treatment of wounds within the meaning of §1862(a)(1)(A) of the Social Security Act and will not be covered by Medicare.

65-1 HYDROPHILIC CONTACT LENSES

Hydrophilic contact lenses are eyeglasses within the meaning of the exclusion in §1862(a)(7) of the law and are not covered when used in the treatment of nondiseased eyes with spherical ametrophia, refractive astigmatism, and/or corneal astigmatism. Payment may be made under the prosthetic device benefit, however, for hydrophilic contact lenses when prescribed for an aphakic patient.

Contractors are authorized to accept an FDA letter of approval or other FDA published material as evidence of FDA approval.

(See §45-7 for coverage of a hydrophilic lens as a corneal bandage.) Cross-reference: Intermediary Manual, §§3110.3, 3110.4, 3151, and 3157; Carriers Manual, §§2130, 2320; Hospital Manual, §§228.3, 228.4, 260.1 and 260.7.

65-3 SCLERAL SHELL

Scleral shell (or shield) is a catchall term for different types of hard scleral contact lenses.

A scleral shell fits over the entire exposed surface of the eye as opposed to a corneal contact lens which covers only the central non-white area encompassing the pupil and iris. Where an eye has been rendered sightless and shrunken by inflammatory disease, a scleral shell may, among other things, obviate the need for surgical enucleation and prosthetic implant and act to support the surrounding orbital tissue.

In such a case, the device serves essentially as an artificial eye. In this situation, payment may be made for a scleral shell under §1861(s)(8) of the law.

Scleral shells are occasionally used in combination with artificial tears in the treatment of "dry eye" of diverse etiology. Tears ordinarily dry at a rapid rate, and are continually replaced by the lacrimal gland. When the lacrimal gland fails, the half-life of artificial tears may be greatly prolonged by the use of the scleral contact lens as a protective barrier against the drying action of the atmosphere. Thus, the difficult and sometimes hazardous process of frequent installation of artificial tears may be avoided. The lens acts in this instance to substitute, in part, for the functioning of the diseased lacrimal gland and would be covered as a prosthetic device in the rare case when it is used in the treatment of "dry eye."

Cross-reference: HCFA-Pub. 13-3, §§3110.4, 3110.5; HCFA-Pub. 14-3, §§2130, 2133; HCFA- Pub. 10, §§210.4, 211

65-5 ELECTRONIC SPEECH AIDS

Electronic speech aids are covered under Part B as prosthetic devices when the patient has had a laryngectomy or his larynx is permanently inoperative. There are two types of speech aids. One operates by placing a vibrating head against the throat; the other amplifies sound waves through a tube which is inserted into the user's mouth. A patient who has had radical neck surgery and/or extensive radiation to the anterior part of the neck would generally be able to use only the "oral tube" model or one of the more sensitive and more expensive "throat contact" devices.

Cross-reference: HCFA-Pub. 13-3, §3110.4; HCFA Pub. 14-3, §2130; HCFA-Pub. 10, §228.4

65-7 INTRAOCULAR LENSES (IOLs)

An intraocular lens, or pseudophakos, is an artificial lens which may be implanted to replace the natural lens after cataract surgery. Intraocular lens implantation services, as well as the lens itself, may be covered if reasonable and necessary for the individual. Implantation services may include hospital, surgical, and other medical services, including pre-implantation ultrasound (A-scan) eye measurement of one or both eyes.

Cross-reference: HCFA Pub. 13-3, §§3110.4, 3151, and 3157; HCFA Pub.14-3, §2130; HCFA Pub. 10, §228.4

65-8 ELECTRICAL NERVE STIMULATORS

Two general classifications of electrical nerve stimulators are employed to treat chronic intractable pain: peripheral nerve stimulators and central nervous system stimulators.

A. Implanted Peripheral Nerve Stimulators.—Payment may be made under the prosthetic device benefit for implanted peripheral nerve stimulators. Use of this stimulator involves implantation of electrodes around a selected peripheral nerve. The stimulating electrode is connected by an insulated lead to a receiver unit which is implanted under the skin at a depth not greater than 1/2 inch. Stimulation is induced by a generator connected to an antenna unit which is attached to the skin surface over the receiver unit. Implantation of electrodes requires surgery and usually necessitates an operating room.

NOTE: Peripheral nerve stimulators may also be employed to assess a patient's suitability for continued treatment with an electric nerve stimulator. As explained in §35-46, such use of the stimulator is covered as part of the total diagnostic service furnished to the beneficiary rather than as a prosthesis.

B. Central Nervous System Stimulators (Dorsal Column and Depth Brain Stimulators).—The implantation of central nervous system stimulators may be covered as therapies for the relief of chronic intractable pain, subject to the following conditions:

1. Types of Implantations.—There are two types of implantations covered by this instruction:

   a. Dorsal Column (Spinal Cord) Neurostimulation.—The surgical implantation of neurostimulator electrodes within the dura mater (endodural) or the percutaneous insertion of electrodes in the epidural space is covered.
   b. Depth Brain Neurostimulation.—The stereotactic implantation of electrodes in the deep brain (e.g., thalamus and periaqueductal gray matter) is covered.

2. Conditions for Coverage.—No payment may be made for the implantation of dorsal column or depth brain stimulators or services and supplies related to such implantation, unless all of the conditions listed below have been met:

   a. The implantation of the stimulator is used only as a late resort (if not a last resort) for patients with chronic intractable pain;
   b. With respect to item a, other treatment modalities (pharmacological, surgical, physical, or psychological therapies) have been tried and did not prove satisfactory, or are judged to be unsuitable or contraindicated for the given patient;
   c. Patients have undergone careful screening, evaluation and diagnosis by a multidisciplinary team prior to implantation. (Such screening must include psychological, as well as physical evaluation);
   d. All the facilities, equipment, and professional and support personnel required for the proper diagnosis, treatment training, and followup of the patient (including that required to satisfy item c) must be available; and
   e. Demonstration of pain relief with a temporarily implanted electrode precedes permanent implantation.

Contractors may find it helpful to work with PROs to obtain the information needed to apply these conditions to claims.

See Intermediary Manual, §3110.4 and §§35-20 and 35-27.

65-9 INCONTINENCE CONTROL DEVICE

A. Mechanical/Hydraulic Incontinence Control Devices.—Mechanical/hydraulic incontinence control devices are accepted as safe and effective in the management of urinary incontinence in patients with permanent anatomic and neurologic dysfunctions of the bladder. This class of devices achieves control of urination by compression of the urethra. The materials used and the success rate may vary somewhat from device to device. Such a device is covered when its use is reasonable and necessary for the individual patient.

B. Collagen Implant.—A collagen implant, which is injected into the submucosal tissues of the urethra and/or the bladder neck and into tissues adjacent to the urethra, is a prosthetic device used in the treatment of stress urinary incontinence resulting from intrinsic sphincter deficiency (ISD). ISD is a cause of stress urinary incontinence in which the urethral sphincter is unable to contract and generate sufficient resistance in the bladder, especially during stress maneuvers.

Prior to collagen implant therapy, a skin test for collagen sensitivity must be administered and evaluated over a 4 week period.

In male patients, the evaluation must include a complete history and physical examination and a simple cystometrogram to determine that the bladder fills and stores properly. The patient then is asked to stand upright with a full bladder and to cough or otherwise exert abdominal pressure on his bladder. If the patient leaks, the diagnosis of ISD is established.

In female patients, the evaluation must include a complete history and physical examination (including a pelvic exam) and a simple cystometrogram to rule out abnormalities of bladder compliance and abnormalities of urethral support. Following that determination, an abdominal leak point pressure (ALLP) test is performed. Leak point pressure, stated in cm H2O, is defined as the intra-abdominal pressure at which leakage occurs from the bladder (around a catheter) when the bladder has been filled with a minimum of 150 cc fluid. If the patient has an ALLP of less than 100 cm H2O, the diagnosis of ISD is established.

To use a collagen implant, physicians must have urology training in the use of a cystoscope and must complete a collagen implant training program.

Coverage of a collagen implant, and the procedure to inject it, is limited to the following types of patients with stress urinary incontinence due to ISD:

- Male or female patients with congenital sphincter weakness secondary to conditions such as myelomeningocele or epispadias;
- Male or female patients with acquired sphincter weakness secondary to spinal cord lesions;
- Male patients following trauma, including prostatectomy and/or radiation; and
- Female patients without urethral hypermobility and with abdominal leak point pressures of 100 cm H2O or less.

Patients whose incontinence does not improve with 5 injection procedures (5 separate treatment sessions) are considered treatment failures, and no further treatment of urinary incontinence by collagen implant is covered. Patients who have a reoccurrence of incontinence following successful treatment with collagen implants in the past (e.g., 6-12 months previously) may benefit from additional treatment sessions. Coverage of additional sessions may be allowed but must be supported by medical justification.

See Intermediary Manual, §3110.4.

65-10 ENTERAL AND PARENTERAL NUTRITIONAL THERAPY COVERED AS PROSTHETIC DEVICE (Effective for items and services furnished on or after 07-11-84.)

There are patients who, because of chronic illness or trauma, cannot be sustained through oral feeding. These people must rely on either enteral or parenteral nutritional therapy, depending upon the particular nature of their medical condition.

Coverage of nutritional therapy as a Part B benefit is provided under the prosthetic device benefit provision, which requires that the patient must have a permanently inoperative internal body organ or function thereof (See Intermediary Manual, §3110.4.) Therefore, enteral and parenteral nutritional therapy are not covered under Part B in situations involving temporary impairments. Coverage of such therapy, however, does not require a medical judgment that the impairment giving rise to the therapy will persist throughout the patient's remaining years. If the medical record, including the judgment of the attending physician, indicates that the impairment will be of long and indefinite duration, the test of permanence is considered met.

If the coverage requirements for enteral or parenteral nutritional therapy are met under the prosthetic device benefit provision, related supplies, equipment and nutrients are also covered under the conditions in the following paragraphs and the Intermediary Manual, §3110.4.

65-10.1 Parenteral Nutrition Therapy.—Daily parenteral nutrition is considered reasonable and necessary for a patient with severe pathology of the alimentary tract which does not allow absorption of sufficient nutrients to maintain weight and strength commensurate with the patient's general condition.

Since the alimentary tract of such a patient does not function adequately, an indwelling catheter is placed percutaneously in the subclavian vein and then advanced into the superior vena cava where intravenous infusion of nutrients is given for part of the day. The catheter is then plugged by the patient until the next infusion. Following a period of hospitalization, which is required to initiate parenteral nutrition and to train the patient in catheter care, solution preparation, and infusion technique, the parenteral nutrition can be provided safely and effectively in the patient's home by nonprofessional persons who have undergone special training. However, such persons cannot be paid for their services, nor is payment available for any services furnished by nonphysician professionals except as services furnished incident to a physician's service.

For parenteral nutrition therapy to be covered under Part B, the claim must contain a physician's written order or prescription and sufficient medical documentation to permit an independent conclusion that the requirements of the prosthetic device benefit are met and that parenteral nutrition therapy is medically necessary. An example of a condition that typically qualifies for coverage is a massive small bowel resection resulting in severe nutritional deficiency in spite of adequate oral intake. However, coverage of parenteral nutrition therapy for this and any other condition must be approved on an individual, case-by-case basis initially and at periodic intervals of no more than 3 months by the carrier's medical consultant or specially trained staff, relying on such medical and other documentation as the carrier may require. If the claim involves an infusion pump, sufficient evidence must be provided to support a determination of medical necessity for the pump. Program payment for the pump is based on the reasonable charge for the simplest model that meets the medical needs of the patient as established by medical documentation.

Nutrient solutions for parenteral therapy are routinely covered. However, Medicare pays for no more than one month's supply of nutrients at any one time. Payment for the nutrients is based on the reasonable charge for the solution components unless the medical record, including a signed statement from the attending physician, establishes that the beneficiary, due to his/her physical or mental state, is unable to safely or effectively mix the solution and there is no family member or other person who can do so. Payment will be on the basis of the reasonable charge for more expensive pre-mixed solutions only under the latter circumstances.

65-10.2 Enteral Nutrition Therapy.—Enteral nutrition is considered reasonable and necessary for a patient with a functioning gastrointestinal tract who, due to pathology to or nonfunction of the structures that normally permit food to reach the digestive tract, cannot maintain weight and strength commensurate with his or her general condition. Enteral therapy may be given by nasogastric, jejunostomy, or gastrostomy tubes and can be provided safely and effectively in the home by nonprofessional persons who have undergone special training. However, such persons cannot be paid for their services, nor is payment available for any services furnished by nonphysician professionals except as services furnished incident to a physician's service.

Typical examples of conditions that qualify for coverage are head and neck cancer with reconstructive surgery and central nervous system disease leading to interference with the neuromuscular mechanisms of ingestion of such severity that the beneficiary cannot be maintained with oral feeding. However, claims for Part B coverage of enteral nutrition therapy for these and any other conditions must be approved on an individual, case-by-case basis. Each claim must contain a physician's written order or prescription and sufficient medical documentation (e.g., hospital records, clinical findings from the attending physician) to permit an independent conclusion that the patient's condition meets the requirements of the prosthetic device benefit and that enteral nutrition therapy is medically necessary. Allowed claims are to be reviewed at periodic intervals of no more than 3 months by the contractor's medical consultant or specially trained staff, and additional medical documentation considered necessary is to be obtained as part of this review.

Medicare pays for no more than one month's supply of enteral nutrients at any one time.

If the claim involves a pump, it must be supported by sufficient medical documentation to establish that the pump is medically necessary, i.e., gravity feeding is not satisfactory due to aspiration, diarrhea, dumping syndrome. Program payment for the pump is based on the reasonable charge for the simplest model that meets the medical needs of the patient as established by medical documentation.

65-10.3 Nutritional Supplementation.—Some patients require supplementation of their daily protein and caloric intake. Nutritional supplements are often given as a medicine between meals to boost protein-caloric intake or the mainstay of a daily nutritional plan. Nutritional supplementation is not covered under Medicare Part B.

65-14 COCHLEAR IMPLANTATION

A cochlear implant device is an electronic instrument, part of which is implanted surgically to stimulate auditory nerve fibers, and part of which is worn or carried by the individual to capture, analyze and code sound. Cochlear implant devices are available in single channel and multi-channel models. The purpose of implanting the device is to provide an awareness and identification of sounds and to facilitate communication for persons who are profoundly hearing impaired.
Medicare coverage is provided only for those patients who meet all of the following selection guidelines.

A. General.—

- Diagnosis of bilateral severe-to-profound sensorineural hearing impairment with limited benefit from appropriate hearing (or vibrotactile) aids;
- Cognitive ability to use auditory clues and a willingness to undergo an extended program of rehabilitation;
- Freedom from middle ear infection, an accessible cochlear lumen that is structurally suited to implantation, and freedom from lesions in the auditory nerve and acoustic areas of the central nervous system;
- No contraindications to surgery; and
- The device must be used in accordance with the FDA-approved labeling.

B. Adults.—Cochlear implants may be covered for adults (over age 18) for prelinguistically, perilinguistically, and postlinguistically deafened adults. Postlinguistically deafened adults must demonstrate test scores of 30 percent or less on sentence recognition scores from tape recorded tests in the patient's best listening condition.

C. Children.—Cochlear implants may be covered for prelinguistically and postlinguistically deafened children aged 2 through 17. Bilateral profound sensorineural deafness must be demonstrated by the inability to improve on age appropriate closed-set word identification tasks with amplification.

65-16 TRACHEOSTOMY SPEAKING VALVE

A trachea tube has been determined to satisfy the definition of a prosthetic device, and the tracheostomy speaking valve is an add on to the trachea tube which may be considered a medically necessary accessory that enhances the function of the tube. In other words, it makes the system a better prosthesis. As such, a tracheostomy speaking valve is covered as an element of the trachea tube which makes the tube more effective.

70-1 CORSET USED AS HERNIA SUPPORT

A hernia support (whether in the form of a corset or truss) which meets the definition of a brace is covered under Part B under §1861(s)(9) of the Act.

See Intermediary Manual, §3110.5; Medicare Carriers Manual, §2133; and Hospital Manual, §228.5.

70-2 SYKES HERNIA CONTROL

Based on professional advice, it has been determined that the Sykes hernia control (a spring-type, U-shaped, strapless truss) is not functionally more beneficial than a conventional truss. Make program reimbursement for this device only when an ordinary truss would be covered. (Like all trusses, it is only of benefit when dealing with a reducible hernia). Thus, when a charge for this item is substantially in excess of that which would be reasonable for a conventional truss used for the same condition, base reimbursement on the reasonable charges for the conventional truss.

See Intermediary Manual, §3110.5; Medicare Carriers Manual, §2133; and Hospital Manual, §228.5.

MEDICARE CARRIERS MANUAL (MCM) REFERENCES

The following Medicare references refer to policy issues identified in the main body of the HCPCS code section. Medicare Carriers Manual references are identified with the term MCM: followed by the reference number(s).

2000 COVERED MEDICAL AND OTHER HEALTH SERVICES

The supplementary medical insurance plan covers expenses incurred for the following medical and other health services:

1. Physician's services, including surgery, consultation, and office, and institutional calls, and services and supplies furnished incident to a physician's professional service;
2. Outpatient hospital services furnished incident to physicians services;
3. Outpatient diagnostic services furnished by a hospital;
4. Outpatient physical therapy; outpatient speech pathology services;
5. Diagnostic X-ray tests, laboratory tests, and other diagnostic tests;
6. X-ray, radium, and radioactive isotope therapy;
7. Surgical dressings, and splints, casts, and other devices used for reduction of fractures and dislocations;
8. Rental or purchase of durable medical equipment for use in the patient's home;
9. Ambulance service;
10. Prosthetic devices which replace all or part of an internal body organ;

11. Leg, arm, back and neck braces and artificial legs, arms, and eyes;
12. Certain medical supplies used in connection with home dialysis delivery systems;
13. Rural health clinic (RHC) services.
14. Ambulatory surgical center (ASC) services.

(See §2255 for provisions regarding supplementary medical insurance coverage of certain of these services when furnished to hospital and SNF inpatients.)

Supplementary medical insurance also provides coverage for home health visits for which the intermediary makes payment on the basis of the reasonable cost. Outpatient hospital services are also reimbursed by the intermediary.

Some medical services may be considered for coverage under more than one of the above enumerated categories. For example, EKGs can be covered as physician's services, services incident to a physician's service or as other diagnostic tests. It is sufficient to determine that the requirements for coverage under one category are met to permit payment.

Payment for physician services and medical and other health services rendered to beneficiaries is made on a reasonable charge basis. Make payment to the beneficiary, or the physician or supplier who renders the service, depending on whether the itemized bill or assignment method is used. Payment for medical services performed by a provider-based physician is made to the physician or beneficiary or, when the physician authorizes it, to the provider. When covered medical and other health services are furnished by a nonparticipating skilled nursing facility, make payment to the SNF or to the beneficiary on the basis of the reasonable charge.

An organization which furnishes medical and other health services on a prepayment basis may elect to be paid on the basis of reasonable costs in lieu of reasonable charges.

Payment may not be made under Part B for services furnished an individual if he is entitled to have payment made for those services under Part A. An individual is considered entitled to have payment made under Part A if the expenses incurred were used to satisfy a Part A deductible or coinsurance amount, or if payment would be made under Part A except for the lack of a request for payment or physician certification.

When covered Part B services are furnished by a participating hospital, skilled nursing facility, or home health agency, the intermediary makes payment on a reasonable cost basis to the provider only. Outpatient physical therapy or speech pathology providers are reimbursed on a reasonable cost basis by the designated intermediary or carrier.

Where covered Part B services are furnished by a nonparticipating hospital, the emergency intermediary makes payment on the basis of reasonable charges to the hospital or to the patient.

Membership dues, subscription fees, charges for service policies, insurance premium and other payments analogous to premiums which entitle enrollees to services or to repairs or replacement of devices or equipment or parts therefore without charge or at a reduced charge, are not considered expenses incurred for covered items or services furnished under such contracts or undertakings. Examples of such arrangements are memberships in ambulance companies, insurance for replacement of prosthetic lenses, and service contracts for durable medical equipment.

2005.1 Physicians' Expense for Surgery, Childbirth, and Treatment for Infertility

A. Surgery and Childbirth.—Skilled medical management is appropriate throughout the events of pregnancy, beginning with diagnosis, continuing through delivery and ending after the necessary postnatalcare. Similarly, in the event of termination of pregnancy,regardless of whether terminated spontaneously or for therapeutic reasons (i.e., where the life of the mother would be endangered if the fetus were brought to term), the need for skilled medical management and/or medical services is equally important as in those cases carried to full term.After the infant is delivered and is a separate individual, items and services furnished to the infant are not covered on the basis of the mother's eligibility.

Most surgeons and obstetricians bill patients an all inclusive package charge intended to cover all services associated with the surgical procedure or delivery of the child. All expenses for surgical and obstetrical care, including preoperative/prenatal examinations and tests and postoperative/postnatal services are considered incurred on the date of surgery or delivery, as appropriate. This policy applies whether the physician bills on a package charge basis, or itemizes his/her bill separately for these items.

Occasionally, a physician's bill may include charges for additional services not directly related to the surgical procedure or the delivery. Such charges are considered incurred on the date the additional services are furnished.

The above policy applies only where the charges are imposed by one physician or by a clinic on behalf of a group of physicians. Where charges are imposed by more than one physician for surgical or obstetrical services, all preoperative/prenatal and postoperative/postnatal services performed by the physician who performed the surgery or delivery are considered incurred on the date of the surgery or delivery. Expenses for services rendered by other physicians are considered incurred on the date they were performed.

B. Treatment for Infertility.—Reasonable and necessary services associated with treatment forinfertility are covered under Medicare. Infertility is a condition sufficiently at variance with the usual state of health to make it appropriate for a person who normally is expected to be fertile to seek medical consultation and treatment. Coordinate with PROs to see that utilization guidelines are established for this treatment if inappropriate utilization or abuse is suspected.

2049 DRUGS AND BIOLOGICALS

The Medicare program provides limited benefits for outpatient drugs. The program covers drugs that are furnished "incident to" a physician's service provided that the drugs are not usually self-administered by the patients who take them.

Generally, drugs and biologicals are covered only if all of the following requirements are met:

- They meet the definition of drugs or biologicals (see §2049.1);
- They are of the type that are not usually self-administered by the patients who take them. (See §2049.2);
- They meet all the general requirements for coverage of items as incident to a physician's services (see § §2050.1 and 2050.3);
- They are reasonable and necessary for the diagnosis or treatment of the illness or injury for which they are administered according to accepted standards of medical practice (see §2049.4);

- They are not excluded as immunizations (see §2049.4.B); and
- They have not been determined by the FDA to be less than effective. (See §2049.4 D.)

Drugs that are usually self-administered by the patient, such as those in pill form, or are used for self-injection, are generally not covered by Part B. However, there are a limited number of self-administered drugs that are covered because the Medicare statute explicitly provides coverage. Examples of self-administered drugs that are covered include blood clotting factors, drugs used in immunosuppressive therapy, erythropoietin for dialysis patients, osteoporosis drugs for certain homebound patients, and certain oral cancer drugs.

(See §§2100.5 and 2130.D for coverage of drugs which are necessary to the effective use of DME or prosthetic devices.)

2049.2 Determining Self-Administration of Drug or Biological.—Whether a drug or biological is of a type which cannot be self-administered is based on the usual method of administration of the form of that drug or biological as furnished by the physician.

Whole blood is a biological which cannot be self-administered and is covered when furnished incident to a physician's services. Payment may also be made for blood fractions if all coverage requirements are satisfied. (See §2455 on Part B blood deductible.)

Medicare carriers have discretion in applying the criteria in this instruction in determining whether drugs are subject to this exclusion in their local areas. Carriers are to follow the instructions below when applying the exclusion for drugs that are usually self-administered by the patient. Each individual contractor must make its own individual determination on each drug. Contractors must continue to apply the policy that not only the drug is medically reasonable and necessary for any individual claim, but also that the route of administration is medically reasonable and necessary. That is, if a drug is available in both oral and injectable forms, the injectable form of the drug must be medically reasonable and necessary as compared to using the oral form. (See §2049.4.2)

For certain injectable drugs, it will be apparent due to the nature of the condition(s) for which they are administered or the usual course of treatment for those conditions, they are, or are not, usually self-administered. For example, an injectable drug used to treat migraine headaches is usually self-administered. On the other hand, an injectable drug, administered at the same time as chemotherapy, used to treat anemia secondary to chemotherapy is not usually self-administered.

Administered—The term "administered" refers only to the physical process by which the drug enters the patient's body. It does not refer to whether the process is supervised by a medical professional (for example, to observe proper technique or side-effects of the drug). Only injectable (including intravenous) drugs are eligible for inclusion under the "incident to" benefit. Other routes of administration including, but not limited to, oral drugs, suppositories, topical medications are all considered to be usually self-administered by the patient.

Usually—In arriving at a single determination as to whether a drug is usually self-administered, contractors should make a separate determination for each indication for a drug as to whether that drug is usually self-administered.

After determining whether a drug is usually self-administered for each indication, contractors should determine the relative contribution of each indication to total use of the drug (i.e., weighted average) in order to make an overall determination as to whether the drug is usually self-administered. For example, if a drug has three indications, is not self-administered for the first indication, but is self-administered for the second and third indications, and the first indication makes up 40% of total usage, the second indication makes up 30% of total usage, and the third indication makes up 30% of total usage, then the drug would be considered usually self-administered.

Reliable statistical information on the extent of self-administration by the patient may not always be available. Consequently, we offer the following guidance for each contractor's consideration in making this determination in the absence of such data:

1. Absent evidence to the contrary, drugs delivered intravenously should be presumed to be not usually self-administered by the patient.
2. Absent evidence to the contrary, drugs delivered by intramuscular injection should be presumed to be not usually self-administered by the patient. (For example, interferon beta-1a, tradename Avonex, when delivered by intramuscular injection is not usually self administered by the patient.) The contractor may consider the depth and nature of the particular intramuscular injection in applying this presumption.
3. Absent evidence to the contrary, drugs delivered by subcutaneous injection should be presumed to be self-administered by the patient.

In applying these presumptions, contractors should examine the use of the particular drug and consider the following factors:

A. Acute condition.—For the purposes of determining whether a drug is usually self-administered, an acute condition means a condition that begins over a short time period, is likely to be of short duration and/or the expected course of treatment is for a short, finite interval. A course of treatment consisting of scheduled injections lasting less than two weeks, regardless of frequency or route of administration, is considered acute. Evidence to support this may include Food and Drug administration (FDA) approval language, package inserts, drug compendia, and other information.

B. Frequency of administration.—How often is the injection given? For example, if the drug is administered once per month, it is less likely to be self-administered by the patient. However, if it is administered once or more per week, it is likely that the drug is self-administered by the patient.

By the patient—The term "by the patient" means Medicare beneficiaries as a collective whole. Include only the patients themselves and not other individuals (that is, do not include spouses, friends, or other care-givers). Base your determination on whether the drug is self-administered by the patient a majority of the time that the drug is used on an outpatient basis by Medicare beneficiaries for medically necessary indications. Ignore all instances when the drug is administered on an inpatient basis. Make this determination on a drug-by-drug basis, not on a beneficiary-by-beneficiary basis. In evaluating whether beneficiaries as a collective whole self-administer, do not consider individual beneficiaries who do not have the capacity to self-administer any drug due to a condition other than the condition for which they are taking the drug in question. For example, an individual afflicted with paraplegia or advanced dementia would not have the capacity to self-administer any injectable drug, so such individuals would not be included in the population upon which the determination for self-administration by the patient was based. Note that some individuals afflicted with a less severe stage of an otherwise debilitating condition would be included in the population upon which the determination for "self-administered by the patient" was based; for example, an early onset of dementia.

Evidentiary Criteria —In making a self-administration determination, contractors are only required to consider the following types of evidence: peer reviewed medical literature, standards of medical practice, evidence-based practice guidelines, FDA approved label, and package inserts. Contractors may also consider other evidence submitted by interested individuals or groups subject to their judgment.

Contractors should also use these evidentiary criteria when reviewing requests for making a determination as to whether a drug is usually self-administered, and requests for reconsideration of a pending or published determination.

Please note that prior to August 1, 2002, one of the principal factors used to determine whether a drug was subject to the self-administered exclusion was whether the FDA label contained instructions for self-administration. However, we note that under the standard in effect after August 1, 2002, the fact that the FDA label includes instructions for self-administration is not, by itself, a determining factor that a drug is subject to this exclusion.

Provider Notice of Non-Covered Drugs—Contractors must describe the process they will use to determine whether a drug is usually self-administered and thus does not meet the "incident to" benefit category. Contractors must place a description of the process on their Web site. Contractors must publish a list of the injectable drugs that are subject to the self-administered exclusion on their Web site, including the data and rationale that led to the determination. Contractors will report the workload associated with developing new coverage statements in CAFM 21208.

Contractors must provide notice 45 days prior to the date that these drugs will not be covered. During the 45-day time period, contractors will maintain existing medical review and payment procedures. After the 45-day notice, contractors may deny payment for the drugs subject to the notice.

Contractors must not develop local medical review policies (LMRPs) for this purpose because further elaboration to describe drugs that do not meet the 'incident to' and the 'not usually self-administered' provisions of the statute are unnecessary. Current LMRPs based solely on these provisions must be withdrawn. LMRPs that address the self-administered exclusion and other information may be reissued absent the self-administered drug exclusion material. Contractors will report this workload in CAFM 21206. However, contractors may continue to use and write LMRPs to describe reasonable and necessary uses of drugs that are not usually self-administered.

Conferences Between Contractors—Contractors' Medical Directors may meet and discuss whether a drug is usually self-administered without reaching a formal consensus. Each contractor uses its discretion as to whether or not it will participate in such discussions. Each contractor must make its own individual determinations, except that fiscal intermediaries may, at their discretion, follow the determinations of the local carrier with respect to the self-administered exclusion.

Beneficiary Appeals—If a beneficiary's claim for a particular drug is denied because the drug is subject to the "self-administered drug" exclusion, the beneficiary may appeal the denial. Because it is a "benefit category" denial and not a denial based on medical necessity, an Advance Beneficiary Notice (ABN) is not applicable. A "benefit category" denial (i.e., a denial based on the fact that there is no benefit category under which the drug may be covered) does not trigger the financial liability protection provisions of Limitation On Liability [under §1879 of the Act]. Therefore, physicians or providers may charge the beneficiary for an excluded drug. See Chapter XV of the Medicare Carrier Manual for more detail on the appeals process.

Provider and Physician Appeals—A physician accepting assignment may appeal a denial under the provisions found in §12000 of the Medicare Carriers Manual. See Chapter XV of the Medicare Carrier Manual for more detail on the appeals process.

Reporting Requirements—Each carrier must report to CMS, every September 1 and March 1, its complete list of injectable drugs that the contractor has determined are excluded when furnished incident to a physician's service on the basis that the drug is usually self-administered. We anticipate that contractors will review injectable drugs on a rolling basis and publish their list of excluded drugs as it is developed. For example, contractors should not wait to publish this list until every drug has been reviewed. Contractors must send their exclusion list to the following e-mail address: drugdata@cms.hhs.gov. Below is an example of the Microsoft Excel template that should be submitted to CMS.

Carrier Name	State	Carrier ID #	HCPCS	Descriptor	Effective date of exclusion	End date of exclusion	Comments

2049.3 Incident-to Requirements.—In order for Medicare payment to be made for a drug, the "incident to" requirements are met. "Incident to" a physician's professional service means that the services are furnished as an integral, although incidental, part of the physician's personal professional services in the course of diagnosis or treatment of an illness or injury. See §2050.1 for more detail on incident-to requirements.

In order to meet all the general requirements for coverage under the incident-to provision, an FDA approved drug or biological must be furnished by a physician and administered by him/her or by auxiliary personnel employed by him/her under his/her personal supervision. The charge, if any, for the drug or biological must be included in the physician's bill, and the cost of the drug or biological must represent an expense to the physician. Drugs and biologicals furnished by other health professionals may also meet these requirements. (See §§2154, 2156, 2158 and 2160 for specific instructions.)

2049.4 Reasonableness and Necessity.—Use of the drug or biological must be safe and effective and otherwise reasonable and necessary. (See §2303.) Drugs or biologicals approved for marketing by the Food and Drug Administration (FDA) are considered safe and effective for purposes of this requirement when used for indications specified on the labeling. Therefore, you may pay for the use of an FDA approved drug or biological, if:

- It was injected on or after the date of the FDA's approval;
- It is reasonable and necessary for the individual patient; and
- All other applicable coverage requirements are met.

Deny coverage for drugs and biologicals which have not received final marketing approval by the FDA unless you receive instructions from CMS to the contrary. For specific guidelines on coverage of Group C cancer drugs, see the Coverage Issues Manual.

If there is reason to question whether the FDA has approved a drug or biological for marketing, obtain satisfactory evidence of FDA's approval. Acceptable evidence includes a copy of the FDA's letter to the drug's manufacturer approving the new drug application (NDA); or listing of the drug or biological in the FDA's Approved Drug Products or FDA Drug and Device Product Approvals; or a copy of the manufacturer's package insert, approved by the FDA as part of the labeling of the drug, containing its recommended uses and dosage, as well as possible adverse reactions and recommended precautions in using it. When necessary, the RO may be able to help in obtaining information.

An unlabeled use of a drug is a use that is not included as an indication on the drug's label as approved by the FDA. FDA approved drugs used for indications other than what is indicated on the official label may be covered under Medicare if the carrier determines the use to be medically accepted, taking into consideration the major drug compendia, authoritive medical literature and/or accepted standards of medical practice. In the case of drugs used in an anti-cancer chemotherapeutic regimen, unlabeled uses are covered for a medically accepted indication as defined in §2049.4.C.

Determinations as to whether medication is reasonable and necessary for an individual patient should be made on the same basis as all other such determinations (i.e., with the advice of medical consultants and with reference to accepted standards of medical practice and the medical circumstances of the individual case). The following guidelines identify three categories with specific examples of situations in which medications would not be reasonable and necessary according to accepted standards of medical practice.

1. Not for Particular Illness.—Medications given for a purpose other than the treatment of a particular condition, illness, or injury are not covered (except for certain immunizations). Exclude the charge for medications, e.g., vitamins, given simply for the general good and welfare of the patient and not as accepted therapy for a particular illness.

2. Injection Method Not Indicated.—Medication given by injection (parenterally) is not covered if standard medical practice indicates that the administration of the medication by mouth(orally) is effective and is an accepted or preferred method of administration. For example, the accepted standards of medical practice for the treatment of certain diseases is to initiate therapy with parenteral penicillin and to complete therapy with oral penicillin. Exclude the entire charge for penicillin injections given after the initiation of therapy if oral penicillin is indicated unless there are special medical circumstances which justify additional injections.

3. Excessive Medications.—Medications administered for treatment of a disease which exceed the frequency or duration of injections indicated by accepted standards of medical practice are not covered. For example, the accepted standard of medical practice in the maintenance treatment of pernicious anemia is one vitamin B-12 injection per month. Exclude the entire charge for injections given in excess of this frequency unless there are special medical circumstances which justify additional injections.

Supplement the guidelines as necessary with guidelines concerning appropriate use of specific injections in other situations. Use the guidelines to screen out questionable cases for special review, further development or denial when the injection billed for would not be reasonable and necessary. Coordinate any type of drug treatment review with the PRO.

If a medication is determined not to be reasonable and necessary for diagnosis or treatment of an illness or injury according to these guidelines, exclude the entire charge (i.e., for both the drug and its administration). Also exclude from payment any charges for other services (such as office visits) which were primarily for the purpose of administering a noncovered injection (i.e., an injection that is not reasonable and necessary for the diagnosis or treatment of an illness or injury).

A. Antigens.—Payment may be made for a reasonable supply of antigens that have been prepared for a particular patient if: (1) the antigens are prepared by a physician who is a doctor of medicine or osteopathy, and (2) the physician who prepared the antigens has examined the patient and has determined a plan of treatment and a dosage regimen. Antigens must be administered in accordance with the plan of treatment and by a doctor of medicine or osteopathy or by a properly instructed person (who could be the patient) under the supervision of the doctor. The associations of allergists that HCFA consulted advised that a reasonable supply of antigens is considered to be not more than a 12-week supply of antigens that has been prepared for a particular patient at any one time. The purpose of the reasonable supply limitation is to assure that the antigens retain their potency and effectiveness over the period in which they are to be administered to the patient. (See §§2005.2 and 2050.2.)

B. Immunizations.—Vaccinations or inoculations are excluded as immunizations unless they are directly related to the treatment of an injury or direct exposure to a disease or condition, such as anti-rabies treatment, tetanus antitoxin or booster vaccine, botulin antitoxin, antivenin sera, or immune globulin. In the absence of injury or direct exposure, preventive immunization (vaccination or inoculation) against such diseases as smallpox, polio, diphtheria, etc., is not covered. However, pneumococcal, hepatitis B, and influenza virus vaccines are exceptions to this rule. (See items 1, 2, and 3.) In cases where a vaccination or inoculation is excluded from coverage, deny the entire charge.

1. Furnished on or after May 1, 1981, the Medicare Part B program covers pneumococcal pneumonia vaccine and its administration when furnished in compliance with any applicable State law by any provider of services or any entity or individual with a supplier number. This includes revaccination of patients at highest risk of pneumococcal infection. Typically, these vaccines are administered once in a lifetime except for persons at highest risk. Effective July 1, 2000, Medicare does not require for coverage purposes that the vaccine must be ordered by a doctor of medicine or osteopathy. Therefore, the beneficiary may receive the vaccine upon request without a physician's order and without physician supervision.

An initial vaccine may be administered only to persons at high risk (see below) of pneumococcal disease. Revaccination may be administered only to persons at highest risk of serious Pneumococcal Pneumonia Vaccinations.—Effective for services pneumococcal infection and those likely to have a rapid decline in pneumococcal antibody levels, provided that at least 5 years have passed since receipt of a previous dose of pneumococcal vaccine.

Persons at high risk for whom an initial vaccine may be administered include all people age 65 and older; immunocompetent adults who are at increased risk of pneumococcal disease or its complications because of chronic illness (e.g., cardiovascular disease, pulmonary disease, diabetes mellitus, alcoholism, cirrhosis, or cerebrospinal fluid leaks); and individuals with compromised immune systems (e.g., splenic dysfunction or anatomic asplenia, Hodgkin's disease, lymphoma, multiple myeloma, chronic renal failure, HIV infection, nephrotic syndrome, sickle cell disease, or organ transplantation).

Persons at highest risk and those most likely to have rapid declines in antibody levels are those for whom revaccination may be appropriate. This group includes persons with functional or anatomic asplenia (e.g., sickle cell disease, splenectomy), HIV infection, leukemia, lymphoma, Hodgkin's disease, multiple myeloma, generalized malignancy, chronic renal failure, nephrotic syndrome, or other conditions associated with immunosuppression such as organ or bone marrow transplantation, and those receiving immuno-suppressive chemotherapy. Routine revaccination of people age 65 or older who are not at highest risk is not appropriate.

Those administering the vaccine should not require the patient to present an immunization record prior to administering the pneumococcal vaccine, nor should they feel compelled to review the patient's complete medical record if it is not available. Instead, provided that the patient is competent, it is acceptable for them to rely on the patient's verbal history to determine prior vaccination status. If the patient is uncertain about their vaccination history in the past 5 years, the vaccine should be given. However, if the patient is certain he/she was vaccinated in the last 5 years, the vaccine should not be given. If the patient is certain that the vaccine was given and that more than 5 years have passed since receipt of the previous dose, revaccination is not appropriate unless the patient is at highest risk.

2. Hepatitis B Vaccine.—With the enactment of P.L. 98-369, coverage under Part B was extended to hepatitis B vaccine and its administration, furnished to a Medicare beneficiary who is at high or intermediate risk of contracting hepatitis B. This coverage is effective for services furnished on or after September 1, 1984.

High-risk groups currently identified include (see exception below):

- End stage renal disease (ESRD) patients;
- Hemophiliacs who receive Factor VIII or IX concentrates;
- Clients of institutions for the mentally retarded;
- Persons who live in the same household as an Hepatitis B Virus (HBV) carrier;
- Homosexual men; and
- Illicit injectable drug abusers.

Intermediate risk groups currently identified include:

- Staff in institutions for the mentally retarded; and
- Workers in health care professions who have frequent contact with blood or blood-derived body fluids during routine work.

EXCEPTION: Persons in the above-listed groups would not be considered at high or intermediate risk of contracting hepatitis B, however, if there is laboratory evidence positive for antibodies to hepatitis B. (ESRD patients are routinely tested for hepatitis B antibodies as part of their continuing monitoring and therapy.)

For Medicare program purposes, the vaccine may be administered upon the order of a doctor of medicine or osteopathy by home health agencies, skilled nursing facilities, ESRD facilities, hospital outpatient departments, persons recognized under the incident to physicians' services provision of law, and doctors of medicine and osteopathy.

A charge separate from the ESRD composite rate will be recognized and paid for administration of the vaccine to ESRD patients.

For ESRD laboratory tests, see Coverage Issues Manual, §50-17.

3. Influenza Virus Vaccine.—Effective for services furnished on or after May 1, 1993, the Medicare Part B program covers influenza virus vaccine and its administration when furnished in compliance with any applicable State law by any provider of services or any entity or individual with a supplier number. Typically, these vaccines are administered once a year in the fall or winter. Medicare does not require for coverage purposes that the vaccine must be ordered by a doctor of medicine or osteopathy. Therefore, the beneficiary may receive the vaccine upon request without a physician's order and without physician supervision.

D. Unlabeled Use For Anti-Cancer Drugs.—Effective January 1, 1994, unlabeled uses of FDA approved drugs and biologicals used in an anti-cancer chemotherapeutic regimen for a medically accepted indication are evaluated under the conditions described in this paragraph. A regimen is a combination of anti-cancer agents which has been clinically recognized for the treatment of a specific type of cancer. An example of a drug regimen is: Cyclophosphamide + vincristine + prednisone (CVP) for non-Hodgkin's lymphoma.

In addition to listing the combination of drugs for a type of cancer, there may be a different regimen or combinations which are used at different times in the history of the cancer (induction, prophylaxis of CNS involvement, post remission, and relapsed or refractory disease). A protocol may specify the combination of drugs, doses, and schedules for administration of the drugs. For purposes of this provision, a cancer treatment regimen includes drugs used to treat toxicities or side effects of the cancer treatment regimen when the drug is administered incident to a chemotherapy treatment. Contractors must not deny coverage based solely on the absence of FDA approved labeling for the use, if the use is supported by one of the following and the use is not listed as "not indicated" in any of the three compendia. (See note at the end of this subsection.)

1. American Hospital Formulary Service Drug Information.--Drug monographs are arranged in alphabetical order within therapeutic classifications. Within the text of the monograph, information concerning indications is provided, including both labeled and unlabeled uses. Unlabeled uses are identified with daggers. The text must be analyzed to make a determination whether a particular use is supported.
2. American Medical Association Drug Evaluations.--Drug evaluations are organized into sections and chapters that are based on therapeutic classifications. The evaluation of a drug provides information concerning indications, including both labeled and unlabeled uses. Unlabeled uses are not specifically identified as such. The text must be analyzed to make a determination whether a particular use is supported. In making these determinations, also refer to the AMA Drug Evaluations Subscription, Volume III, section 17 (Oncolytic Drugs), chapter 1 (Principles of Cancer Chemotherapy), tables 1 and 2.

Table 1, Specific Agents Used In Cancer Chemotherapy, lists the anti-neoplastic agents which are currently available for use in various cancers. The indications presented in this table for a particular anti- cancer drug include labeled and unlabeled uses (although they are not identified as such). Any indication appearing in this table is considered to be a medically accepted use.

Table 2, Clinical Responses To Chemotherapy, lists some of the currently preferred regimens for various cancers. The table headings include (1) type of cancer, (2) drugs or regimens currently preferred, (3) alternative or secondary drugs or regimens, and (4) other drugs or regimens with reported activity.

A regimen appearing under the preferred or alternative/secondary headings is considered to be a medically accepted use.

A regimen appearing under the heading "Other Drugs or Regimens With Reported Activity" is considered to be for a medically accepted use provided;

- The preferred and alternative/secondary drugs or regimens are contraindicated; or
- A preferred and/or alternative/secondary drug or regimen was used but was not tolerated or was ineffective; or
- There was tumor progression or recurrence after an initial response.

3. United States Pharmacopoeia Drug Information (USPDI).--Monographs are arranged in alphabetic order by generic or family name. Indications for use appear as accepted, unaccepted, or insufficient data. An indication is considered to be a medically accepted use only if the indication is listed as accepted. Unlabeled uses are identified with brackets. A separate indications index lists all indications included in USPDI along with the medically accepted drugs used in treatment or diagnosis.

4. A Use Supported by Clinical Research That Appears in Peer Reviewed Medical Literature.—This applies only when an unlabeled use does not appear in any of the compendia or is listed as insufficient data or investigational. If an unlabeled use of a drug meets these criteria, contact the compendia to see if a report regarding this use is forthcoming. If a report is forthcoming, use this information as a basis for your decision making. The compendium process for making decisions concerning unlabeled uses is very thorough and continuously updated. Peer reviewed medical literature includes scientific, medical, and pharmaceutical publications in which original manuscripts are published, only after having been critically reviewed for scientific accuracy, validity, and reliability by unbiased independent experts. This does not include in-house publications of pharmaceutical manufacturing companies or abstracts (including meeting abstracts).

In determining whether there is supportive clinical evidence for a particular use of a drug, your medical staff (in consultation with local medical specialty groups) must evaluate the quality of the evidence in published peer reviewed medical literature. When evaluating this literature, consider (among other things) the following:

- The prevalence and life history of the disease when evaluating the adequacy of the number of subjects and the response rate. While a 20 percent response rate may be adequate for highly prevalent disease states, a lower rate may be adequate for rare diseases or highly unresponsive conditions.
- The effect on the patient's well-being and other responses to therapy that indicate effectiveness, e.g., a significant increase in survival rate or life expectancy or an objective and significant decrease in the size of the tumor or a reduction in symptoms related to the tumor. Stabilization is not considered a response to therapy.
- The appropriateness of the study design. Consider:

1. Whether the experimental design in light of the drugs and conditions under investigation is appropriate to address the investigative question. (For example, in some clinical studies, it may be unnecessary or not feasible to use randomization, double blind trials, placebos, or crossover.);
2. That nonrandomized clinical trials with a significant number of subjects may be a basis for supportive clinical evidence for determining accepted uses of drugs; and
3. That case reports are generally considered uncontrolled and anecdotal information and do not provide adequate supportive clinical evidence for determining accepted uses of drugs.

Use peer reviewed medical literature appearing in the following publications:

- *American Journal of Medicine;*
- *Annals of Internal Medicine;*
- *The Journal of the American Medical Association;*
- *Journal of Clinical Oncology;*
- *Blood;*
- *Journal of the National Cancer Institute;*
- *The New England Journal of Medicine;*
- *British Journal of Cancer;*
- *British Journal of Hematology;*
- *British Medical Journal;*
- *Cancer;*
- *Drugs;*
- *European Journal of Cancer* (formerly *European Journal of Cancer and Clinical Oncology*);

- *Lancet*; or
- *Leukemia.*

You are not required to maintain copies of these publications. If a claim raises a question about the use of a drug for a purpose not included in the FDA approved labeling or the compendia, ask the physician to submit copies of relevant supporting literature.

4. Unlabeled uses may also be considered medically accepted if determined by you to be medically accepted generally as safe and effective for the particular use.

NOTE: If a use is identified as not indicated by HCFA or the FDA or if a use is specifically identified as not indicated in one or more of the three compendia mentioned or if you determine based on peer reviewed medical literature that a particular use of a drug is not safe and effective, the off- label usage is not supported and, therefore, the drug is not covered.

5. Less Than Effective Drug.—This is a drug that has been determined by the Food and Drug Administration (FDA) to lack substantial evidence of effectiveness for all labeled indications. Also, a drug that has been the subject of a Notice of an Opportunity for a Hearing (NOOH) published in the *Federal Register* before being withdrawn from the market, and for which the Secretary has not determined there is a compelling justification for its medical need, is considered less than effective. This includes any other drug product that is identical, similar, or related. Payment may not be made for a less than effective drug.

Because the FDA has not yet completed its identification of drug products that are still on the market,existing FDA efficacy decisions must be applied to all similar products once they are identified.

6. Denial of Medicare Payment for Compounded Drugs Produced in Violation of Federal Food, Drug, and Cosmetic Act.—The Food and Drug Administration (FDA) has found that, from time to time, firms established as retail pharmacies engage in mass production of compounded drugs, beyond the normal scope of pharmaceutical practice, in violation of the Federal Food, Drug, and Cosmetic Act (FFDCA). By compounding drugs on a large scale, a company may be operating as a drug manufacturer within the meaning of the FFDCA, without complying with requirements of that law. Such companies may be manufacturing drugs which are subject to the new drug application (NDA) requirements of the FFDCA, but for which FDA has not approved an NDA or which are misbranded or adulterated. If the manufacturing and processing procedures used by these facilities have not been approved by the FDA, the FDA has no assurance that the drugs these companies are producing are safe and effective. The safety and effectiveness issues pertain to such factors as chemical stability, purity, strength, bioequivalency, and biovailability.

Section 1862(a)(1)(A) of the Act requires that drugs must be reasonable and necessary in order to by covered under Medicare. This means, in the case of drugs, they must have been approved for marketing by the FDA. Section 2049.4 instructs carriers to deny coverage for drugs that have not received final marketing approval by the FDA, unless instructed otherwise by HCFA. Section 2300.1 instructs carriers to deny coverage of services related to the use of noncovered drugs as well. Hence, if DME or a prosthetic device is used to administer a noncovered drug, coverage is denied for both the nonapproved drug and the DME or prosthetic device.

In those cases in which the FDA has determined that a company is producing compounded drugs in violation of the FFDCA, Medicare does not pay for the drugs because they do not meet the FDA approval requirements of the Medicare program. In addition, Medicare does not pay for the DME or prosthetic device used to administer such a drug if FDA determines that a required NDA has not been approved or that the drug is misbranded or adulterated.

HCFA will notify you when the FDA has determined that compounded drugs are being produced in violation of the FFDCA. Do not stop Medicare payment for such a drug unless you are notified that it is appropriate to do so through a subsequent instruction. In addition, if you or ROs become aware that other companies are possibly operating in violation of the FFDCA, notify:

Health Care Financing Administration
Bureau of Policy Development
Office of Physician and Ambulatory Care Policy
Baltimore, MD 21244-1850

2049.5 Self-Administered Drugs and Biologicals.—Drugs that are self-administered are not covered by Medicare Part B unless the statute provides for such coverage. This includes blood clotting factors, drugs used in immunosuppressive therapy, erythropoietin for dialysis patients, certain oral anti-cancer drugs, and oral anti-nausea drugs when used in certain situations.

A. Immunosuppressive Drugs.—Until January 1, 1995, immunosuppressive drugs are covered under Part B for a period of one year following discharge from a hospital for a Medicare covered organ transplant. HCFA interprets the 1-year period after the date of the transplant procedure to mean 365 days from the day on which an inpatient is discharged from the hospital. Beneficiaries are eligible to receive additional Part B coverage within 18 months after the discharge date for drugs furnished in 1995; within 24 months for drugs furnished in 1996; within 30 months for drugs furnished in 1997; and within 36 months for drugs furnished after 1997.

Covered drugs include those immunosuppressive drugs that have been specifically labeled as such and approved for marketing by the FDA, as well as those prescription drugs, such as prednisone, that are used in conjunction with immunosuppressive drugs as part of a therapeutic regimen reflected in FDA approved labeling for immunosuppressive drugs. Therefore, antibiotics, hypertensives, and other drugs that are not directly related to rejection are not covered. The FDA had identified and approved for marketing five specifically labeled immunosuppressive drugs. They are Sandimmune (cyclosporine), Sandoz Pharmaceutical; Imuran (azathioprine), Burroughs Wellcome; Atgam (antithymocyte globulin), Upjohn; and Orthoclone OKT3 (Muromonab-CD3), Ortho Pharmaceutical and, Prograf (tacrolimus), Fujisawa USA, Inc. You are expected to keep informed of FDA additions to the list of the immunosuppressive drugs.

B. Erythropoietin (EPO).—The statute provides that EPO is covered for the treatment of anemia for patients with chronic renal failure who are on dialysis. Coverage is available regardless of whether the drug is administered by the patient or the patient's caregiver. EPO is a biologically engineered protein which stimulates the bone marrow to make new red blood cells.

NOTE: Non-ESRD patients who are receiving EPO to treat anemia induced by other conditions such as chemotherapy or the drug zidovudine (commonly called AZT) must meet the coverage requirements in §2049.

EPO is covered for the treatment of anemia for patients with chronic renal failure who are on dialysis when:

- It is administered in the renal dialysis facility; or
- It is self-administered in the home by any dialysis patient (or patient caregiver) who is determined competent to use the drug and meets the other conditions detailed below.

NOTE: Payment may not be made for EPO under the incident to provision when EPO is administered in the renal dialysis facility. (See §5202.4.)

Medicare covers EPO and items related to its administration for dialysis patients who use EPO in the home when the following conditions are met.

1. Patient Care Plan.—A dialysis patient who uses EPO in the home must have a current care plan (a copy of which must be maintained by the designated back-up facility for Method II patients) for monitoring home use of EPO which includes the following:

   a. Review of diet and fluid intake for aberrations as indicated by hyperkalemia and elevated blood pressure secondary to volume overload;
   b. Review of medications to ensure adequate provision of supplemental iron;
   c. Ongoing evaluations of hematocrit and iron stores;
   d. Reevaluation of the dialysis prescription taking into account the patient's increased appetite and red blood cell volume;
   e. Method for physician and facility (including back-up facility for Method II patients) follow-up on blood tests and a mechanism (such as a patient log) for keeping the physician informed of the results;
   f. Training of the patient to identify the signs and symptoms of hypotension and hypertension; and
   g. The decrease or discontinuance of EPO if hypertension is uncontrollable.

2. Patient Selection.—The dialysis facility, or the physician responsible for all dialysis-related services furnished to the patient, must make a comprehensive assessment that includes the following:

   a. Pre-selection monitoring. The patient's hematocrit (or hemoglobin), serum iron, transferrin saturation, serum ferritin, and blood pressure must be measured.
   b. Conditions the patient must meet. The assessment must find that the patient meets the following conditions:

   (1) Is a dialysis patient;
   (2) Has a hematocrit (or comparable hemoglobin level) that is as follows:

   (a) For a patient who is initiating EPO treatment, no higher than 30 percent unless there is medical documentation showing the need for EPO despite a hematocrit (or comparable hemoglobin level) higher than 30 percent. Patients with severe angina, severe pulmonary distress, or severe hypotension may require EPO to prevent adverse symptoms even if they have higher hematocrit or hemoglobin levels.
   (b) For a patient who has been receiving EPO from the facility or the physician, between 30 and 36 percent; and

3. Is under the care of:

   a. A physician who is responsible for all dialysis-related services and who prescribes the EPO and follows the drug labeling instructions when monitoring the EPO home therapy; and
   b. A renal dialysis facility that establishes the plan of care and monitors the progress of the home EPO therapy.
   c. The assessment must find that the patient or a caregiver meets the following conditions:
   (1) Is trained by the facility to inject EPO and is capable of carrying out the procedure;
   (2) Is capable of reading and understanding the drug labeling; and
   (3) Is trained in, and capable of observing, aseptic techniques.
   d. Care and storage of drug. The assessment must find that EPO can be stored in the patient's residence under refrigeration and that the patient is aware of the potential hazard of a child's having access to the drug and syringes.

4. Responsibilities of Physician or Dialysis Facility.—The patient's physician or dialysis facility must:

   a. Develop a protocol that follows the drug label instructions;
   b. Make the protocol available to the patient to ensure safe and effective home use of EPO;
   c. Through the amounts prescribed, ensure that the drug on hand at any time does not exceed a 2-month supply; and
   d. Maintain adequate records to allow quality assurance for review by the network and State survey agencies. For Method II patients, current records must be provided to and maintained by the designated back-up facility.

See §5202.4 for information on EPO payment.

Submit claims for EPO in accordance with §§4273.1 and 4273.2.

C. Oral Anti-Cancer Drugs.—Effective January 1, 1994, Medicare Part B coverage is extended to include oral anti-cancer drugs that are prescribed as anti-cancer chemotherapeutic agents providing they have the same active ingredients and are used for the same indications as anti-cancer chemotherapeutic agents which would be covered if they were not self administered and they were furnished incident to a physician's service as drugs and biologicals.

This provision applies only to the coverage of anti-neoplastic chemotherapeutic agents. It does not apply to oral drugs and/or biologicals used to treat toxicity or side effects such as nausea or bone marrow depression. Medicare will cover anti-neoplastic chemotherapeutic agents, the primary drugs which directly fight the cancer, and self-administered antiemetics which are necessary for the administration and absorption of the anti-neoplastic chemotherapeutic agents when a high likelihood of vomiting exists. The substitution of an oral form of an anti-neoplastic drug requires that the drug be retained for absorption. The antiemetics drug is covered as a necessary means for administration of the oral drug (similar to a syringe and needle necessary for injectable administration). Oral drugs prescribed for use with the primary drug which enhance the anti-neoplastic effect of the primary drug or permit the patient to tolerate the primary anti-neoplastic drug in higher doses for longer periods are not covered. Self-administered antiemetics to reduce the side effects of nausea and vomiting brought on by the primary drug are not included beyond the administration necessary to achieve drug absorption.

In order to assure uniform coverage policy, regional carriers and FIs must be apprised of local carriers'anti-cancer drug medical review policies which may impact on future medical review policy development. Local carrier's current and proposed anti cancer drug medical review polices should be provided by local carrier medical directors to regional carrier or FI medical directors, upon request.

For an oral anti-cancer drug to be covered under Part B, it must:

- Be prescribed by a physician or other practitioner licensed under State law to prescribe such drugs as anti-cancer chemotherapeutic agents;
- Be a drug or biological that has been approved by the Food and Drug Administration (FDA);
- Have the same active ingredients as a non-self-administrable anti-cancer chemotherapeutic drug or biological that is covered when furnished incident to a physician's service. The oral anti-cancer drug and the non-self-administrable drug must have the same chemical/generic name as indicated by the FDA's Approved Drug Products (Orange Book), Physician's Desk Reference (PDR), or an authoritative drug compendium; —or, effective January 1, 1999, be a prodrug—an oral drug ingested into the body that metabolizes into the same active ingredient that is found in the non-self-administrable form of the drug;
- Be used for the same indications, including unlabeled uses, as the non-self-administrable version of the drug; and
- Be reasonable and necessary for the individual patient.

D. Oral Anti-Nausea Drugs—Section 4557 of the Balanced Budget Act of 1997 amends §1861(s)(2) by extending the coverage of oral anti-emetic drugs under the following conditions:

- Coverage is provided only for oral drugs approved by FDA for use as anti-emetics;
- The oral anti-emetic(s) must either be administered by the treating physician or in accordance with a written order from the physician as part of a cancer chemotherapy regimen;
- Oral anti-emetic drug(s) administered with a particular chemotherapy treatment must be initiated within 2 hours of the administration of the chemotherapeutic agent and may be continued for a period not to exceed 48 hours from that time.
- The oral anti-emetic drug(s) provided must be used as a full therapeutic replacement for the intravenous anti-emetic drugs that would have otherwise been administered at the time of the chemotherapy treatment.

629

Only drugs pursuant to a physician's order at the time of the chemotherapy treatment qualify for this benefit. The dispensed number of dosage units may not exceed a loading dose administered within 2 hours of that treatment, plus a supply of additional dosage units not to exceed 48 hours of therapy. However, more than one oral anti-emetic drug may be prescribed and will be covered for concurrent usage within these parameters if more than one oral drug is needed to fully replace the intravenous drugs that would otherwise have been given.

Oral drugs that are not approved by the FDA for use as anti-emetics and which are used by treating physicians adjunctively in a manner incidental to cancer chemotherapy are not covered by this benefit and are not reimbursable within the scope of this benefit.

It is recognized that a limited number of patients will fail on oral anti-emetic drugs. Intravenous anti-emetics may be covered (subject to the rules of medical necessity) when furnished to patients who fail on oral anti-emetic therapy.

This coverage, effective for services on or after January 1, 1998, is subject to regular Medicare Part B coinsurance and deductible provisions.

NOTE: Existing coverage policies authorizing the administration of suppositories to prevent vomiting when oral cancer drugs are used are unchanged by this new coverage.

E. Hemophilia Clotting Factors.—Section 1861(s)(2)(I) of the Act provides Medicare coverage of blood clotting factors for hemophilia patients competent to use such factors to control bleeding without medical supervision, and items related to the administration of such factors. Hemophilia, a blood disorder characterized by prolonged coagulation time, Is caused by deficiency of a factor in plasma necessary for blood to clot. (The discovery in 1964 of a cryoprecipitate rich in antihemophilic factor activity facilitated management of acute bleeding episodes.) For purposes of Medicare Part B coverage, hemophilia encompasses the following conditions:

- Factor VIII deficiency (classic hemophilia);
- Factor IX deficiency (also termed plasma thromboplastin component (PTC) or Christmas factor deficiency); and
- Von Willebrand's disease.

Claims for blood clotting factors for hemophilia patients with these diagnoses may be covered if the patient is competent to use such factors without medical supervision.

The amount of clotting factors determined to be necessary to have on hand and thus covered under this provision is based on the historical utilization pattern or profile developed by the carrier for each patient. It is expected that the treating source; e.g., a family physician or comprehensive hemophilia diagnostic and treatment center, has such information. From this data, the contractor is able to make reasonable projections concerning the quantity of clotting factors anticipated to be needed by the patient over a specific period of time. Unanticipated occurrences involving extraordinary events, such as automobile accidents of inpatient hospital stays, will change this base line data and should be appropriately considered. In addition, changes in a patient's medical needs over a period of time require adjustments in the profile. (See §5245 for payment policies.)

2070.1   Independent Laboratories.—Diagnostic laboratory services furnished by an independent laboratory are covered under medical insurance if the laboratory is an approved Independent Clinical Laboratory. (However, as is the case of all diagnostic services, in order to be covered these services must be related to a patient's illness or injury (or symptom or complaint) and ordered by a physician. See §2020.1 for the definition of a "physician".)

A. Definition of Independent.—An independent laboratory is one which is independent both of an attending or consulting physician's office and of a hospital which meets at least the requirements to qualify as an emergency hospital as defined in section 1861(e) of the Act. (A consulting physician is one whose services include history taking, examination of the patient, and, in each case, furnishing to the attending physician an opinion regarding diagnosis or treatment. A physician providing clinical laboratory services for patients of other physicians is not considered to be a consulting physician.)

A laboratory which is operated by or under the supervision of a hospital (or the organized medical staff of the hospital) which does not meet at least the definition of an emergency hospital is considered to be an independent laboratory. However, a laboratory serving hospital patients and operated on the premises of a hospital which meets the definition of an emergency hospital is presumed to be subject to the supervision of the hospital or its organized medical staff and is not an independent laboratory. A laboratory which a physician or group of physicians maintains for performing diagnostic tests in connection with his own or the group practice is also not considered to be an independent laboratory.

An out-of-hospital laboratory is ordinarily presumed to be independent unless there is written evidence establishing that it is operated by or under the supervision of a hospital which meets at least the definition of an emergency hospital or of the organized medical staff of such a hospital.

Where a laboratory operated on hospital premises is claimed to be independent or where an out-of-hospital facility is designated as a hospital laboratory, the RO makes the determination concerning the laboratory's status.

B. Clinical Defined.—A clinical laboratory is a laboratory where microbiological, serological, chemical, hematological, radiobioassay, cytological, immuno-hematological, or pathological examinations are performed on materials derived from the human body, to provide information for the diagnosis, prevention, or treatment of a disease or assessment of a medical condition.

C. Approval of Laboratories.—An approved independent clinical laboratory is one which is approved by the Secretary of Health, Education, and Welfare as meeting the specific conditions for coverage under the program. These require that: (1) where State or applicable local law provides for licensing of independent clinical laboratories, the laboratory is either licensed under such law or it is approved as meeting the requirements for licensing laboratories; and (2) such laboratories also meet the health and safety requirements prescribed by the Secretary of Health, Education, and Welfare. See "Conditions for Coverage of Services of Independent Laboratories. (HIRM 1 Subpart M)

Diagnostic laboratory tests performed by a laboratory of a nonparticipating hospital which meet the statutory definition of an emergency hospital are covered only if the laboratory meets the requirements set forth in the regulations for hospital laboratories.

Services rendered by an independent clinical laboratory are covered under medical insurance only if the laboratory has been approved under the program. Carriers are furnished lists of approved laboratories and their approved specialties by HCFA. If you have any reason to question the lists concerning additions or deletions of particular laboratories or specialties, clarifying information should be requested from the RO.

Laboratory Certification and Decertification

You must notify your physicians of the initial certification of the laboratories in your service areas and also furnished certification information about laboratories outside your service area upon request from individual physicians or clinics. This information is available from the RO (see § 2070.1D below). Where there are any changes in the certification of a laboratory, i.e., addition or deletion of tests for which the laboratory is certified, notify the physicians in your service areas of these changes.

When some or all of the services of an independent laboratory no longer meet the conditions for coverage, inform all physicians having an interest in the laboratory's certification status of the effective date of decertification, reasons for the decertification, and the applicability of the determination to the various categories of diagnostic tests performed by the independent laboratory. Notification to the physicians must be made prior to the termination date since you cannot honor any bill for services performed after the termination date.

If you issue a monthly bulletin or newsletter to physicians in your service area you may wish to use this vehicle to inform the physicians involved. If, in a particular instance, timely notification cannot be made by use of the regular monthly bulletin or newsletter, a special bulletin will be necessary. In cases where there are a limited number of physicians in a remote area, a notification to all physicians in your service area may not be necessary. In these situations, you may wish to limit the scope of the notification and use means other than the monthly newsletter. You must secure the prior approval of the regional office for limited notification.

For notices of decertification, you will receive a copy of the decertification letter to the laboratory from the RO. Language suitable for use in the carrier notices to physicians concerning the reasons for the decertification will also be supplied. The following information will be included in the notification:

1. Name and address of laboratory;
2. Effective date of decertification;
3. Which services are not covered (all or particular specialty(ies); and
4. Reason for decertification.

Your notification to the physicians should contain a statement that no payment can be made under title XVIII on behalf of Medicare patients receiving these services from the laboratory on or after the effective decertification dates.

A copy of all notifications to physicians concerning laboratory decertifications, whether by regular monthly newsletter or by a special bulletin, should be sent to the RO Contractor Operations Staff on the date of issuance.

NOTE: The notification to physicians also applies to services performed by suppliers of portable X-ray services (see §2070.4B).

D. The Specialty Provision.—One of the conditions for coverage of services of independent laboratories is that the laboratory agrees to perform tests for Medicare beneficiaries only in the specialties for which it is certified. Clinical laboratory services rendered in a specialty for which an independent laboratory is not certified are not covered and claims for payment of benefits for these services must be denied.

HCFA furnishes lists to the carriers showing specialties and subspecialties in which each laboratory has been certified. The lists are updated quarterly. Each carrier receives two lists showing the independent laboratories located in its service area: one list by provider number and the other list alphabetical. For information on laboratories not located within a carrier's service area, the RO's maintain national lists showing all approved laboratories. A key is furnished for interpreting the codes on the lists. See §§ 4110ff. for additional information.

Following is a list of covered clinical laboratory test procedures and calculations by specialty and subspecialty that may be performed by independent laboratories participating in the Medicare program (hospital laboratories are not currently approved by specialty/subspecialty). The list contains most of the common test procedures but is not considered all inclusive. Test procedures and calculations that may be performed in more than one specialty/subspecialty are asterisked and cross-referred.

This list is also used by State agencies of certification of the laboratories in the various specialty and subspecialty categories.

2079 SURGICAL DRESSINGS, AND SPLINTS, CASTS, AND OTHER DEVICES USED FOR REDUCTIONS OF FRACTURES AND DISLOCATIONS

Surgical dressings are limited to primary and secondary dressings required for the treatment of a wound caused by, or treated by, a surgical procedure that has been performed by a physician or other health care professional to the extent permissible under State law. In addition, surgical dressings required after debridement of a wound are also covered, irrespective of the type of debridement, as long as the debridement was reasonable and necessary and was performed by a health care professional who was acting within the scope of his or her legal authority when performing this function. Surgical dressings are covered for as long as they are medically necessary.

Primary dressings are therapeutic or protective coverings applied directly to wounds or lesions either on the skin or caused by an opening to the skin. Secondary dressing materials that serve a therapeutic or protective function and that are needed to secure a primary dressing are also covered. Items such as adhesive tape, roll gauze, bandages, and disposable compression material are examples of secondary dressings. Elastic stockings, support hose, foot coverings, leotards, knee supports, surgical leggings, gauntlets, and pressure garments for the arms and hands are examples of items that are not ordinarily covered as surgical dressings. Some items, such as transparent film, may be used as a primary or secondary dressing.

If a physician, certified nurse midwife, physician assistant, nurse practitioner, or clinical nurse specialist applies surgical dressings as part of a professional service that is billed to Medicare, the surgical dressings are considered incident to the professional services of the health care practitioner. (See sections 2050.1, 2154, 2156, 2158, and 2160.) When surgical dressings are not covered incident to the services of a health care practitioner and are obtained by the patient from a supplier (e.g., a drugstore, physician, or other health care practitioner that qualifies as a supplier) on an order from a physician or other health care professional authorized under State law or regulation to make such an order, the surgical dressings are covered separately under Part B.

2125 COVERAGE GUIDELINES FOR AMBULANCE SERVICE CLAIMS

Reimbursement may be made for expenses incurred by a patient for ambulance service provided the following conditions have been met:

A. Patient was transported by an approved supplier of ambulance services.

B. The patient was suffering from an illness or injury which contraindicated transportation by other means. (section 2120.2A)

C. The patient was transported from and to points listed below.(section 2120.3)

1. From patient's residence (or other place where need arose) to hospital or skilled nursing home.
2. Skilled nursing home to a hospital or hospital to a skilled nursing home.
3. Hospital to hospital or skilled nursing home to skilled nursing home.
4. From a hospital or skilled nursing home to patient's residence.
5. Round trip for hospital or participating skilled nursing facility inpatients to the nearest hospital or nonhospital treatment facility

A patient's residence is the place where he makes his home and dwells permanently, or for an extended period of time. A skilled nursing home is one which is listed in the Directory of Medical Facilities as a participating SNF or as an institution which meets section 1861(j)(1) of the law. Ambulance service to a physician's office or a physician-directed clinic is not covered. (See section 2120.3G where a stop is made at a physician's office enroute to a hospital and 2120.3C for additional exceptions.)

2133 LEG, ARM, BACK, AND NECK BRACES, TRUSSES, AND ARTIFICIAL LEGS, ARMS, AND EYES

These appliances are covered when furnished incident to physicians' services or on a physician's order. A brace includes rigid and semi-rigid devices which are used for the purpose of supporting a weak or deformed body member or restricting or eliminating motion in a diseased or injured part of the body. Elastic stockings, garter belts, and similar devices do not come within the scope of the definition of a brace. Back braces include, but are not limited to, special corsets, e.g., sacroiliac, sacrolumbar, dorsolumbar corsets and belts. A terminal device (e.g., hand or hook) is covered under this provision whether an artificial limb is required by the patient. (See §2323.) Stump stockings and harnesses (including replacements) are also covered when these appliances are essential to the effective use of the artificial limb.

Adjustments to an artificial limb or other appliance required by wear or by a change in the patient's condition are covered when ordered by a physician. To the extent applicable, follow the provisions in §2100.4 relating to the repair and replacement of durable medical equipment for the repair and replacement of artificial limbs, braces, etc. Adjustments, repairs and replacements are covered even when the item had been in use before the user enrolled in Part B of the program so long as the device continues to be medically required.

2134 THERAPEUTIC SHOES FOR INDIVIDUALS WITH DIABETES

Coverage of therapeutic shoes (depth or custom-molded) along with inserts for individuals with diabetes is available as of May 1, 1993. These diabetic shoes are covered if the requirements as specified in this section concerning certification and prescription are fulfilled. In addition, this benefit provides for a pair of diabetic shoes even if only one foot suffers from diabetic foot disease. Each shoe is equally equipped so that the affected limb, as well as the remaining limb, is protected.

Claims for therapeutic shoes for diabetics are processed by the Durable Medical Equipment Regional Carriers (DMERCs.)

A. Definitions.—The following items may be covered under the diabetic shoe benefit:

1. Custom-Molded Shoes.—Custom-molded shoes are shoes that are:

- Constructed over a positive model of the patient's foot;
- Made from leather or other suitable material of equal quality;
- Have removable inserts that can be altered or replaced as the patient's condition warrants; and
- Have some form of shoe closure.

2. Depth Shoes.—Depth shoes are shoes that:

- Have a full length, heel-to-toe filler that, when removed, provides a minimum of 3/16 inch of additional depth used to accommodate custom-molded or customized inserts;
- Are made from leather or other suitable material of equal quality;
- Have some form of shoe closure; and
- Are available in full and half sizes with a minimum of 3 widths so that the sole is graded to the size and width of the upper portions of the shoes according to the American standard last sizing schedule or its equivalent. (The American standard last sizing schedule is the numerical shoe sizing system used for shoes sold in the United States.)

3. Inserts.—Inserts are total contact, multiple density, removable inlays that are directly molded to the patient's foot or a model of the patient's foot and that are made of a suitable material with regard to the patient's condition.

B. Coverage.—

1. Limitations.—For each individual, coverage of the footwear and inserts is limited to one of the following within one calendar year:

- No more than one pair of custom-molded shoes (including inserts provided with such shoes) and two additional pairs of inserts; or
- No more than one pair of depth shoes and three pairs of inserts (not including the non-customized removable inserts provided with such shoes).

2. Coverage of Diabetic Shoes and Brace.—Orthopedic shoes, as stated in §2323.D, generally are not covered. This exclusion does not apply to orthopedic shoes that are an integral part of a leg brace. In situations in which an individual qualifies for both diabetic shoes and a leg brace, these items are covered separately. Thus, the diabetic shoes may be covered if the requirements for this section are met, while the brace may be covered if the requirements of section 2133 are met.

3. Substitution of Modifications for Inserts.—An individual may substitute modification(s) of custom-molded or depth shoes instead of obtaining a pair(s) of inserts in any combination. Payment for the modification(s) may not exceed the limit set for the inserts for which the individual is entitled. The following is a list of the most common shoe modifications available, but it is not meant as an exhaustive list of the modifications available for diabetic shoes:

- Rigid Rocker Bottoms. These are exterior elevations with apex positions for 51 percent to 75 percent distance measured from the back end of the heel. The apex is a narrowed or pointed end of an anatomical structure. The apex must be positioned behind the metatarsal heads and tapering off sharply to the front tip of the sole. Apex height helps to eliminate pressure at the metatarsal heads. Rigidity is ensured by the steel in the shoe. The heel of the shoe tapers off in the back in order to cause the heel to strike in the middle of the heel.
- Roller Bottoms (Sole or Bar). These are the same as rocker bottoms, but the heel is tapered from the apex to the front tip of the sole.
- Metatarsal Bars.—An exterior bar is placed behind the metatarsal heads in order to remove pressure from the metatarsal heads. The bars are of various shapes, heights, and construction depending on the exact purpose.
- Wedges (Posting). Wedges are either of hind foot, fore foot, or both and may be in the middle or to the side. The function is to shift or transfer weight bearing upon standing or during ambulation to the opposite side for added support, stabilization, equalized weight distribution, or balance.
- Offset Heels. This is a heel flanged at its base either in the middle, to the side, or a combination, that is then extended upward to the shoe in order to stabilize extreme positions of the hind foot.

Other modifications to diabetic shoes include, but are not limited to:

- Flared heels;
- Velcro closures; and
- Inserts for missing toes.

4. Separate Inserts. Inserts may be covered and dispensed independently of diabetic shoes if the supplier of the shoes verifies in writing that the patient has appropriate footwear into which the insert can be placed. This footwear must meet the definitions found above for depth shoes and custom-molded shoes.

C. Certification. The need for diabetic shoes must be certified by a physician who is a doctor of medicine or a doctor of osteopathy and who is responsible for diagnosing and treating the patient's diabetic systemic condition through a comprehensive plan of care. This managing physician must:

- Document in the patient's medical record that the patient has diabetes;
- Certify that the patient is being treated under a comprehensive plan of care for his or her diabetes, and that he or she needs diabetic shoes; and
- Document in the patient's record that the patient has one or more of the following conditions:

  - Peripheral neuropathy with evidence of callus formation;
  - History of pre-ulcerative calluses;
  - History of previous ulceration;
  - Foot deformity;
  - Previous amputation of the foot or part of the foot; or
  - Poor circulation.

D. Prescription. Following certification by the physician managing the patient's systemic diabetic condition, a podiatrist or other qualified physician who is knowledgeable in the fitting of diabetic shoes and inserts may prescribe the particular type of footwear necessary.

E. Furnishing Footwear. The footwear must be fitted and furnished by a podiatrist or other qualified individual such as a pedorthist, an orthotist, or a prosthetist. The certifying physician may not furnish the diabetic shoes unless he or she is the only qualified individual in the area. It is left to the discretion of each carrier to determine the meaning of "in the area."

F. Payment. For 1994, payment for diabetic shoes and inserts is limited to 80 percent of the reasonable charge, up to a limit of $348 for one pair of custom-molded shoes including any initial inserts, $59 for each additional pair of custom-molded shoe inserts, $116 for one pair of depth shoes, and $59 for each pair of depth shoe inserts. These limits are based on 1988 amounts that were set forth in §1833(o) of the Act and then adjusted by the same percentage increases allowed for DME for fee screen limits by applying the same update factor that is applied to DME fees, except that if the updated limit is not a multiple of $1, it is rounded to the nearest multiple of $1. Although percentage increase in payment for diabetic shoes are the same percentage increases that are used for payment of DME through the DME fee schedule, the shoes are not subject to DME coverage rules or the DME fee schedule. In addition, diabetic shoes are neither considered DME nor orthotics, but a separate category of coverage under Medicare Part B. (See §1861(s)(12) and §1833(o) of the Act.)

Payment for the certification of diabetic shoes and for the prescription of the shoes is considered to be included in the payment for the visit or consultation during which these services are provided. If the sole purpose of an encounter with the beneficiary is to dispense or fit the shoes, then no payment may be made for a visit or consultation provided on the same day by the same physician. Thus, a separate payment is not made for certification of the need for diabetic shoes, the prescribing of diabetic shoes, or the fitting of diabetic shoes unless the physician documents that these services were not the sole purpose of the visit or consultation.

2136 DENTAL SERVICES

As indicated under the general exclusions from coverage, items, and services in connection with the care, treatment, filling, removal, or replacement of teeth or structures directly supporting the teeth are not covered. Structures directly supporting the teeth means the periodontium, which includes the gingivae, dentogingival junction, periodontal membrane, cementum of the teeth, and alveolar process.

In addition to the following, see section 2020.3 and Coverage Issues Manual, section 50-26 for specific services which may be covered when furnished by a dentist. If an otherwise noncovered procedure or service is performed by a dentist as incident to and as an integral part of a covered procedure or service performed by him/her, the total service performed by the dentist on such an occasion is covered.

Example 1: The reconstruction of a ridge performed primarily to prepare the mouth for dentures is a noncovered procedure. However, when the reconstruction of a ridge is performed as a result of and at the same time as the surgical removal of a tumor (for other than dental purposes), the totality of surgical procedures is a covered service.

Example 2: Make payment for the wiring of teeth when this is done in connection with the reduction of a jaw fracture.

The extraction of teeth to prepare the jaw for radiation treatment of neoplastic disease is also covered. This is an exception to the requirement that to be covered, a noncovered procedure or service performed by a dentist must be an incident to and an integral part of a covered procedure or service performed by him/her. Ordinarily, the dentist extracts the patient's teeth, but another physician, e.g., a radiologist, administers the radiation treatments.

When an excluded service is the primary procedure involved, it is not covered, regardless of its complexity or difficulty. For example, the extraction of an impacted tooth is not covered. Similarly, an alveoplasty (the surgical improvement of the shape and condition of the alveolar process) and a frenectomy are excluded from coverage when either of these procedures is performed in connection with an excluded service, e.g., the preparation of the mouth for dentures. In a like manner, the removal of a torus palatinus (a bony protuberance of the hard palate) may be a covered service. However, with rare exception, this surgery is performed in connection with an excluded service, i.e., the preparation of the mouth for dentures. Under such circumstances, do not pay for this procedure.

Whether such services as the administration of anesthesia, diagnostic X-rays, and other related procedures are covered depends upon whether the primary procedure being performed by the dentist is itself covered. Thus, an X-ray taken in connection with the reduction of a fracture of the jaw or facial bone is covered. However, a single X-ray or X-ray survey taken in connection with the care or treatment of teeth or the periodontium is not covered.

Make payment for a covered dental procedure no matter where the service is performed. The hospitalization or nonhospitalization of a patient has no direct bearing on the coverage or exclusion of a given dental procedure. Payment may also be made for services and supplies furnished incident to covered dental services. For example, the services of a dental technician or nurse who is under the direct supervision of the dentist or physician are covered if the services are included in the dentist's or physician's bill.

Rev. 1495/Page 2-86.1

2150 CLINICAL PSYCHOLOGIST SERVICES

Section 6113(a) of OBRA 1989 (P. L. 101-239) eliminates the restriction on clinical psychologist (CP) services imposed by prior law, which required that, to be paid for directly, the services be furnished at community mental health centers (CMHCs) or offsite at a CMHC for those who are institutionalized or are physically or mentally impaired.

A CMHC is an institution that provides the mental health services required by section 1916(c)(4) of the PHS Act and is certified by the appropriate State authorities as meeting such requirements.

Services furnished by a CP and services furnished incident to the services of a CP to hospital patients during the period July 1, 1990, through December 31, 1990, were bundled. Therefore, Medicare made payment to the hospital for these services. However, as a result of the enactment of section 4157 of OBRA 1990, effective January 1, 1991, professional CP services furnished to hospital patients are no longer bundled under 42 CFR 411.15(m). Section 4157 amended section 1862(a)(14) of the Act to permit direct payment to CPs under Medicare Part B for such services. However, services furnished incident to the professional services of CPs to hospital patients remain bundled. Therefore, payment must continue to be made to the hospital for such "incident to" services.

The diagnostic services of psychologists who are not clinical psychologists, and who are practicing independently, are discussed in section 2070.2.

A. Clinical Psychologist Defined.—To qualify as a CP, a practitioner must meet the following requirements:

- Hold a doctoral degree in psychology;
- Be licensed or certified, on the basis of the doctoral degree in psychology, by the State in which he or she practices, at the independent practice level of psychology to furnish diagnostic, assessment, preventive, and therapeutic services directly to individuals.

B. Qualified Clinical Psychologist Services Defined.—Effective July 1, 1990, the diagnostic and therapeutic services of CPs and services and supplies furnished incident to such services are covered as the services furnished by a physician or as incident to physician's services are covered. However, the CP must be legally authorized to perform the services under applicable licensure laws of the State in which they are furnished.

C. Types of Clinical Psychologist Services That May Be Covered.—CPs may provide the following services:

- Diagnostic and therapeutic services that the CP is legally authorized to perform in accordance with State law and/or regulation. Pay all qualified CPs based on the fee schedule for their diagnostic and therapeutic services. Also, pay those practitioners who do not meet the requirements for a CP on the basis of the physician fee schedule for the provision of diagnostic services under section 2070.2.
- Services and supplies furnished incident to a CP's services are covered if the requirements that apply to services incident to a physician's services, as described in section 2050.1 are met. These services must be:

    -Mental health services that are commonly furnished in CPs' offices;
    -An integral, although incidental, part of professional services performed by the CP;
    -Performed under the direct personal supervision of the CP, i.e., the CP must be physically present and immediately available; and
    -Furnished without charge or included in the CP's bill.

Any person involved in performing the service must be an employee of the CP (or an employee of the legal entity that employs the supervising CP) under the common law control test of the Act, as set forth in 20 CFR 404.1007 and section RS 2101.020 of the Retirement and Survivors Insurance part of the Social Security Program Operations Manual System.

Be familiar with appropriate State laws and/or regulations governing a CP's scope of practice. The development of lists of appropriate services may prove useful.

D. Noncovered Services. The services of CPs are not covered if they are otherwise excluded from Medicare coverage even though a clinical psychologist is authorized by State law to perform them. For example, section 1862(a)(1)(A) of the Act excludes from coverage services that are not "reasonable and necessary for the diagnosis or treatment of an illness or injury or to improve the functioning of a malformed body member." Therefore, even though the services are authorized by State law, the services of a CP that are determined to be not reasonable and necessary are not covered. Additionally, any therapeutic services that are billed by CPs under CPT psychotherapy codes that include medical evaluation and management services are not covered.

E. Requirement for Consultation.—When applying for a Medicare provider number, a CP must submit to the carrier a signed Medicare provider/supplier enrollment form that indicates an agreement to the effect that, contingent upon the patient's consent, he or she will attempt to consult with the patient's attending or primary care physician in accordance with accepted professional ethical norms, taking into consideration patient confidentiality.

If the patient assents to the consultation, the CP must attempt to consult with the patient's physician within a reasonable time after receiving the consent. If the CP's attempts to consult directly with the physician are not successful, the CP must notify the physician within a reasonable time that he or she is furnishing services to the patient. Additionally, the CP must document, in the patient's medical record, the date the patient consented or declined consent to consultations, the date of consultation, or, if attempts to consult did not succeed, that date and manner of notification to the physician.

The only exception to the consultation requirement for CPs is in cases where the patient's primary care or attending physician refers the patient to the CP. Also, neither a CP nor a primary care or attending physician may bill Medicare or the patient for this required consultation.

See H.R. Conf. Rep. No. 386, 101st Cong., 1st Sess. 789 (1989).

F. Payment Methodology Limitation.—Payment for the services of CPs is made on the basis of a fee schedule or the actual charge, whichever is less, and only on the basis of assignment.

G. Outpatient Mental Health Services Limitation.—All covered therapeutic services furnished by qualified CPs are subject to the outpatient mental health services limitation in section 2470ff (i.e., only 62 1/2 percent of expenses for these services are considered incurred expenses for Medicare purposes). The limitation does not apply to diagnostic services. (See section 2472.4.C.)

H. Assignment Requirement.—Make all claims for covered services rendered by CPs on an assignment basis.

2152 CLINICAL SOCIAL WORKER SERVICES

Medical and other health services include the services provided by a clinical social worker (CSW). Payment is made only under assignment. The amount payable cannot exceed 80 percent of the lesser of the actual charge for the services or 75 percent of the amount paid to a psychologist for the same service. See §5112 for the payment guidelines and subsection F for application of the mental health payment limitation.

A. Clinical Social Worker Defined.—Section 1861(hh) of the Act defines a "clinical social worker" as an individual who:

- Possesses a master's or doctor's degree in social work;
- Has performed at least 2 years of supervised clinical social work; and
- either;

  - Is licensed or certified as a clinical social worker by the State in which the services are performed; or

  - In the case of an individual in a State that does not provide for licensure or certification, has completed at least 2 years or 3,000 hours of post master's degree supervised clinical social work practice under the supervision of a master's level social worker in an appropriate setting such as a hospital, SNF, or clinic.

B. Clinical Social Worker Services Defined.—Section 1861(hh)(2) of the Act defines "clinical social worker services" as those services that the CSW is legally authorized to perform under State law (or the State regulatory mechanism provided by State law) of the State in which such services are performed for the diagnosis and treatment of mental illnesses. Services furnished to an inpatient of a hospital or an inpatient of a SNF that the SNF is required to provide as a requirement for participation are not included. The services that are covered are those that are otherwise covered if furnished by a physician or as an incident to a physician's professional service.

C. Covered Services.—Coverage is limited to the services a CSW is legally authorized to perform in accordance with State law (or State regulatory mechanism established by State law). The services of a CSW may be covered under Part B if they are:

- The type of services that are otherwise covered if furnished by a physician, or as incident to a physician's service. (See §2020 for a description of physicians' services and section 2020.2 for the definition of a physician.);
- Performed by a person who meets the definition of a CSW (see subsection A); and
- Not otherwise excluded from coverage.

Become familiar with the State law or regulatory mechanism governing a CSW's scope of practice in your service area. The development of a list of services within the scope of practice may prove useful.

D. Noncovered Services.—Services of a CSW are not covered when furnished to inpatients of a hospital or to inpatients of a SNF if the services furnished in the SNF are those that the SNF is required to furnish as a condition of participation in Medicare. In addition, CSW services are not covered if they are otherwise excluded from Medicare coverage even though a CSW is authorized by State law to perform them. For example, the Medicare law excludes from coverage services that are not "reasonable and necessary for the diagnosis or treatment of an illness or injury or to improve the functioning of a malformed body member."

E. Outpatient Mental Health Services Limitation.—All covered therapeutic services furnished by qualified CSWs are subject to the outpatient psychiatric services limitation in §2470ff (i.e., only 62 1/2 percent of expenses for these services are considered incurred expenses for Medicare purposes). The limitation does not apply to diagnostic services. (See §2476.5.)

GLOSSARY OF LABORATORY TESTS AND CALCULATIONS LISTED BY CATEGORY
010 Historcompatibility Testing (Tissue Typing)
Antiglobulin Crossmatch for Transplantation
Antiglobulin microcytotoxicity Technique
Capillary Agglutination
Cell-mediated lympholysis Test

HLA Typing - Platelet Complement Fixation (FLCF)
HLA Typing - Lymphocyte Complement Fixation
HLA Typing - B27, specific B lymphocyte antigen
HLA Typing - Total
Leukocyte Aggregation Test (LAT)
Leukoagglutination or Phytohemagglutination
Lymphocyte Antibody Lymphocytolytic Interaction (LALI)
Lymphocyte - dependent antibody-mediated lysis (LDA)
Mixed Leukocyte Culture
Mixed Lymphocyte Reaction (Mixed Lymphocyte Culture)-MLR, MLC
Screening Sera for HLA antibodies
Detection of Leukocyte antibodies by the Complement Consumption Test
Separation of multiple HLA antibody specificities by platelet absorption and acid elution
Other techniques: Target Cells
(terminology used) Killer Cells

100 MICROBIOLOGY
110 Bacteriology (with antimicrobial susceptibility
Acid-fast culture, primary isolation
Acid-fast culture, identification
Acid-fast smear
Antimicrobial susceptibility test (mycobacteriology)
Antimicrobial susceptibility test (general bacteriology)
Antogenous vaccine
Culture, primary isolation
Culture, identification
Culture, for Mycoplasma pneumoniae
Gram Smear
Leptospirosis (Blood, Urine and CSF)
PKU (Guthrie only)
Pyrogen test
Pyrogen test (Samples containing protein)
*Streptococcus MG agglutination-220
*Tularemia agglutination-220
120 Mycology
*Coccidiomycosis, Precipitin-220
Culture for Fungi Identification
Abscess
Blood
Bone Marrow
CSF (cerebrospinal fluid)
Eye
Skin, Hair, Nail
Sputum
Tissue Section
Vaginal
Culture, Primary isolation
*Histoplasma agglutionation-220
Mycelia Direct Examination--fungal smear
130 Parasitology
Blood Specimen for Filariasis
*Blood Specimen for Malaria-400
Purged Stool for Amebiasis
Routine Stool for Ova and Parasite
Scotch Tape Test for Enterobius Vermicularis
Stool, urine for Schistosomiasis toxoplasmosis
*Toxoplasmosis agglutionation-220
*Trichina agglutionation-130
Vaginal Swab for Trichomonas vaginalis
140 Virology (including Rickettsiae and chlamydiae)
(isolation and identification)
150 Other
*Febrile Group-220
Fluorescent stains for bacterial identification
*Immunoflourescence Methods - 220
Phage typing for staphylococci/other bacterial organisms

200 SEROLOGY
210 Syphilis
Automated reagin test (ART)
Dark field Examination
Flourescent treponemal antibodies (FTA)
Kolmer, qual.
Kolmer, quant.
Rapid Plasma Reagin test (RPR Card Test)
Reagin Screen Test (RST)
Spinal Fluid, VDRL
VDRL (Venereal Disease Research Laboratory), qualitative slide
220 Serology-Other
Non-syphilis serology (Diagnostic Immunology)
Alpha - 1 - antitrypsin
Alpha - 1 - fetoprotein (AFP) - 330
Anti-deoxuribonuclease (ADNase)
Anti-mitrochonorial antibody
Anti-nuclear antibodies (ANA)
Anti-parietal cell antibody
Anti-skeltal muscle antibody
Anti-smooth muscle antibody
Anti-streptococcalhyaluronidase (ASH)
Anti-streptolysin O (ASO) Test
Anti-thyroglobulin antibodies
Anti-toxoplasmosis antibody
Beta-lc/Beta la globulin
Brucella Agglutination
*Carcinoembryonic Antigen Assay (CEA) - 330
*Coccidiomycosis, Precipitin-120
Cold Agglutinin
Complement, (Total Serum (C') & C'3 and components
C-reactive protein (CRP)
Free DNA Antibody
Free DNA Antigen
*Febrile group (Brucella, typhoid Q & H, OX-l9, OX-K and OX-2)-150
Gamma globulin, by salt pptn.
*Glucose-6 Phosphate Dehydrogenase (G-6-PD) - 130, 400
*Hepatitis B Antigen (HBsAg) - 330, 540
*Hepatitis B Antibody (Anti-HBs-330, 540
Heterophile antibodies (Presumptive)
Heterophile with absorptions (Differential)
*Histoplasma aggluatination - 120
l-Immunoglobulin Quantitation - See serum specific proteins
*Immunofluorescence Methods (Flourescent Antibody Techniques- Identification of Group A streptococci; Neisseria gonorrhoeae, etc) - 150
Infectious Mononucleosis
Leptospira agglutination
Lupus erythematosus - latex agglutination (LE)
*Mycoplasma pneumoniae CF test - ll0
Ox cell hemolysin test
Q-Fever, Agglutination Titre
Q-Fever, Complement Fixation
Radioallergo Sorbent Test (RAST Test)
Rheumatoid Arthritis-latex fixation (RA)
Rose test
Rubella CF antibody
Bubella HI antibody
Serum Specific Proteins - Immunoglobulin quantitation (IgG; IgA; IgM; IgD; IgE)
Sheep Cell Agglutination test for RA
*Streptococcus MG agglutination - ll0
Thyroid auto-antibodies
*Trichina agglutination - 130
*Toxoplasmosis Agglutination - 130
*Tularemia agglutination - ll0

300 CLINICAL CHEMISTRY - ROUTINE
310 Clinical Chemistry - Routine
Blood Urine, Stool, Cerebro-Spinal Fluid Chemistry (includes electrophoresis and enzymes

Acetone-acetoacetic acid-serum
Acid mucopolysaccharides, qualitative
Acid phosphatase
Acidity, titration
Albumin
Albumin-globulin (A/G) ratio (calculation)
Aldolase
Alkaline phospahtase, serum
Alpha-hydroxybutyric dehydrogenasc (IIED)
Alpha-amino acid nitrogen
Delta-aminolevulinic acid (ALA)
Amino acids, fractionated quant.
p-aminohippuric acid (PAH)
Aminophylline
Ammonia, Blood Urine
Amylase, Serum, Urine
Arterial Blood pH
Ascorbic Acid (Vitamin C)
Atyherogenic Index (AI)
Bicarbonate
Bile Acids, fractionated
Bilirubin, total
Bilirubin, Total and Direct
Blood gas and pH (calculation) (Pco2; po2; % 02 saturation; base-total)
Boric Acid
Bromide
Bromsulfalcin, dye analysis only (BSP) - Sulfobromphthalein   Excretion - Liver
BUN (Blood Urea Nitrogen)
Calcium, Serum, Urine, Feces
Carbon Dioxide Content
Carotene
Cephalin Flocculation
Ceruloplasmin
Chloride
Cholesterol, total
Cholesterol, total and esters
Cholinesterase, serum, plasma, RBC
Chondroitin sulfate, qual.
Cltric acid, serum, urine
C02-combining power
Creatine phosphokinase (CPK) - also known as creatine kinase
Creatine, urine, serum
Creatinine, urine, serum
Creatinine Clearance
Cryoglobulins
Cystine
Diastase
Electrolytes (Na, K, Cl) - sodium, potassium, chloride
FATS, serum or stool
Fatty acids, unesterified
Folate, RBC, serum
Free Fatty acids
Galactose, by chromatography
Gamma glutamyl transpetidase (Gamma-GTP)
Globulins, total
Glucose
Glucose tolerance
*Glucose-6-Phosphate Dehydrogenase-220,400
Glutathione Reductase
Glycoprotein
Guanase
Haptoglobin
*Hemoglobin electrophoresis - 400
Hexosamine
Hippuric acid quant.
Histamine
Homogentisic acid quant.
Icterus index (calculation)

Indocyanine green excretion-liver dye test
Iron, total, serum, urine
*More than one specialty category
Iron-binding capacity and total iron
Unsaturated iron binding capacity-UIBEL
Isocitric dehydrogenase (ICD)
Kynurenic and Xanthurenic acids
Lactic acid
Lactose tolerance test
LDH (lactic dehydrogenase), serum, CSF
LDH (fractionated)
LDH Isoenzymes by electrophoresis
Leucine aminopeptidase (LAP), serum, urine
Lipase
Lipid Profile-Phospholipids, cholesterol, triglycerides
Lipids, total and fractionated, serum
Lipids, total, feces
Lipids, total and split fat, feces
Lipids per dry weight, feces
B-Liporpotein screening
Lipoproteins by electrophoresis
Lipoproteins, phenotyping
Lipoproteins by ultracentrigufation
Lithium
Macroglobulin by ultracentrifugation
Magnesium, serum
Magnesium, urine
Manganese
Melanin, qualitative
Methylmalonic acid
Mucopolysaccharides, acid, qual.
Mucoprotein
Nitrogen, total, Urine, Feces
Non-esterified fatty acids (NEFA)
Non-protein nitrogen (NPN)
5'-Nucleotidase
Orinase Tolerance Test (Tolbutamide)
Ornithine carbamyl transferase (OCT)
Osmolatity by freezing point depression
Oxalate
Paraldehyde (as acetaldehyde)
PCO2
Pepsinogen
pH
Phenylpyruvic acid, qual.
Phosphoethanolamine by column chromatography
Phosphogalactose transferase
Phospholipids
Phospholipids, cholesterol, triglycerides
Phosphorus, Serum & Urine
Rev. 754/Page 2-32.4
PKU (exluding Guthrie method)
P02
Potassium, Serum, Urine, Feces
Protein, total
Protein, quant., urine, CSF
Protein fractionation by electrophoresis
Protoporphyrin, REC
Pyruvic acid
Reducing sugars by chromatography, qual., blood
Salicylates, serum, urine - 330
SGOT (Serum glutamic - oxalacetic transaminase) - also known as aspartate amino transferase
SGPT (Serum glutamic - pyruvic transaminase) - also know as alanine amino transferase
Silica, in lung tissue
Sodium, Serum, Urine, Feces
Spinal Fluid, Chlorides
Spinal Fluid, Sugar
Spinal Fluid, Total Protein

Split fat and total lipids, feces
Stercobilinogen
Sugars, qual., by paper chromatography
Sulfa level
Sulfate
Sweat Chlorides
Thiocyanate
Thymol Turbidity
Trichloracetic acid (TCA)
Trichlorethanol
Triglycerides
Triglycerides, phospholipids, cholesterol, total lipids
Tryspin
Tryptamine
Tryrosine
Urea clearance
Uric acid (phosphotungstate method)
Uropepsin
Vitamin A
Vitamin B2
*Vitamin Bl2-400
Xanthurenic and kynurenic acids
Xylose (for tolerance test)
320 Urinalysis (Routine and Calculi)-Clinical Microscopy
Acetone-acetoacetic acid (urine) Addis Count
Basic chemical profile
Qualitative glucose
Qualitative bile
Qualitative Ketone bodies
Qualitative blood
Qualitative nitrate
Qualitative protein (predominantly albumin)
pH
Specific gravity
Color and appearance
Bile, urine
Calculi, qualitative
Coproporphyrin
Diagnex Blue (Tubeless gastric)
Galactose (for tolerance test)
Hippuric acid
Homogentisic acid, qualitative
Microscopic examination of urine sediment (cells, casts)
Myoglobin, semi-quantitive
Para-aminohippuric acid (PAH)
Pentose Sugar in urine (qual) screening
Phenosulfonphthalein excretion test-
renal function test (P.S.P.)
Porphobilinogen, quant.
Porphyrins, urine
Porphyrins, feces
Protein, Bence-Jones
Protoporphyrin
Reducing sugars by chromatography, qual., urine
*Serotonin, urine - 5HIAA - 330
Urinalysis (including Microscopic)
Urobilinogen, urine, feces
Uroporphyrin
320 Chemistry - Other (including Toxiocology)
Alkaloids and other organic bases
*Alpha-l-fetoprotein - 220
Amphetamine
Anti-convulsant group
Antimony
Arsenic, quantitative
Barbiturates
Barbiturates, tissue, quant.
Beryllium

Bismuth
Blood Alcohol ethyl)
Bromides, serum
Bromides, urine
Cadmium
Carbon Monoxide (Carboxyhemoglobin)
*Carcinoembryonic Antigen Assay (CEA) - 220
Chloramphenicol (Chloromycetin)
Chromium
Codeine, urine
Copper, Serum, Urine
Cyanide
Darvon
Dicumarol
Digitalis
Digitoxin
Digoxin
Dilantin
Doriden (glutethimide)
Elavil
Ethyl Alcohol (ethanol)
Fluoride
Gentamicin (by RIA)
Gold
Heavy metals (arsenic, lead, mercury) - Reinsch Test
*Hepatitis B Antigen (HBsAg) - 220, 540
*Hepatitis B Antibody (Anti-HBs) - 220, 540
Hypnotic and Tranquilizer Screen
Lead
Librium
Meprobamate (Miltown, Equanil)
Mercury
Methaqualone
Minerals
Nickel
Nicotine
Phenacetin
Phenols
Phenothiazines
Quinidine
Reinsch Test
*Salicylates, serum, urine - 310
Selenium
Strychnine
Thallium
Theophylline
Trace Elements
Trofranil - Imipramine)
*More than one specialty category
Rev. 620Page 2-32.7
Valium
Volatiles by gas chromatography (Acetaldehyde, acetone, ethanol, diethyl ether, isopropanol, methanol; other may be detected)
Zinc
330 Chemistry - Other (Endrocrinology)
Adrenocorticotrophic hormone
Anti-diuretic hormone
Andrenaline-noradrenaline, total
Adrenaline-noradrenaline fractionation
A/E/DHA, by chromatography
Aldosterone
Calcitonin
Catecholamines, total
Chorionic gonadotropin, quant. BIOASSAY
Chorionic gonadodotropin, quant., IMMUNOASSAY
Cortiosol, plasma
11-Deoxy: 11-oxy ratio of 17-KGS
Dehydroepiandrosterone (DHA)

Estradiol receptor assay
Estriol, placental
Estrogens, total
Estrogens, fractionated (Brown method)
Estrogen receptor assay
Etiocholanolone, dehydroepiandrosterone, androsterone and total 17-Ketosteriods (A/E/DHA)
Ferminiminoglutamic acid (FIGLU)
Free thyroxine (Includes T4-by-column)
FSH (Follicle stimulating Hormone)
Gastrin
Growth hormone (GH OR HGH)
5-HIAA (5 OH-indoleacetic acid, serotonin metabolite)
Homovanillic Acid (HVA)
Human growth hormone (HGH)
Hydroxbutyric dehydrogenase (HBD)
17-Hydroxycorticosteroids, plasma (cortisol by fluorescence method)
17-Hydroxycorticosteroids, urine
11-R-Hydroxylase inhibition test
Hydroxyproline, free
Hydroxyproline, total
5-Hydroxytryptamine
Indole-3-Acetic Acid
Insulin
Insulin (for clearance test)
Inulin
Iodine, T4-by-column chromatography
Iodine, total, fluids, feces
Iodine, total inorganic and PBI
17-Ketosteroids, total, plasma, urine
17-Ketosteroids, beta: alpha ratio
17-Ketosteroids, separated by chromatography (7 compounds)
17-Ketogenic steroids (l7KGS)
Long-acting thyroid stimulator and Thyroid stimulating hormone (LATS and TSH)
Luteinizing hormone (LH)
Metanephrines (total)
11-Oxysteroids
Parathyroid hormone
PBI
PBI, total and inorganic iodine
Phenylalanine
Phenylketonuria (PKU) screening
Pituitary gonadotropins (FSH)
Placental estroil
Placidyl
Plasma cortisol
Pregnanediol
Pragnanetriol
Progesterone
Prolactin
Renin activity
Serotonin, Blood - 5HIAA, 5-hydroxyindoleacetic acid
*Serotonin metabolite, urine - 320
Testosterone
Tetrahydro compound S (THS)
Thyroid stimulating hormone
Thyroxine by column chromatography (T4)
Thyroxine, Free (T4)
Thyroxine by Murphy-Pattee method (T4)
Thyroxine-binding globulin (TBG)
Thyroxine-binding globulin (TBG) without T4 test)
Triiodothyronine (T3)
Vanillyl mandelic acid (VMA)

400   HEMATOLOGY
A2 hemoglobin
A2 and fetal hemoglobin
Basophillic stippling
*Blood specimen for malaria - 130

Cell count - spinal fluid
Complete Blood Count with Differential
Differential
Eosinophile Count
Erythrocyte Sedimentation Rate, Sed Rate
*Folate, R.B.C., Serum - 310
Fragility Test, erythrocytes
*More than one specialty category
*G-6-PD (Glucose-6-Phosphate dehydrogenase) - 220, 310
Hemoglobin A2
Hemoglobin, Fetal
Hemoglobin, Fetal and A2
Hemoglobin-binding protein
*Hemoglobin electrophoresis - 310
Hematocrit
Hemoglobin (cyanmethemoglobin method)
Hemoglobin (iron assay)
Hemoglobin, plasma, urine
Indices, Wintrobe (calculation)
Methemalbumin (Schumm Test)
Platelet Count
Red Blood Count (Erythrocyte Count, RBC)
Reticulocyte Count
Screening test for DIC - Disseminated Intravascular Coagulation
Sickle Cell Preparation
Sulfhemoglobin, methemoglobin, and total Hgb
*Vitamin B-12 - 310
White Blood Count (Leukocyte Count, WBC)
Coagulation Studies Hematology
Bleeding time (Duke) or Ivy and Clotting time (Lee and White)
Complete Coagulation Study
Factor Assays (Factor VIII, IX, VII, XI)
Fibrin-Fibrinogen l egradation Products
Fibrinogen
Partial Thromboplastin Time (APTT, PTT)
Prothrombin Time (Pro time, PT)
Prothrombin Consumption
Prothrombin Utilization
Tests for Circulating Anticoagulants
Cellular Study Hematology
Bone Marrow Aspirate
Eosinophile Smear
Leukocyte Alkaline Phosphatase
Lupus crythematosus Preparation (L.E. Pre)
*Blood Specimen for malaria - See 130 and for other parasites
Molecular abnormality studies
Hemoglobinopathy
Synovial Fluid - Cell Count or Differential

500 IMMUNOHEMATOLOGY
510 A Subgrouping
Blood Grouping, A., B, O, and AB
Rh factor Including Du
Rh Cenotype (C, D, E, c, e)
*M+N Type - 540
*Husband's red cell genotype - 540
*More than one specialty category
520 Antibody Indentification
*Antibody screening test - Indirect Coombs - 540
Antibody titration
Rh antibody titer and blocking antibodies
530 Compatibility Testing - Crossmatch
540 Blood Typing for paternity tests
Direct Coomb's Test
*Hepatitis B Antigen (HBsAg) - 220, 330
*Hepatitis B Antibody (Anti-HBs) - 220, 330
*Husband's Red Cell Genotype - 510
*Indirect Coombs - Antibody screening test - 520

*M + N typing - 510
Rho Gam Workup

600 PATHOLOGY
601 Histopathology
Tissue Decalcification
Bone Marrow Biopsy
Tissue Pathology
Surgical pathology
Frozen sections
Autopsy and sections
620 Oral Pathology
630 Exfoliative Cytology
Cytology - Female Genital Tract
Cytology - nongynecological fluid cytologies

700 PHYSIOLOGICAL TESTING
710 EKG Services

800 RADIOBIOASSAY and NUCLIDES RADIOBIOASSAY
Blood volume - RBC Mass (Cr 51)
1131 Therapy
Polonium
Schilling test (Cobalt 60 - labelled B-12)
Thyroid function studies (1131 Uptake) (IST-3)
Tritium

900 ALL SPECIALTIES AND SUBSPECIALTIES

*More than one specialty category

E. Certification Changes.--Each page of the lists of approved specialties also includes a column "Certification Changed" in which the following codes are used:

- C" indicates a change in the laboratory's approved certification since the preceding listing.
- A" discloses an accretion.
- "TERM" - Laboratory not approved for payment after the indicated date which follows the code.

The reason for termination also is given in the following codes:

1. Involuntary termination - no longer meets requirements
2. Voluntary withdrawal
3. Laboratory closed, merged with other interests, or organizational change
4. Ownership change with new ownership participating under different name
5. Ownership change with new owner not participating
6. Change in ownership - new provider number assigned
7. Involuntary termination - failure to abide by agreement
8. Former "emergency" hospital now fully participating

F. Carrier Contacts With Independent Clinical Laboratories.--An important role of the carrier is as a communicant of necessary information to independent clinical laboratories. Experience has shown that the failure to inform laboratories of Medicare regulations and claims processing procedures may have an adverse effect on prosecution of laboratories suspected of fraudulent activities with respect to tests performed by, or billed on behalf of, independent laboratories. United Stated Attorneys often have to prosecute under a handicap or may simply refuse to prosecute cases where there is no evidence that a laboratory has been specifically informed of Medicare regulations and claims processing procedures.

To assure that laboratories are aware of Medicare regulations and carrier's policy, carrier newsletters should be sent to independent laboratories when any changes are made in coverage policy or claims processing procedures. Additionally, to completely document efforts to fully inform independent laboratories of Medicare policy and their responsibilities, previously issued newsletters should be periodically re-issued to remind laboratories of existing requirements. Some items which should be discussed are the requirements to have the same fee schedule for Medicare and private patients, to specify whether the tests are manual or automated, to indicate the numeric designation 6 or 12 when billing for SMA tests, to document fully the medical necessity for pick-up of specimens from a skilled nursing facility or a beneficiary's home, and, in cases when a laboratory service is referred from one independent laboratory to another independent laboratory, to identify the laboratory actually performing the test.

Additionally, when carrier professional relations representatives make personal contacts with particular laboratories, they should prepare and retain reports of contact indicating dates, persons present, and issues discussed.

G. Independent Laboratory Service to a Patient in His Home or an Institution.--Where it is medically necessary for an independent laboratory to visit a patient to obtain a specimen or to perform EKGs, the service would be covered in the following circumstances:

1. Patient Confined to His Home.--If a patient is confined to his home or other place of residence used as his home, (see §2051.1 for the definition of a "homebound patient"), medical necessity would exist, for example, where a laboratory technician draws a blood specimen or takes an EKG tracing. However, where the specimen is a type which would require only the services of a messenger and would not require the skills of a laboratory technician, e.g., urine or sputum, a specimen pickup service would not be considered medically necessary.

2. Place of Residence is an Institution.--Medical necessity could also exist where the patient's place of residence is an institution including a skilled nursing facility, that does not perform venipunctures. This would apply even though the institution meets the basic definition of a skilled nursing facility and would not ordinarily be considered a beneficiary's home under the rules in § 2100.3. (This policy is intended for independent laboratories only and does not expand the range of coverage of services to homebound patients under the incident to provision.) A trip by an independent laboratory technician to a facility (other than a hospital) for the purpose of performing a venipuncture or taking an EKG tracing is considered medically necessary only if (a) the patient was confined to the facility, and (b) the facility did not have on duty personnel qualified to perform this service. When facility personnel actually obtained and prepared the specimens for the independent laboratory to pick them up, the laboratory provides this pickup service as a service to the facility in the same manner as it does for physicians.

2070.4 Coverage of Portable X-ray Services Not Under the Direct Supervision of a Physician.--
A. Diagnostic X-ray Tests.--Diagnostic x-ray services furnished by a portable x-ray supplier are covered under Part B when furnished in a place or residence used as the patient's home and in nonparticipating institutions. These services must be performed under the general supervision of a physician and certain conditions relating to health and safety (as prescribed by the Secretary) must be met.

Diagnostic portable x-ray services are also covered under Part B when provided in participating SNFs and hospitals, under circumstances in which they cannot be covered under hospital insurance, i.e., the services are not furnished by the participating institution either directly or under arrangements that provide for the institution to bill for the services. (See §2255 for reimbursement for Part B services furnished to inpatients of participating and nonparticipating institutions.)

B. Applicability of Health and Safety Standards.--The health and safety standards apply to all suppliers of portable x-ray services, except physicians who provide immediate personal supervision during the administration of diagnostic x-ray services. Payment is made only for services of approved suppliers who have been found to meet the standards. Notice of the coverage dates for services of approved suppliers are given to carriers by the RO.

When the services of a supplier of portable x-ray services no longer meet the conditions of coverage, physicians having an interest in the supplier's certification status must be notified. The notification action regarding suppliers of portable x-ray equipment is the same as required for decertification of independent laboratories, and the procedures explained in §2070.lC should be followed.

C. Scope of Portable X-Ray Benefit.--In order to avoid payment for services which are inadequate or hazardous to the patient, the scope of the covered portable x-ray benefit is defined as:

• Skeletal films involving arms and legs, pelvis, vertebral column, and skull;
• Chest films which do not involve the use of contrast media (except routine screening procedures and tests in connection with routine physical examinations); and
• Abdominal films which do not involve the use of contrast media.

D. Exclusions From Coverage as Portable X-Ray Services.--Procedures and examinations which are not covered under the portable x-ray provision include the following:

• Procedures involving fluoroscopy;
• Procedures involving the use of contrast media;

- Procedures requiring the administration of a substance to the patient or injection of a substance into the patient and/or special manipulation of the patient;
- Procedures which require special medical skill or knowledge possessed by a doctor of medicine or doctor of osteopathy or which require that medical judgment be exercised;
- Procedures requiring special technical competency and/or special equipment or materials;
- Routine screening procedures; and
- Procedures which are not of a diagnostic nature.

E. Reimbursement Procedure.--
1. Name of Ordering Physician.--Assure that portable x-ray tests have been provided on the written order of a physician. Accordingly, if a bill does not include the name of the physician who ordered the service, that information must be obtained before payment may be made.
2. Reason Chest X-Ray Ordered.--Because all routine screening procedures and tests in connection with routine physical examinations are excluded from coverage under Medicare, all bills for portable x-ray services involving the chest contain, in addition to the name of the physician who ordered the service, the reason an x-ray test was required. If this information is not shown, it is obtained from either the supplier or the physician. If the test was for an excluded routine service, no payment may be made.

See also §§4110 ff. for additional instructions on reviewing bills involving portable x-ray.

F. Electrocardiograms.--The taking of an electrocardiogram tracing by an approved supplier of portable x-ray services may be covered as an "other diagnostic test." The health and safety standards referred to in §2070.4B are thus also applicable to such diagnostic EKG services, e.g., the technician must meet the personnel qualification requirements in the Conditions for Coverage of Portable x-ray Services. (See §50-15 (Electrocardiographic Services) in the Coverage Issues Manual.)

2100 DURABLE MEDICAL EQUIPMENT - GENERAL

Expenses incurred by a beneficiary for the rental or purchase of durable medical equipment (DME) are reimbursable if the following three requirements are met. The decision whether to rent or purchase an item of equipment resides with the beneficiary.

A. The equipment meets the definition of DME (§2100.1); and
B. The equipment is necessary and reasonable for the treatment of the patient's illness or injury or to improve the functioning of his malformed body member (§2100.2); and
C. The equipment is used in the patient's home (§2100.3).

Payment may also be made under this provision for repairs, maintenance, and delivery of equipment as well as for expendable and nonreusable items essential to the effective use of the equipment subject to the conditions in §2100.4.

See §2105 and its appendix for coverage guidelines and screening list of DME. See §4105.3 for models of payment: decisions as to rental or purchase, lump sum and periodic payments, etc. Where covered DME is furnished to a beneficiary by a supplier of services other than a provider of services, reimbursement is made by the carrier on the basis of the reasonable charge. If the equipment is furnished by a provider of services, reimbursement is made to the provider by the intermediary on a reasonable cost basis; see Coverage Issues Appendix 25-1 for hemodialysis equipment and supplies.

2100.1 Definition of Durable Medical Equipment.--Durable medical equipment is equipment which a) can withstand repeated use, and b) is primarily and customarily used to serve a medical purpose, and c) generally is not useful to a person in the absence of an illness or injury; and d) is appropriate for use in the home.

All requirements of the definition must be met before an item can be considered to be durable medical equipment.

A. Durability.--An item is considered durable if it can withstand repeated use, i.e., the type of item which could normally be rented. Medical supplies of an expendable nature such as, incontinent pads, lambs wool pads, catheters, ace bandages, elastic stockings, surgical face masks, irrigating kits, sheets and bags are not considered "durable" within the meaning of the definition. There are other items which, although durable in nature, may fall into other coverage categories such as braces, prosthetic devices, artificial arms, legs, and eyes.

B. Medical Equipment.--Medical equipment is equipment which is primarily and customarily used for medical purposes and is not generally useful in the absence of illness or injury. In most instances, no development will be needed to determine whether a specific item of equipment is medical in nature. However, some cases will require development to determine whether the item constitutes medical equipment. This development would include the advice of local medical organizations (hospitals, medical schools, medical societies) and specialists in the field of physical medicine and rehabilitation. If the equipment is new on the market, it may be necessary, prior to seeking professional advice, to obtain information from the supplier or manufacturer explaining the design, purpose, effectiveness and method of using the equipment in the home as well as the results of any tests or clinical studies that have been conducted.

1. Equipment Presumptively Medical.--Items such as hospital beds, wheelchairs, hemodialysis equipment, iron lungs, respirators, intermittent positive pressure breathing machines, medical regulators, oxygen tents, crutches, canes, trapeze bars, walkers, inhalators, nebulizers, commodes, suction machines and traction equipment presumptively constitute medical equipment. (Although hemodialysis equipment is a prosthetic device (§ 2130), it also meets the definition of DME, and reimbursement for the rental or purchase of such equipment for use in the beneficiary's home will be made only under the provisions for payment applicable to DME. See 25-1 and 25-2 of the Coverage Issues Appendix for coverage of home use of hemodialysis.)

NOTE: There is a wide variety in type of respirators and suction machines. The carrier's medical staff should determine whether the apparatus specified in the claim is appropriate for home use.

2. Equipment Presumptively Nonmedical.--Equipment which is primarily and customarily used for a nonmedical purpose may not be considered "medical" equipment for which payment can be made under the medical insurance program. This is true even though the item has some remote medically related use. For example, in the case of a cardiac patient, an air conditioner might possibly be used to lower room temperature to reduce fluid loss in the patient and to restore an environment conducive to maintenance of the proper fluid balance. Nevertheless, because the primary and customary use of an air conditioner is a nonmedical one, the air conditioner cannot be deemed to be medical equipment for which payment can be made.

Other devices and equipment used for environmental control or to enhance the environmental setting in which the beneficiary is placed are not considered covered DME. These include, for example, room heaters, humidifiers, dehumidifiers, and electric air cleaners. Equipment which basically serves comfort or convenience functions or is primarily for the convenience of a person caring for the patient, such as elevators, stairway elevators, and posture chairs do not constitute medical equipment. Similarly,physical fitness equipment, e.g., an exercycle; first-aid or precautionary-type equipment, e.g., present portable oxygen units; self-help devices, e.g., safety grab bars; and training equipment, e.g., speech teaching machines and braille training texts, are considered nonmedical in nature.

3. Special Exception Items.--Specified items of equipment may be covered under certain conditions even though they do not meet the definition of DME because they are not primarily and customarily used to serve a medical purpose and/or are generally useful in the absence of illness or injury. These items would be covered when it is clearly established that they serve a therapeutic purpose in an individual case and would include:

a. Gel pads and pressure and water mattresses (which generally serve a preventive purpose) when prescribed for a patient who had bed sores or there is medical evidence indicating that he is highly susceptible to such ulceration; and

b. Heat lamps for a medical rather than a soothing or cosmetic purpose, e.g., where the need for heat therapy has been established.

In establishing medical necessity (§2100.2) for the above items, the evidence must show that the item is included in the physician's course of treatment and a physician is supervising its use. (See also Appendix to § 2105.)

NOTE: The above items represent special exceptions and no extension of coverage to other items should be inferred.

2100.4 Repairs, Maintenance, Replacement, and Delivery.--Under the circumstances specified below, payment may be made for repair, maintenance, and replacement of medically required DME, including equipment which had been in use before the user enrolled in Part B of the program. However, do not pay for repair, maintenance, or replacement of equipment in the frequent and substantial servicing or oxygen equipment payment categories. In addition, payments for repair and maintenance may not include payment for parts and labor covered under a manufacturer's or supplier's warranty.

A. Repairs.-- To repair means to fix or mend and to put the equipment back in good condition after damage or wear. Repairs to equipment which a beneficiary owns are covered when necessary to make the equipment serviceable. However, do not pay for repair of previously denied equipment or equipment in the frequent and substantial servicing or oxygen equipment payment categories. If the expense for repairs exceeds the estimated expense of purchasing or renting another item of equipment for the remaining period of medical need, no payment can be made for the amount of the excess. (See subsection C where claims for repairs suggest malicious damage or culpable neglect.)

Since renters of equipment recover from the rental charge the expenses they incur in maintaining in working order the equipment they rent out, separately itemized charges for repair of rented equipment are not covered. This includes items in the frequent and substantial servicing, oxygen equipment, capped rental, and inexpensive or routinely purchased payment categories which are being rented.

A new Certificate of Medical Necessity (CMN) and/or physician's order is not needed for repairs.

For replacement items, see Subsection C below.

B. Maintenance.--Routine periodic maintenance, such as testing, cleaning, regulating and checking of the beneficiary's equipment is not covered. Such routine maintenance is generally expected to be done by the owner rather than by a retailer or some other person who charges the beneficiary. Normally, purchasers of DME are given operating manuals which describe the type of servicing an owner may perform to properly maintain the equipment. It is reasonable to expect that beneficiaries will perform this maintenance. Thus, hiring a third party to do such work is for the convenience of the beneficiary and is not covered.

However, more extensive maintenance which, based on the manufacturers' recommendations, is to be performed by authorized technicians, is covered as repairs for medically necessary equipment which a beneficiary owns. This might include, for example, breaking down sealed components and performing tests which require specialized testing equipment not available to the beneficiary. Do not pay for maintenance of purchased items that require frequent and substantial servicing or oxygen equipment. See §5102.2.G.

Since renters of equipment recover from the rental charge the expenses they incur in maintaining in working order the equipment they rent out, separately itemized charges for maintenance of rented equipment are generally not covered. Payment may not be made for maintenance of rented equipment other than the maintenance and servicing fee established for capped rental items in §5102.1.E.4.

A new CMN and/or physician's order is not needed for covered maintenance.

C. Replacement.--Replacement refers to the provision of an identical or nearly identical item. Situations involving the provision of a different item because of a change in medical condition are not addressed in this section.

Equipment which the beneficiary owns or is a capped rental item may be replaced in cases of loss or irreparable damage. Irreparable damage refers to a specific accident or to a natural disaster (e.g., fire, flood, etc.). A physician's order and/or new Certificate of Medical Necessity (CMN), when required, is needed to reaffirm the medical necessity of the item.

Irreparable wear refers to deterioration sustained from day-to-day usage over time and a specific event cannot be identified. Replacement of equipment due to irreparable wear takes into consideration the reasonable useful lifetime of the equipment. If the item of equipment has been in continuous use by the patient on either a rental or purchase basis for the equipment's useful lifetime, the beneficiary may elect to obtain a new piece of equipment. Replacement may be reimbursed when a new physician order and/or new CMN, when required, is needed to reaffirm the medical necessity of the item.

The reasonable useful lifetime of durable medical equipment is determined through program instructions. In the absence of program instructions, carriers may determine the reasonable useful lifetime of equipment, but in no case can it be less than 5 years. Computation of the useful lifetime is based on when the equipment is delivered to the beneficiary, not the age of the equipment. Replacement due to wear is not covered during the reasonable useful lifetime of the equipment. During the reasonable useful lifetime, Medicare does cover repair up to the cost of replacement (but not actual replacement) for medically necessary equipment owned by the beneficiary. (See subsection A.)

Charges for the replacement of oxygen equipment, items that require frequent and substantial servicing or inexpensive or routinely purchased items which are being rented are not covered.

Cases suggesting malicious damage, culpable neglect or wrongful disposition of equipment as discussed in §2100.6 should be investigated and denied where the DMERC/Carrier determines that it is unreasonable to make program payment under the circumstances.

D. Delivery.--Payment for delivery of DME whether rented or purchased is generally included in the fee schedule allowance for the item. See §5105 for the rules that apply to making reimbursement for exceptional cases.

E. Leased Renal Dialysis Equipment.--Generally, where renal dialysis equipment is leased directly from the manufacturer, the rental charge is closely related to the manufacturer's cost of the equipment which means it does not include a margin for recovering the cost of repairs beyond the initial warranty period.

In view of physical distance and other factors which may make it impractical for the manufacturer to perform repairs, it is not feasible to make the manufacturer responsible for all repairs and include a margin for the additional costs. Therefore, reimbursement may be made for the repair and maintenance of home dialysis equipment leased directly from the manufacturer (or other party acting essentially as an intermediary between the patient and the manufacturer for the purpose of assuming the financial risk) if the rental charge does not include a margin to recover these costs, and then only when the patient is free to secure repairs locally in the most economical manner.

Where, on the other hand, a third party is in the business of medical equipment retail supply and rental, the presumption that there is a margin in the rental charge for dialysis equipment to cover the costs of repair services will be retained. The exclusion from coverage of separately itemized repair charges will, therefore, continue to be applied in these situations, and the patient must look to the supplier to perform (or cover the cost of) necessary repairs, maintenance, and replacement of the home dialysis equipment.

In all cases, whether the dialysis equipment is being purchased, is owned outright, or is being leased, Medicare payment is to be made only after the initial warranty period has expired. Generally, reimbursement for repairs, maintenance, and replacement parts for medically necessary home dialysis equipment may be made in a lump sum payment. However, where extensive repairs are required and the charge for repairing the item represents a substantial proportion of the purchase price of a replacement system, exercise judgment with respect to a possible need to make periodic payments, instead of a lump-sum payment, for repair of such equipment.

As in the case of the maintenance of purchased DME, routine periodic servicing of leased dialysis equipment, including most testing and cleaning, is not covered. While reimbursement will be made for more extensive maintenance and necessary repairs of leased dialysis equipment, the patient or family member is expected to perform those services for which the training for home or self-dialysis would have qualified them, e.g., replacement of a light bulb.

Reasonable charges for travel expenses related to the repair of leased dialysis equipment are covered if the repairman customarily charges for travel and this is a common practice among other repairman in the area. When a repair charge includes an element for travel, however, the location of other suitably qualified repairmen will be considered in determining the allowance for travel.

NOTE: The above coverage instructions pertain to a special case and no extension of such coverage with respect to other items should be inferred.

2100.5   Coverage of Supplies and Accessories.--Reimbursement may be made for supplies, e.g., oxygen (see §60-4 in the Coverage Issues Manual for the coverage of oxygen in the home), that are necessary for the effective use of durable medical equipment. Such supplies include those drugs and biologicals which must be put directly into the equipment in order to achieve the therapeutic benefit of the durable medical equipment or to assure the proper functioning of the equipment, e.g., tumor chemotherapy agents used with an infusion pump or heparin used with a home dialysis system. However, the coverage of such drugs or biologicals does not preclude the need for a determination that the drug or biological itself is reasonable and necessary for treatment of the illness or injury or to improve the functioning of a malformed body member.

In the case of prescription drugs, other than oxygen, used in conjunction with durable medical equipment, prosthetic, orthotics, and supplies (DMEPOS) or prosthetic devices, the entity that dispenses the drug must furnish it directly to the patient for whom a prescription is written. The entity that dispenses the drugs must have a Medicare supplier number, must possess a current license.

2120.1   Vehicle and Crew Requirement

A. The Vehicle.--The vehicle must be a specially designed and equipped automobile or other vehicle (in some areas of the United States this might be a boat or plane) for transporting the sick or injured. It must have customary patient care equipment including a stretcher, clean linens, first aid supplies, oxygen equipment, and it must also have such other safety and lifesaving equipment as is required by State or local authorities.

B. The Crew.--The ambulance crew must consist of at least two members. Those crew members charged with the care or handling of the patient must include one individual with adequate first aid training, i.e., training at least equivalent to that provided by the standard and advanced Red Cross first aid courses. Training "equivalent" to the standard and advanced Red Cross first aid training courses included ambulance service training and experience acquired in military service, successful completion by the individual of a comparable first aid course furnished by or under the sponsorship of State or local authorities, an educational institution, a fire department, a hospital, a professional organization, or other such qualified organization. On-the-job training involving the administration of first aid under the supervision of or in conjunction with trained first aid personnel for a period of time sufficient to assure the trainee's proficiency in handling the wide range of patient care services that may have to be performed by a qualified attendant can also be considered as "equivalent training."

C. Verification of Compliance.--In determining whether the vehicles and personnel of each supplier meet all of the above requirements, carriers may accept the supplier's statement (absent information to the contrary) that its vehicles and personnel meet all of the requirements if (l) the statement describes the first aid, safety, and other patient care items with which the vehicles are equipped, (2) the statement shows the extent of first aid training acquired by the personnel assigned to those vehicles, (3) the statement contains the supplier's agreement to notify the carrier of any change in operation which could affect the coverage of his ambulance services, and (4) the information provided indicates that the requirements are met. The statement must be accompanied by documentary evidence that the ambulance has the equipment required by State and local authorities. Documentary evidence could include a letter from such authorities, a copy of a license, permit certificate, etc., issued by the authorities. The statement and supporting documentation would be kept on file by the carrier.

When a supplier does not submit such a statement or whenever there is a question about a supplier's compliance with any of the above requirements for vehicle and crew (including suppliers who have completed the statement), carriers should take appropriate action including, where necessary, on-site inspection of the vehicles and verification of the qualifications of personnel to determine whether the ambulance service qualifies for reimbursement under Medicare. Since the requirements described above for coverage of ambulance services are applicable to the overall operation of the ambulance supplier's service, it is not required that information regarding personnel and vehicles be obtained on an individual trip basis.

D. Ambulance of Providers of Services.--The Part A intermediary is responsible for the processing of claims for ambulance service furnished by participating hospitals, skilled nursing facilities and home health agencies and has the responsibility to determine the compliance of provider's ambulance and crew. Since provider ambulance services furnished "under arrangements" with suppliers can be covered only if the supplier meets the above requirements, the Part A intermediary may ask the carrier to identify those suppliers who meet the requirements.

E. Equipment and Supplies.--As mentioned above, the ambulance must have customary patient care equipment and first aid supplies. Reusable devices and equipment such as backboards, neckboards and inflatable leg and arm splints are considered part of the general ambulance service and would be included in the charge for the trip. On the other hand, separate reasonable charge based on actual quantities used may be recognized for nonreusable items and disposable supplies such as oxygen, gauze and dressings required in the care of the patient during his trip.

2130 PROSTHETIC DEVICES

A. General.--Prosthetic devices (other than dental) which replace all or part of an internal body organ (including contiguous tissue), or replace all or part of the function of a permanently inoperative or malfunctioning internal body organ are covered when furnished on a physician's order. This does not require a determination that there is no possibility that the patient's condition may improve sometime in the future. If the medical record, including the judgment of the attending physician, indicates the condition is of long and indefinite duration, the test of permanence is considered met. (Such a device may also be covered under §2050.l as a supply when furnished incident to a physician's service.)

Examples of prosthetic devices include cardiac pacemakers, prosthetic lenses (see subsection B), breast prostheses (including a surgical brassiere) for postmastectomy patients, maxillofacial devices and devices which replace all or part of the ear or nose. A urinary collection and retention system with or without a tube is a prosthetic device replacing bladder function in case of permanent urinary incontinence. The Foley catheter is also considered a prosthetic device when ordered for a patient with permanent urinary incontinence. However, chucks, diapers, rubber sheets, etc., are supplies that are not covered under this provision. (Although hemodialysis equipment is a prosthetic device, payment for the rental or purchase of such equipment for use in the home is made only under the provisions for payment applicable to durable medical equipment (see §4105ff) or the special rules that apply to the ESRD program.)

NOTE: Medicare does not cover a prosthetic device dispensed to a patient prior to the time at which the patient undergoes the procedure that makes necessary the use of the device. For example, do not make a separate Part B payment for an intraocular lens (IOL) or pacemaker that a physician, during an office visit prior to the actual surgery, dispenses to the patient for his/her use. Dispensing a prosthetic device in this manner raises health and safety issues. Moreover, the need for the device cannot be clearly established until the procedure that makes its use possible is successfully performed. Therefore, dispensing a prosthetic device in this manner is not considered reasonable and necessary for the treatment of the patient's condition.

Colostomy (and other ostomy) bags and necessary accouterments required for attachment are covered as prosthetic devices. This coverage also includes irrigation and flushing equipment and other items and supplies directly related to ostomy care, whether the attachment of a bag is required.

Accessories and/or supplies which are used directly with an enteral or parenteral device to achieve the therapeutic benefit of the prosthesis or to assure the proper functioning of the device are covered under the prosthetic device benefit subject to the additional guidelines in the Coverage Issues Manual §§65-10 - 65-10.3.

Covered items include catheters, filters, extension tubing, infusion bottles, pumps (either food or infusion), intravenous (I.V.) pole, needles, syringes, dressings, tape, Heparin Sodium (parenteral only), volumetric monitors (parenteral only), and parenteral and enteral nutrient solutions. Baby food and other regular grocery products that can be blenderized and used with the enteral system are not covered. Note that some of these items, e.g., a food pump and an I.V. pole, qualify as DME. Although coverage of the enteral and parenteral nutritional therapy systems is provided on the basis of the prosthetic device benefit, the payment rules relating to rental or purchase of DME apply to such items. (See §4105.3.) Code claims in accordance with the HCFA Common Procedure Coding System (HCPCS).

The coverage of prosthetic devices includes replacement of and repairs to such devices as explained in subsection D.

B. Prosthetic Lenses.--The term "internal body organ" includes the lens of an eye. Prostheses replacing the lens of an eye include post-surgical lenses customarily used during convalescence from eye surgery in which the lens of the eye was removed. In addition, permanent lenses are also covered when required by an individual lacking the organic lens of the eye because of surgical removal or congenital absence. Prosthetic lenses obtained on or after the beneficiary's date of entitlement to supplementary medical insurance benefits may be covered even though the surgical removal of the crystalline lens occurred before entitlement.

    1. Prosthetic Cataract Lenses.--Make payment for one of the following prosthetic lenses or combinations of prosthetic lenses when determined to be medically necessary by a physician (see §2020.25 for coverage of prosthetic lenses prescribed by a doctor of optometry) to restore essentially the vision provided by the crystalline lens of the eye:

        • prosthetic bifocal lenses in frames;
        • prosthetic lenses in frames for far vision, and prosthetic lenses in frames for near vision; or
        • when a prosthetic contact lens(es) for far vision is prescribed (including cases of binocular and monocular aphakia), make payment for the contact lens(es) and prosthetic lenses in frames for near vision to be worn at the same time as the contact lens(es), and prosthetic lenses in frames to be worn when the contacts have been removed.

Make payment for lenses which have ultraviolet absorbing or reflecting properties, in lieu of payment for regular (untinted) lenses, if it has been determined that such lenses are medically reasonable and necessary for the individual patient.

Do not make payment for cataract sunglasses obtained in addition to the regular (untinted) prosthetic lenses since the sunglasses duplicate the restoration of vision function performed by the regular prosthetic lenses.

2. Payment for IOLs Furnished in Ambulatory Surgical Centers (ASCs). Effective for services furnished on or after March 12, 1990, payment for IOLs inserted during or subsequent to cataract surgery in a Medicare certified ASC is included with the payment for facility services that are furnished in connection with the covered surgery. Section 5243.3 explains payment procedures for ASC facility services and the IOL allowance.

3. Limitation on Coverage of Conventional Lenses.--Make payment for no more than one pair of conventional eyeglasses or conventional contact lenses furnished after each cataract surgery with insertion of an IOL.

C. Dentures.--Dentures are excluded from coverage. However, when a denture or a portion thereof is an integral part (built-in) of a covered prosthesis (e.g., an obturator to fill an opening in the palate), it is covered as part of that prosthesis.

D. Supplies, Repairs, Adjustments, and Replacement.--Make payment for supplies that are necessary for the effective use of a prosthetic device (e.g., the batteries needed to operate an artificial larynx). Adjustment of prosthetic devices required by wear or by a change in the patient's condition is covered when ordered by a physician. To the extent applicable, follow the provisions relating to the repair and replacement of durable medical equipment in §2100.4 for the repair and replacement of prosthetic devices. (See §2306.D in regard to payment for devices replaced under a warranty.) Regardless of the date that the original eyewear was furnished (i.e., whether before, on, or after January 1, 1991), do not pay for replacement of conventional eyeglasses or contact lenses covered under subsection B.3.

Necessary supplies, adjustments, repairs, and replacements are covered even when the device had been in use before the user enrolled in Part B of the program, so long as the device continues to be medically required.

2210.3 Application of Guidelines.--The following discussion illustrates the application of the above guidelines to some of the more common physical therapy modalities and procedures utilized in the treatment of patients:

1. Hot Pack, Hydrocollator, Infra-Red Treatments, Paraffin Baths and Whirlpool Baths.--Heat treatments of this type and whirlpool baths do not ordinarily require the skills of a qualified physical therapist. However, in a particular case the skills, knowledge, and judgment of a qualified physical therapist might be required in such treatments or baths, e.g., where the patient's condition is complicated by circulatory deficiency, areas of desensitization, open wounds, or other complications. Also, if such treatments are given prior to but as an integral part of a skilled physical therapy procedure, they would be considered part of the physical therapy service.

2. Gait Training.--Gait evaluation and training furnished a patient whose ability to walk has been impaired by neurological, muscular, or skeletal abnormality require the skills of a qualified physical therapist. However, if gait evaluation and training cannot reasonably be expected to improve significantly the patient's ability to walk, such services would not be considered reasonable and necessary. Repetitive exercises to improve gait or maintain strength and endurance, and assistive walking, such as provided in support for feeble or unstable patients, are appropriately provided by supportive personnel, e.g., aides or nursing personnel and do not require the skills of a qualified physical therapist.

3. Ultrasound, Shortwave, and Microwave Diathermy Treatments.--These modalities must always be performed by or under the supervision of a qualified physical therapist, and therefore, such treatments constitute physical therapy.

4. Range of Motion Tests.--Only the qualified physical therapist may perform range of motion tests and, therefore, such tests would constitute physical therapy.

5. Therapeutic Exercises.--Therapeutic exercises which must be performed by or under the supervision of a qualified physical therapist due either to the type of exercise employed or to the condition of the patient would constitute physical therapy. Range of motion exercises require the skills of a qualified physical therapist only when they are part of the active treatment of a specific disease which has resulted in a loss or restriction of mobility (as evidenced by physical therapy notes showing the degree of motion lost and the degree to be restored) and such exercises, either because of their nature or the condition of the patient, may only be performed safely and effectively by or

under the supervision of a qualified physical therapist. Generally, range of motion exercises which are not related to the restoration of a specific loss of function but rather are related to the maintenance of function (see §2210.2) do not require the skills of a qualified physical therapist.

2230 TREATMENT OF END- STAGE RENAL DISEASE

2230.1 Definition of Terms.--

A. End-Stage Renal Disease (ESRD).--The term "end- stage renal disease" means that stage of kidney impairment that appears irreversible and permanent and requires a regular course of dialysis or kidney transplantation to maintain life.

B. Dialysis.--A process by which waste products are removed from the body by diffusion from one fluid compartment to another across a semi-permeable membrane. There are two types of renal dialysis in common clinical usage, hemodialysis and peritoneal dialysis. Both hemodialysis and peritoneal dialysis are acceptable modes of treatment of chronic renal disease.

- Hemodialysis.--Where blood is passed through an artificial kidney machine and the waste products diffuse across a man-made membrane into a bath solution known as dialysate after which the cleansed blood is returned to the patient's body.
- Peritoneal Dialysis.--Where the waste products pass from the patient's body through the peritoneal membrane into the peritoneal (abdominal) cavity where the bath solution (dialysate) is introduced and removed periodically.
- Peritoneal dialysis is particularly suited for:
  * patients without family members to assist in self-hemodialysis;
  * children;
  * patients with no peripheral sites available for fistula or cannula placement;
  * patients who have difficulty learning the more complex hemodialysis technique; and
  * elderly patients with cardiovascular disease who are unable to tolerate intravascular fluid shifts associated with hemodialysis.

Peritoneal dialysis may involve the use of a machine as in the case of intermittent or continuous cycling peritoneal dialysis, or it may not as in the case of continuous ambulatory peritoneal dialysis (CAPD). See §2231 for a discussion of CAPD.

C. Maintenance Dialysis.--The usual periodic dialysis treatments which are given to a patient who has end-stage renal disease in order to sustain life and ameliorate uremic symptoms. Maintenance peritoneal and hemodialysis is generally required two to three times per week, but less frequent treatments are sometimes adequate. In addition, greater frequency may be covered upon review of evidence which establishes medical necessity.

D. Acute Dialysis.--Dialysis given to patients who are not ESRD patients, but who require dialysis because of temporary kidney failure due to a sudden trauma; e.g., traffic accident or ingestion of certain drugs.

E. Self-Dialysis.--Dialysis performed, with little or no professional assistance, by an ESRD patient who has completed an appropriate training course. The patient may perform self-dialysis at home or in an outpatient facility.

F. Back-Up Dialysis.-- Dialysis given to patients under special circumstances, in a situation other than the patients' usual dialysis environment. Examples are dialysis of a home dialysis patient in a dialysis facility when his equipment fails, inpatient dialysis when the patient's illness requires more comprehensive care on an inpatient basis, and pre- and postoperative dialysis provided to transplant patients.

G. Inpatient Dialysis.--Dialysis furnished to an ESRD patient who is a hospital inpatient.

H. Hemofiltration.--A safe and effective technique for the treatment of ESRD patients and an alternative to peritoneal dialysis and hemodialysis. Hemofiltration (which is also known as diafiltration) removes fluid, electrolytes and other low molecular weight toxic substances from the blood by filtration through hollow artificial membranes and may be routinely performed in 3 weekly sessions. In contrast to both hemodialysis and peritoneal dialysis treatments, which eliminate dissolved substances via diffusion across semipermeable membranes, hemofiltration mimics the filtration process of the normal kidney. The technique requires an arteriovenous access. Hemofiltration may be performed either in facility or at home.

The procedure is most advantageous when applied to high-risk unstable patients, such as older patients with cardiovascular diseases or diabetes, because there are fewer side effects such as hypotension, hypertension or volume overload.

I. Hemoperfusion.--Hemoperfusion is a process which removes substances from the blood through the dialysis membrane by using a charcoal or resin artificial kidney. When used in the treatment of life threatening drug overdose, hemoperfusion is a covered service for patients with or without renal dialysis. Hemoperfusion is also covered when used in conjunction with DFO to treat aluminum toxicity. However, hemoperfusion is not covered when used to improve the results of hemodialysis nor when used in conjunction with deferoxamine (DFO) to remove iron overload.

2230.2 Approved Dialysis Settings

A. Facility.--Maintenance dialysis may be furnished in a provider-based or independently operated ESRD facility approved under the ESRD program.

B. Home--Patients who have been appropriately trained can dialyze at home. They may or may not require the assistance of another person who has also been appropriately trained. In the home setting all home dialysis supplies and equipment are covered, as well as home dialysis support services furnished by an ESRD facility approved under the ESRD program.

2230.3 Physician's Services--General.--Payment for physician's services generally is subject to the guidelines in §2020. Basically, physician's services furnished to a renal dialysis patient are covered if determined to be reasonable and necessary. Pay physician's services furnished in connection with dialysis sessions for outpatients who are on maintenance dialysis in a facility or at home by the monthly capitation payment method or the initial method. (See §§4272, 4273, 5037, and 5211.1 for payment instructions.)

2230.4 Physician's Services to an Inpatient.--Physicians' services furnished to ESRD patients who require inpatient hospital care in connection with the renal condition or any other condition are covered if you determine the services to be reasonable and necessary.

(See §5211.1 for a discussion of paying for ESRD physician services to ESRD inpatients.)

2230.5 Physician's Services - Outpatient Maintenance Dialysis.--A physician's service furnished to dialysis patients who are treated as outpatients are divided into two major categories: direct patient care and administrative. (See §§4272, 4273 and 5037 for payment instructions.)

A. Direct Patient Care Services--These services are part of the medical treatment furnished to an individual patient that:

1. Are personally furnished by a physician to an individual patient;
2. Contribute directly to the diagnosis or treatment of an individual patient; and
3. Ordinarily must be performed by a physician.

They include:

- Visits to the patient during dialysis, in conjunction with review of laboratory test results, nurses' notes and any other medical documentation, as a basis for:
    * Adjustment of the patient's medication or diet or the dialysis procedure;
    * Prescription of medical supplies; and
    * Evaluation of the patient's psychosocial status and the appropriateness of the treatment modality.
- Medical direction of staff in delivering services to a patient during a dialysis session.
- Pre- and post-dialysis examinations where medically appropriate;
- Insertions of a catheter for patients on maintenance peritoneal dialysis who are not provided an indwelling catheter;
- Services which must be furnished at a time other than during the dialysis procedure; e.g., monthly and semi-annual examinations to review health status and treatment;
- Other services furnished during dialysis; e.g., declotting of shunts, needle insertions into fistulae, care during immediately life-threatening complications related to the dialysis procedure, and care of nonrenal conditions.

B. Administrative Services.--A component of the facility's cost or charge for dialysis is for "administrative services" furnished by physicians. Administrative services are differentiated from physicians' direct patient care services because they constitute supervision of staff or are not directly related to the care of an individual patient, but benefit all patients and the facility as a whole. The administrative type of physician's service are services that are supportive of the facility as a whole

657

and of benefit to patients in general. Examples of such services include participation in management of the facility, advice on and procurement of facility equipment and supplies, supervision of staff, staff training and staff conferences. Disallow all claims for these services with an explanation that such services are paid as part of the dialysis services which are included in the facility charge for dialysis.

2230.6   Physician's Services During Self-Dialysis Training.--
A. Initial Training.--All physician's services required to create the capacity for self-dialysis are covered. For example,

1. Direction of, and participation in, training of dialysis patients.
2. Review of family and home status, environment and counseling and training of family members.
3. Review of training progress.

See §5037.6 for reimbursement instructions for physician's training services.

B. Subsequent Training.-- Occasionally, it is necessary to furnish additional training to an ESRD self-dialysis beneficiary after the initial training course is completed; e.g., because of a change from hemodialysis to peritoneal dialysis, a change in equipment. The amount of additional training required depends upon the transferability of the skills the patient has already learned; subsequent training would normally be very limited. Physicians' training services furnished during subsequent training of an ESRD beneficiary are covered and reimbursed in addition to the initial training fee. Base the payment for subsequent training sessions on the amount of $20 per training session. The total payment for a course of subsequent training may not be based on an amount that exceeds $500.

Subsequent training sessions that are reimbursable under this rule must be distinguished from the ongoing services for which the original training fee is considered payment in full; e.g., answering the patient's questions arising after home dialysis has begun about the machine the patient has already been trained to use. No additional payment is made after the initial training course unless the subsequent training is required because of a change from the patient's treatment machine to a machine that he had not been trained to use in the initial training course, a change in the type of dialysis, or a change in setting or dialysis partner.

2300 GENERAL EXCLUSIONS

No payment can be made under either the hospital insurance or supplementary medical insurance programs for certain items and services.

A. Not reasonable and necessary (§2303);
B. No legal obligation to pay for or provide services (§2306);
C. Furnished or paid for by government instrumentalities (§2309);
D. Not provided within United States (§2312);
E. Resulting from war (§2315);
F. Personal comfort (§2318);
G. Routine services and appliances (§2320);
H. Supportive devices for feet (§2323);
I. Custodial care (§2326);
J. Cosmetic surgery (§2329);
K. Charges by immediate relatives or members of household (§2332);
L. Dental services (§2336);
M. Paid or expected to be paid under worker's compensation (§2370).
N. Nonphysician services provided to a hospital inpatient which were not provided directly or arranged for by the hospital (§2390).

2300.1 Services Related to and Required as a Result of Services Which Are Not Covered Under Medicare
A.   Medical and hospital services are sometimes required to treat a condition that arises as a result of services which are not covered because they are determined to be not reasonable and necessary or because they are excluded from coverage for other reasons. Services "related to" noncovered services (e.g., cosmetic surgery, noncovered organ transplants, noncovered artificial organ implants, etc.), including services related to followup care and complications of noncovered services which require treatment during a hospital stay in which the noncovered service was performed, are not covered services under Medicare. Services "not related to" noncovered services are covered under Medicare.

B. Identify which services are related to noncovered services and which are not. Following are some examples of services "related to" and "not related to" noncovered services while the beneficiary is an inpatient:

1. A beneficiary was hospitalized for a noncovered service and broke a leg while in the hospital. Services related to care of the broken leg during this stay is a clear cut example of "not related to" services and are covered under Medicare.

2. A beneficiary was admitted to the hospital for covered services, but during the course of hospitalization became a candidate for a noncovered transplant or implant and actually received the transplant or implant during that hospital stay. When the original admission was entirely unrelated to the diagnosis that led to a recommendation for a noncovered transplant or implant, the services related to the admitting condition would be covered.

3. A beneficiary was admitted to the hospital for covered services related to a condition which ultimately led to identification of a need for transplant and receipt of a transplant during the same hospital stay. If, on the basis of the nature of the services and a comparison of the date they are received with the date on which the beneficiary is identified as a transplant candidate, the services could reasonably be attributed to preparation for the noncovered transplant, the services would be "related to" noncovered services and would also be noncovered.

C. After a beneficiary has been discharged from the hospital stay in which he received noncovered services, medical and hospital services required to treat a condition or complication that arises as a result of the prior noncovered services may be covered when they are reasonable and necessary in all other respects. Thus, coverage could be provided for subsequent inpatient stays or outpatient treatment ordinarily covered by Medicare, even if the need for treatment arose because of a previous noncovered procedure. Some examples of services that may be found to be covered under this policy are the reversal of intestinal bypass surgery for obesity, repair of complications from transsexual surgery or from cosmetic surgery, removal of a noncovered bladder stimulator, or treatment of any infection at the surgical site of a noncovered transplant that occurred following discharge from the hospital.

However, any subsequent services that could be expected to have been incorporated into a global fee should be denied. Thus, where a patient undergoes cosmetic surgery and the treatment regimen calls for a series of postoperative visits to the surgeon for evaluating the patient's progress, these visits should be denied.

(See Intermediary Manual, §3637.15 and Hospital Manual, §415.18 for billing procedures.)

2303 SERVICES NOT REASONABLE AND NECESSARY

Items and services which are not reasonable and necessary for the diagnosis or treatment of illness or injury, or to improve the functioning of a malformed body member; e.g., payment cannot be made for the rental of a special hospital bed to be used by the patient in his home unless it was a reasonable and necessary part of the patient's treatment. See also §2318.

2320 ROUTINE SERVICES AND APPLIANCES

Routine physical checkups; eyeglasses, contact lenses, and eye examinations for the purpose of prescribing, fitting or changing eyeglasses; eye refractions; hearing aids and examinations for hearing aids; and immunizations are not covered.

The routine physical checkup exclusion applies to (a) examinations performed without relationship to treatment or diagnosis for a specific illness, symptom, complaint, or injury, and (b) examinations required by third parties such as insurance companies, business establishments, or Government agencies.

(If the claim is for a diagnostic test or examination performed solely for the purpose of establishing a claim under title IV of Public Law 91-173 (Black Lung Benefits), advise the claimant to contact his/her Social Security office regarding the filing of a claim for reimbursement under that program.)

The exclusions apply to eyeglasses or contact lenses and eye examinations for the purpose of prescribing, fitting, or changing eyeglasses or contact lenses for refractive errors. The exclusions do not apply to physician services (and services incident to a physician's service) performed in conjunction with an eye disease (e.g., glaucoma or cataracts) or to postsurgical prosthetic lenses which are customarily used during convalescence from eye surgery in which the lens of the eye was removed or to permanent prosthetic lenses required by an individual lacking the organic lens of the eye, whether by surgical removal or congenital disease. Such prosthetic lens is a replacement for an internal body organ (the lens of the eye). (See §2130.)

The coverage of services rendered by an ophthalmologist is dependent on the purpose of the examination rather than on the ultimate diagnosis of the patient's condition. When a beneficiary goes to an ophthalmologist with a complaint or symptoms of an eye disease or injury, the ophthalmologist's services (except for eye refractions) are covered regardless of the fact that only eyeglasses were prescribed. However, when a beneficiary goes to his/her ophthalmologist for an eye examination with no specific complaint, the expenses for the examination are not covered even though as a result of such examination the doctor discovered a pathologic condition.

In the absence of evidence to the contrary, you may carrier may assume that an eye examination performed by an ophthalmologist on the basis of a complaint by the beneficiary or symptoms of an eye disease was not for the purpose of prescribing, fitting, or changing eyeglasses.

Expenses for all refractive procedures, whether performed by an ophthalmologist (or any other physician) or an optometrist and without regard to the reason for performance of the refraction, are excluded from coverage. (See §§4125 and 5217 for claims review and reimbursement instructions concerning refractive services.)

With the exception of vaccinations for pneumococcal pneumonia, hepatitis B, and influenza, which are specifically covered under the law, vaccinations or inoculations are generally excluded as immunizations unless they are directly related to the treatment of an injury or direct exposure such as antirabies treatment, tetanus antitoxin or booster vaccine, botulin antitoxin, antivenin, or immune globulin.

2323 FOOT CARE AND SUPPORTIVE DEVICES FOR FEET

NOTE: See §4281 for the relationship between foot care and the coverage and billing of the diagnosis and treatment of peripheral neuropathy with loss of protective sensation (LOPS) in people with diabetes.

A. Exclusion of Coverage.--The following foot care services are generally excluded from coverage under both Part A and Part B. Exceptions to this general exclusion for limited treatment of routine foot care services are described in subsections A.2 and B. (See §4120 for procedural instructions in applying foot care exclusions.)

    1. Treatment of Flat Foot.--The term "flat foot" is defined as a condition in which one or more arches of the foot have flattened out. Services or devices directed toward the care or correction of such conditions, including the prescription of supportive devices, are not covered.
    2. Treatment of Subluxation of Foot.--Subluxations of the foot are defined as partial dislocations or displacements of joint surfaces, tendons ligaments, or muscles of the foot. Surgical or nonsurgical treatments undertaken for the sole purpose of correcting a subluxated structure in the foot as an isolated entity are not covered.

This exclusion does not apply to medical or surgical treatment of subluxation of the ankle joint (talo-crural joint). In addition, reasonable and necessary medical or surgical services, diagnosis, or treatment for medical conditions that have resulted from or are associated with partial displacement of structures is covered. For example, if a patient has osteoarthritis that has resulted in a partial displacement of joints in the foot, and the primary treatment is for the osteoarthritis, coverage is provided.

    3. Routine Foot Care.--Except as provided in subsection B, routine foot care is excluded from coverage. Services that normally are considered routine and not covered by Medicare include the following:

- The cutting or removal of corns and calluses;
- The trimming, cutting, clipping, or debriding of nails; and
- Other hygienic and preventive maintenance care, such as cleaning and soaking the feet, the use of skin creams to maintain skin tone of either ambulatory or bedfast patients, and any other service performed in the absence of localized illness, injury, or symptoms involving the foot.

B. Exceptions to Routine Foot Care Exclusion.--
    1. Necessary and Integral Part of Otherwise Covered Services.--In certain circumstances, services ordinarily considered to be routine may be covered if they are performed as a necessary and integral part of otherwise covered services, such as diagnosis and treatment of ulcers, wounds, or infections.
    2. Treatment of Warts on Foot.--The treatment of warts (including plantar warts) on the foot is covered to the same extent as services provided for the treatment of warts located elsewhere on the body.
    3. Presence of Systemic Condition.--The presence of a systemic condition such as metabolic, neurologic, or peripheral vascular disease may require scrupulous foot care by a professional that in the absence of such condition(s) would be considered routine (and, therefore, excluded from

coverage). Accordingly, foot care that would otherwise be considered routine may be covered when systemic condition(s) result in severe circulatory embarrassment or areas of diminished sensation in the individual's legs or feet. (See subsection C.)

In these instances, certain foot care procedures that otherwise are considered routine (e.g., cutting or removing corns and calluses, or trimming, cutting, clipping, or debriding nails) may pose a hazard when performed by a nonprofessional person on patients with such systemic conditions. (See §4120 for procedural instructions.)

4. Mycotic Nails.--In the absence of a systemic condition, treatment of mycotic nails may be covered.

The treatment of mycotic nails for an ambulatory patient is covered only when the physician attending the patient's mycotic condition documents that (1) there is clinical evidence of mycosis of the toenail, and (2) the patient has marked limitation of ambulation, pain, or secondary infection resulting from the thickening and dystrophy of the infected toenail plate.

The treatment of mycotic nails for a nonambulatory patient is covered only when the physician attending the patient's mycotic condition documents that (1) there is clinical evidence of mycosis of the toenail, and (2) the patient suffers from pain or secondary infection resulting from the thickening and dystrophy of the infected toenail plate.

For the purpose of these requirements, documentation means any written information that is required by the carrier in order for services to be covered. Thus, the information submitted with claims must be substantiated by information found in the patient's medical record. Any information, including that contained in a form letter, used for documentation purposes is subject to carrier verification in order to ensure that the information adequately justifies coverage of the treatment of mycotic nails. (See §4120 for claims processing criteria.)

C.   Systemic Conditions.--Although not intended as a comprehensive list, the following metabolic, neurologic, and peripheral vascular diseases (with synonyms in parentheses) most commonly represent the underlying conditions that might justify coverage for routine foot care.

   *Diabetes mellitus
   Arteriosclerosis obliterans (arteriosclerosis of extremities, occlusive peripheral arteriosclerosis)
   Buerger's disease (thromboangiitis obliterans)
   *Chronic thrombophlebitis

Peripheral neuropathies involving the feet -

   *Associated with malnutrition and vitamin deficiency
   Malnutrition (general, pellagra)
   Alcoholism
   Malabsorption (celiac disease, tropical sprue)
   Pernicious anemia
   *Associated with carcinoma
   *Associated with diabetes mellitus
   *Associated with drugs and toxins
   *Associated with multiple sclerosis
   *Associated with uremia (chronic renal disease)
   Associated with traumatic injury
   Associated with leprosy or neurosyphilis
   Associated with hereditary disorders -
   Hereditary sensory radicular neuropathy
   Angiokeratoma corporis diffusum (Fabry's)
   Amyloid neuropathy

When the patient's condition is one of those designated by an asterisk (*), routine procedures are covered only if the patient is under the active care of a doctor of medicine or osteopathy who documents the condition.

D. Supportive Devices for Feet.--Orthopedic shoes and other supportive devices for the feet generally are not covered. However, this exclusion does not apply to such a shoe if it is an integral part of a leg brace (see §2133), and its expense is included as part of the cost of the brace. Also, this exclusion does not apply to therapeutic shoes furnished to diabetics. (See §2134.)

E. Coding.--You are responsible for informing all medical specialties that codes and policies for routine foot care and supportive devices for the feet are not exclusively for the use of podiatrists. These codes must be used to report foot care services regardless of the specialty of the physician who furnishes the services. Instruct physicians to use the most appropriate code available when billing for routine foot care.

2336 DENTAL SERVICES AND EXCLUSION

Items and services in connection with the care, treatment, filling, removal, or replacement of teeth, or structures directly supporting the teeth are not covered. "Structures directly supporting the teeth" means the periodontium, which includes the gingivae, dentogingival junction, periodontal membrane, cementum, and alveolar process. However, payment may be made for other services of a dentist. (See §§2020.3, 2136 and Coverage Issues Manual §50-26.)

The hospitalization or nonhospitalization of a patient has no direct bearing on the coverage or exclusion of a given dental procedure. (See also §§2020.3 and 2136 for additional information on dental services.)

2455 MEDICAL INSURANCE BLOOD DEDUCTIBLE

A. General.--Program payment under Part B may not be made for the first three units of whole blood, or packed red cells, received by a beneficiary in a calendar year. For purpose of the blood deductible, a unit of whole blood means a pint of whole blood. The term whole blood means human blood from which none of the liquid or cellular components has been removed. Where packed red cells are furnished, a unit of packed red cells is considered equivalent to a pint of whole blood. After the three unit deductible has been satisfied, payment may be made for all blood charges, subject to the normal coverage and reasonable charge criteria.

NOTE: Blood is a biological and can be covered under Part B only when furnished incident to a physician's services. (See §§2050.1ff. for a more complete explanation of services rendered "incident to a physician's services.")

B. Application of the Blood Deductible.--The blood deductible applies only to whole blood or packed red cells. Other components of blood such as platelets, fibrinogen, plasma, gamma globulin, and serum albumin are not subject to the blood deductible. These components of blood are covered biologicals.

The blood deductible involves only the charges for the blood (or packed red cells). Charges for the administration of blood or packed cells are not subject to the blood deductible. Accordingly, although payment may not be made for the first three pints of blood and/or units of packed red cells furnished to a beneficiary in a calendar year, payment may be made (subject to the cash deductible) for the administration charges for all covered pints or units including the first three furnished in a calendar year.

The blood deductible applies only to the first three pints and/or units furnished in a calendar year, even though more than one physician or clinic furnished blood. Furthermore, to count toward the deductible, the blood must be covered with respect to all applicable criteria (i.e., it must be medically necessary, it must be furnished incident to a physician's services, etc.). (See §2050.5.)

C. Physician or Supplier Right to Charge for Deductible Blood.--A physician or other supplier who accepts assignment may bill a beneficiary the reasonable charge for unreplaced deductible blood (i.e., any of the first three units in a calendar year) but may not charge for blood which has been replaced.

Once a physician or supplier accepts a replacement unit of whole blood or packed red cells from a beneficiary or another individual acting on his behalf, the beneficiary may not be charged for the blood.

When a supplier accepts blood donated in advance, in anticipation of need by a specific beneficiary, whether the beneficiary's own blood, that is, an autologous donation, or blood furnished by another individual or blood assurance group, such donations are considered replacement for units subsequently furnished the beneficiary.

D. Distinction Between Blood Charges and Blood Administration Charges.--Since the blood deductible applies only to charges for blood and does not apply to charges for blood administration, these two charges must be considered separately. Where a bill for unreplaced blood shows only a single blood charge, break down the charge between blood and blood administration in accordance with the supplier's customary charges for these items. If the supplier does not customarily bill separately for blood and for blood administration, the portion of the single charge that is considered to be a charge for blood is determined by reference to the established reasonable charge in the locality as it applies to blood. The remainder of the charge is considered a blood administration charge.

E. Relationship to Other Deductibles.--Part B payment for all blood administration charges and for blood charges after the beneficiary has received three pints and/or units in a calendar year is subject to the annual cash deductible and coinsurance provisions. Expenses incurred in meeting the Part B blood deductible do not count as incurred expenses under Part B for purposes of meeting the cash deductible or for purposes of payment.

There is also a Part A blood deductible applicable to the first three pints of whole blood or equivalent units of packed red cells received by a beneficiary in a benefit period. The Part A and Part B blood deductibles are applied separately.

F. Example of Application of the Part B Blood Deductible.--In 1991, a beneficiary received three pints of blood from a physician for which the total charge is $100 per pint. (The physician does not specify how much of the charge is for blood, and how much is for blood administration.) The physician accepted assignment and submitted a claim for Part B payment.

Determine that the beneficiary has not met any part of the Part B blood deductible and has met only $40 of the cash deductible. You determine that the physician's customary charge for blood administration is $50 per unit and that it is reasonable. Consequently, charges for blood administration are $50 per unit or a total of $150 for the three units furnished and charges for blood are $50 per unit or a total of $150 for the three units furnished. The beneficiary replaces one pint of blood. Since the beneficiary had not met any of the Part B blood deductible, none of the $150 in blood charges are payable nor may any of such charges be applied to satisfy the annual cash deductible ($100). Of the $150 in blood administration charges, $60 is applied to satisfy the beneficiary's unmet cash deductible and a payment of $72 is made on the remaining $90 in charges ($90 x 80%). Since the physician accepted assignment and since the beneficiary replaced one pint of blood, the physician may charge the beneficiary the reasonable charge only for the two remaining deductible pints.

3045.4 Effect of Assignment Upon Purchase of Cataract Glasses from Participating Physician or Supplier.--A pair of cataract glasses is comprised of two distinct products: a professional product (the prescribed lenses) and a retail commercial product (the frames). The frames serve not only as a holder of lenses but also as an article of personal apparel. As such, they are usually selected on the basis of personal taste and style. Although Medicare will pay only for standard frames, most patients want deluxe frames. Participating physicians and suppliers cannot profitably furnish such deluxe frames unless they can make an extra (non-covered) charge for the frames even though they accept assignment.

Therefore, a participating physician or supplier (whether an ophthalmologist, optometrist, or optician) who accepts assignment on cataract glasses with deluxe frames may charge the Medicare patient the difference between his usual charge to private pay patients for glasses with standard frames and his usual charge to such patients for glasses with deluxe frames, in addition to the applicable deductible and coinsurance on glasses with standard frames, if all of the following requirements are met:

A. The participating physician or supplier has standard frames available, offers them for sale to the patient, and explains to the patient the price and other differences between standard and deluxe frames.
B. The participating physician or supplier obtains from the patient (or his representative) and keeps on file the following signed and dated statement:

Name of Patient   Medicare Claim Number

Having been informed that an extra charge is being made by the physician or supplier for deluxe frames, that this extra charge is not covered by Medicare, and that standard frames are available for purchase from the physician or supplier at no extra charge, I have chosen to purchase deluxe frames.

_____   _____
Signature   Date

C. The participating physician or supplier itemizes on his claim his actual charge for the lenses, his actual charge for the standard frames, and his actual extra charge for the deluxe frames (charge differential).

Once the assigned claim for deluxe frames has been processed, the carrier will explain the extra charge for the deluxe frames on the EOMB, as indicated in the following example.

		BILLED	**APPROVED**
CATARACT LENSES	JULY 20, 1985	$200.00	$175.00

APPROVED AMOUNT LIMITED BY ITEM 5C ON BACK

STANDARD FRAMES	JULY 20, 1985	$ 20.00	$ 15.00

APPROVED AMOUNT LIMITED BY ITEM 5C ON BACK DR. JONES AGREED TO CHARGE NO MORE FOR THE ABOVE SERVICES THAN THE AMOUNT APPROVED BY MEDICARE.

EXTRA CHARGE DELUXE	JULY 20, 1985	$ 35.00	$ 00.00

MEDICARE DOES NOT PAY THE EXTRA CHARGE FOR DELUXE FRAMES.

TOTAL APPROVED AMOUNT $190.00
MEDICARE PAYMENT (80% OF THE APPROVED AMOUNT) $152.00

WE ARE PAYING A TOTAL OF $152.00 TO DR. JONES FOR THE ABOVE SERVICES. YOU ARE RESPONSIBLE FOR THE DIFFERENCE OF $38.00 BETWEEN THE APPROVED AMOUNT AND THE MEDICARE PAYMENT, PLUS THE EXTRA CHARGE OF $35.00 FOR DELUXE FRAMES.

3045.7 Mandatory Assignment and Other Requirements for Home Dialysis Supplies and Equipment Paid Under Method II.--

A. General.--Durable Medical Equipment Regional Carriers (DMERCs) must pay only on an assignment basis for home dialysis supplies and equipment furnished a beneficiary who has selected Method II. There is also a monthly payment limitation: $1974.45 for continuous cycling peritoneal dialysis (CCPD) and $1490.85 for all other methods of dialysis. (Note, however, that beneficiaries are permitted to have on hand one month's emergency reserve supplies.) This payment may be made to only one supplier per beneficiary. (See §§4270-4271.)

B. Billing Instructions.--Suppliers of Method II home dialysis supplies and equipment must complete their claims as follows:

- Submit claims to the appropriate DMERC on a monthly basis for one month's worth of supplies and equipment;
- Enter appropriate Healthcare Common Procedure Coding System (HCPCS) codes for each supply or piece of equipment provided, with a "KX" modifier on each line item to signify that the supplier has a valid agreement with an appropriate support service facility; and
- Use modifier "EM" to designate each HCPCS code for emergency reserve supplies. This allows the DMERC to identify situations in which the payment limit for a given month may be exceeded if an emergency reserve is billed for in addition to regular monthly supplies. It also allows DMERCs to ensure that emergency supplies are not purchased more frequently than once in a beneficiary's lifetime per mode of dialysis. Suppliers must bill for all emergency dialysis supplies in the same calendar month.

C. Processing Claims.--The monthly limit applies to all home dialysis supplies and equipment furnished to the beneficiary. Since more than one supply or piece of equipment may be furnished for a given month, apply the limit to the supplies in the order in which they are billed by the sole supplier.

If a claim identifies the beneficiary as a CCPD patient, apply the higher monthly limit.

If two different suppliers submit bills for the same month for the same beneficiary, pay only the first supplier that submits a bill.

DMERCs must deny payment for home dialysis supplies and equipment if any of the following conditions are met:

- The supplier has not accepted assignment;
- The supplies were furnished by a second supplier;
- The monthly limit has been paid;
- The beneficiary filed the claim;
- The beneficiary has elected Method I for the date of service on the claim;
- The DMERC finds that the supplier does not have a valid written agreement with a support service facility, or
- The supplier did not use the "KX" modifier on each line item to indicate that it has a valid written backup agreement with a support service facility (see §4270).

3060.6 Payment Under Reciprocal Billing Arrangements.--
A. General.--The patient's regular physician may submit the claim, and (if assignment is accepted) receive the Part B payment, for covered visit services (including emergency visits and related services) which the regular physician arranges to be provided by a substitute physician on an occasional reciprocal basis, if:

- The regular physician is unavailable to provide the visit services;
- The Medicare patient has arranged or seeks to receive the visit services from the regular physician;
- The substitute physician does not provide the visit services to Medicare patients over a continuous period of longer than 60 days; and
- The regular physician identifies the services as substitute physician services meeting the requirements of this section by entering in item 24d of Form CMS-1500 HCPCS Q5 modifier (service furnished by a substitute physician under a reciprocal billing arrangement) after the
- The regular physician identifies the services as substitute physician services meeting the requirements of this section by entering in item 24d of Form CMS 1500 HCPCS Q5 modifier (service furnished by a substitute physician under a reciprocal billing arrangement) after the procedure code. When Form CMS-1500 is next revised, provision will be made to identify the substitute physician by entering his/her unique physician identification number (UPIN) on the form and cross-referring the entry to the appropriate service line item(s) by number(s). Until further notice, the regular physician must keep on file a record of each service provided by the substitute physician, associated with the substitute physician's UPIN, and make this record available to you upon request.

If the only substitution services a physician performs in connection with an operation are post-operative services furnished during the period covered by the global fee, these services need not be identified on the claim as substitution services.

A physician may have reciprocal arrangements with more than one physician. The arrangements need not be in writing.

B. Definitions.--
1. Covered Visit Service.--The term "covered visit service" includes not only those services ordinarily characterized as a covered physician visit, but also any other covered items and services furnished by the substitute physician or by others as incident to his/her services.
Items and services furnished by the staff of the substitute physician covered as incident to his/her services if billed by him/her are still covered if billed by the regular physician under this section.
Items and services furnished by the staff of the regular physician covered as incident to his/her services if furnished under his/her supervision are still covered if furnished under the supervision of the substitute physician.
2. Continuous Period of Covered Visit Services.--A continuous period of covered visit services begins with the first day on which the substitute physician provides covered visit services to Medicare Part B patients of the regular physician, and it ends with the last day on which the substitute physician provides these services to these patients before the regular physician returns to work. This period continues without interruption on days on which no covered visit services are

provided to patients on behalf of the regular physician or are furnished by some other substitute physician on behalf of the regular physician. A new period of covered visit services can begin after the regular physician has returned to work.

EXAMPLE: The regular physician goes on vacation on June 30, 1992, and returns to work on September 4, 1992. A substitute physician provides services to Medicare Part B patients of the regular physician on July 2, 1992, and at various times thereafter, including August 30th and September 2, 1992. The continuous period of covered visit services begins on July 2nd and runs through September 2nd, a period of 63 days. Since the September 2nd services are furnished after the expiration of 60 days of the period, the regular physician is not entitled to bill and receive direct payment for them. The substitute physician must bill for these services in his/her own name. The regular physician may, however, bill and receive payment for the services which the substitute physician provides on his/her behalf in the period July 2nd through August 30th.

C. Unassigned Claims Under Reciprocal Billing Arrangements.--The requirements for the submission of claims under reciprocal billing arrangements are the same for assigned and unassigned claims.

D. Medical Group Claims Under Reciprocal Billing Arrangements.--The requirements of this section generally do not apply to the substitution arrangements among physicians in the same medical group where claims are submitted in the name of the group. On claims submitted by the group, the group physician who actually performed the service must be identified in the manner described in §3060.9, with one exception. When a group member provides services on behalf of another group member who is the designated attending physician for a hospice patient, the Q5 modifier may be used by the designated attending physician to bill for services related to a hospice patient's terminal illness that were performed by another group member.

For a medical group to submit assigned and unassigned claims for the covered visit services of a substitute physician who is not a member of the group, the requirements of subsection A must be met. The medical group must enter in item 24d of Form CMS-1500 the HCPCS modifier Q5 after the procedure code. Until further notice, the medical group must keep on file a record of each service provided by the substitute physician, associated with the substitute physician's UPIN, and make this record available to you upon request. In addition, the medical group physician for whom the substitution services are furnished must be identified by his/her provider identification number (PIN) in block 24k of the appropriate line item.

For an independent physician to submit assigned and unassigned claims for the substitution services of a physician who is a member of a medical group, the requirements of subsection A must be met. The independent physician must enter in item 24 of Form CMS-1500 HCPCS modifier Q5 after the procedure code. Until further notice, the independent physician must keep on file a record of each service provided by the substitute medical group physician, associated with the substitute physician's UPIN, and make this record available to you upon request.

Physicians who are members of a group but who bill in their own names are treated as independent physicians for purposes of applying the requirements of this section.

E. Guidance to Physicians--Inform physicians of the requirements of this section. Advise physicians and, if necessary, remind them that, in entering the code Q5 modifier, the regular physician (or the medical group, where applicable) is certifying that the services are covered visit services furnished by the substitute physician identified in a record of the regular physician which is available for inspection, and are services for which the regular physician (or group) is entitled under this section to submit the claim. Mention the possible penalties under subsection F for false certifications.

F. Penalties.--A physician or other person who falsely certifies that the requirements of this section are met may be subject to possible civil and criminal penalties for fraud. Also, the physician's right to receive payment or to submit claims under this section or even to accept any assignments may be revoked. The revocation procedures are set forth in §14025.

G. Claims Review.--If a line item includes the code Q5 certification, assume that the claim meets the requirements of this section in the absence of evidence to the contrary. You need not track the 60-day period or validate the billing arrangement on a prepayment basis, absent postpayment findings which indicate that the certifications by a particular physician may not be valid.

H. Payment Amount.--When you make Part B payment under this section, you determine the payment amount as though the regular physician or his/her staff provided the services. The identification of the substitute physician is primarily for purposes of providing an audit trail to verify that the services were furnished, not for purposes of the payment or the limiting charge. Also, notices of noncoverage under §§7300ff. and 7330ff. are to be given in the name of the regular physician.

3060.7 Payment Under Locum Tenens Arrangements.--
A. Background.--It is a longstanding and widespread practice for physicians to retain substitute physicians to take over their professional practices when the regular physicians are absent for reasons such as illness, pregnancy, vacation, or continuing medical education, and for the regular physician to bill and receive payment for the substitute physician's services as though he/she performed them himself/herself. The substitute physician generally has no practice of his/her own and moves from area to area as needed. The regular physician generally pays the substitute physician a fixed amount per diem, with the substitute physician having the status of an independent contractor rather than of an employee. These substitute physicians are generally called "locum tenens" physicians.

Section 125(b) of the Social Security Act Amendments of 1994 makes this procedure available on a permanent basis. Thus, beginning January 1, 1995, a regular physician may bill for the services of Alocum tenens@ physicians. A regular physician is the physician that is normally scheduled to see a patient. Thus, a regular physician may include physician specialists (such as, a cardiologist, oncologist, urologist, etc.).

B. Payment Procedure--A patient's regular physician may submit the claim, and (if assignment is accepted) receive the Part B payment, for covered visit services (including emergency visits and related services) of a locum tenens physician who is not an employee of the regular physician and whose services for patients of the regular physician are not restricted to the regular physician's offices, if:

- The regular physician is unavailable to provide the visit services;
- The Medicare beneficiary has arranged or seeks to receive the visit services from the regular physician;
- The regular physician pays the locum tenens for his/her services on a per diem or similar fee-for-time basis;
- The substitute physician does not provide the visit services to Medicare patients over a continuous period of longer than 60 days; and
- The regular physician identifies the services as substitute physician services meeting the requirements of this section by entering HCPCS Q6 modifier (service furnished by a locum tenens physician) after the procedure code. When Form CMS-1500 is next revised, provision will be made to identify the substitute physician by entering his/her unique physician identification number (UPIN) to you upon request.

See §3060.6B for definitions of covered visit services and continuous period of covered visit services.

If the only substitution services a physician performs in connection with an operation are post-operative services furnished during the period covered by the global fee, these services need not be identified on the claim as substitution services.

C. Unassigned Claims Under Locum Tenens Arrangements.--The requirements for the submission of claims under reciprocal billing arrangements are the same for assigned and unassigned claims.

D. Medical Group Claims Under Locum Tenens Arrangements.--For a medical group to submit assigned and unassigned claims for the services a locum tenens physician provides for patients of the regular physician who is a member of the group, the requirements of subsection B must be met. For purposes of these requirements, per diem or similar fee-for-time compensation which the group pays the locum tenens physician is considered paid by the regular physician. Also, a physician who has left the group and for whom the group has engaged a locum tenens physician as a temporary replacement may still be considered a member of the group until a permanent replacement is obtained. The group must enter in item 24d of Form CMS-1500 the HCPCS Q6 modifier after the procedure code. Until further notice, the group must keep on file a record of each service provided by the substitute physician, associated with the substitute physician's UPIN, and make this record available to you upon request. In addition, the medical group physician for whom the substitution services are furnished must be identified by his/her provider identification number (PIN) on block 24k of the appropriate line item.

Physicians who are members of a group but who bill in their own names are generally treated as independent physicians for purposes of applying the requirements of subsection A for payment for locum tenens physician services. Compensation paid by the group to the locum tenens physician is considered paid by the regular physician for purposes of those requirements. The term "regular physician" includes a physician who has left the group and for whom the group has hired the locum tenens physician as a replacement.

E. Guidance to Physicians, Penalties, Claims Review and Payment Amount.--In regard to guidance for physicians, possible penalties, claims review, and payment amounts, proceed as in §3060.6.

3312 EVIDENCE OF MEDICAL NECESSITY FOR DURABLE MEDICAL EQUIPMENT

Section 3312 has been moved to Chapter 5 of the Program Integrity Manual, which can be found at http://cms.hhs.gov/manuals/108_pim/pim83c05.asp.

3350.3 Claims Coding Requirements.--Physicians must indicate that their services were provided in an incentive-eligible rural or urban HPSA by using one of the following modifiers:

- QB - physician providing a service in a rural HPSA; or
- QU - physician providing a service in an urban HPSA.

3350.5 Services Eligible for HPSA Bonus Payments.--
A. Information in the Professional Component/Technical Component (PC/TC) Indicator Field of the Medicare Physician Fee Schedule Database.--Use the information in the Professional Component/Technical Component (PC/TC) indicator field of the Medicare Physician Fee Schedule Database to identify professional services eligible for HPSA bonus payments. The following are the rules to apply in determining whether to pay the bonus on services furnished within a geographic HPSA and billed with a QB or QU modifier, as appropriate.

PC/TC	HPSA Payment Policy
0	Pay the HPSA bonus.
1	Globally billed. Only the professional component of this service qualifies for the HPSA bonus payment. The HPSA bonus cannot be paid on the technical component of globally-billed services. ACTION: Return the service as unprocessable. Instruct the provider to re-bill the service as two components with separate charges for the professional component (billed with the "26" and "HPSA" modifiers) and the technical component (billed with the "TC" modifier but not the "HPSA" modifier). (See §3350.6(A).)
1	Professional Component (modifier 26). Pay the bonus.
1	Technical Component (modifier TC). Do not pay the bonus. (See §3350.6(B).)
2	Professional Component only. Pay the bonus.
3	Technical Component only. Do not pay the bonus. (See §3350.6(B).)
4	Global test only. Only the professional component of this service qualifies for the HPSA bonus payment. ACTION: Return the service as unprocessable. Instruct the provider to re-bill the service as separate professional and technical component procedure codes. The HPSA modifier should only be used with the professional component code. (See §3350.6(A).)
5	Incident to codes. Do not pay the bonus. (See §3350.6(B).)
6	Laboratory physician interpretation codes. Pay the bonus.
7	Physical therapy service. Do not pay the bonus. (See §3350.6(B).)
8	Physician interpretation codes. Pay the bonus.
9	Concept of PC/TC does not apply. Do not pay the bonus. (See §3350.6(B).)

B. Anesthesia Codes (CPT Codes 00100 Through 01999) Which Do Not Appear on the MFSDB.--Anesthesia codes (CPT codes 00100 through 01999) do not appear on the MFSDB. However, when a medically necessary anesthesia service is furnished within a HPSA area by a physician, a HPSA bonus is payable. In addition to using the MFSDB PC/TC indicator to identify HPSA services, pay physicians the HPSA bonus when CPT codes 00100 through 01999 are billed with the following modifiers: QY, QK, AD, AA, or GC. These modifiers signify that the anesthesia service was performed by a physician.

NOTE: Codes that have a status of "X" on the Medicare Physician Fee Schedule Database (MFSDB) have been assigned PC/TC indicator 9 and are not considered physician services for MFSDB payment purposes. Therefore, the HPSA bonus payment will not be paid for these codes.

4107 DURABLE MEDICAL EQUIPMENT - BILLING AND PAYMENT CONSIDERATIONS UNDER THE FEE SCHEDULE

The Omnibus Budget Reconciliation Act of 1987 requires that payment for DME, prosthetics and orthotics be made under fee schedules effective January 1, 1989. The allowable charge is limited to the lower of the actual charge for the equipment, or the fee schedule amount. The equipment is categorized into one of six classes:

* Inexpensive or other routinely purchased DME;
* Items requiring frequent and substantial servicing;
* Customized items;
* Prosthetic and orthotic devices;
* Capped rental items; or
* Oxygen and oxygen equipment.

The fee schedule allowances for each class are determined in accord with §§5102ff.

4107.6 Written Order Prior to Delivery.--Ensure that your system will pay for the equipment listed below only when the supplier has a written order in hand prior to delivery. Otherwise, do not pay for that item even if a written order is subsequently furnished. However, you can pay for a similar item if it is subsequently provided by an unrelated supplier which has a written order in hand prior to delivery. The HCPCS codes for the equipment requiring a written order are:

B0180
B0181
B0182
B0183
B0184
B0185
B0188
B0189
B0190
B0192
B0195
B0620
B0720
B0730
B1230

4107.8 EOMB Messages.--The following EOMB messages are suggested: (See §§7012ff. for other applicable messages.)
A. General.--
* "This is the maximum approved amount for this item." (Use when payment is reduced for a line item.)
B. Inexpensive/Frequently Purchased Equipment.--
* "The total approved amount for this item is _____ whether this item is purchased or rented." (Use in first month.)
* "This is your next to last rental payment."
* "This is your last rental payment."
* "This item has been rented up to the Medicare payment limit."
* "The approved amount has been reduced by the previously approved rental amounts."
C. Items Requiring Frequent and Substantial Servicing.--Use the general rental messages in §4107.8A, if applicable. If the beneficiary has purchased the item prior to June 1, 1989, follow §7014.6. If the beneficiary purchase an item in this category on or after June 1, 1989, use the following message:

- "This equipment can only be paid for on a rental basis."

D. Customized Items and Other Prosthetic and Orthotic Devices.--

- "The total approved amount for this item is _____."

E. Capped Rental Items.--

- "Under a provision of Medicare law, monthly rental payments for this item can continue for up to 15 months from the first rental month or until the equipment is no longer needed, whichever comes first."
- "If you no longer are using this equipment or have recently moved and will rent this item from a different supplier, please contact our office." (Use on beneficiary's EOMB.)
- "This is your next to last rental payment."
- "This is your last rental payment."
- "This item has been rented up to the 15 month Medicare payment limit."
- "Your equipment supplier must supply and service this item for as long as you continue to need it."
- "Medicare cannot pay for maintenance and/or servicing of this item until 6 months have elapsed since the end of the 15th paid rental month."
- If the beneficiary purchased a capped rental item prior to June 1, 1989, follow §7014.6. If the beneficiary purchased a capped rental item on or after June 1, 1989, use the following denial message:
- "This equipment can only be paid for on a rental basis."

F. Oxygen and Oxygen Equipment.--

- "The monthly allowance includes payment for all covered oxygen contents and supplies."
- "Payment for the amount of oxygen supplied has been reduced or denied based on the patient's medical condition." (To supplier after medical review.)
- "The approved amount has been reduced to the amount allowable for medically necessary oxygen therapy." (To beneficiary.)
- "Payment denied because the allowance for this item is included in the monthly payment amount."
- "Payment denied because Medicare oxygen coverage requirements are not met."

If the beneficiary purchased an oxygen system prior to June 1, 1989, follow §7014.6. If the beneficiary purchased an oxygen system on or after June 1, 1989, use the following denial message:

- "This item can only be paid for on a rental basis."

G. Items Requiring a Written Order Prior to Delivery.--

- "Payment is denied because the supplier did not obtain a written order from your doctor prior to the delivery of this item."

4107.9 Oxygen HCPCS Codes Effective 1/1/89.--

NEW	OLD	DEFINITION
Q0036 notes (1) and (8)	E1377-E1385, E1397	Oxygen concentrator, See High humidity
Q0038 See note (2)	E0400, E0405	Oxygen contents, gaseous, per unit (for use with owned gaseous stationary systems or when both a stationary and portable gaseous system are owned; 1 unit = 50 cubic ft.)
Q0039 See note (2)	E0410, E0415O	Oxygen contents, liquid, per unit, (for use with owned stationary liquid systems or when both a stationary and portable liquid system are owned; 1 unit = 10 lbs.)

Q0040 See note (2)	E0416	Portable oxygen contents, per unit (for use only with portable gaseous systems when no stationary gas system is used; 1 unit = 5 cubic ft.)
Q0041 See note (2)	None	Portable oxygen contents, liquid, per unit (for use only with portable liquid systems when no stationary liquid system is used; 1 unit = 1 lb.)
Q0042	E0425	Stationary compressed See note (3)gas system rental, includes contents (per unit), regulator with flow gauge, humidifier, nebulizer, cannula or mask & tubing; 1 unit = 50 cubic ft.
E0425 See notes (4) and (8)	Same	No change
E0430 See notes (8) and (9)	Same	No change
E0435 See notes (7) and 8	Same	No change in terminology, but and (8)see note (7).
Q0043	E0440	Stationary liquid (see note (3) oxygen system rental), includes contents (per unit), use of reservoir, contents indicator, flowmeter, humidifier, nebulizer, cannula or mask and tubing; 1 unit of contents = 10 lbs.
B0440 See note (4)	Same	No change
E0455	Same	No change See note (6)
E0555 See note (6)	Same	No change
E0580	Same	No change See note (6)
E1351	Same	No change See note (6)
E1352 See note (6)	Same	No change
E1353	Same See notes (6) and (8)	No change
E1354 See note (6)	Same	No change
E1371	Same See note (6)	No change
E1374 See note (6)	Same	No change
E1400 See note (1) and (8)	E1388-E1396	Same as Q0014
E1401 See notes (1) and (8)	E1388-E1396	Same as Q0015
E1402	Same	No change

E1403	Same	No change
E1404	Same	No change
E1405	Q0037	Combine the fee See note (10)schedule amounts for the stationary oxygen system and the nebulizer with a compressor and heater (code E0585) to determine the fee schedule amount to apply to oxygen enrichers with a heater (code E1405)
E1406	Q0037	Combine the fee schedule amounts for the stationary oxygen system and the nebulizer with only a compressor (i.e., without a heater, code E0570) to determine the fee schedule amount to apply to oxygen enrichers without a heater (code E1406)

4120 FOOT CARE

NOTE: See §4281 for the relationship between foot care and the coverage and billing of the diagnosis and treatment of peripheral neuropathy with loss of protective sensation (LOPS) in people with diabetes.

4120.1 Application of Foot Care Exclusions to Physicians' Services.--The exclusion of foot care is determined by the nature of the service (§2323). Thus, reimbursement for an excluded service should be denied whether performed by a podiatrist, osteopath, or a doctor of medicine, and without regard to the difficulty or complexity of the procedure.

When an itemized bill shows both covered services and noncovered services not integrally related to the covered service, the portion of charges attributable to the noncovered services should be denied. (For example, if an itemized bill shows surgery for an ingrown toenail and also removal of calluses not necessary for the performance of toe surgery, any additional charge attributable to removal of the calluses should be denied.)

In reviewing claims involving foot care, the carrier should be alert to the following exceptional situations:

1. Payment may be made for incidental noncovered services performed as a necessary and integral part of, and secondary to, a covered procedure. For example, if trimming of toenails is required for application of a cast to a fractured foot, the carrier need not allocate and deny a portion of the charge for the trimming of the nails. However, a separately itemized charge for such excluded service should be disallowed. When the primary procedure is covered the administration of anesthesia necessary for the performance of such procedure is also covered.
2. Payment may be made for initial diagnostic services performed in connection with a specific symptom or complaint if it seems likely that its treatment would be covered even though the resulting diagnosis may be one requiring only noncovered care.

4173 POSITRON EMISSION TOMOGRAPHY (PET) SCANS

BACKGROUND:

For dates of service on or after March 14, 1995, Medicare covers one use of PET scans, imaging of the perfusion of the heart using Rubidium 82 (Rb 82).

For dates of service on or after January 1, 1998, Medicare expanded coverage of PET scans for the characterization of solitary pulmonary nodules and for the initial staging of lung cancer, conditioned upon its ability to effect the management and treatment of patients with either suspected or demonstrated lung cancer. All other uses of PET scans remain not covered by Medicare.

Beginning for dates of service on or after July 1, 1999, Medicare will cover PET scans for evaluation of recurrent colorectal cancer in patients with levels of carinoembryonic antigen (CEA), staging lymphoma (both Hodgkins and non-Hodgkins) in place of a Gallium study or lymphangiogram, and for the staging of recurrent melanoma prior to surgery.

See Coverage Issues Manual §50-36 for specific coverage criteria for PET scans.

Regardless of any other terms or conditions, all uses of PET scans, in order to be covered by Medicare program, must meet the following conditions:

- Scans must be performed using PET scanners that have either been approved or cleared for marketing by the FDA as PET scanners;
- Submission of claims for payment must include any information Medicare requires to assure that the PET scans performed were: (a) reasonable and necessary; (b) did not unnecessarily duplicate other covered diagnostic tests, and (c) did not involve investigational drugs or procedures using investigational drugs, as determined by the Food and Drug Administration (FDA); and
- The PET scan entity submitting claims for payment must keep such patient records as Medicare requires on file for each patient for whom a PET scan claim is made.

4173.1   Conditions for Medicare Coverage of PET Scans for Noninvasive Imaging of the Perfusion of the Heart.--Pet scans done at rest or with pharmacological stress used for noninvasive imaging of the perfusion of the heart for the diagnosis management of patients with known or suspected coronary artery disease using the FDA-approved radiopharmaceutical Rubidium 82 (Rb 82) are covered for services performed on or after March 15, 1995, provided such scans meet either of the two following conditions:

- The PET scan, whether rest alone or rest with stress, is used in place of, but not in addition to, a single photon emission computed tomography (SPECT); or
- The PET scan, whether rest alone or rest with stress, is used following a SPECT that was found inconclusive. In these cases, the PET scan must have been considered necessary in order to determine what medical or surgical intervention is required to treat the patient. (For purposes of this requirement, an inconclusive test is a test whose results are equivocal, technically uninterpretable, or discordant with a patient's other clinical data.)

NOTE: PET scans using Rubidium 82, whether rest or stress are not covered by Medicare for routine screening of asymptomatic patients, regardless of the level of risk factors applicable to such patients.

4173.2 Conditions of Coverage of PET Scans for Characterization of Solitary Pulmonary Nodules (SPNs) and PET Scans Using FDG to Initially Stage Lung Cancer

PET scans using the glucose analog 2-[fluorine-18]-fluoro-2-deoxy-D-glucose(FDG) are covered for services on or after January 1, 1998, subject to the condition and limitations described in CIM 50-36.

NOTE: A Tissue Sampling Procedure (TSP) should not be routinely covered in the case of a negative PET scan for characterization of SPNs, since the patient is presumed not to have a malignant lesion, based upon the PET scan results. Claims for a TSP after a negative PET must be submitted with documentation in order to determine if the TSP is reasonable and necessary in spite of a negative PET. Claims submitted for a TSP after a negative PET without documentation should be denied. Physicians should discuss with their patients the implications of this decision, both with respect to the patient's responsibility for payment for such a biopsy if desired, as well as the confidence the physician has in the results of such PET scans, prior to ordering such scans for this purpose. This physician-patient decision should occur with a clear discussion and understanding of the sensitivity and specificity trade-offs between a computerized tomography (CT) and PET scans. In cases where a TSP is performed, it is the responsibility of the physician ordering the TSP to provide sufficient documentation of the reasonableness and necessity for such procedure or procedures. Such documentation should include, but is not necessarily limited to, a description of the features of the PET scan that call into question whether it is an accurate representation of the patient's condition, the existence of other factors in the patient's condition that call into question the accuracy of the PET scan, and such other information as the contractor deems necessary to determine whether the claim for the TSP should be covered and paid.

In cases of serial evaluation of SPNs using both CT and regional PET chest scanning, such PET scans will not be covered if repeated within 90 days following a negative PET scan.

4173.3 Conditions of Coverage of PET Scans for Recurrence of Colorectal Cancer, Staging and Characterization of Lymphoma, and Recurrence of Melanoma

Medicare adds coverage for these three new indications for PET, one for evaluation of recurrent colorectal cancer in patients with rising levels of carcinoembryonic antigen (CEA), one for staging of lymphoma (both Hodgkins and non-Hodgkins) when the PET scan substitutes for a Gallium scan, and one for the detection of recurrent melanoma, provided certain conditions are met. All three indications are covered only when using the radiopharmaceutical FDA (2-[fluorine-18]-fluoro-2-deoxy-D-glucose), and are further predicated on the legal availability of FDG for use in such scans.

4173.4 Billing Requirements for PET Scans.--

A. Effective for Services on or After January 1, 1998, Claims for Characterizing SPNs Should Include.--

NOTE: PET scans are not covered by Medicare for routine screening of asymptomatic patients, regardless of the level of risk factors applicable to such patients.

B. Effective for services on or after January 1, 1998, claims for staging metastatic non-small-cell lung carcinoma (NSCLC) must include:

- Since this service is covered only in those cases in which a primary cancerous lung tumor has been confirmed, claims for PET must show evidence of the detection of such primary lung tumor. For example, a diagnosis code indicating the existence of a primary tumor or any other evidence you deem appropriate. A surgical pathology report which documents the presence of an NSCLC must be kept on file with the provider. If you deem it necessary, contact the provider for a copy of this documentation.
- Whole body PET scan results and results of concurrent CT and follow-up lymph node biopsy. In order to ensure that the PET scan is properly coordinated with other diagnostic modalities, claims must include both (1) the results of concurrent thoracic CT, which is necessary for anatomic information, and (2) the results of any lymph node biopsy performed to finalize whether the patient will be a surgical candidate.

NOTE: A lymph node biopsy is not covered in the case of a negative CT and negative PET where the patient is considered a surgical candidate, given the presumed absence of metastatic NSCLC.

C. Effective for Dates of Service on or After July 1, 1999 PET Claims For the Following Conditions Must Include:

- Recurring colorectal cancer with rising CEA:
  --A statement or other evidence of previous colorectal tumor;
  --The results of the concurrent CT, which is necessary for anatomic information; and
  --The necessary procedure codes and/or modifiers.
- Staging or restaging of lymphoma in place of a Gallium study or lymphangiogram:
  --A statement or other evidence of previously-made diagnosis of lymphoma;
  --The results of the concurrent CT, which is necessary for anatomic information; and
  --The date of the last Gallium scan or lymphangiogram when done in the same facility as the PET scan.
- Recurrent Melanoma prior to surgery:
  --A statement or other evidence of previous melanoma;
  --The results of the concurrent CT, which is necessary for anatomic information; and
  --The date of the last Gallium scan when done in the same facility as the PET scan.

As with any claim but particularly in view of the limitations on this coverage, you may decide to conduct post-payment reviews to determine that the use of PET scans is consistent with this instruction. PET scan facilities must keep patient record information on file for each Medicare patient for whom a PET scan claim is made. These medical records will be used in any post-payment reviews and must include the information necessary to substantial the need for the PET scan.

4173.5 HCPCS and Modifiers for PET Scans.--Providers should use HCPCS codes G0030 through G0047 to indicate the conditions under which a PET scan was done for imaging of the perfusion of the heart. These codes represent the global service, so providers performing just the technical or professional component of the test should use modifier TC or 26, respectively. The following codes should be reported for PET scans used for the imaging of the lungs:

- G0125--PET lung imaging of solitary pulmonary nodules using 2-[fluorine-18]-fluoro-2-deoxy-D-glucose (FDG), following CT (71250/71260 or 71270); or
- G0126--PET lung imaging of solitary pulmonary nodules using 2-[fluorine-18]-fluoro-2-deoxy-D-glucose (FDG), following CT (71250/71260 or 71270); for initial staging of pathologically diagnosed NSCLC, or
- G0163--Positron Emission Tomography (PET), whole body, for recurrence of colorectal or colorectal metastatic cancer; or
- G0164--Positron Emission Tomography (PET), whole body, for staging and characterization of lymphoma; or
- G0165--Positron Emission Tomography (PET), whole body, for recurrence of melanoma or melanoma metastic cancer

NOTE: The payment for the radio tracer, or radio pharmaceutical is included in the relative value units of the technical components of the above procedure codes. Do not make any separate payments for these agents for PET scans.

In addition, providers must indicate the results of the PET scan and the previous test using a two digit modifier. (The modifier is not required for technical component-only billings or billings to the intermediary.) The first character should indicate the result of the PET scan; the second character should indicate the results of the prior test. Depending on the procedure codes with which the modifiers are used, the meaning of the modifier will be apparent. The test result modifiers and their descriptions are as follows:

Modifier	Description
N	Negative;
E	Equivocal;
P	Positive, but not suggestive of, extensive ischemia or not suggestive of malignant single pulmonary nodule; and
S	Positive and suggestive of; extensive ischemia (greater than 20 percent of the left ventricle) or malignant single pulmonary nodule.

These modifiers may be used in any combination.

4173.6 Claims Processing Instructions for PET Scan Claims.--
A. FDA Approval.--PET scans are covered only when performed at a PET imaging center with a PET scanner that has been approved or cleared by the FDA. When submitting the claim, the provider is certifying this and must be able to produce a copy of this approval upon request. An official approval letter need not be submitted with the claim.

You may consider conducting a review on a post-payment basis to verify, based on a sample of PET scan claims, that the PET scan was performed at a center with a PET scanner which was approved or cleared for marketing.

B. EOMB and Remittance Messages.--Providers must indicate the results of the PET scan and the previous test using a two-digit modifier as specified in §4173.4. Deny assigned claims received prior to April 1, 1996 without such modifier, using the following EOMB message:

C. "Your service was denied because information required to make payment was missing. We have asked your provider to resubmit a claim with the missing information so that it may be reprocessed." (Message 9.33)

Deny unassigned claims received prior to April 1, 1996, without the two-digit modifier using the following EOMB message:

"Medicare cannot pay for this service because the claim is missing information/documentation. Please ask your provider to submit a new, complete claim to us." (Messages 9.8 and 9.15)

Claims received on or after April 1, 1996, without the two-digit modifier must be returned as unprocessable. (See §3005.)

Use the following remittance message for assigned claims:

"The procedure code is inconsistent with the modifier used, or a required modifier is missing." (Reason Code 4)

Assigned claims for dates of service on or after January 1, 1998, without the proper documentation must be denied using the following EOMB message:

C. "Your service was denied because information required to make payment was missing. We have asked your provider to resubmit a claim with the missing information so that it may be reprocessed." (Message 9.33)

D. Type of Service.--The type of service for the PET scan codes in the "G" range is 4, Diagnostic Radiology.

4175.5 Medicare Summary Notices (MSNs) and Explanation of Medicare Benefits (EOMB) and Remittance Advise Messages.--Use the following MSN or EOMB messages where appropriate.

If a claim is denied because it was submitted by a physician, other than the hospice patient's designated attending physician, who treated the beneficiary for the terminal condition use:

- MSN #27.13, "According to Medicare hospice requirements this service is not covered because the service was provided by a non-attending physician."
- EOMB #20.4, "According to Medicare hospice requirements this service is not covered because the service was provided by a non-attending physician."
- The Spanish version of the above message is:
- Según requisitos de hospicio de Medicare este servicio no se cubre debido a que el servicio fue proporcionado por un médico no primario.
- When the claim is being denied per the above reason, use the following code in the remittance advice message.
- Remark Code N90, "Covered only when performed by the attending physician."

4182 PROSTATE CANCER SCREENING TESTS AND PROCEDURES

The following sections summarize coverage requirements and detail claims processing procedures for prostate cancer screening tests and procedures.

4182.1 Coverage Summary.--Sections 1861(s)(2)(P) and 1861(oo) of the Social Security Act (as added by §4103 of the Balanced Budget Act of 1997), provide for coverage of certain prostate cancer screening tests and procedures subject to certain coverage, frequency, and payment limitations. Effective for services furnished on or after January 1, 2000, Medicare will cover prostate cancer screening tests and procedures for the early detection of prostate cancer. Coverage currently consists of the following tests and procedures furnished to an individual for the early detection of prostate cancer:

A. Screening Digital Rectal Examination.--This test is a clinical examination of an individual's prostate for nodules or other abnormalities of the prostate; and
B. Screening Prostate Specific Antigen (PSA) Blood Test.--This test detects the marker for adenocarcinoma of the prostate.

For more information regarding coverage of prostate cancer screening tests and procedures, refer to §50-55 of the Coverage Issues Manual.

4182.2 Requirements for Submitting Claims.--Submit claims for prostate cancer screening tests on Health Insurance Claim Form HCFA-1500 or electronic equivalent. Follow the general instructions in §2010, Purpose of Health Insurance Claim Form HCFA1500, Medicare Carriers Manual, Part 4, Chapter 2.

4182.3 HCPCS Codes and Payment Requirements.--The following table lists coverable codes and services for prostate cancer screening tests and procedures. Pay for these services according to the appropriate fee schedule when all of the requirements noted are met.

HCPCS (TOS)	Description	Requirements	Methodology/ Fee Schedule
G0102; TOS=1	Prostate cancer screening; digital rectal exam	1. Performed on a male Medicare beneficiary over 50 years of age (i.e., for services starting at least one day after the beneficiary attained age 50).	Refer to the Physician's fee schedule. 1. Apply deductible and coinsurance.
		2. Performed by one of the following, who is authorized under State law to perform the examination, is fully knowledgeable about the beneficiary, and is responsible for explaining the results of the examination to the beneficiary: a. Doctor of medicine or osteopathy b. Qualified physician assistant c. Qualified nurse practitioner d. Qualified clinical nurse specialist e. Qualified certified nurse midwife 3. Performed at a frequency no greater than once every 12 months (See §4182.4).	2. Claims from physicians for these examinations where assignment was not taken are subject to the Medicare limiting charge. (See §7555.) 3. Correct Coding Initiative requirements apply. See §4182.6.

G0103; TOS=5	Prostate cancer screening; PSA test	1. Performed on a male Medicare beneficiary over 50 years of age (i.e., for services starting at least one day after the beneficiary attained age 50)	1. Refer to the clinical laboratory fee schedule; payment for this test is the same as for code "84153, PSA; total."
		2. Ordered by one of the following, who is authorized under State law to perform the examination, is fully knowledgeable about the beneficiary, and is responsible for explaining the results of the examination to the beneficiary: a. Physician (doctor of medicine or osteopathy) b. Qualified physician assistant c. Qualified nurse practitioner d. Qualified clinical nurse specialist e. Qualified certified nurse midwife 3. Performed at a frequency no greater than once every 12 months. (See §4182.4.)	2. Do not apply deductible and coinsurance.

4182.4   Calculating the Frequency.--Once a beneficiary has received any (or all) of the covered prostate cancer screening test/procedures, he may receive another (or all) of such test/procedures after 11 full months have passed. To determine the 11-month period, start your count beginning with the month after the month in which any (or all) of the previous covered screening test/procedures was performed.

EXAMPLE: The beneficiary received a screening PSA test on February 25, 2000. Start your count beginning March 2000. The beneficiary is eligible to receive another screening PSA test on February 1, 2001 (the month after 11 months have passed.)

4182.5 CWF Edits.--CWF will edit prostate cancer screening tests and procedures for age, frequency, sex, and valid HCPCS code.

4182.6 Correct Coding Requirements.--Billing and payment for a Digital Rectal Exam (DRE) (G0102) is to be bundled into the payment for a covered E/M service (CPT codes 99201-99456 and 99499) when the two services are furnished to a patient on the same day. If the DRE is the only service or is provided as part of an otherwise noncovered service, HCPCS code G0102 would be payable separately if all other coverage requirements are met.

4182.7 Diagnosis Coding Requirements.--There are no specific diagnosis requirements for prostate screening tests and procedures. However, prostate cancer screening digital rectal examinations and screening Prostate Specific Antigen (PSA) blood tests must be billed using screening ("V") code V76.44 (Special Screening for Malignant Neoplasms, Prostate).

4182.8 Denial Messages.--
A. Remittance Advice Notices.--If the claim for a screening prostate antigen test or screening digital rectal examination is being denied because the patient is not over 50 years of age, use existing American National Standard Institute (ANSI) X12-835 claim adjustment reason code 6 "the procedure code is inconsistent with the patient's age", at the line level along with line level Remark Code M140 "Service not covered until after the patient's 50th birthday, i.e., no coverage prior to the day after the patient's 50th birthday"

If the claim for a screening prostate antigen test or screening digital rectal examination is being denied because the time period between the test/procedure has not passed, use existing ANSI X12-835 claim adjustment reason code 119 "Benefit maximum for this time period has been reached" at the line level.

If the claim for a screening prostate antigen test or screening digital rectal examination is being denied due to the absence of diagnosis code V76.44 on the claim, use existing ANSI X-12-835 claim adjustment reason code 47, "This (these) diagnosis (es) is (are) not covered, missing, or invalid."

B. Medicare Summary Notice (MSN) and Explanation of Your Medicare Benefits (EOMB) Messages.--If the claim for a screening prostate specific antigen test or screening digital rectal examination is being denied because the patient is not over 50 years of age, the following new line (May 2000) MSN or EOMB message:

C. "This service is not covered until after the beneficiary's 50th birthday." (MSN Message 18.19, EOMB Message 18.27)

The Spanish version of this MSN or EOMB message should read:

"Este servicio no está cubierto hasta después de que el beneficiario cumpla 50 años."

If a claim for screening prostate specific antigen test or screening digital rectal examination is being denied because the minimum time period between the same test or procedure has not elapsed, use the following MSN or EOMB message:

"Service is being denied because it has not been [12/24/48] months since your last [test/procedure] of this kind." (MSN Message 18.14, EOMB Message 18.23)

The Spanish version of this MSN or EOMB message should read:

"Este servicio está siendo denegado ya que no han transcurrido [12, 24, 48] meses desde el último [examen/procedimiento] de esta clase."

4270 ESRD BILL PROCESSING PROCEDURES

Physicians, independent laboratories, and beneficiaries must submit claims (Form CMS-1500, Form CMS-1490Sor electronic equivalent) to their local carrier for services furnished to end stage renal disease (ESRD) beneficiaries. Suppliers of Method II dialysis equipment and supplies will submit their claims (Form CMS-1500 or electronic equivalent) to the appropriate Durable Medical Equipment Regional Carriers (DMERCs). All ESRD facilities must submit their claims to their appropriate fiscal intermediary (FI).

4270.2 Bill Review of Laboratory Services.--See §5114.1 for a detailed description of payment for outpatient clinical diagnostic laboratory tests using fee schedules and for specimen collection fees.

All laboratory tests not included under the ESRD composite rate payment and performed by an independent laboratory for dialysis patients of independent dialysis facilities must be billed by the independent laboratory to carriers. The fee schedule applies to all clinical diagnostic tests except for tests already included under the ESRD composite rate payment. These tests are reimbursed only through the composite rate paid by the intermediary.

Laboratory tests not included under the ESRD composite rate payment, including all laboratory tests furnished to home dialysis patients who have selected payment Method II (see §4271), are billed to and paid by you at the fee schedule, if the tests are performed by an independent laboratory for an independent dialysis facility patient.

For purposes of the fee schedule, clinical diagnostic laboratory services include all laboratory tests listed in codes 80002-89399 of the Current Procedural Terminology Fourth Edition (CPT-4) with the following exceptions:

85095-85109: Codes dealing with bone marrow smears and biopsies
85120: Bone marrow transplant
88000-88130: Certain cytopathology services
88160-88199: Certain cytopathology services
88260-88299: Cytogenetic studies
88300-88399: Surgical pathology services

Where tests not included in the composite rate are performed, the lab includes all tests (both those included in the composite rate and those that meet the frequency guidelines) on the bill. The tests listed below are included in the composite rate if their frequency does not exceed that which is indicated. Do not pay for tests up to the frequency described as they are paid under the composite rate. Tests in excess of the frequency may be paid unless you determine they are not medically necessary. Medical documentation is required to substantiate the frequency. A diagnosis of renal disease is not sufficient. The nature of the illness or injury (diagnosis, complaint, or symptom) requiring the performance of the test(s) must be present on the claim. A diagnosis from the ICD-9-CM coding system may be shown in lieu of a narrative description.

1. Laboratory Tests For Hemodialysis, Peritoneal Dialysis, and CCPD Included in the Composite Rate
2. Per Treatment
All hematocrit or hemoglobin and clotting time tests furnished incident to dialysis treatments.
3. Weekly
 • Prothrombin time for patients on anti-coagulant therapy
 • Serum Creatinine
 • Weekly or Thirteen Per Quarter
 • BUN
4. Monthly

Serum Calcium	Serum Bicarbonate	Alkaline Phosphatase
Serum Chloride	Serum Phosphorous	AST, SGOT
Total Protein	Serum Potassium	LDH
CBC	Serum Albumin	

Monthly
Laboratory Tests For CAPD Included in the Composite Rate

BUN	Magnesium	Alkaline Phosphatase
Creatinine	Phosphate	LDH
Sodium	Potassium	AST, SGOT
CO2	Total Protein	HCT
Calcium	Albumin	Hgb Dialysate Protein

A. Automated Profile Tests.--Clinical laboratory tests can be performed individually or in groups on automated profile equipment. If a clinical laboratory test is performed individually, it is paid in accordance with §§5114ff. If clinical laboratory tests are performed as part of an automated profile, then the following procedure applies:

1. Determine which of the laboratory tests in the automated profile are included under the composite rate and which are separately billable ESRD laboratory tests.

2. Determine the payment allowance of the automated profile by comparing it to the total payment allowances of the covered laboratory tests in the automated profile when the medically necessary tests in the profile are performed individually. The payment allowance of the automated profile is the lower of these two amounts. (See §5114.1.L.) If the payment allowance for the automated profile containing only the medically necessary tests is lower, you must determine the percentage of covered tests included under the composite rate payment. If 50 percent or more of the covered tests are included under the composite rate payment, then the entire profile is included within the composite payment. In this case, no separate payment in addition to the composite rate is made for any of the separately billable tests. If more than 50 percent of the covered tests are separately billable, the entire automated profile is considered separately billable. In this case, the entire automated profile is paid for in addition to the ESRD composite rate.

If the lower payment allowance is the payment allowance of the laboratory tests taken individually, the tests may be billed individually. In this case, the tests included under the composite rate are not billed or paid separately, and the tests that are not included under the composite rate are billed and paid separately.

B. Separately Billable Tests Furnished by Hospital-Based Facilities.--Hospital-based facilities are paid for the separately billable ESRD laboratory tests furnished to their outpatients following the same rules that apply to all other Medicare covered outpatient laboratory services furnished by a hospital.

C. Separately Billable Tests Furnished to Patients of Independent Dialysis Facilities.--All separately billable ESRD clinical laboratory services furnished to patients of independent dialysis facilities must be billed by and reimbursed to the person or entity that performs the laboratory test in accordance with usual Medicare program rules. Independent dialysis facilities with the appropriate clinical laboratory certification may perform and bill their intermediary for separately billable laboratory services. Independent dialysis facilities are paid for separately billable clinical laboratory tests according to the Medicare laboratory fee schedule for independent laboratories.

Following are tests not included in the composite rate which may be paid at the frequency shown without medical documentation. Tests in excess of that frequency require medical documentation. A diagnosis of ESRD alone is not sufficient medical documentation. The nature of the illness or injury (diagnosis, complaint, or symptom) requiring the performance of the test(s) must be present on the claim. A diagnosis from the ICD-9-CM coding system may be shown in lieu of a narrative description.

Guidelines for Separately Billable Tests for Hemodialysis, IPD, and CCPD

• Serum Aluminum: one every 3 months
• Serum Ferritin: one every 3 months

Guidelines for CAPD (every 3 months)

• WBC
• RBC
• Platelet count

4273 CLAIMS FOR PAYMENT FOR EPOETIN ALFA (EPO)

Effective June 1, 1989, the drug EPO is covered under Part B if administered incident to a physician's services. EPO is used to treat anemia associated with chronic renal failure, including patients on dialysis and those who are not on dialysis.

4273.1 Completion of Initial Claim for EPO.--The following information is required. Due to space limitations, some items must be documented on a separate form. Therefore, initial claims are generally submitted on paper unless your electronic billers are able to submit supplemental documentation with EMC claims. Return incomplete assigned claims in accordance with §3311. Develop incomplete unassigned claims.

A. Diagnoses.--The diagnoses must be submitted according to ICD-9-CM and correlated to the procedure. This information is in Items 23A and 24D, of the Form HCFA-1500.
B. Hematocrit (HCT)/Hemoglobin (Hgb).--There are special HCPCS codes for reporting the injection of EPO. These allow the simultaneous reporting of the patient's latest HCT or Hgb reading before administration of EPO.

Instruct the physician and/or staff to enter a separate line item for injections of EPO at different HCT/Hgb levels. The Q code for each line items is entered in Item 24C.

1. Code Q9920 - Injection of EPO, per 1,000 units, at patient HCT of 20 or less/Hgb of 6.8 or less.
2. Codes Q9921 through Q9939 - Injection of EPO, per 1,000 units, at patient HCT of 21 to 39/Hgb of 6.9 to 13.1. For HCT levels of 21 or more, up to a HCT of 39/Hgb of 6.9 to 13.1, a Q code that includes the actual HCT levels is used. To convert actual Hgb to corresponding HCT values for Q code reporting, multiply the Hgb value by 3 and round to the nearest whole number. Use the whole number to determine the appropriate Q code.
EXAMPLES: If the patient's HCT is 25/Hgb is 8.2-8.4, Q9925 must be entered on the claim. If the patient's HCT is 39/Hgb is 12.9-13.1, Q9939 is entered.
3. Code Q9940 - Injection of EPO, per 1,000 units at patient HCT of 40 or above.

A single line item may include multiple doses of EPO administered while the patient's HCT level remained the same.

C. Units Administered.--The standard unit of EPO is 1,000. The number of 1,000 units administered per line item is included on the claim. The physician's office enters 1 in the units field for each multiple of 1,000 units. For example, if 12,000 units are administered, 12 is entered. This information is shown in Item 24F (Days/Units) on Form HCFA-1500.
In some cases, the dosage for a single line item does not total an even multiple of 1,000. If this occurs, the physician's office rounds down supplemental dosages of 0 to 499 units to the prior 1,000 units. Supplemental dosages of 500 to 999 are rounded up to the next 1,000 units.
EXAMPLES: A patient's HCT reading on August 6 was 22/Hgb was 7.3. The patient received 5,000 units of EPO on August 7, August 9 and August 11, for a total of 15,000 units. The first line of Item 24 of Form HCFA-1500 shows:

Dates of Service	Procedure Code	Days or Units
8/7-8/11	Q9922	15

On September 13, the patient's HCT reading increased to 27/Hgb increased to 9. The patient received 5,100 units of EPO on September 13, September 15, and September 17, for a total of 15,300 units. Since less than 15,500 units were given, the figure is rounded down to 15,000. This line on the claim form shows:

Dates of Service	Procedure Code	Days or Units
9/13-9/17	Q9927	15

On October 16, the HCT level increased to 33/Hgb increased to 11. The patient received doses of 4,850 units on October 16, October 18, and October 20 for a total of 14,550 units. Since more than 14,500 units were administered, the figure is rounded up to 15,000. Form HCFA-1500 shows:

Dates of Service	Procedure Code	Days or Units
10/16-10/20	Q9933	15

D. Date of the patient's most recent HCT or Hgb.
E. Most recent HCT or Hgb level prior to initiation of EPO therapy.
F. Date of most recent HCT or Hgb level prior to initiation of EPO therapy.
G. Patient's most recent serum creatinine, within the last month, prior to initiation of EPO therapy.
H. Date of most recent serum creatinine prior to initiation of EPO therapy.

I. Patient's weight in kilograms.

J. Patient's starting dose per kilogram. (The usual starting dose is 50-100 units per kilogram.)

When a claim is submitted on Form HCFA-1500, these items are submitted on a separate document. It is not necessary to enter them into your claims processing system. This information is used in utilization review.

4273.2 Completion of Subsequent Claims for EPO.--Subsequent claims include the following:
A. Diagnoses.

B. Hematocrit or Hemoglobin.--This is indicated by the appropriate Q code. Claims include a EJ modifier to the Q code. This allows you to identify subsequent claims which do not require as much information as initial claims and prevent unnecessary development.

C. Number of units administered.--See §4273.1 for a description of these items. Subsequent claims may be submitted electronically. See §3023.7 for including the number of units in standard format EMC claims.

4450 PARENTERAL AND ENTERAL NUTRITION (PEN)

PEN coverage is determined by information provided by the attending physician and the PEN supplier. A certification of medical necessity (CMN) contains pertinent information needed to ensure consistent coverage and payment determinations nationally. A completed CMN must accompany and support the claims for PEN to establish whether coverage criteria are met and to ensure that the PEN provided is consistent with the attending physician's prescription.

The medical and prescription information on a PEN CMN can be completed most appropriately by the attending physician, or from information in the patient's records by an employee of the physician for the physician's review and signature. Although PEN suppliers may assist in providing PEN items they cannot complete the CMN since they do not have the same access to patient information needed to properly enter medical or prescription information.

A. Scheduling and Documenting Certifications and Recertifications of Medical Necessity for PEN.--A PEN CMN must accompany the initial claim submitted. The initial certification is valid for three months. Establish the schedule on a case-by-case basis for recertifying the need for PEN therapy. A change in prescription for a beneficiary past the initial certification period does not restart the certification process. A period of medical necessity ends when PEN is not medically required for two consecutive months. The entire certification process, if required, begins after the period of two consecutive months have elapsed.

B. Initial Certifications.--In reviewing the claim and the supporting data on the CMN, compare certain items, especially pertinent dates of treatment. For example, the start date of PEN coverage cannot precede the date of physician certification. The estimated duration of therapy must be contained on the CMN. Use this information to verify that the test of permanence is met. Once coverage is established, the estimated length of need at the start of PEN services will determine the recertification schedule. (See §4450 A.)

Verify that the information shown on the certification supports the need for PEN supplies as billed. A diagnosis must show a functional impairment that precludes the enteral patient from swallowing and the parenteral patient from absorbing nutrients.

The attending physician and/or his/her designated employee are in a position to accurately complete the patient's medical information including:

- The patient's general condition, estimated duration of therapy, and other treatments or therapies (see §3329 B.2.);
- The patient's clinical assessment relating to the need for PEN therapy (see §3329 B.3.); and
- The nutritional support therapy (i.e., the enteral or parenteral formulation). (See §3329 B.4.)

Initial assigned claims with the following conditions can be denied without development:

- Inappropriate or missing diagnosis or functional impairment;
- Estimated duration of therapy is less than 90 consecutive days;
- Duration of therapy is not listed;
- Supplies have not been provided;
- Supplies were provided prior to onset date of therapy; and
- Stamped physician's signature.

Develop unassigned claims for missing or incomplete information. (See §3329 C.)

Review all claims with initial certifications and recertifications before payment is authorized.

C.   Revised Certifications/Change in Prescription.--Remind suppliers to submit revised certifications if the attending physician changes the PEN prescription. A revised certification is appropriate when:

- There is a change in the attending physician's orders in the category of nutrients and/or calories prescribed;
- There is a change by more than one liter in the daily volume of parenteral solutions;
- There is a change from home-mix to pre-mix or pre-mix to home-mix parenteral solutions;
- There is a change from enteral to parenteral or parenteral to enteral therapy; or
- There is a change in the method of infusion (e.g., from gravity-fed to pump-fed).

Do not adjust payments on PEN claims unless a revised or renewed certification documents the necessity for the change. Adjust payments timely, if necessary, for supplies since the PEN prescription was changed.

Do not exceed payment levels for the most current certification or recertification if a prescription change is not documented by a new recertification.

Adjust your diary for scheduled recertifications. When the revised certification has been considered, reschedule the next recertification according to the recertification schedule. (See § 4450 A.)

D. Items Requiring Special Attention.--
1.   Nutrients.--Category IB of enteral nutrients contains products that are natural intact protein/protein isolates commonly known as blenderized nutrients. Additional documentation is required to justify the necessity of Category IB nutrients. The attending physician must provide sufficient information to indicate that the patient:

- Has an intolerance to nutritionally equivalent (semi-synthetic) products;
- Had a severe allergic reaction to a nutritionally equivalent (semi-synthetic) product; or
- Was changed to a blenderized nutrient to alleviate adverse symptoms expected to be of permanent duration with continued use of semi-synthetic products.

Also, enteral nutrient categories III through VI require additional medical justification for coverage.

Parenteral nutrition may be either "self-mixed" (i.e., the patient is taught to prepare the nutrient solution aseptically) or "pre-mixed" (i.e., the nutrient solution is prepared by trained professionals employed or contracted by the PEN supplier). The attending physician must provide information to justify the reason for "pre-mixed" parenteral nutrient solutions.

2. Prospective Billing.--Pay for no more than a one-month supply of parenteral or enteral nutrients for any one prospective billing period. Claims submitted retroactively may include multiple months.
3. Pumps.--Enteral nutrition may be administered by syringe, gravity, or pump. The attending physician must specify the reason that necessitates the use of an enteral feeding pump. Ensure that the equipment for which payment is claimed is consistent with that prescribed (e.g., expect a claim for an I.V. pole, if a pump is used).

Effective April 1, 1990, claims for parenteral and enteral pumps are limited to rental payments for a total of 15 months during a period of medical need. A period of medical need ends when enteral or parenteral nutrients are not medically necessary for two consecutive months.

Do not allow additional rental payments once the 15-month limit is reached, unless the attending physician changes the prescription between parenteral and enteral nutrients.

Do not continue rental payments after a pump is purchased unless the attending physician changes the prescription between parenteral and enteral nutrients.

Do not begin a new 15-month rental period when a patient changes suppliers. The new supplier is entitled to the balance remaining on the 15-month rental period.

Effective October 1, 1990, necessary maintenance and servicing of pumps after the 15-month rental limit is reached, includes repairs and extensive maintenance that involves the breaking down of sealed components or performing tests that require specialized testing equipment not available to the beneficiary or nursing home.

4. Supplies.--Enteral care kits contain all the necessary supplies for the enteral patient using the syringe, gravity, or pump method of nutrient administration. Parenteral nutrition care kits and their components are considered all inclusive items necessary to administer therapy during a monthly period.

- Compare the enteral feeding care kits on the claim with the method of administration indicated on the CMN.
- Reduce the allowance to the amount paid for a gravity-fed care kit when billed for a pump feeding kit in the absence of documentation or unacceptable documentation for a pump.
- Limit payment to a one-month supply.
- Deny payment for additional components included as part of the PEN supply kit.

5. Attending Physician Identification.--A CMN must contain the attending physician's Unique Physician Identification Number (UPIN) and be signed and dated by the attending physician. A stamped signature is unacceptable.

Deny certifications and recertifications altered by "whiting out" or "pasting over" and entering new data. Consider suppliers that show a pattern of altering CMNs for educational contact and/or audit.

Be alert to certifications from suppliers who have questionable utilization or billing practices or who are under sanction. Consider an audit of any such situations

4471 PAYMENT FOR IMMUNOSUPPRESSIVE DRUGS

Beginning January 1, 1987, Medicare pays for FDA approved immunosuppressive drugs and for drugs used in immunosuppressive therapy. (See §2050.5.) Generally, pay for self-administered immunosuppressive drugs that are specifically labeled and approved for marketing as such by the FDA, or identified in FDA-approved labeling for use in conjunction with immunosuppressive drug therapy. This benefit is subject to the Part B deductible and coinsurance provision and is limited to the 1-year period after the date of the transplant. Pay for immunosuppressive drugs which are provided outside the 1-year period if they are covered under another provision of the law (e.g., as inpatient hospital services or are furnished incident to a physician's service).

"One-year period after the date of the transplant" means 365 days from the day on which an inpatient is discharged from the hospital. From surgery until hospital discharge, payment for these drugs is included in Medicare's Part A payment to the hospital. If the same patient receives a subsequent transplant operation within 365 days, the period begins anew.

Prescriptions generally should be nonrefillable and limited to a 30 day supply. The 30 day guideline is necessary because dosage frequently diminishes over a period of time, and further, it is not uncommon for the physician to change the prescription from one drug to another. Also, these drugs are expensive and the coinsurance liability on unused drugs could be a financial burden to the beneficiary. Unless there are special circumstances, do not consider a supply of drugs in excess of 30 days to be reasonable and necessary.

5102.3 Transition to Fee Schedule-Relationship to Prior Rules.--
A. Comparability and Inherent Reasonableness Limitations.--Effective January 1, 1989, until further notice, you may no longer apply the comparable circumstances provision contained in §5026. Between January 1, 1989 and December 31, 1990, you may not apply the special limitations provision contained in §5246.

B. Purchase of Items Requiring Frequent and Substantial Servicing or Capped Rental Items.--
1. Purchase Prior to January 1, 1989.--If the beneficiary purchased an item of equipment in either of these two categories (see §5102.1.B or E) prior to January 1, 1989, pay the reasonable and necessary charges for maintenance and servicing of this equipment. In the event the item of equipment needs to be replaced on or after June 1, 1989, pay on a rental basis according to the instructions in §5102.1.B. or E.

If the beneficiary purchased the equipment even though you determined that rental was more economical under the rent/purchase guidelines, or if the beneficiary made an approved purchase on an installment plan, make payment on an installment basis until the purchase price has been reached or medical necessity terminated. If the purchase price has not been reached by January 1, 1989, continue paying on an installment basis but at the monthly fee schedule amount until the purchase price is reached, the purchase price fee schedule calculated under prior instructions is reached, or the medical necessity ends, whichever occurs first. The limitation on total payments to 15 months rental (as described in §5102.1.E) does not apply.

2. Purchase On Or After June 1, 1989.--If a beneficiary purchased an item of equipment that requires frequent and substantial servicing on or after June 1, 1989, do not make payment. Also, do not make payment for maintenance and servicing or for replacement of items in either category that are purchased on or after June 1, 1989.

If a beneficiary purchased an item of equipment in the capped rental category between June 1, 1989 and April 30, 1991, do not make payment. Also, do not make payment for maintenance and servicing. However, see §5102.1.E.5 or 6 for payment of purchase options after April 30, 1991 and for payment of replacement of items purchased between June 1, 1989 and April 30, 1991.

3. Purchase Between January 1, 1989 and June 1, 1989.--If a beneficiary purchased an item of equipment in either category after December 31, 1988, but before June 1, 1989, pay monthly installments equivalent to the rental fee schedule amounts until the medical necessity ends, the purchase price fee schedule calculated under prior instructions is reached, or the actual purchase charge has been reached, whichever occurs first. Pay the reasonable and necessary charges for maintenance and servicing of this equipment. In the event the item of equipment needs to be replaced on or after June 1, 1989, pay on a rental basis according to the instructions in §5102.1.B. or E. Payment may be made for purchase even if the purchase was preceded by a period of rental. However, total payments for rental plus purchase of capped rental items may not exceed the amount that would have been paid had the equipment been continuously rented for 15 months. (Therefore, if a purchase occurs during a period of continuous use after 15 months of rentals have been paid, no payment may be made other than the reasonable and necessary charges for servicing as described in §5102.1.E.4.)

C. Purchase of Oxygen Equipment.--
1. Purchase Prior to June 1, 1989.--If the beneficiary purchased stationary or portable oxygen equipment (see §5102.1.F) prior to June 1, 1989, pay the reasonable and necessary charges for maintenance and servicing of this equipment. In the event the item of equipment needs to be replaced on or after June 1, 1989, pay on a rental basis according to the instructions in §5102.1.F.

If the beneficiary purchased the equipment even though you determined that rental was more economical under the rent/purchase guidelines, or if the beneficiary made an approved purchase on an installment plan, make payment on an installment basis until the purchase price had been reached or medical necessity terminated. If the purchase price has not been reached by June 1, 1989, continue paying on an installment basis (see §5102.1.F.9) but at the monthly fee schedule amount until the purchase price is reached or the medical necessity ends, whichever occurs first.

2. Purchase On Or After June 1, 1989.--If a beneficiary purchased stationary or portable oxygen equipment on or after June 1, 1989, do not make payment for the equipment. However, make payment for the contents in accordance with §5102.1.F.4 or 5. Also, do not make payment for maintenance and servicing or for replacement of oxygen equipment that is purchased on or after June 1, 1989.

D. 15-Month Ceiling.--For purposes of computing the 10-month purchase option or the 15-month period for capped rental items, begin counting the first month that the beneficiary continuously rented the equipment. For example, if the beneficiary began renting the equipment in July 1988, the rental month which begins in January 1989 is counted as the beneficiary's 7th month of rental. Therefore, if the equipment has been continuously rented prior to October 2, 1987, no further rental payments are made since the 15-month period is terminated before January 1, 1989. The maintenance and service provision in §5102.1.E.4 begins July 1, 1989.

If the beneficiary has reached (on a date of service prior to January 1989) the purchase price limitation on a rental claim, do not make any further purchase or rental payments until the useful life has elapsed according to the instructions in §5102.1.E.7. However, for capped rental items previously rented that have reached the purchase cap under the rent/purchase rules, pay claims for maintenance and servicing fees in accordance with §5102.1.E.4 effective July 1, 1989.

E. Oxygen.--Claims for oxygen contents provided after May 31, 1989, but prior to the start of the June equipment rental month, may be paid in either of the following two ways. Either continue paying the reasonable charge payment amount for contents through the end of the May monthly rental period; or pay the reasonable charge payment amount for contents through the end of May and pay the actual charge for contents up to the fee schedule allowance for oxygen contents only, as prorated for the period June 1 through the end of the May rental period. Begin paying the appropriate full fee schedule amount at the beginning of the new rental period. For example, a beneficiary's rental period began May 15, 1989. Pay on a reasonable charge basis from May 15 through June 14; or pay on a reasonable charge basis from May 15 through May 31, 1989 and pay the actual charge up to 14/31 of the oxygen contents fee (established in §5102.1.F.4) from June 1 through June 14, 1989. Pay the lesser of the full fee schedule amount or actual charge beginning June 15, 1989.

F. Purchase Options For Capped Rental Items.--
    1. Electric Wheelchairs.--If the beneficiary purchases an electric wheelchair prior to May 1, 1991, pay for the wheelchair as a routinely purchased item in accordance with §5102.1.A. If the beneficiary elects to rent an electric wheelchair prior to May 1, 1991, pay the rental fee schedule amount not to exceed the purchase price in accordance with §5102.1.A. If, on May 1,1991, the purchase price has not been reached, convert the monthly fee schedule amount from routinely purchased to capped rental. As such, each month's rental before and after conversion must be counted toward the 10 month purchase option in §5102.1.E.6 and the 15 month rental cap in §5102.1.E.2.
    2. All Other Capped Rental Items.--If the beneficiary purchased a capped rental item prior to May 1, 1991, do not make payment. If the beneficiary rented a capped rental item prior to May 1, 1991, pay the rental fee schedule amount not to exceed the 15 month rental cap in accordance with §5102.1.E.2. Each month's rental must be counted toward the 10 month purchase option in §5102.1.E.6 and the 15 month rental cap in §5102.1.E.2.

5112 PAYMENT TO PSYCHOLOGISTS

The methodology used for determining payment to psychologists varies according to the professional classification of the psychologist: clinical psychologist (CP) or a psychologist other than a clinical psychologist. (See §2150 and §2070.2.)

5112.1 Clinical Psychologists.--Payment for all services rendered by CPs in community mental health centers (CMHCs) on or after July 1, 1988 and in all settings on or after July 1, 1990 is:

- based on the lower of the actual charge or a fee schedule;
- made only on an assignment-related basis; and
- subject to the outpatient mental health services limitation. (See §2470ff.)

A. Fee Schedule to be Used for Payment of CP Services.--Although a uniform fee schedule methodology is in development, it is not yet approved and will be the subject of rulemaking. In the absence of an approved fee schedule, establish your own fees based on an evaluation of all available charge data and any other relevant factors. The following summarizes the research completed to date and is provided for your information and guidance. It represents the best judgment at this time of what the final approach will be for Medicare payment to CPs.

In order to minimize any disruption which may occur when the final regulations and guidelines are issued, you are urged to adopt this approach. If you have alternate sources of data available as a result of your own Medicare or private plan experience which convinces you of a better approach or more appropriate level of payment, use your own analysis as a guide. So that the rulemaking process can benefit from your findings, if you choose a different approach, carefully document your analyses and data sources and send a copy of that documentation to the Division of Medical Services Payment, Office of Payment Policy, Bureau of Policy Development, 6325 Security Blvd., Baltimore, MD 21207.

In developing an appropriate fee schedule, HCFA is focusing on information readily available from the mental health services marketplace, including the private sector, Medicare and other large Federal programs.

The fee schedule for CPs, provided for in OBRA of 1987, became effective July 1, 1988. The methodology discussed below is applicable for establishing initial (1988) fees. For subsequent years, update the fee schedule by applying the same factor used to adjust the inflation-indexed charge, i.e., CPI-U.

    1. Fees for Therapeutic Services.--Since there is Medicare Part B charge data only for psychiatrists and not for psychologists (other than a very limited volume of diagnostic testing by psychologists in independent practice), we compared psychiatrist and psychologist charging patterns for both the overall mental health services marketplace and the Civilian Health and Medical Program of the Uniformed Services (CHAMPUS) administered by the Department of Defense to develop a fee schedule for therapeutic services.

For the overall market, information on fees for psychotherapy services performed by psychiatrists and psychologists was based on 1985 and 1986 data reported in Medical Economics (issue of September 1986) and Psychotherapy Finances (1986 Survey Report). In 1985, the median psychiatrist fee for individual psychotherapy was $81 per hour (i.e, a 45-50 minute session). To provide comparability with 1986 charge data for psychologists, HCFA updated the $81 by the 1986

Medicare Economic Index (MEI) of 1.0315, which resulted in an estimated 1986 median fee of $83.55 for psychiatrists. During that same year, the median psychologist fee for individual psychotherapy was $70, or 84 percent of the estimated psychiatrist fee.

A review of 1988 CHAMPUS program data shows that psychiatrist prevailing charges for a 1-hour psychotherapy session range from a low of $70 to a high of $130, with a median charge of $90. For psychologists, prevailing charges range from $65 to $114.40 hourly, with a median charge of $80. The fee differential between the two professions is 11 percent, i.e., the median psychologist prevailing charge amounts to approximately 89 percent of the median psychiatrist fee.

Another factor to be considered in developing a Medicare fee schedule is the relationship of Medicare allowances to prevailing charges. Due to the reasonable charge methodology, e.g., the use of customary charges, the average Medicare allowance is lower than the prevailing charge. In attempting to determine the appropriate prevailing charge reduction factor for Medicare, HCFA found that reliable Part B charge data for therapeutic services by psychiatrists do not exist, since application of the outpatient mental health services limitation against Medicare claims artificially deflates the average amount allowed. Because Part B Medicare Annual Data System (BMAD) data shows that the average allowance in proportion to adjusted prevailing charges is uniformly low for psychotherapy services (in some cases, as low as 6 percent), it was not possible to use these data to establish an accurate relationship between prevailing and allowed charges.

As a result, HCFA reviewed 1985 BMAD Medicare charge data for other cognitive services, since this category of service is the most likely to provide a comparable basis for analysis. A limited office visit (CPT code 90050) was selected for analysis because it represents the office medical service with the highest volume--over 36 percent of the total of 213 million frequencies. To minimize specialty- specific bias, HCFA analyzed collective charge data for three large physician specialties: general practice, general surgery, and internal medicine. The review found that the average allowance for code 90050 amounts to 91 percent of the adjusted prevailing charge.

HCFA also reviewed charge data for intermediate office visits (CPT code 90060), which account for another 30 percent of the 213 million frequencies for office medical services, for the internal medicine specialty. This analysis found that the average allowance for intermediate office visits amounts to 88 percent of the adjusted prevailing charge.

The results of these findings lead to the conclusion that the combined effect of the professional fee differential and the relationship between the adjusted prevailing and allowed charges could yield a fair CP fee schedule for therapeutic services. Depending on the variables, the resultant psychologist fee lies between 74 percent (derived by applying the highest fee differential against the greatest prevailing charge reduction) and 81 percent (the lowest fee differential multiplied by the lowest prevailing charge reduction factor) of the adjusted prevailing charge for participating psychiatrists.

Therefore, a fee schedule methodology of setting psychologist fees for therapeutic services at 80 percent of participating psychiatrists' adjusted prevailing charges for corresponding services in the locality is reasonable and allows for the maximum margin of error.

2. Fees for Diagnostic Services.--A limited volume of Medicare charge data exists for diagnostic services, i.e., psychological testing performed by qualified psychologists in independent practice. As a result, there was no need to refer to psychiatrists' charging patterns to develop a fee schedule for such services. However, the 9-11 percent prevailing charge reduction factor found in the office medical service codes discussed in §5112.A.1. must still be taken into account.

Therefore, a fee schedule methodology of setting fees for diagnostic services by CPs at 90 percent of the current adjusted prevailing charge for psychologists practicing independently in the locality is considered reasonable.

B. Payment Limitation.--All CP services (other than diagnostic services--see §2476.5) rendered outside of the hospital inpatient setting are subject to the outpatient mental health services limitation in §1833(c) of the Act and in §2470ff. Apply the limitation of 62.5 percent (see §2472) to the lesser of the actual charge or fee schedule amount.

C. Coinsurance and Deductible.--The annual deductible and the 20 percent Part B coinsurance apply to CP services.

D. Assignment Requirement.--All claims for CP services must be made on an assignment- related basis, i.e., the CP must accept assignment, claim direct Medicare payment after the death of the beneficiary, or submit the claim under the indirect payment procedure in §7065.

E. Coding.--Use the professional specialty code number 68 for CPs. Use HCPCS code M0601 for diagnostic services and HCPCS codes H5010-H5030 for therapeutic services billed by CPs in independent practice. Where the CP is not practicing independently, and is employed by a provider, physician or supplier who bills for the CP, the claims for services M0601 and H5010- H5030 must be submitted with modifier QP.

EXAMPLE: A beneficiary who has met his annual deductible begins receiving psychotherapy during April 1990. He visits the psychologist's office once weekly and the charge for each session is $75. The adjusted prevailing charge for the same service rendered by participating psychiatrists in the locality is $90. Therefore, the fee schedule amount for the CP is set at 80 percent of $90, or $72. This fee schedule amount is lower than the actual charge and effectively represents the reasonable charge for the psychologist's service. Multiply $72 by the outpatient mental health limitation of 62.5 percent to obtain the net Medicare allowed amount of $45. Since the annual deductible has previously been satisfied, no further subtraction needs to be made from the net allowed amount. Multiply $45 by 80 percent to calculate the Medicare amount payable to the psychologist. The difference between the Medicare payment of $36 and the fee schedule amount of $72 is the financial responsibility of the beneficiary.

5112.2 Psychological Tests Performed by Psychologists Who Are Not Clinical Psychologists.--Payment for diagnostic services rendered by independent psychologists who are not CPs (see §2070.2) is:

* made on the basis of the reasonable charge for the service;
* not subject to the outpatient mental health services limitation (see §2476.5); and
* not subject to assignment.

The time involved in the service is the principal factor when determining the reasonable charge where the psychologist ordinarily bills on a time-unit basis. Thus, where the bill is based on the number and length of testing sessions involved, use the psychologist's customary half-hour and hourly rates and the prevailing half-hour and hourly rates for comparable services in the locality in making the reasonable charge determinations.

Consider the time expended by a psychologist in the preparation of the report an integral part of the diagnostic testing services, not a separate covered service.

If the psychologist customarily bases his or her fee on factors other than time, apply the usual criteria for the determination of reasonable charges to the specific diagnostic procedure performed.

Use supplier specialty code 62 for psychologists who are not CPs and use HCPCS code M0601 to identify diagnostic services.

5113 PAYMENT TO CLINICAL SOCIAL WORKERS

Effective July 1, 1990, direct payment may be made to clinical social workers for covered diagnostic and therapeutic services. (See §2152 for coverage guidelines.) Payment for all covered services is based on the lower of the actual charge or a fee schedule.

A. Fee Schedule to be Used for Payment of Clinical Social Worker Services.--The fee schedule for clinical social worker services is set at 75 percent of the fee schedule for comparable services furnished by clinical psychologists.

B. Payment Limitation.--Clinical social worker services are subject to the outpatient mental health services limitation in §1833(c) of the Act and in §2470ff. Apply the limitation of 62.5 percent (see §2472) to the lesser of the actual charge or fee schedule amount. Diagnostic services are not subject to the limitation. (See §2476.5.)

C. Assignment Requirement.--All claims for clinical social worker services must be made on an assignment-related basis, i.e., the social worker must accept assignment, claim direct Medicare payment after the death of the beneficiary, or submit the claim under the indirect payment procedure in §7065.

D. Coinsurance and Deductible.--The annual deductible and the 20 percent Part B coinsurance apply to clinical social worker services.

E. Coding.--Use professional specialty code 80 for clinical social workers. Use HCPCS procedure codes M0601 for diagnostic services and H5010-H5030 for therapeutic services billed by clinical social workers in independent practice. Where the social worker is not practicing independently and is employed by a provider, physician or supplier who bills for the social worker, claims for services M0601 and H5010-H5030 must be submitted with modifier QS.

See §4162 for billing instructions for CSW services in outpatient settings.

5114 PAYMENT FOR DIAGNOSTIC LABORATORY SERVICES

This section sets out payment rules for diagnostic laboratory services, i.e., (1) outpatient clinical diagnostic laboratory tests subject to the fee schedule, and (2) other diagnostic laboratory tests.

Regardless of whether a diagnostic laboratory test is performed in a physician's office, by an independent laboratory, or by a hospital laboratory for its outpatients or nonpatients, it is considered a laboratory service. When a hospital laboratory performs diagnostic laboratory tests for nonhospital patients, the laboratory is functioning as an independent laboratory. Also, when physicians and laboratories perform the same test, whether manually or with automated equipment, the services are deemed similar.

The laboratory services for which this instruction applies are those listed in §2070.1.D. The tests are not subject to the economic index under the guidelines in §5020.3.A. Any test not listed in §2070.1.D is considered a physicians' service, is subject to the economic index as described in §5020.3.A, and is not considered in implementing this instruction. The only exceptions are as specified in §5020.3.A. For example, the taking of an EKG is a laboratory service when billed separately; but an EKG interpretation alone, as well as the taking of an EKG billed with interpretation, is a physician service subject to the economic index. Similarly, clinical laboratory services not subject to the fee schedule (see §5114.1) included in office visits for which a single prevailing charge screen is maintained are subject to the economic index.

Clinical diagnostic laboratory tests subject to the fee schedule are specifically delineated in §5114.1.B.

Other diagnostic laboratory tests are laboratory tests other than clinical diagnostic laboratory tests subject to fee schedule reimbursement. Such tests include EKGs and physiological testing.

Payment for clinical diagnostic laboratory tests subject to the fee schedule is made in accordance with the instructions in §5114.1.

Generally, payment for other diagnostic laboratory tests is made in accordance with the reasonable charge methodology. Special payment rules for physicians who do not personally perform or supervise other diagnostic laboratory tests but who bill for such tests are referenced in §5258. In accordance with §5262, payment for diagnostic radiology tests is made on a fee schedule basis.

D. Specimen Collection Fee.--Separate charges made by physicians (except for services furnished to dialysis patients as indicated below), independent laboratories (except for services furnished to dialysis patients as indicated below), or hospital laboratories for drawing or collecting specimens are allowed up to $3 whether the specimens are referred to physicians or other laboratories for testing. This fee is not paid to anyone who has not actually extracted the specimen from the patient. Only one collection fee is allowed for each patient encounter, regardless of the number of specimens drawn. When a series of specimens is required to complete a single test (e.g., glucose tolerance test), the series is treated as a single encounter. A specimen collection fee is allowed in circumstances such as drawing a blood sample through venipuncture (i.e., inserting into a vein a needle with syringe or vacutainer to draw the specimen) or collecting a urine sample by catheterization.

A specimen collection fee for physicians is allowed only when (1) it is the accepted and prevailing practice among physicians in the locality to make separate charges for drawing or collecting a specimen, and (2) it is the customary practice of the physician performing such services to bill separate charges for them.

A specimen collection fee is not allowed when the cost of collecting the specimen is minimal, such as a throat culture or a routine capillary puncture for clotting or bleeding time. Stool specimen collection for an occult blood test is usually done by the patients at home, and a fee for such collection is not allowed. When a stool specimen is collected during a rectal examination, the collection is an incidental byproduct of that examination. Costs such as gloves are related to the rectal examination and compensated for in the payment for the visit. Payment for performing the test is separate from the specimen collection fee. Costs such as media (e.g., the slides) and labor are included in the payment for the test.

You no longer have authority to make payment for routine handling charges where a specimen is referred by one laboratory to another. Preparatory services, e.g., where a referring laboratory prepares a specimen before transfer to a reference laboratory, are considered an integral part of the testing process, and the costs of such services are included in the charge for the total testing service.

A specimen collection fee is allowed when it is medically necessary for a laboratory technician to draw a specimen from either a nursing home patient or homebound patient. The technician must personally draw the specimen, e.g., venipuncture or urine sample by catheterization. A specimen collection fee is not allowed in situations where a patient is not in a nursing facility or confined to his or her home. When a laboratory performs the specimen collection, it may receive payment both for the draw and for the associated travel to obtain the specimen(s) for testing. Payment may be made to the laboratory even if the nursing facility has on- duty personnel qualified to perform the specimen collection. When the nursing home performs the specimen collection, it may only receive payment for the draw. Specimen collection performed by nursing home personnel for patients covered under Part A is paid for as part of the facility's payment for its reasonable costs, not on the basis of the specimen collection fee.

Special rules apply when services are furnished to dialysis patients. ESRD facilities are only paid by intermediaries. Therefore, never pay a specimen collection fee to an ESRD facility. The specimen collection fee is not allowed when a physician or one of the physician's employees draws the specimen from the dialysis patient because it is included in the Monthly Capitation Payment (MCP). (See §5037.) Independent laboratories are not paid the specimen collection fee for specimens collected that are used in performing a laboratory test reimbursed under the composite rate. If a home dialysis patient selects reimbursement Method II (see §4271) and all other criteria for payment are met, pay an independent laboratory the specimen collection fee for specimens collected from the patient.

The coinsurance and deductible provisions do not apply to the specimen collection fee where 100 percent of the fee schedule amount is payable on the basis of an assignment to the persons or entities drawing the specimen. For services (including specimen collection) rendered on or after January 1, 1987, payment to laboratories or physicians is only made on the basis of an assignment. For services rendered prior to January 1, 1987, acceptance of an assignment is optional for physicians. However, the coinsurance and deductible is applied to the specimen collection fee where a physician collects the specimen and does not accept assignment.

Complex vascular injection procedures, such as arterial punctures and venesections, are not subject either to this specimen collection policy or to the assignment provisions.

K. Travel Allowance.--In addition to a specimen collection fee allowed under §5114.1.D, a travel allowance can also be made to cover the costs of travel to collect a specimen from a nursing home or homebound patient. The additional allowance can be made only where a specimen collection fee is also payable, i.e., no travel allowance is made where the technician merely performs a messenger service to pick up a specimen drawn by a physician or nursing home personnel. The travel allowance may not be paid to a physician unless the trip to the home or nursing home was solely for the purpose of drawing a specimen. Otherwise travel costs are considered to be associated with the other purposes of the trip. Since a travel allowance can now be paid routinely, the differential specimen collection amount formerly allowed when a specimen is collected from a single patient rather than multiple patients (i.e., $5 rather than $3) is discontinued.

The allowance is intended to cover the estimated travel costs of collecting a specimen and is an allowance reflecting the technician's salary and travel costs. The following HCPCS codes are used for travel allowances:

- P9603--Travel allowance - one way, in connection with medically necessary laboratory specimen collection drawn from homebound or nursing home bound patient; prorated miles actually traveled (carrier allowance on per mile basis); or
- P9604--Travel allowance - one way, in connection with medically necessary laboratory specimen collection drawn from homebound or nursing home bound patient; prorated trip charge (carrier allowance on flat fee basis).

Identify round trip travel by use of modifier LR.

If you determine that it results in equitable payment, you may extend your former payment allowances for additional travel (such as to a distant rural nursing home) to all circumstances where travel is required. This might be appropriate, for example, if your former payment allowance was on a per mile basis. Otherwise you must establish an appropriate allowance. If you decide to establish a new allowance, one method is to consider developing a travel allowance consisting of:

- The current Federal mileage allowance for operating personal automobiles, plus
- A personnel allowance per mile to cover personnel costs based on an estimate of average hourly wages and average driving speed.

For your convenience, a chronology of mileage rates from July 1, 1984 to date is listed below:

- 20.5 cents: July 1, 1984 - July 31, 1987
- 21.0 cents: August 1, 1987 - August 13, 1988
- 22.5 cents: August 14, 1988 - September 16, 1989
- 24.0 cents: September 17, 1989 - June 29, 1991
- 25.0 cents: June 30, 1991 - Present

Travel allowance amounts claimed by suppliers are prorated by the total number of patients (including Medicare and non Medicare patients) from whom specimens are drawn or picked up on a given trip.

EXAMPLE 1: On October 1, 1989, a carrier determines that the average technician is paid $9 per hour and estimates 45 miles per hour as the average speed driven or $.20 per mile. This amount plus the Federal mileage allowance of $0.24 per mile results in a total allowance of $0.44 per mile. A laboratory technician makes a trip to two nursing homes involving a total mileage of 20 miles and draws specimens from three patients, Medicare as well as non- Medicare patients. In addition, specimens that were not drawn by the technician are picked up from two patients. A travel allowance per Medicare claim of $1.76 can be made (20 miles round trip x $0.44 per mile divided by 5). The supplier bills 4 miles (20 miles .5) under code P9603LR.

EXAMPLE 2: The carrier, through a review of the laboratory records, estimates that on average four specimens are drawn or picked up each trip, and that the average trip is 30 miles including both round trips and one way trips. Assuming the same facts as Example 1 (i.e., $9 per hour and 45 miles per hour), the carrier establishes a flat travel allowance of $3.30. Suppliers bill code P9604 and are paid $3.30 regardless of actual distance or number of patients served.

In keeping with the principles of §5024 and §5200, a payment in addition to the routine travel allowance determined under this section may be allowed to cover the additional costs of travel to collect a specimen from a nursing home or homebound patient when clinical diagnostic laboratory tests are needed on an emergency basis outside the general business hours of the laboratory making the collection.

5249 PAYMENT FOR IMMUNOSUPPRESSIVE DRUGS FURNISHED TO TRANSPLANT PATIENTS

A. General.--Beginning January 1, 1987, Medicare pays for FDA approved Immunosuppressive drugs. (For coverage, see §2050.5.) Generally under this benefit, payment is made for self-administered immunosuppressive drugs that are specifically labeled and approved for marketing as such by the FDA as well as those prescription drugs, such as prednisone, that are used in conjunction with immunosuppressive drugs as part of a therapeutic regimen reflected in FDA approved labeling for immunosuppressive drugs. This benefit is subject to the Part B deductible and coinsurance provision and is limited to the 1-year period after the date of the transplant procedure. Medicare pays for immunosuppressive drugs which are provided outside the 1-year period if the drugs are covered under some other provision of the law (e.g., when the drugs are covered as inpatient hospital services or are furnished incident to a physician's service).

We interpret "1-year period after the date of the transplant procedure" to mean 365 days from the day on which an inpatient is discharged from the hospital; from surgery until hospital discharge, payment for these drugs is included in Medicare's Part A payment to the hospital. If the same patient receives a subsequent transplant operation within 365 days, the period for this benefit begins anew.

When you receive the initial claim for a beneficiary, process it and make payment but contact the patient's physician and ask him/her to, in the future, furnish the patient with a non-refillable 30-day prescription for the immunosuppressive drugs. Also, ask the physician the date of that patient's discharge from the hospital and to indicate discharge information on the first immunosuppressive drug prescription for subsequent transplant patients. Use this date for benefit limitation purposes. This is because the dosage of these drugs frequently diminishes over a period of time and, further it is not uncommon for the physician to change the prescription from one drug to another because of the patient's needs. Also, these drugs are expensive and the coinsurance liability on unused drugs could be a financial burden to the beneficiary. Unless there are special circumstances, do not consider a supply of drugs in excess of 30 days to be reasonable and necessary and limit payment accordingly.

B. Payment.--Payment is made on a reasonable cost basis if the beneficiary is the outpatient of a participating hospital. In all other cases, payment is made on a reasonable charge basis.

C. FDA Approved Drugs.--Some of the most commonly prescribed immuno-suppressive drugs are:

- Sandimmune (cyclosporine), Sandoz Pharmaceutical (oral or parenteral);
- Imuran(azathioprine), Burroughs Wellcome Vial (oral);
- Atgam (antithymocyte/globulin), Upjohn (parenteral); and
- Orthoclone OKT3 (muromonab - CD3) Ortho Pharmaceutical (parenteral).

In addition, prescription drugs used in conjunction with immunosuppressive drugs as part of a therapeutic regimen reflected in FDA-approved labeling for immuno-suppressive drugs are also covered.

Limit the payment for the drug to the cost of the frequently administered dosage of the drug (adjusted for medical factors as determined by the physician).

Consult such sources as the Drug Topics Red Book, American Druggists Blue Book, and Medispan, realizing that substantial discounts are available.

15018 PAYMENT CONDITIONS FOR ANESTHESIOLOGY SERVICES

H. Monitored Anesthesia Care.--Pay for reasonable and medically necessary monitored anesthesia care services on the same basis as other anesthesia services. Instruct anesthesiologists to use modifier QS to report monitored anesthesia care cases. Monitored anesthesia care involves the intraoperative monitoring by a physician or qualified individual under the medical direction of a physician or of the patient's vital physiological signs in anticipation of the need for administration of general anesthesia or of the development of adverse physiological patient reaction to the surgical procedure. It also includes the performance of a pre-anesthetic examination and evaluation, prescription of the anesthesia care required, administration of any necessary oral or parenteral medications (e.g., etropine, demerol, valium) and provision of indicated post-operative anesthesia care.

15022 PAYMENT CONDITIONS FOR RADIOLOGY SERVICES

A. Professional Component (PC).--Pay for the PC of radiology services furnished by a physician to an individual patient in all settings under the fee schedule for physician services regardless of the specialty of the physician who performs the service. For services furnished to hospital patients, pay only if the services meet the conditions for fee schedule payment in §15014.C.1 and are identifiable, direct, and discrete diagnostic or therapeutic services to an individual patient, such as an interpretation of diagnostic procedures and the PC of therapeutic procedures. The interpretation of a diagnostic procedure includes a written report.

B. Technical Component TC).--
1. Hospital Patients.--Do not pay for the TC of radiology services furnished to Hospital patients. Payments for physicians' radiological services to the hospital, e.g., Aministrative orsupervisory services, and for provider services needed to produce the radiology service is made by the intermediary as provider services through various payment mechanisms.
2. Services Not Furnished in Hospitals.--Pay under the fee schedule for the TC of radiology services furnished to beneficiaries who are not patients of any hospital in a physician's office, a freestanding imaging or radiation oncology center, or other setting that is not part of a hospital.
3. Services Furnished in Leased Departments.--In the case of procedures furnished in a leased hospital radiology department to a beneficiary who is neither an inpatient nor an outpatient of any hospital, e.g., the patient is referred by an outside physician and is not registered as a hospital outpatient, both the PC and the TC of the services are payable under the fee schedule.
4. Purchased TC Services.--Apply the purchased services limitation as set forth in §15048 to the TC of radiologic services other than screening mammography procedures.
5. Computerized Axial Tomography (CT) Procedures.--Do not reduce or deny payment for medically necessary multiple CT scans of different areas of the body that are performed on the same day.

The TC RVUs for CT procedures that specify "with contrast" include payment for high osmolar contrast media. When separate payment is made for low osmolar contrast media under the conditions set forth in subsection F.1, reduce payment for the contrast media as set forth in subsection F.2.

6. Magnetic Resonance Imaging (MRI) Procedures.--Do not make additional payments for 3 or more MRI sequences. The RVUs reflect payment levels for 2 sequences.

The TC RVUs for MRI procedures that specify "with contrast" include payment for paramagnetic contrast media. Do not make separate payment under code A4647.
A diagnostic technique has been developed under which an MRI of the brain or spine is first performed without contrast material, then another MRI is performed with a standard (0.1mmol/kg) dose of contrast material and, based on the need to achieve a better image, a third MRI is performed with an additional double dosage (0.2mmol/kg) of contrast material. When the high-dose contrast technique is utilized:

- Do not pay separately for the contrast material used in the second MRI procedure;
- Pay for the contrast material given for the third MRI procedure through supply code A4643 when billed with CPT codes 70553, 72156, 72157, and 72158;
- Do not pay for the third MRI procedure. For example, in the case of an MRI of the brain, if CPT code 70553 (without contrast material, followed by with contrast material(s) and further sequences) is billed, make no payment for CPT code 70551 (without contrast material(s)), the additional procedure given for the purpose of administering the double dosage, furnished during the same session. Medicare does not pay for the third procedure (as distinguished from the contrast material) because the CPT definition of code 70553 includes all further sequences; and
- Do not apply the payment criteria for low osmolar contrast media in subsection F to billings for code A4643.

7. Stressing Agent.--Make separate payment under code J1245 for pharmacologic stressing agents used in connection with nuclear medicine and cardiovascular stress testing procedures furnished to beneficiaries in settings in which TCs are payable. Such an agent is classified as a supply and covered as an integral part of the diagnostic test. However, pay for code J1245 under the policy for determining payments for "incident to" drugs.

D. Nuclear Medicine (CPT 78000 Through 79999).--
7. Payments for Radionuclides.--The TC RVUs for nuclear medicine procedures (CPT codes 78XXX for diagnostic nuclear medicine, and codes 79XXX for therapeutic nuclear medicine) do not include the radionuclide used in connection with the procedure. These substances are separately billed under codes A4641 and A4642 for diagnostic procedures and code 79900 for therapeutic procedures and are paid on a "By Report" basis depending on the substance used. In addition, CPT code 79000 is separately payable in connection with certain clinical brachytherapy procedures. (See subsection D.3.)
8. Application of Multiple Procedure Policy (CPT Modifier 51).--Apply the multiple procedure reduction as set forth in §15038 to the following nuclear medicine diagnostic procedures: codes 78306, 78320, 78803, 78806, and 78807.
9. Generation and Interperetation of Automated Data.--Payment for CPT codes 78890 and 78891 is bundled into payments for the primary procedure.
10. Positron Emission Tomography (PET) Scans (HCPCS Codes G0030-G0047).--For procedures furnished on or after March 14, 1995, pay for PET procedure of the heart under the limited coverage policy set forth in §50-36 of the Coverage Issues Manual (HCFA Pub. 6) using the billing instructions in §4173 of the Medicare Carriers Manual.

D. Radiation Oncology (Therapeutic Radiology) (CPT 77261-77799).--
1. Weekly Radiation Therapy Management (CPT 77419-77430).--Pay for a physician's weekly treatment management services under codes 77419, 77420, 77425, and 77430. Instruct billing entities to indicate on each claim the number of fractions for which payment is sought.

A weekly unit of treatment management is equal to five fractions or treatment sessions. A week for the purpose of making payments under these codes is comprised of five fractions regardless of the actual time period in which the services are furnished. It is not necessary that the radiation therapist personally examine the patient during each fraction for the weekly treatment management code to be payable. Multiple fractions representing two or more treatment sessions furnished on the same day may be counted as long as there has been a distinct break in therapy sessions, and the fractions are of the character usually furnished on different days. If, at the final billing of the treatment course, there are three or four fractions beyond a multiple of five, those three or four fractions are paid for as a week. If there are one or two fractions beyond a multiple of five, consider payment for these services as having been made through prior payments.

EXAMPLE:
18 fractions = 4 weekly services
62 fractions = 12 weekly services
8 fractions = 2 weekly services
6 fractions = 1 weekly service

If billings have occurred which indicate that the treatment course has ended (and, therefore, the number of residual fractions has been determined), but treatments resume, adjust your payments for the additional services consistent with the above policy.

EXAMPLE:
8 fractions = payment for 2 weeks

2 additional fractions are furnished by the same physician. No additional Medicare payment is made for the 2 additional fractions.

There are situations in which beneficiaries receive a mixture of simple (code 77420), intermediate (code 77425), and complex (code 77430) treatment management services during a course of treatment. In such cases, pay under the weekly treatment management code that represents the more frequent of the fractions furnished during the five-fraction week. For example, an intermediate weekly treatment management service is payable when, in a grouping of five fractions, a beneficiary receives three intermediate and two simple fractions.

2. Services Bundled Into Treatment Management Codes.--Make no separate payment for any of the following services rendered by the radiation oncologists or in conjunction with radiation therapy:

11920: Tattooing, intradermal introduction of insoluble opaque pigments to correct color defects of skin; 6.0 sq. cm or less
11921: 6.1 to 20.0 sq. cm
11922: each additional 20.0 sq. cm
16000: Initial treatment, first degree burn, when no more than local treatment is required
16010: Dressings and/or debridement, initial or subsequent; under anesthesia, small
16015: under anesthesia, medium or large, or with major debridement
16020: without anesthesia, office or hospital, small
16025: without anesthesia, medium (e.g., whole face or whole extremity)
16030: without ancsthesia, large (e.g., more than one extremity)
36425: Venipuncture, cut down age 1 or over
53670: Catheterization, urethra; simple
53675: complicated (may include difficult removal of balloon catheter)
99211: Office or other outpatient visit, established patient; Level I
99212: Level II
99213: Level III
99214: Level IV
99215: Level V
99238: Hospital discharge day management
99281: Emergency department visit, new or established patient; Level I
99282: Level II
99283: Level III
99284: Level IV
99285: Level V
90780: IV infusion therapy, administered by physician or under direct supervision of physician; up to one hour
90781: each additional hour, up to eight (8) hours
90841: Individual medical psychotherapy by a physician, with continuing medical diagnostic evaluation, and drug management when indicated, including psychoanalysis, insight oriented, behavior modifying or supportive psychotherapy; time unspecified
90843: approximately 20 to 30 minutes
90844: approximately 45 to 50 minutes
90847: Family medical psychotherapy (conjoint psychotherapy) by a physician, with continuing medical diagnostic evaluation, and drug management when indicated
99050: Services requested after office hours in addition to basic service
99052: Services requested between 10:00 PM and 8:00 AM in addition to basic service
99054: Services requested on Sundays and holidays in addition to basic service
99058: Office services provided on an emergency basis
99071: Educational supplies, such as books, tapes, and pamphlets, provided by the physician for the patient's education at cost to physician
99090: Analysis of information data stored in computers (e.g., ECG, blood pressures, hematologic data)

99150: Prolonged physician attendance requiring physician detention beyond usual service (e.g., operative standby, monitoring ECG, EEG, intrathoracic pressures, intravascular pressures, blood gases during surgery, standby for newborn care following caesarean section); 30 minutes to one hour

99151: more than one hour

99180: Hyperbaric oxygen therapy initial

99182: Subsequent

99185: Hypothermia; regional

99371: Telephone call by a physician to patient or for consultation or medical management or for coordinating medical management with other health care professionals; simple or brief (e.g., to report on tests and/or laboratory results, to clarify or alter previous instructions, to integrate new information from other health professionals into the medical treatment plan, or to adjust therapy)

99372: intermediate (e.g., to provide advice to an established patient on a new problem, to initiate therapy that can be handled by telephone, to discuss test results in detail, to coordinate medical management of a new problem in an established patient, to discuss and evaluate new information and details, or to initiate a new plan of care)

99373: complex or lengthy (e.g., lengthy counseling session with anxious or distraught patient, detailed or prolonged discussion with family members regarding seriously ill patient, lengthy communication necessary to coordinate complex services or several different health professionals working on different aspects of the total patient care plan)

- Anesthesia (whatever code billed)
- Care of Infected Skin (whatever code billed)
- Checking of Treatment Charts
- Verification of Dosage, As Needed (whatever code billed)
- Continued Patient
- Evaluation, Examination, Written Progress Notes, As Needed (whatever code billed)
- Final Physical
- Examination (whatever code billed)
- Medical Prescription Writing (whatever code billed)
- Nutritional
- Pain Management (whatever code billed)
- Review & Revision of Treatment Plan (whatever code billed)
- Routine Medical Management of Unrelated Problem (whatever code billed)
- Special Care of Ostomy (whatever code billed)
- Written Reports, Progress Note (whatever code billed)
- Follow-up Examination and Care for 90 Days After Last Treatment (whatever code billed)

3. Radiation Treatment Delivery (CPT 77401-77417).--Pay for these TC services on a daily basis under CPT codes 77401-77416 for radiation treatment delivery. Do not use local codes and RVUs in paying for the TC of radiation oncology services. Multiple treatment sessions on the same day are payable as long as there has been a distinct break in therapy services, and the individual sessions are of the character usually furnished on different days. Pay for CPT code 77417 (Therapeutic radiology port film(s)) on a weekly (5 fractions) basis.

4. Clinical Brachytherapy (CPT Codes 77750-77799).--Apply the bundled services policy in §15022.D.2. to procedures in this family of codes other than CPT code 77776. For procedures furnished in settings in which you make TC payments, pay separately for the expendable source associated with these procedures under CPT code 79900 except in the case of remote afterloading high intensity brachytherapy procedures (CPT codes 77781-77784). In the 4 codes cited, the expendable source is included in the RVUs for the TC of the procedures.

5. Radiation Physics Services (CPT Codes 77300-77399).--Until further notice, pay for the PC and TC of CPT codes 77300-77334 and 77739 on the same basis as you pay for radiologic services generally. For PC billings in all settings, presume that the radiologist participated in the provision of the service, e.g., reviewed/validated the physicist's calculation. CPT codes 77336 and 77370 are technical services only codes that are payable by carriers only in settings in which TCs are payable.

F. Supervision and Interpretation (S&I) Codes and Interventional Radiology.--

4. Physician Presence.--Radiologic S&I codes are used to describe the personal supervision of the performance of the radiologic portion of a procedure by one or more physicians and the interpretation of the findings. In order to bill for the supervision aspect of the procedure, the physician must be present during its performance. This kind of personal supervision of the performance of the procedure is a service to an individual beneficiary and differs from the type of general supervision of the radiologic procedures performed in a hospital for which intermediaries pay the costs as physician services to the hospital. The interpretation of the procedure may be performed later by another physician. In situations in which a cardiologist, for example, bills for the supervision (the "S") of the S&I code, and a radiologist bills for the interpretation (the "I") of

the code, both physicians should use a -52 modifier indicating a reduced service, e.g., the interpretation only. Pay no more for the fragmented S&I code than you would if a single physician furnished both aspects of the procedure.

5. Multiple Procedure Reduction.--Make no multiple procedure reductions in the S&I or primary nonradiologic codes in these types of procedures, or in any procedure codes for which the descriptor and RVUs reflect a multiple service reduction. For additional procedure codes that do not reflect such a reduction, apply the multiple procedure reductions set forth in §15038.

G. Low Osmolar Contrast Media (LOCM) (HCPCS Codes A4644-A4646).--
1. Payment Criteria.--Make separate payments for LOCM (HCPCS codes A4644, A4645, and A4646) in the case of all medically necessary intrathecal radiologic procedures furnished to nonhospital patients. In the case of intraarterial and intravenous radiologic procedures, pay separately for LOCM only when it is used for nonhospital patients with one or more of the following characteristics:

- A history of previous adverse reaction to contrast material, with the exception of a sensation of heat, flushing, or a single episode of nausea or vomiting;
- A history of asthma or allergy;
- Significant cardiac dysfunction including recent or imminent cardiac decompensation, severe arrhythmia, unstable angina pectoris, recent myocardial infarction, and pulmonary hypertension;
- Generalized severe debilitation; or
- Sickle cell disease.

If the beneficiary does not meet any of these criteria, the payment for contrast media is considered to be bundled into the TC of the procedure, and the beneficiary may not be billed for LOCM.
2. Payment Level.--A LOCM pharmaceutical is considered to be a supply which is an integral part of the diagnostic test. However, determine payment in the same manner as for a drug furnished incident to a physician's service with the following additional requirement. Reduce the lower of the estimated actual acquisition cost or the national average wholesale price by 8 percent to take into account the fact that the TC RVUs of the procedure codes reflect less expensive contrast media.

H. Services of Portable X-Ray Suppliers.--Services furnished by portable X-ray suppliers (see §2070.4) may have as many as four components.
1. Professional Component.--Pay the PC of radiologic services furnished by portable X-ray suppliers on the same basis as other physician fee schedule services.
2. Technical Component.--Pay the TC of radiology services furnished by portable X-ray suppliers under the fee schedule on the same basis as TC services generally.
3. Transportation Component (HCPCS Codes R0070-R0076).--This component represents the transportation of the equipment to the patient. Establish local RVUs for the transportation R codes based on your knowledge of the nature of the service furnished. Allow only a single transportation payment for each trip the portable X-ray supplier makes to a particular location. When more than one Medicare patient is X-rayed at the same location, e.g., a nursing home, prorate the single fee schedule transportation payment among all patients receiving the services. For example, if two patients at the same location receive X-rays, make one-half of the transportation payment for each.

Use any information regarding the number of patients X-rayed in each location that the supplier visits during each trip that the supplier of the X-ray may volunteer on the bill or claim for payment. If such information is not indicated, assume that at least four patients were X-rayed at the same location, and pay only one-fourth of the fee schedule payment amount for any one patient. Advise the suppliers in your area regarding the way in which you use this information.

NOTE: No transportation charge is payable unless the portable X-ray equipment used was actually transported to the location where the X-ray was taken. For example, do not allow a transportation charge when the X-ray equipment is stored in a nursing home for use as needed. However, a set-up payment (see subsection G.4) is payable in such situations. Further, for services furnished on or after January 1, 1997, make no separate payment under HCPCS code R0076 for the transportation of EKG equipment by portable X-ray suppliers or any other entity.

4. Set-Up Component (HCPCS Code Q0092).--Pay a set-up component for each radiologic procedure (other than retakes of the same procedure) during both single patient and multiple patient trips under Level II HCPCS code Q0092. Do not make the set-up payment for EKG services furnished by the portable X-ray supplier.

15030 SUPPLIES

Make a separate payment for supplies furnished in connection with a procedure only when one of the two following conditions exists:

A. HCPCS codes A4550, A4200, and A4263 are billed in conjunction with the appropriate procedure in the Medicare Physician Fee Schedule Data Base (place of service is physician's office); or

B. The supply is a pharmaceutical or radiopharmaceutical diagnostic imaging agent (including codes A4641 through A4647); pharmacologic stressing agent (code J1245); or therapeutic radionuclide (CPT code 79900). The procedures performed are:

- Diagnostic radiologic procedures (including diagnostic nuclear medicine) requiring pharmaceutical or radiopharmaceutical contrast media and/or pharmocological stressing agent,
- Other diagnostic tests requiring a pharmacological stressing agent,
- Clinical brachytherapy procedures (other than remote afterloading high intensity brachytherapy procedures (CPT codes 77781 through 77784) for which the expendable source is included in the TC RVUs), or
- Therapeutic nuclear medicine procedures.

15360 ECHOCARDIOGRAPHY SERVICES (CODES 93303 - 93350)

Separate Payment for Contrast Media.--Effective October 1, 2000, physicians may separately bill for contrast agents used in echocardiography. Physicians should use HCPCS Code A9700 (Supply of injectable contrast material for use in echocardiography, per study). The type of service code is 9. This code will be carrier-priced.

INDEX

A

Abarelix J0128
Abciximab. J0130
Abdomen
    dressing holder/binder A4462
    pad low profile. L1270
    supports, pendulous. L0920, L0930
Abduction control, each. L2624
Abduction rotation bar, foot L3140-L3170
Absorption dressing A6251-A6256
Access system. A4301
Accessories
    ambulation devices. E0153-E0159
    artificial kidney and machine (see also ESRD) . . . E1510-E1699
    beds E0271-E0280, E0300-E0326
    wheelchairs E0950-E1030, E1050-E1298, E2300-E2399,
    . . . . K0001-K0109
Acetazolamide sodium J1120
Acetylcysteine, inhalation solution J7608
Acetylcysteine, injection. J0132
Acyclovir J0133
Adalimumab J0135
Adenosine J0150, J0152
Adhesive A4364
    disc or foam pad A5126
    remover A4365, A4455
    support, breast prosthesis A4280
    tape. A4454, A6265
Administrative, Miscellaneous and Investigational. A9000-A9999
Adrenalin J0170
Aerosol
    compressor E0571, E0572
    compressor filter. K0178-K0179
    mask K0180

INDEX

AFO E1815, E1830, L1900-L1990, L4392, L4396

Agalsidase beta. J0180

Aggrastat. J3245

A-hydroCort. J1710

Air ambulance (see also Ambulance) A0030, A0040

Air bubble detector, dialysis. E1530

Air fluidized bed E0194

Air pressure pad/mattress E0176, E0186, E0197

Air travel and non-emergency transportation A0140

Alarm, pressure, dialysis E1540

Alatrofloxacin mesylate J0200

Albumin, human P9041, P9042

Albuterol, all formulations, inhalation solution, concentrated . . . J7611

Albuterol, all formulations, inhalation solution, unit dose J7613

Albuterol, all formulations, inhalation solution J7620

Alcohol A4244

Alcohol wipes. A4245

Aldesleukin (IL2) J9015

Alefacept. J0215

Alemtuzumab. J9010

Alert device A9280

Alginate dressing A6196-A6199

Alglucerase J0205

Alpha-1-proteinase inhibitor, human J0256

Alprostadil, injection J0270

Alprostadil, urethral suppository. J0275

Alteplase recombinant J2997

Alternating pressure mattress/pad A4640, E0180, E0181, E0277

Alveoloplasty D7310-D7320

Amalgam dental restoration D2110-D2161

Ambulance A0021-A0999

    air A0430, A0431, A0435, A0436

    disposable supplies A0382-A0398

    oxygen A0422

Ambulation device E0100-E0159

Amikacin Sulfate J0278

Aminolevulinic acid HCL. J7308

Aminophylline J0280

Amiodarone Hcl J0282

Amitriptyline HCI. J1320
Ammonia N-13 . . . . A9526
Ammonia test paper A4774
Amniotic membrane V2790
Amobarbital. J0300
Amphotericin B J0285
Amphotericin B Lipid Complex J0287-J0289
Ampicillin sodium. J0290
Ampicillin sodium/sulbactam sodium J0295
Amputee
    adapter, wheelchair E0959
    prosthesis. L5000-L7510, L7520, L7900, L8400-L8465
    stump sock. L8470-L8490
    wheelchair. E1170-E1190, E1200, K0100
Amygdalin. J3570
Analgesia, dental D9230
Ancsthesia
    dental D7110-D7130, D7210-D7250, D9210-D9240
    dialysis A4735
Anistreplase. J0350
Ankle splint, recumbent. K0126-K0130
Ankle-foot orthosis (AFO)
    . . . . L1900-L1990, L2106-L2116, L4392, L4396
Anterior-posterior-lateral orthosis
    . . . . L0520, L0550-L0565, L0700, L0710
Anterior-posterior-lateral-rotary orthosis. L0340-L0440
Anterior-posterior orthosis L0320, L0330, L0530
Anti-emetic, oral. Q0163-Q0181, J8498, J8597
Anti-hemophilic factor (Factor VIII) J7190-J7192
Anti-inhibitors, per I.U. J7198
Anti-neoplastic drug, NOC J9999
Antithrombin III J7197
Antral fistula closure, oral D7260
Apexification, dental. D3351-D3353
Apicoectomy. D3410-D3426
Apnea monitor. E0608
Appliance
    cleaner A5131
    pneumatic. E0655-E0673

Aprotinin. J0365
Aqueous
    shunt L8612
    sterile J7051
Arbutamine HCL J0395
Arch support L3040-L3100
    intralesional J3302
Arm, wheelchair E0973
Arsenic trioxide J9017
Artificial
    cornea. L8609
    kidney machines and accessories (see also Dialysis)
    . . . . E1510-E1699
    larynx. L8500
Asparaginase J9020
Assessment
    audiologic V5008-V5020
    cardiac output M0302
    speech. V5362-V5364
Astramorph J2275
Atropine, inhalation solution, concentrated. J7635
Atropine, inhalation solution, unit dose J7636
Atropine sulfate J0460
Audiologic assessment V5008-V5020
Auricular prosthesis. D5914, D5927
Aurothioglucose J2910
Azacitidine J9025
Azathioprine. J7500, J7501
Azithromycin injection. J0456

B

Back supports L0500-L0960
Baclofen J0475, J0476
Bacterial sensitivity study. P7001
Bag
    drainage A4357
    irrigation supply A4398

Bag—*continued*

    urinary A5112, A4358

Bandage A4441-A4456

Basiliximab J0480

Bathtub

    chair E0240

    stool or bench E0245, E0247-E0248

    transfer rail E0246

    wall rail E0241, E0242

Battery K0082-K0087, L7360, L7364-L7368

    charger E1066, K0088, K0089, L7362, L7366

    replacement for blood glucose monitor A4233-A4234

    replacement for cochlear implant device L8623-L8624

    replacement for TENS A4630

    ventilator A4611-A4613

    wheelchair A4631

BCG live, intravesical J9031

Beclomethasone inhalation solution J7622

Bed

    air fluidized E0194

    cradle, any type E0280

    drainage bag, bottle A4357, A5102

    hospital E0250-E0270, E0298-E0301

    pan E0275, E0276

    rail E0305, E0310

    safety enclosure frame/canopy E0316

Below knee suspension sleeve L5674, L5675

Belt

    extremity E0945

    ostomy A4367

    pelvic E0944

    safety K0031

    wheelchair E0978, E0979

Bench, bathtub (see also Bathtub) E0245

Benefix, see Factor IX Q0161

Benesch boot L3212-L3214

Benztropine J0515

Betadine A4246, A4247

Betameth J0704

Betamethasone inhalation solution J7624
Betamethasone acetate and betamethasone sodium phosphate. . . J0702
Betamethasone sodium phosphate. J0704
Bethanechol chloride J0520
Bevacizumab J9035
Bicarbonate dialysate A4705
Bicuspid (excluding final restoration). D3320
    retreatment, by report D3347
    surgery, first root D3421
Bifocal, glass or plastic. V2200-V2299
Bilirubin (phototherapy) light E0202
Binder A4465
Biofeedback device. E0746
Bioimpedance, electrical, cardiac output. M0302
Biperiden lactate. J0190
Bitewing. D0270-D0274
Bitolterol mesylate, inhalation solution, concentrated J7628
Bitolterol mesylate, inhalation solution, unit dose J7629
Bivalirudin. J0583
Bladder calculi irrigation solution Q2004
Bladder capacity test, ultrasound. G0050
Bleaching tooth D3960
Bleomycin sulfate J9040
Blood
    Congo red P2029
    fresh frozen plasma P9017
    glucose monitor E0607, E2100, E2101
    glucose test A4253
    granulocytes, pheresis. P9050
    leak detector, dialysis. E1560
    leukocyte poor P9016
    mucoprotein P2038
    platelets. P9019
    platelets, irradiated. P9032
    platelets, leukocytes reduced P9031
    platelets, leukocytes reduced, irradiated P9033
    platelets, pheresis P9034
    platelets, pheresis, irradiated P9036
    platelets, pheresis, leukocytes reduced P9035

Blood—*continued*

    platelets, pheresis, leukocytes reduced, irradiated P9037

    pressure monitor A4660, A4663, A4670

    pump, dialysis E1620

    red blood cells, deglycerolized P9039

    red blood cells, irradiated P9038

    red blood cells, leukocytes reduced P9016

    red blood cells, leukocytes reduced, irradiated P9040

    red blood cells, washed P9022

    strips A4253

    supply P9010-P9022

    testing supplies A4770

    tubing A4750, A4755

Blood collection devices accessory A4257, E0620

Body jacket

    lumbar-sacral orthosis (spinal) L0500-L0565, L0600, L0610

    scoliosis L1300, L1310

Body sock L0984

Bond or cement, ostomy skin A4364

Bone mineral density study G0062, G0063

Boot

    pelvic E0944

    surgical, ambulatory L3260

Bortezomib J9041

Botulinum toxin type A J0585

Botulinum toxin type B J0587

Brachytherapy radioelements Q3001

Brachytherapy source A9670

Breast prosthesis L8000-L8035, L8600

Breast prosthesis, adhesive skin support A4280

Breast pump

    accessories A4281-A4286

    electric, any type E0603

    heavy duty, hospital grade E0604

    manual, any type E0602

Breathing circuit A4618

Bridge

    recement D6930

    repair, by report D6980

Brompheniramine maleate. J0945
Budesonide inhalation solution J7626, J7627, J7633
Buprenorphine hydrochloride. J0592
Bus, non-emergency transportation A0110
Butorphanol tartrate. J0595

C

Cabergoline, oral. J8515
Caffeine citrate. J0706
Calcitriol. J0636
Calcitonin-salmon J0630
Calcium disodium edetate. J0600
Calcium gluconate. J0610
Calcium glycerophosphate and calcium lactate J0620
Calcium lactate and calcium glycerophosphate J0620
Calcium leucovorin J0640
Calibrator solution A4256
Cane E0100, E0105
        accessory A4636, A4637
Canister, disposable, used with suction pump A7000
Canister, non-disposable, used with suction pump A7001
Cannula, nasal. A4615
Capecitabine, oral J8520, J8521
Carbon filter A4680
Carboplatin J9045
Cardia Event, recorder, implantable E0616
Cardiokymography Q0035
Cardiovascular services M0300-M0302
Carmustine J9050
Caries susceptibility test D0425
Case management T1016, T1017
Caspofungin acetate. J0637
Cast
        diagnostic, dental D0470
        hand restoration. L6900-L6915
        materials, special A4590
        plaster. L2102, L2122

Cast—*continued*

supplies A4580, A4590, Q4001-Q4051

synthetic L2104, L2124

thermoplastic L2106, L2126

Caster, front, for power wheelchair K0099

Caster, wheelchair E0997, E0998

Catheter A4300-A4365

anchoring device A5200, A4333, A4334

cap, disposable (dialysis) A4860

external collection device . A4327-A4330, A4347, K0410, K0411

implanted A7042, A7043

indwelling A4338-A4346

indwelling, insertion of G0002

insertion tray A4354

intermittent with insertion supplics A4353

irrigation supplies A4355, K0409

male external A4324, A4325, A4348

oropharyngeal suction A4628

starter set A4329

trachea (suction) A4609, A4610, A4624

transtracheal oxygen A4608

Catheterization, specimen collection P9612, P9615

Ccfazolin sodium J0690

Cefepime HCL J0692

Cefotaxime sodium J0698

Ceftazidime J0713

Ceftizoxime sodium J0715

Ceftriaxone sodium J0696

Cefuroxime sodium J0697

CellCept K0412

Cellular therapy M0075

Cement, ostomy A4364

Centrifuge A4650

Cephalin flocculation, blood P2028

Cephalothin sodium J1890

Cephapirin sodium J0710

Cervical

halo L0810-L0830

head harness/halter E0942

Cervical—*continued*

   orthosis L0100-L0200

   pillow E0943

   traction E0855

Cervical cap contraceptive A4261

Cervical-thoracic-lumbar-sacral orthosis (CTLSO) L0700, L0710

Cetuximab J9055

Chair

   adjustable, dialysis E1570

   commode with seat lift E0169

   lift E0627

   rollabout E1031

   sitz bath E0160-E0162

Chelation therapy M0300

Chemical endarterectomy M0300

Chemistry and toxicology tests P2028-P3001

Chemotherapy

   administration (hospital reporting only) Q0083-Q0085

   drug, oral, not otherwise classified J8999

   drugs (see also drug by name) J9000-J9999

Chest shell (cuirass) E0457

Chest Wall Oscillation System E0483

   hose, replacement A7026

   vest, replacement A7025

Chest wrap E0459

Chin cup, cervical L0150

Chin strap (for positive airway pressure device) K0186

Chloramphenicol sodium succinate J0720

Chlordiazepoxide HCL J1990

Chloromycetin Sodium Succinate J0720

Chloroprocaine HCL J2400

Chloroquine HCL J0390

Chlorothiazide sodium J1205

Chlorpromazine HCL J3230

Chorionic gonadotropin J0725

Chromic phosphate P32 suspension A9564

Chromium CR-51 sodium chromate A9553

Cidofovir J0740

Cilastatin sodium, imipenem J0743

Ciprofloxacin, for intravenous infusion J0744
Cisplatin J9060, J9062
Cladribine J9065
Clamp
    dialysis A4910, A4918, A4920
    external urethral A4356
Cleanser, wound A6260
Cleansing agent, dialysis equipment. A4790
Clofarabine J9027
Clonidine J0735
Clotting time tube A4771
Clubfoot wedge L3380
Cochlear prosthetic implant L8614
    accessories L8615-L8617
    batteries L8620-L8622
    replacement L8619
Codeine phosphate J0745
Colchicine J0760
Colistimethate sodium J0770
Collagen
    skin test G0025
    urinary tract implant L8603
    wound dressing. A6020-A6024
Collar, cervical
    multiple post. L0180-L0200
    nonadjust (foam). L0120
Collection device for nebulizer K0177
Coly-Mycin M J0770
Comfort items. A9190
Commode E0160-E0175
    chair E0170-E0171
    lift E0625, E0172
    pail. E0167
    seat, wheelchair E0968
Composite dressing. A6200-A6205
Compressed gas system E0424-E0480, L3902
Compression bandage A4460
Compression burn garment. A6501-A6512
Compression stockings A6530-A6549

Compressor E0565, E0570, E0571, E0572, E0650-E0652, E1375
    filter, aerosol K0178-K0179
Concentrator, oxygen. E1377-E1385
Conductivity meter, bath, dialysis E1550
Congo red, blood P2029
Contact layer. A6206-A6208
Contact lens V2500-V2599
Continent device A5081, A5082
Continuous positive airway pressure (CPAP) device E0601
    compressor K0269
    intermittent assist E0452
    nasal application accessories K0184
Contraceptive
    cervical cap A4261
    condoms. A4267, A4268
    diaphragm A4266
    intrauterine, copper. J7300
    intrauterine, levonorgestrel releasing. J7302
    levonorgestrel, implants and supplies A4260
    patch. J7304
    spermicide. A4269
    vaginal ring J7303
Contracts, maintenance, ESRD A4890
Contrast material
    injection during MRI. A4643
    low osmolar. A4644-A4646
Corneal tissue processing. V2785
Corrugated tubing, used with nebulizer K0175, K0176
Corset, spinal orthosis L0970-L0976
Corticorelin ovine triflutate J0795
Corticotropin J0800
Corvert, see Ibutilide fumarate
Cosyntropin J0835
Cough stimulating device. E0482
Counseling for control of dental disease D1310, D1320
Cover, wound
    alginate dressing. A6196-A6198
    collagen dressing A6020
    foam dressing. A6209-A6214

Cover, wound—*continued*

  hydrocolloid dressing. K0234-K0239

  hydrogel dressing A0242-A0248

  non-contact wound warming cover, and accessory
  . . . . A6000, E0231, E0232

  specialty absorptive dressing A6251-A6256

CPAP (continuous positive airway pressure) device. E0601

  chin strap K0186

  compressor K0269

  filter K0188, K0189

  headgear. K0185

  humidifier A7046, K0193, K0268

  intermittent assist E0452, K0194

  nasal application accessories. K0183, K0184

  tubing. K0187

Cradle, bed. E0280

Crib. E0300

Cromolyn sodium, inhalation solution, unit dose. J7631

Crowns. D2710-D2810, D2930-D2933, D4249, D6720-D6792

Crutches E0110-E0118

  accessories A4635-A4637, K0102

Cryoprecipitate, each unit. P9012

CTLSO L1000-L1120, L0700, L0710

Cuirass. E0457

Culture sensitivity study. P7001

Cushion, wheelchair E0962-E0965, E0977

Cyanocobalamin Cobalt C057 . . . . A9559

Cycler dialysis machine. E1594

Cyclophosphamide J9070-J9092

Cyclophosphamide, lyophilized J9093-J9097

Cyclophosphamide, oral J8530

Cyclosporine. J7502, J7515, J7516

Cylinder tank carrier. K0104

Cytarabine. J9110

Cytarabine liposome J9098

Cytomegalovirus immune globulin (human) J0850

D

Dacarbazine J9130, J9140
Daclizumab J7513
Dactinomycin J9120
Dalalone J1100
Dalteparin sodium J1645
Daptomycin J0878
Darbepoetin Alfa J0881-J0882
Daunorubicin Citrate J9151
Daunorubicin HCL J9150
DaunoXome, see Daunorubicin citrate
Decubitus care equipment E0176-E0199
Deferoxamine mesylate J0895
Defibrillator, external E0617, K0606
    battery K0607
    electrode K0609
    garment K0608
Deionizer, water purification system E1615
Delivery/set-up/dispensing A9901
Denileukin diftitox J9160
Dental procedures
    adjunctive general services D9000-D9999
    alveoloplasty D7310-D7320
    analgesia D9230
    diagnostic D0100-D0999
    endodontics D3000-D3999
    implant services D6000-D6199
    maxillofacial D5900-D5999
    orthodontics D8000-D8999
    periodontics D4000-D4999
    preventive D1000-D1999
    prosthodontics, fixed D6200-D6999
    prosthodontics, removable D5000-D5999
    restorative D2000-D2999
Dentures D5110-D5899
Depo-estradiol cypionate J1000
Desmopressin acetate J2597

Detector, blood leak, dialysis E1560
Device, water collection (for nebulizer) K0177
Dexamethasone acetate. J1094
Dexamethasone, inhalation solution, concentrated J7637
Dexamethasone, inhalation solution, unit dose J7638
Dexamethasone, oral J8540
Dexamethasone sodium phosphate J1100
Dextran. J7100
Dextrose
    saline (normal) J7042
    water J7060, J7070
Dextrostick. A4772
Diagnostic
    dental services D0100-D0999
    radiology services R0070-R5999
Dialysate concentrate additives A4765
Dialysate solution A4700, A4705, A4728
Dialysate testing solution. A4760
Dialysis
    air bubble detector. E1530
    bath conductivity, meter E1550
    chemicals/antiseptics solution A4674
    continuous ambulatory peritoneal dialysis (CAPD) supply kit
    . . . . A4900
    continuous cycling peritoneal dialysis (CCPD) supply kit . A4901
    disposable cycler set A4671
    equipment E1510-E1702
    extension line. A4672-A4673
    filter. A4680
    fluid barrier E1575
    forceps A4910
    kit. A4820, A4914
    measuring cylinder A4921
    pressure alarm E1540
    shunt A4740
    supplies. A4650-A4927
    thermometer. A4910
    tourniquet A4910
    unipuncture control system E1580

Dialysis—*continued*

venous pressure clamp A4918
Dialyzer A4690
  holder A4919
Diaper T1500, T4521-T4540
Diaper, adult incontinence garment A4520
Diazepam J3360
Diazoxide J1730
Dicyclomine HCL J0500
Diethylstilbestrol diphosphate J9165
Digoxin J1160
Digoxin immune fab (ovine) J1162
Dihydroergotamine mesylate J1110
Dimenhydrinate J1240
Dimercaprol J0470
Dimethyl sulfoxide (DMSO) J1212
Diphenhydramine HCL J1200
Dipyridamole J1245
Disarticulation
  lower extremities, prosthesis L5000-L5999
  upper extremities, prosthesis L6000-L6692
Disposable supplies, ambulance A0382, A0384, A0392- A0398
Distilled water (for nebulizer) K0182
DMSO J1212
Dobutamine HCL J1250
Docetaxel J9170
Dolasetron mesylate J1260
Dome and mouthpiece (for nebulizer) A7016
Dopamine HCL J1265
Dornase alpha, inhalation solution, unit dose form J7639
Doxercalciferol J1270
Doxil J9001
Doxorubicin HCL J9000, J9001
Drainage
  bag A4347, A4357, A4358
  board, postural E0606
  bottle A5102
Dressing (see also Bandage) A6020-A6406
  alginate A6196-A6199

Dressing—*continued*

collagen A6020-A6024

composite A6200-A6205

contact layer A6206-A6208

foam. A6209-A6215

gauze A6216-A6230, A6402-A6406

holder/binder A4462

hydrocolloid. A6234-A6241

hydrogel A6242-A6248

specialty absorptive A6251-A6256

tape. A4454, A6265

transparent film. A6257-A6259

tubular A6457

Droperidol. J1790

and fentanyl citrate. J1810

Dropper. A4649

Drugs (see also Table of Drugs)

administered through a metered dose inhaler J3535

chemotherapy J8500-J9999

dispensing fee for DME drugs. E0590

disposable delivery system, 5 ml or less per hour A4306

disposable delivery system, 50 ml or greater per hour . . . A4305

immunosuppressive J7500-J7599

infusion supplies A4230-A4232, A4221, A4222

inhalation solutions J7608-J7699

not otherwise classified J3490, J7599, J7699, J7799, J8499,

. . . . J8999, J9999

prescription, oral. J8499, J8999

Dry pressure pad/mattress E0179, E0184, E0199

Durable medical equipment (DME). . . . . E0100-E1830, K Codes

Duraclon, see Clonidine

Dyphylline. J1180

E

Ear mold V5264

Echocardiography injectable contrast material A9700

Edetate calcium disodium. J0600

Edetate disodium J3520
Egg crate dry pressure pad/mattress E0179, E0184, E0199
Elastic
    bandage A4460
    gauze. A6263, A6405
Elbow
    disarticulation, endoskeletal. L6450
    orthosis (EO) E1800, L3700-L3740, L3760
    protector E0191
Electrical work, dialysis equipment A4870
Electrocardiogram strips,
    monitoring. G0004-G0007
    physician interpretation G0016
    tracing G0015
    transmission G0015, G0016
Electrodes, per pair A4556
Elevating leg rest. K0195
Elliott's b solution. J9175
EMG. E0746
Eminase J0350
Endarterectomy, chemical M0300
Endodontic procedures D3000-D3999
    periapical services. D3410-D3470
    pulp capping. D3110, D3120
    root canal therapy D3310-D3353
Endoscope sheath. A4270
Endoskeletal system, addition L5848, L5856-L5857, L5925
Enoxaparin sodium J1650
Enteral
    feeding supply kit (syringe) (pump) (gravity) B4034-B4036
    formulae B4149-B4156
    nutrition infusion pump (with alarm) (without). . . B9000, B9002
Epinephrine. J0170
Epirubicin HCL J9178
Epoetin alpha J0885-J0886
Epoprostenol J1325
Ergonovine maleate. J1330
Ertapenem sodium. J1335
Erythromycin lactobionate J1364

ESRD (End Stage Renal Disease; see also Dialysis)

 machines and accessories E1500-E1699

 plumbing. A4870

 supplies. A4651-A4929

Estrogen conjugated. J1410

Estrone (5, Aqueous). J1435

Ethanolamine oleate J1430

Etidronate disodium. J1436

Etoposide. J9181, J9182

Etoposide, oral J8560

Examination, oral. D0120-D0160

Exercise equipment A9300

External

 ambulatory infusion pump E0781, E0784

 power, battery components. L7360-L7499

 power, elbow L7160-L7191

 urinary supplies A4356-A4359

Extractions (see also Dental procedures) D7110-D7130, D7250

Extraoral films D0250, D0260

Extremity belt/harness. E0945

Eye

 case V2756

 lens (contact) (spectacle) V2100-V2615

 pad. A4610-A4612

 prosthetic V2623, V2629

 service (miscellaneous). V2700-V2799

F

Faceplate, ostomy A4361, K0428

Face tent, oxygen. A4619

Factor VIIA coagulation factor, recombinant J7189

Factor VIII, anti-hemophilic factor. J7190-J7192

Factor IX J7193, J7194, J7195

Family Planning Education H1010

Fecal leukocyte examination. G0026

Fentanyl citrate. J3010

Fentanyl citrate and droperidol J1810

Fern test. Q0114
Filgrastim (G-CSF) J1440, J1441
Filler, wound
    alginate dressing. A6199
    foam dressing. A6215
    hydrocolloid dressing A6240, A6241
    hydrogel dressing A6248
    not elsewhere classified. A6261, A6262
Film, transparent (for dressing). A6257-A6259
Filter
    aerosol compressor A7014
    CPAP device. K0188, K0189
    dialysis carbon A4680
    ostomy A4368
    tracheostoma A4481
    ultrasonic generator. A7014
Fistula cannulation set A4730
Flowmeter E0440, E0555, E0580
Floxuridine J9200
Fluconazole, injection J1450
Fludarabine phosphate J9185
Fluid barrier, dialysis E1575
Flunisolide inhalation solution. J7641
Fluoride treatment D1201-D1205
Fluorodeoxyglucose F-18 FDG. A9552
Fluorouracil. J9190
Foam dressing. A6209-A6215
Foam pad adhesive. A5126
Folding walker E0135, E0143
Foley catheter. A4312-A4316, A4338-A4346
Fomepizole J1451
Fomivirsen sodium intraocular. J1452
Fondaparinux sodium. J1652
Footdrop splint L4398
Footplate E0175, E0970, L3031
Footwear, orthopedic. L3201-L3265
Forceps, dialysis A4910
Forearm crutches. E0110, E0111
Formoterol. J7640

Foscarnet sodium J1455
Fosphenytoin. Q2009
Fracture
    bedpan E0276
    frame E0920, E0930, E0946-E0948
    orthosis L2102-L2136, L3980-L3986
    orthotic additions. L2180-L2192, L3995
Fragmin, see Dalteparin sodium
Frames (spectacles) V2020, V2025
Fulvestrant. J9395
Furosemide J1940

G

Gadolinium. A4647
Gait trainer E8000-E8002
Gallium Ga67 . . . . A9556
Gallium nitrate. J1457
Gamma globulin J1460-J1561
Ganciclovir, implant J7310
Ganciclovir sodium J1570
Garamycin. J1580
Gas system
    compressed E0424, E0425
    gaseous E0430, E0431, E0441, E0443
    liquid E0434-E0440, E0442, E0444
Gastrostomy/jejunostomy tubing B4084
Gastrostomy tube. B4085
Gatifloxacin. J1590
Gauze (see also Bandage)
    elastic A6263, A6405
    impregnated A6222-A6230, A6231-A6233, A6266
    nonelastic. A6264, A6406
    nonimpregnated A6216-A6221, A6402-A6404
Gefitinib J8565
Gel
    conductive. A4558
    pressure pad E0178, E0185, E0196

Gemcitabine HCL J9201
Gemtuzumab ozogamicin J9300
Generator
    implantable neurostimulator E0751
    ultrasonic with nebulizer E0574
Gentamicin (Sulfate) J1580
Gingival procedures D4210-D4240
Glasses
    air conduction V5070
    binaural V5120-V5150
    bone conduction V5080
    frames V2020, V2025
    hearing aid V5230
Glatiramer acetate Q2010
Gloves A4927
Glucagon HCL J1610
Glucose monitor with integrated lancing/blood sample collection
. . . . E2101
Glucose monitor with integrated voice synthesizer E2100
Glucose test strips A4253, A4772
Gluteal pad L2650
Glycopyrrolate, inhalation solution, concentrated J7642
Glycopyrrolate, inhalation solution, unit dose J7643
Gold foil dental restoration D2410-D2430
Gold sodium thiomalate J1600
Gomco drain bottle A4912
Gonadorelin HCL J1620
Goserelin acetate implant (see also Implant) J9202
Grab bar, trapeze E0910, E0940
Grade-aid, wheelchair E0974
Granisetron HCL J1626
Gravity traction device E0941
Gravlee jet washer A4470

H

Hair analysis (excluding arsenic) P2031
Hallus-Valgus dynamic splint L3100

Hallux prosthetic implant. L8642
Haloperidol J1630
    decanoate J1631
Halo procedures L0810-L0860
Halter, cervical head. E0942
Hand finger orthosis, prefabricated. L3923
Hand restoration. L6900-L6915
    partial prosthesis L6000-L6020
    orthosis (WHFO). . . E1805, E1825, L3800-L3805, L3900-L3954
    rims, wheelchair E0967
Handgrip (cane, crutch, walker) A4636
Harness. E0942, E0944, E0945
Harvard pressure clamp, dialysis. A4920
Headgear (for positive airway pressure device) K0185
Hearing devices. V5000-V5299, L8614
Heat
    application E0200-E0239
    lamp. E0200, E0205
    infrared heating pad system A4639, E0221
    pad E0210, E0215, E0237, E0238, E0249
Heater (nebulizer). E1372
Heel
    elevator, air E0370
    protector E0191
    shoe L3430-L3485
    stabilizer L3170
Helicopter, ambulance (see also Ambulance)
Helmet, cervical L0100, L0110
Helmet, head. E0701
Hemin J1640
Hemi-wheelchair. E1083-E1086
Hemipelvectomy prosthesis L5280, L5340
Hemodialysis
    kit A4820
    machine. E1590
Hemodialyzer, portable E1635
Hemofil M J7190
Hemoglobin Q0116
Hemophilia clotting factor J7190-J7198

Hemophilia clotting factor, NOC J7199
Hemostats. A4850
Hemostix A4773
Heparin infusion pump, dialysis E1520
Heparin lock flush J1642
Heparin sodium A4800, J1644
Hepatitis B vaccine Q3021-Q3023
Hep-Lock (U/P) J1642
Hexalite A4590
High osmolar contrast material Q9958-Q9964
Hip
      disarticulation prosthesis L5250, L5270, L5330
      orthosis (HO) L1600-L1690
Hip-knee-ankle-foot orthosis (HKAFO) L2040-L2090
Histrelin acetate J1675
Histrelin implant. J9225
HKAFO L2040-L2090
Home Health Agency Services T0221
Hot water bottle. E0220
Humidifier A7046, E0550-E0563
Hyaluronate, sodium J7317
Hyaluronidase J3470
Hyaluronidase, ovine. J3471-J3472
Hydralazine HCL J0360
Hydraulic patient lift. E0630
Hydrocollator E0225, E0239
Hydrocolloid dressing A6234-A6241
Hydrocortisone
      acetate J1700
      sodium phosphate. J1710
      sodium succinate J1720
Hydrogel dressing A6242-A6248, A6231-A6233
Hydromorphone J1170
Hydroxyzine HCL. J3410
Hylan G-F 20. . . . . J7320
Hyoscyamine Sulfate J1980
Hyperbaric oxygen chamber, topical A4575
Hypertonic saline solution. J7130

I

Ibutilide Fumarate. J1742
Ice
    cap. E0230
    collar E0230
Idarubicin HCL J9211
Ifosfamide. J9208
Imiglucerase. J1785
Immune globulin intravenous J1566-J1567
Immunosuppressive drug, not otherwise classified J7599
Implant
    access system. A4301
    aqueous shunt. L8612
    breast L8600
    cochlear L8614, L8619
    collagen, urinary tract L8603
    contraceptive A4260
    ganciclovir J7310
    hallux L8642
    indium III-in Pentetreotide Q3008
    infusion pump, programmable E0783, E0786
    joint. L8630, L8641, L8658
    lacrimal duct. A4262, A4263
    maintenance procedures D6080
    maxillofacial D5913-D5937
    metacarpophalangeal joint. L8630
    metatarsal joint. L8641
    neurostimulator electrode E0752
    neurostimulator pulse generator E0756, L8681-L8688
    neurostimulator radiofrequency receiver E0757
    not otherwise specified. L8699
    ocular L8610
    ossicular L8613
    osteogenesis stimulator. E0749
    percutaneous access system. A4301
    removal, dental. D6100
    repair, dental D6090

Implant—*continued*

    replacement implantable intraspinal catheter E0785

    synthetic, urinary. L8606

    urinary tract. L8603, L8606

    vascular graft L8670

Impregnated gauze dressing. A6222-A6230, K0535-K0537

Incontinence

    appliances and supplies. A4310-A4355, A4356-A4360,

    . . . . A5071-A5075, A5102-A5114, K0280, K0281

    products A4521-A4538

    treatment system E0740

Indium in-111

    carpromab pendetide A9507

    ibritumomab tiuxetan. A9542

    oxyquinoline A9547

    pentetate A9548

    pentetreotide A9565

    satumomab A4642

Indwelling catheter insertion G0002

Infliximab injection. J1745

Infusion pump

    ambulatory, with administrative equipment,. E0781

    heparin, dialysis E1520

    implantable E0782, E0783

    implantable, refill kit. A4220

    insulin. E0784

    mechanical, reusable E0779, E0780

    uninterrupted infusion of Epiprostenol. K0455

Infusion supplies A4221, A4222, A4230-A4232

Infusion therapy, other than chemotherapeutic drugs Q0081

Inhalation solution (see also drug name). J7608-J7699

Injections (see also drug name). J0120-J7320

    contrast material, during MRI A4643

    dental service D9610, D9630

    supplies for self-administered A4211

Inlay/onlay dental restoration D2510-D2664

Insertion, indwelling catheter G0002

Insertion tray. A4310-A4316

Insulin. J1815, J1817

Insulin lispro. K0548
Interferon
    Alpha J9212-J9215
    Beta-1 a J1825, Q3025-Q3026
    Beta- 1 b J1830
    Gamma J9216
Intermittent
    assist device with continuous positive airway pressure device
    . . . . E0470-E0472
    peritoneal dialysis system E1592
    positive pressure breathing (IPPB) machine E0500
Interphalangeal joint, prosthetic implant L8658, L8659
Interscapular thoracic prosthesis
    endoskeletal L6570
    upper limb L6350-L6370
Intraconazole J1835
Intraocular lenses. V2630-V2632
Intraoral radiographs, dental. D0210-D0240
Intrapulmonary percussive ventilation system. E0481
Intrauterine copper contraceptive J7300
Iodine Iobenguane sulfate I-131 . . . . A9508
Iodine I-123 sodium iodide. A9516, A9517
Iodine I-125 serum albumin. A9532
Iodine I-125 sodium iothalamate. A9554
Iodine I-131 iodinated serum albumin A9524
Iodine I-131 sodium iodide capsule. A9528
Iodine I-131 sodium iodide solution. A9529-A9531
Iodine I-131 tositumomab A9544-A9545
Iodine swabs/wipes. A4247
IPD
    supply kit A4905
    system. E1592
IPPB machine E0500
Ipratropium bromide, inhalation solution, unit dose J7644
Irinotecan J9206
Iron Dextran. J1751, J1752
Iron sucrose. J1756

Irrigation/evacuation system, bowel
    control unit E0350
    disposable supplies for E0352
Irrigation solution for bladder calculi. Q2004
Irrigation supplies A4320-A4323, A4355, A4397-A4400
Isoetharine HCL, inhalation solution, concentrated. J7648
Isoetharine HCL, inhalation solution, unit dose. J7649
Isolates B4150, B4152
Isoproterenol HCL, inhalation solution, concentrated J7658
Isoproterenol HCL, inhalation solution, unit dose J7659
IV pole, each E0776, K0105

J

Jacket
    body (LSO) (spinal), ... L0500-L0565
    scoliosis, ... L1300, L1310
Jenamicin, ... J1580
Joint supportive device/garment, ... A4464

K

Kanamycin sulfate. J1840, J1850
Kartop patient lift, toilet or bathroom (see also Lift). E0625
Ketorolac thomethamine. J1885
Kidney
    ESRD supply A4650-A4927
    system. E1510
    wearable artificial E1632
Kits
    continuous ambulatory peritoneal dialysis (CAPD) A4900
    continuous cycling peritoneal dialysis (CCPD) A4901
    dialysis. A4910
    enteral feeding supply (syringe) (pump) (gravity). . B4034-B4036
    fistula cannulation (set) A4730
    intermittent peritoneal dialysis (IPD) supply. A4905
    parenteral nutrition. B4220-B4224
    surgical dressing (tray). A4550

Kits—*continued*

    tracheostomy A4625

Knee

    disarticulation, prosthesis L5150, L5160

    joint, miniature L5826

    orthosis (KO) E1810, L1800-L1885

Knee-ankle-foot orthosis (KAFO). L2000-L2039, L2126-L2136

Knee-ankle-foot orthosis (KAFO) addition, high strength,
    lightweight material. L2755

Kutapressin J1910

Kyphosis pad L1020, L1025

L

Laboratory tests

    chemistry P2028-P2038

    microbiology P7001

    miscellaneous P9010-P9615, Q0111-Q0115

    toxicology P3000-P3001, Q0091

    permanent A4263

    temporary A4262

Lactated Ringer's infusion J7120

Laetrile J3570

Lancet. A4258, A4259

Laronidase. J1931

Larynx, artificial L8500

Laser blood collection device and accessory E0620, A4257

Lead investigation T1029

Lead wires, per pair. A4557

Leg

    bag. A4358, A5105, A5112

    extensions for walker. E0158

    rest, elevating. K0195

    rest, wheelchair. E0990

    strap, replacement A5113-A5114

Legg Perthes orthosis L1700-L1755

Lens

    aniseikonic V2118, V2318

    contact V2500-V2599

Lens—*continued*

    eye V2100-V2615, V2700-V2799

    intraocular V2630-V2632

    low vision V2600-V2615

    progressive V2781

Lepirudin J1945

Leucovorin calcium J0640

Leukocyte examination, fecal G0026

Leukocyte poor blood, each unit P9016

Leuprolide acetate J9217, J9218, J9219, J1950

Levalbuterol, all formulations, inhalation solution J7617

Levalbuterol, all formulations, inhalation solution, concentrated . J7612

Levalbuterol, all formulations, inhalation solution, unit dose . . . J7614

Levocarnitine J1955

Levofloxacin J1956

Levonorgestrel, (contraceptive), implants and supplies J7306

Levorphanol tartrate. J1960

Lidocaine HCL. J2001

Lift

    patient (includes seat lift) E0621-E0635

    shoe L3300-L3334

Lincomycin HCL J2010

Linezolid. J2020

Liquid barrier, ostomy A4363

Lodging, recipient, escort non-emergency transport . . . A0180, A0200

Lorazepam. J2060

Low osmolar contrast material Q9945-Q9951

LSO. L0621-L0640

Lubricant. A4402, A4332

Lumbar flexion L0540

Lumbar-sacral orthosis (LSO) L0621-L0640

Lymphocyte immune globulin J7504, J7511

M

Magnesium sulphate J3475

Maintenance contract, ESRD A4890

Manipulation of spine, chiropractic A2000

Mannitol J2150
Mask
    aerosol K0180
    oxygen. A4620, A4621
Mastectomy
    bra. L8000
    form. L8020
    prosthesis L8030, L8600
    sleeve L8010
Mattress
    air pressure E0186
    alternating pressure E0277
    dry pressure. E0184
    gel pressure E0196
    hospital bed. E0271, E0272
    non-powered, pressure reducing E0373
    overlay. E0371-E0372
    powered, pressure reducing E0277
    water pressure E0187
Measuring cylinder, dialysis. A4921
Mechlorethamine HCL. J9230
Medical and surgical supplies. A4206-A8999
Medroxyprogesterone acetate. J1051, J1055
Medroxyprogesterone acetate/estradiol cypionate J1056
Melphalan HCL J9245
Melphalan, oral J8600
Meperidine J2175
Meperidine and promethazine J2180
Mepivacaine HCL. J0670
Meropenem. J2185
Mesna. J9209
Metabolically active tissue. Q0184
Metabolically active D/E tissue. Q0185
Metacarpophalangeal joint, prosthetic implant L8630, L8631
Metaproterenol sulfate, inhalation solution, concentrated. J7668
Metaproterenol sulfate, inhalation solution, unit dose J7669
Metaraminol bitartrate J0380
Metatarsal joint, prosthetic implant L8641
Meter, bath conductivity, dialysis. E1550

Methacholine chloride J7674
Methadone HCL. J1230
Methocarbamol. J2800
Methotrexate, oral J8610
Methotrexate sodium J9250, J9260
Methyldopate HCL J0210
Methylene blue A9535
Methylergonovine maleate J2210
Methylprednisolone
    acetate. J1020-J1040
    oral J7509
    sodium succinate J2920, J2930
Metoclopramide HCL J2765
Microbiology test P7001
Midazolam HCL. J2250
Mileage, ambulance A0380, A0390
Mini-bus, non-emergency transportation A0120
Milrinone lactate. J2260
Mitomycin J9280-J9291
Mitoxantrone HCL J9293
Modalities, with office visit. M0005-M0008
Moisture exchanger for use with invasive mechanical
    ventilation. A4483
Moisturizer, skin A6250
Monitor
    apnea E0608
    blood glucose. E0607, E0609
    blood pressure A4670
    pacemaker E0610, E0615
Monitoring and recording, EKG G0004-G0007
Monoclonal antibodies J7505
Mononine. Q0160
Morphine sulfate. J2270, J2271
    sterile, preservative-free. J2275
Mouthpiece (for respiratory equipment) A4617
    and dome (for nebulizer) K0181
Moxifloxacin J2280
MRI contrast material. A4643
Mucoprotein, blood. P2038

Multiaxial ankle. L5986
Multidisciplinary services. H2000-H2001, T1023-T1028
Multiple post collar, cervical. L0180-L0200
Multi-Podus type AFO L4396
Muromonab-CD3 . . . . J7505
Mycophenolate mofetil. J7517
Mycophenolic acid J7518

N

Nalbuphine HCL. J2300
Naloxone HCL. J2310
Nandrolone decanoate J2320-J2322
Narrowing device, wheelchair. E0969
Nasal application device K0183
Nasal pillows/seals (for nasal application device) K0184
Nasal vaccine inhalation. J3530
Nasogastric tubing. B4081, B4082
Natalizumab Q4079
Nebulizer E0570-E0585
        aerosol compressor E0571
        aerosol mask A7015
        corrugated tubing, disposable. A7010
        corrugated tubing, non-disposable. A7011
        distilled water K0182
        drug dispensing fee E0590
        filter, disposable A7013
        filter, non-disposable A7014
        heater E1372
        large volume, disposable, pre-filled. A7008
        large volume, disposable, unfilled. A7007
        not used with oxygen, durable, glass A7017
        pneumatic, administration set A7003, A7005, A7006
        pneumatic, non-filtered. A7004
        portable. E0570
        small volume A7003-A7005
        ultrasonic. E0575
        ultrasonic, dome and mouthpiece A7016

Nebulizer—*continued*

    ultrasonic, reservoir bottle, non-disposable A7009

    water collection device, large volume nebulizer. A7012

Needle. A4215

    dialysis. A4655

    non-coring. A4212

    with syringe. A4206-A4209

Negative pressure wound therapy pump E2402

    accessories. A6550

Neonatal transport, ambulance, base rate A0225

Neostigmine methylsulfate J2710

Nerve stimulator with batteries E0765

Nesiritide injection J2324

Neuromuscular stimulator E0745

Neurostimulator

    electrodes E0753

    programmer E0754

    pulse generator E0756, L8681-L8688

    receiver. E0757

    transmitter E0758

Nitrogen N-13 ammonia A9526

Nonchemotherapy drug, oral, NOS. J8499

Noncovered services. A9270

Nonelastic gauze. A6264, A6406

Non-emergency transportation. A0080-A0210

Nonimpregnated gauze dressing A6216-A6221, A6402-A6404

Nonmetabolic active tissue. Q0183

Nonprescription drug A9150

Not otherwise classified drug

    . . . . . . J3490, J7599, J7699, J7799, J8499, J8999, J9999, Q0181

NPH. J1820

NTIOL category 1 . . . . Q1001

NTIOL category 2 . . . . Q1002

NTIOL category 3 . . . . Q1003

NTIOL category 4 . . . . Q1004

NTIOL category 5 . . . . Q1005

Nursing care T1030-T1031

Nutrition

    counseling, dental. D1310, D1320

Nutrition—*continued*
    enteral infusion pump B9000, B9002
    parenteral infusion pump B9004, B9006
    parenteral solution B4164-B5200

O

Obturator prosthesis
    definitive. D5932
    interim D5936
    surgical. D5931
Occipital/mandibular support, cervical L0160
Octafluoropropane Q9956
Octreotide acetate J2353, J2354
Ocular prosthetic implant. L8610
Omalizumab. J2357
Ondansetron HCL. J2405
One arm, drive attachment. K0101
Oprelvekin. J2355
O & P supply/accessory/service L9900
Oral and maxillofacial surgery D7000-D7999
Oral device/appliance. E0485-E0486
Oral examination D0120-D0160
Oropharyngeal suction catheter. A4628
Orphenadrine J2360
Orthodontics D8000-D8999
Orthopedic shoes
    arch support L3040-L3100
    footwear L3201-L3265
    insert. L3000-L3030
    lift L3300-L3334
    miscellaneous additions. L3500-L3595
    positioning device L3140-L3170
    transfer L3600-L3649
    wedge L3340-L3420
Orthotic additions
    carbon graphite lamination L2755
    fracture L2180-L2192, L3995

Orthotic additions—*continued*

halo L0860

lower extremity L2200-L2999, L4320

ratchet lock L2430

scoliosis L1010-L1120, L1210-L1290

shoe L3300-L3595, L3649

spinal L0970-L0984

upper extremity joint L3956

upper limb L3810-L3890, L3970-L3974, L3995

Orthotic devices

ankle-foot (AFO; see also Orthopedic shoes)

. . . . E1815, E1816, E1830,

. . . . L1900-L1990, L2102-L2116, L3160

anterior-posterior L0320, L0330, L0530

anterior-posterior-lateral . . . L0520, L0550-L0565, L0700, L0710

anterior-posterior-lateral-rotary L0340-L0440

cervical L0100-L0200

cervical-thoracic-lumbar-sacral (CTLSO) L0700, L0710

elbow (EO) E1800, E1801, L3700-L3740

fracture L2102-L2136, L3980-L3986

halo L0810-L0830

hand, finger, prefabricated L3923

hand, (WHFO)

. . . . . . E1805, E1825, L3800, L3805, L3807, L3900-L3954

hip (HO) L1600-L1690

hip-knee-ankle-foot (HKAFO) L2040-L2090

interface material E1820

knee (KO) E1810, E1811, L1800-L1885

knee-ankle-foot (KAFO; see also Orthopedic shoes)

. . . . L2000-L2038, L2122-L2136

Legg Perthes L1700-L1755

lumbar flexion L0540

lumbar-sacral (LSO) L0500-L0565

multiple post collar L0180-L0200

not otherwise specified . . . L0999, L1499, L2999, L3999, L5999,

. . . . L7499, L8039, L8239

pneumatic splint L4350-L4380

pronation/supination E1818

repair or replacement L4000-L4210

Orthotic devices—*continued*

    replace soft interface material. L4390-L4394

    sacroiliac L0600-L0620

    scoliosis. . . . . L1000 - L1499

    shoe, see Orthopedic shoes

    shoulder (SO). L1840, L3650-L3677

    shoulder-elbow-wrist-hand (SEWHO). L3960-L3978

    side bar disconnect L2768

    spinal, cervical L0100-L0200

    spinal, DME. K0112-K0116

    thoracic. L0210

    thoracic-hip-knee-ankle (THKO) L1500-L1520

    thoracic-lumbar-sacral (TLSO) L0300-L0440

    toe E1830

    torso supports L0900-L0960

    wrist-hand-finger (WHFO) E1805, E1806, E1825, L3800,

    . . . . L3805, L3900-L3954

Ossicula prosthetic implant. L8613

Osteogenesis stimulator E0747-E0749, E0760

Osteotomy, segmented or subapical D7944

Ostomy

    accessories. A5093

    belt A4396

    pouches. A4416-A4434

    skin barrier A4401-A4449

    supplies A4361-A4421, A5051-A5149

Oxacillin sodium. J2700

Oxaliplatin. J9263

Oximeter devices. E0454, A4609

Oxygen

    ambulance A0422

    catheter, transtracheal. A7018

    chamber, hyperbaric, topical A4575

    concentrator E1390-E1391

    mask A4620, A4621

    medication supplies A4611-A4627

    rack/stand E1355

    regulator E1353

    respiratory equipment/supplies A4611-A4627, E0424-E0480

Oxygen—*continued*

    supplies and equipment. E0425-E0444, E0455

    tent. E0455

    tubing. A4616

    water vapor enriching system E1405, E1406

Oxymorphone HCL. J2410

Oxytetracycline HCL. J2460

Oxytocin. J2590

P

Pacemaker monitor. E0610, E0615

Paclitaxel. J9265

Paclitaxel protein-bound particles. J9264

Pad

    gel pressure. E0178, E0185, E0196

    heat. E0210, E0215, E0217, E0238, E0249

    orthotic device interface E1820

    sheepskin E0188, E0189

    water circulating cold with pump E0218

    water circulating heat with pump E0217

    water circulating heat unit. E0249

    wheelchair, low pressure & positioning E0192

Pail, for use with commode chair E0167

Palate, prosthetic implant. L8618

Palifermin J2425

Palonosetron HCL. J2469

Pamidronate disodium J2430

Pan, for use with commode chair E0167

Papanicolaou (Pap) screening smear P3000, P3001, Q0091

Papaverine HCL. J2440

Paraffin A4265

Paraffin bath unit E0235

Paramagnetic contrast material, (Gadolinium) A4647

Paramedic intercept, rural Q0186

Parenteral nutrition

    administration kit B4224

    pump B9004, B9006

Parenteral nutrition—*continued*
  solution B4164-B5200
  supply kit B4220, B4222
Paricalcitol. J2501
Parking fee, non-emergency transport. A0170
Paste, conductive A4558
Patella, prosthetic implant L8640
Pathology and laboratory tests, miscellaneous P9010-P9615
Patient support system. E0636
PEFR, peak expiratory flow rate meter. A4614
Pegademase bovine J2504
Pegaptanib. J2503
Pegaspargase J9266
Pegfilgrastim J2505
Pelvic belt/harness/boot E0944
Pemetrexed J9305
Penicillin
    G benzathine/G benzathine and penicillin G procaine
        . . . . J0530-J0580
    G potassium J2540
    G procaine, aqueous. J2510
Pentamidine isethionate J2545
Pentastarch, 10% solution. J2513
Pentazocine HCL J3070
Pentobarbital sodium J2515
Pentostatin. J9268
Percussor E0480
Percutaneous access system A4301
Perflexane lipid microspheres. Q9955
Perflutren lipid microspheres Q9957
Periapical service. D3410-D3470
Periodontal procedures D4000-D4999
Peroneal strap L0980
Peroxide. A4244
Perphenazine J3310
Personal care services T1019-T1021
Personal comfort item. A9190
Pessary A4561, A4562
PET myocardial perfusion imaging G0030-G0047

Phenobarbital sodium. J2560
Phentolamine mesylate. J2760
Phenylephrine HCL. J2370
Phenytoin sodium J1165
Phisohex solution. A4246
Photofrin, see Porfimer sodium
Phototherapy light E0202
Phytonadione J3430
Pillow, cervical E0943
Pin retention (per tooth) D2951
Pinworm examination Q0113
Plasma
    protein fraction P9018
    single donor, fresh frozen P9017
    multiple donor, pooled, frozen P9023
Plastazote. L3002, L3252, L3253, L3265, L5654-L5658
Platelet
    concentrate, each unit. P9019
    rich plasma, each unit P9020
Platform attachment
    forearm crutch E0153
    walker. E0154
Plicamycin. J9270
Plumbing, for home ESRD equipment A4870
Pneumatic
    appliance E0655-E0673, L4350-L4380
    compressor. E0650-E0652
    splint. L4350-L4380
    tire, wheelchair. E0953
    ventricular assist device Q0480-Q0505
Pneumatic nebulizer
    administration set, small volume, filtered. A7006
    administration set, small volume, non-filtered. A7003
    administration set, small volume, non-filtered,
        non-disposable A7005
    small volume, disposable A7004
Pontics D6210-D6252
Porfimer J9600

Portable

    equipment transfer R0070-R0076

    hemodialyzer system E1635

    nebulizer E1375

    x-ray equipment Q0092

Positioning seat T5001

Positive airway pressure device, accessories A7030-A7039,

    . . . . E0561-E0562

Positive expiratory pressure device. E0484

Post-coital examination Q0115

Post-voiding residual, ultrasound. G0050

Postural drainage board E0606

Potassium chloride J3480

Potassium hydroxide (KOH) preparation. Q0112

Pouch

    fecal collection. A4330

    ostomy. A4375-A4378, A5051-A5054, A5061-A5065

    urinary A4379-A4383, A5071-A5075

Pralidoxime chloride J2730

Prednisolone

    acetate . . . . , ... J2650

    oral J7506, J7510

Prednisone. J7506

Prefabricated crown D2930-D2933

Preparation kits, dialysis A4914

Preparatory prosthesis L5510-L5595

    chemotherapy J8999

    non-chemotherapy J8499

Pressure

    alarm, dialysis E1540

    pad. A4640, E0176-E0199

    ventilator E0454

Preventive dental procedures. D1000-D1999

Procainamide HCL J2690

Prochlorperazine. J0780

Prolotherapy. M0076

Promazine HCL J2950

Promethazine HCL J2550

Promethazine and meperidine J2180

Propranolol HCL J1800
Prosthesis
    artificial larynx battery/accessory L8505
    auricular D5914
    breast L8000-L8035, L8600
    eye L8610, L8611, V2623-V2629
    fitting L5400-L5460, L6380-L6388
    foot/ankle one piece system. L5979
    hand L6000-L6020, L6025
    implants. L8600-L8690
    larynx L8500
    lower extremity L5700-L5999, L8640-L8642
    mandible L8617
    maxilla L8616
    maxillofacial, provided by a non-physician L8040-L8048
    miscellaneous service. L8499
    obturator. D5931-D5933, D5936
    ocular. V2623-V2629
    repair of L7520, L8049
    socks (shrinker, sheath, stump sock) L8400-L8485
    taxes, orthotic/prosthetic/other L9999
    tracheo-esophageal L8507-L8509
    upper extremity L6000-L6999
    vacuum erection system L7900
    voice amplifier E1904
Prosthetic additions
    lower extremity L5610-L5999
    upper extremity L6600-L7405
Prosthodontic procedure
    fixed. D6200-D6999
    removable D5000-D5899
Protamine sulfate J2720
Protectant, skin A6250
Protector, heel or elbow. E0191
Protirelin. J2725
Pulp capping D3110, D3120
Pulpotomy D3220
    vitality test D0460
Pulse generator E2120

Pump

    alternating pressure pad E0182

    ambulatory infusion E0781

    ambulatory insulin E0784

    blood dialysis E1620

    breast E0602-E0604

    enteral infusion B9000, B9002

    external infusion E0779

    heparin infusion E1520

    implantable infusion E0782, E0783

    implantable infusion, refill kit A4220

    infusion, supplies A4230, A4232, K0110-K0111

    negative pressure wound therapy K0538

    parenteral infusion B9004, B9006

    suction, portable E0600

    suction, supplies K0190-K0192

    water circulating pad E0236

Purification system A4880, E1610, E1615

Pyridoxine HCL J3415

Q

Quad cane E0105

Quinupristin/dalfopristin J2770

R

Rack/stand, oxygen E1355

Radial head, prosthetic implant L8620

Radioelements for brachytherapy Q3001

Radiofrequency transmitter E0758, E0759

Radiograph, dental D0210-D0340

Radiology service R0070-R0076

Radiopharmaceutical diagnostic imaging agent A4641, A4642,

    . . . . A9500-A9507, A9512-A9532, Q3002-Q3004

Radiopharmaceutical, therapeutic A9600, A9605

Rail

    bathtub E0241, E0242, E0246

Rail—*continued*

    bed E0305, E0310

    toilet. E0243

Rasburicase J2783

Reaching/grabbing device A9281

Recement

    crown. D2920

    inlay. D2910

Reciprocating peritoneal dialysis system E1630

Red blood cells P9021, P9022

Reduction pneumoplasty G0061

Regular insulin. J1820

Regulator, oxygen. E1353

Repair

    contract, ESRD. A4890

    durable medical equipment E1340

    maxillofacial prosthesis. L8049

    orthosis L4000-L4130

    prosthetic L7500, L7510, K0285

Replacement

    battery. A4254, A4630, A4631

    components, ESRD machine E1640

    pad (alternating pressure) A4640

    tanks, dialysis. A4880

    tip for cane, crutches, walker A4637

    underarm pad for crutches A4635

Reservoir bottle (for ultrasonic nebulizer) K0174

Resin dental restoration. D2330-D2387

RespiGam, see Respiratory syncytial virus immune globulin

Respiratory

    Heated humidifier used with PAP. K0531

    Invasive assist with backup. K0534

    Noninvasive assist with backup K0533

    Noninvasive assist without backup K0532

Respiratory syncytial virus immune globulin J1565

Restorative dental procedure. D2000-D2999

Restraint, any type E0710

Reteplase. J2993

Rho(D) immune globulin, human J2788, J2790, J2792

Rib belt, thoracic A4572, L0210, L0220
Ringers lactate infusion J7120
Ring, ostomy A4404
Risperidone J2794
Rituximab J9310
Robin-Aids L6000, L6010, L6020, L6855, L6860
Rocking bed E0462
Rollabout chair E1031
Root canal therapy D3310-D3353
Ropivacaine HCL J2795
Rubidium Rb-82 . . . . A9555

S

Sacral nerve stimulation test lead A4290
Sacroiliac orthosis L0600-L0620
Safety belt/pelvic strap, each K0031
Safety equipment E0700
    vest, wheelchair E0980
Saline
    hypertonic J7130
    solution J7030-J7050, A4216-A4218
Samarium SM 153 Lexidronamm A9605
Sandimmune K0418
Sargramostim (GM-CSF) J2820
Scale, dialysis A4910
Scissors, dialysis A4910
Scoliosis L1000-L1499
    additions L1010-L1120, L1210-L1290
Sealant
    skin A6250
    tooth D1351
Seat
    attachment, walker E0156
    insert, wheelchair E0992
    lift (patient) E0621, E0627-E0629
    upholstery, wheelchair E0975
Secobarbital sodium J2860

Secretin. J2850
Semen analysis G0027
Sensitivity study. P7001
Sermorelin acetate Q0515
Serum clotting time tube. A4771
SEWHO L3960-L3974
Sheepskin pad. E0188, E0189
Shoes
    arch support L3040-L3100
    for diabetics. A5500-A5508
    insert. L3000-L3030
    lift L3300-L3334
    miscellaneous additions. L3500-L3595
    orthopedic L3201-L3265
    positioning device L3140-L3170
    transfer L3600-L3649
    wedge L3340-L3485
Shoulder
    disarticulation, prosthetic. L6300-L6320, L6550
    orthosis (SO) L3650-L3675
    spinal, cervical L0100-L0200
    spinal, DME. K0112-K0116
Shoulder-elbow-wrist-hand orthosis (SEWHO) L3960-L3969
Shunt accessory for dialysis. A4740
    aqueous. L8612
Sigmoidoscopy, cancer screening G0104, G0106
Silicate dental restoration. D2210
Sincalide. J2805
Sirolimus. J7520
Sitz bath E0160-E0162
Skin
    barrier, ostomy
      . . . . . . A4362, A4363, A4369-A4374, A4385-A4386, A5120
    bond or cement, ostomy. A4364
    sealant, protectant, moisturizer. A6250
    test, collagen G0025
Sling. A4565
    patient lift. E0621, E0630, E0635
Social worker, non-emergency transport A0160

Sock

    body sock L0984

    prosthetic sock L8420-L8435, L8470, L8480, L8485

    stump sock L8470-L8485

Sodium

    chloride injection J2912

    ferric gluconate complex in sucrose J2916

    hyaluronate J7315, J7317

    phosphate P32 . . . . A9563

    succinate J1720

Solution,

    calibrator A4256

    dialysate A4700, A4705, A4760

    Elliott's b J9175

    enteral formulae B4149-B4156

    irrigation A4323

    parenteral nutrition B4164-B5200

Somatrem J2940

Somatropin J2941

Sorbent cartridge, ESRD E1636

Specialty absorptive dressing A6251-A6256

Spectinomycin HCL J3320

Speech assessment V5362-V5364

Speech generating device E2500-E2599

Spinal orthosis,

    anterior-posterior L0320, L0330, L0530

    anterior-posterior-lateral L0520, L0550-L0565

    anterior-posterior-lateral-rotary L0340-L0440

    cervical L0100-L0200

    cervical-thoracic-lumbar-sacral (CTLSO) L0700, L0710

    DME K0112-K0116

    halo L0810-L0830

    lumbar flexion L0540

    lumbar-sacral (LSO) L0500-L0565

    multiple post collar L0180-L0200

    sacroiliac L0600-L0620

    scoliosis L1000-L1499

    torso supports L0900-L0960

Splint A4570, L3100, L4350-L4380
    ankle L4390-L4398
    dynamic . . E1800, E1805, E1810, E1815, E1825, E1830, E1840
    footdrop L4398
Spoke protectors, each K0065
Static progressive stretch
    . . . . E1801, E1806, E1811, E1816, E1818, E1821
Sterile cefuroxime sodium J0697
Sterile water A4216-A4217
Stimulators
    neuromuscular E0744, E0745
    osteogenesis, electrical E0747-E0749
    salivary reflex E0755
    ultrasound E0760
Stomach tube B4083
Streptokinase J2995
Streptomycin J3000
Streptozocin J9320
Strip, blood glucose test A4253, A4772
    urine reagent A4250
Strontium-89 chloride, supply of A9600
Stump sock L8470-L8485
Stylet A4212
Succinylcholine chloride J0330
Suction pump
    canister K0190-K0191
    gastric, home model E2000
    portable E0600
    respiratory, home model E0600
    tubing K0192
Sumatriptan succinate J3030
Supply/accessory/service A9900
Support
    arch L3040-L3090
    cervical L0100-L0200
    spinal L0900-L0960
    stockings L8100-L8239
    suspension sleeve, BK L5674, L5675
Surgery, oral D7000-D7999

Surgical
  boot L3208-L3211
  brush, dialysis A4910
  dressing A6196-A6406, Q0183-Q0185
  stocking A4490-A4510
  supplies. A4649
  tray A4550
Swabs, betadine or iodine A4247
Syringe A4213
  dialysis. A4655
  with needle A4206-A4209

T

Tables, bed. E0274, E0315
Tacrolimus, oral J7507
Tacrolimus, parenteral J7515
Tape A4454, A6265, K0265
Taxi, non-emergency transportation A0100
Technetium TC 99M
  Arcitumomab. A9549
  Bicisate. A9557
  Depreotide. A9536
  Disofenin A9510
  Exametazine. A9521
  Fanolesomab A9566
  Glucepatate A9550
  Labeled red blood cells A9560
  Macroaggregated albumin. A9540
  Mebrofenin A9537
  Mertiatide A9562
  Oxidronate. A9561
  Pentetate. A9539, A9567
  Pertechnetate A9512
  Pyrophosphate A9538
  Sestamibi A9500
  Succimer. A9551
  Sulfur colloid. A9541

TEEV J0900
Telehealth. Q3014
Telehealth transmission T1014
Temozolmide, oral. J8700
Temporomandibular joint D0320, D0321
Tenecteplase. J3100
Teniposide Q2017
TENS A4595, E0720-E0749
Tent, oxygen E0455
Terbutaline sulfate. J3105
Terbutaline sulfate, inhalation solution, concentrated J7680
Terbutaline sulfate, inhalation solution, unit dose. J7681
Teriparatide J3110
Terminal devices. L6700-L6895
Testosterone
    aqueous J3140
    cypionate and estradiol cypionate J1060
    enanthate J3120, J3130
    enanthate and estradiol valerate. J0900
    propionate J3150
    suspension J3140
Tetanus immune globulin, human. J1670
Tetracycline J0120
Thallous Chloride TL 201 . . . . A9505
Theophylline J2810
Therapeutic lightbox. A4634, E0203
Therapy
    activity Q0082
    occupational. H5300
    physical (evaluation/treatment). Q0086
Thermometer. A4931-A4932
Thermometer, dialysis. A4910
Thiamine HCL J3411
Thiethylperazine maleate J3280
Thiotepa J9340
Thoracic-hip-knee-ankle (THKAO). L1500-L1520
Thoracic-lumbar-sacral orthosis (TLSO)
    scoliosis. L1200-L1290
    spinal K0618-K0619, L0430-L0492

Thoracic orthosis L0210
Thymol turbidity, blood P2033
Thyrotropin Alfa J3240
Tinzarparin sodium J1655
Tip (cane, crutch, walker) replacement A4637
Tire, wheelchair E0996, E0999, E1000
Tirofiban J3246
Tissue-based surgical dressings Q0183-Q0185
Tissue of human origin J7340, J7342, J7350
TLSO L0430-L0492, L1200-L1290
Tobramycin, inhalation solution, unit dose J7682
Tobramycin sulfate J3260
Toilet accessories E0167-E0179, E0243, E0244, E0625
Tolazoline HCL J2670
Toll, non-emergency transport A0170
Tomographic radiograph, dental D0322
Tool kit, dialysis A4910
Topical hyperbaric oxygen chamber A4575
Topotecan J9350
Torsemide J3265
Torso support L0900-L0960
Tourniquet, dialysis A4910
Tracheostoma heat moisture exchange system A7501-A7509
Tracheostomy
    care kit A4629
    filter A4481
    speaking valve L8501
    supplies A4623, A4629, A7523-A7524
    tube A7520-A7522
Tracheotomy mask or collar A7525-A7526
Traction device, ambulatory E0830
Traction equipment E0840-E0948
Transcutaneous electrical nerve stimulator (TENS) E0720-E0749
Transducer protector, dialysis E1575
Transfer board or device E0972
Transfer (shoe orthosis) L3600-L3640
Transfer system with seat E1035
Transparent film (for dressing) A6257-A6259

Transportation
    ambulance A0021-A0999, Q3019, Q3020
    corneal tissue V2785
    EKG (portable) R0076
    handicapped A0130
    non-emergency A0080-A0210, T2001-T2005
    service, including ambulance A0021-A0999, T2006
    taxi, non-emergency A0100
    toll, non-emergency A0170
    volunteer, non-emergency A0080, A0090
    x-ray (portable) R0070, R0075
Transtracheal oxygen catheter A7018
Trapeze bar E0910-E0912, E0940
Trapezium, prosthetic implant L8625
Tray
    insertion A4310-A4316
    irrigation A4320
    surgical (see also kits) A4550
    wheelchair E0950
Treprostinil J3285
Triamcinolone J3301-J3303
    acetonide J3301
    diacetate J3302
    hexacetonide J3303
    inhalation solution, concentrated J7683
    inhalation solution, unit dose J7684
Triflupromazine HCI J3400
Trifocal, glass or plastic V2300-V2399
Trigeminal division block anesthesia D9212
Trimethobenzamide HCL J3250
Trimetrexate glucuoronate J3305
Triptorelin pamoate J3315
Trismus appliance D5937
Truss L8300-L8330
Tube/Tubing
    anchoring device A5200
    blood A4750, A4755
    corrugated, for nebulizer K0175, K0176
    CPAP device K0187

Tube/Tubing—*continued*

    drainage extension. A4331

    gastrostomy. B4084, B4085, B4086

    irrigation. A4355

    larynectomy. A4622

    nasogastric B4081, B4082

    oxygen A4616

    serum clotting time. A4771

    stomach. B4083

    suction pump, each A7002

    tire. K0064, K0068, K0078, K0091, K0093, K0095, K0097

    tracheostomy A4622

    urinary drainage K0280

U

Ultrasonic nebulizer E0575

Ultrasonic nebulizer reservoir bottle. K0174

Ultrasound bladder capacity test G0050

Ultrasound bone mineral study. G0133

Ultraviolet cabinet E0690

Ultraviolet light therapy system. A4633, E0691-E0694

Unclassified drug J3490

Unipuncture control system, dialysis E1580

Upper extremity addition, locking elbow. L6693

Upper extremity fracture orthosis. L3980-L3999

Upper limb prosthesis L6000-L7499

Urea. J3350

Ureterostomy supplies. A4454-A4590

Urethral suppository, Alprostadil J0275

Urinal E0325, E0326

Urinary

    catheter. A4338-A4346, A4351-A4353, K0410, K0411

    collection and retention (supplies)

    . . . . A4310-A4359, K0407,K0408, K0410, K0411

    tract implant, collagen L8603

    tract implant, synthetic. L8606

Urine

    sensitivity study P7001

    tests A4250

Urofollitropin J3355

Urokinase J3364, J3365

U-V lens V2755

V

Vabra aspirator A4480

Vaccination, administration

    hepatitis B G0010

    influenza virus G0008

    pneumococcal G0009

Vancomycin HCL J3370

Vaporizer E0605

Vascular

    catheter (appliances and supplies) A4300-A4306

    graft material, synthetic L8670

Vasoxyl J3390

Venipuncture, routine specimen collection G0001

Venous pressure clamp, dialysis A4918

Ventilator

    battery A4611-A4613

    moisture exchanger, disposable A4483

    negative pressure E0460

    volume, stationary or portable E0450, E0461-E0464

Ventricular assist device Q0480-Q0505

Verteporfin J3396

Vest, safety, wheelchair E0980

Vinblastine sulfate J9360

Vincristine sulfate J9370-J9380

Vinorelbine tartrate J9390

Vision service V2020-V2799

Vitamin B-12 cyanocobalamin J3420

Vitamin K J3430

Voice amplifier L8510

Voice prosthesis L8511-L8514

Von Willebrand Factor Complex, human J7188
Voriconazole J3465

W

Waiver T2012-T2050
Walker E0130-E0149
    accessories A4636, A4637
    attachments. E0153-E0159
Walking splint. L4386
Water
    collection device (for nebulizer). K0177
    distilled (for nebulizer). A7018
    pressure pad/mattress. E0177, E0187, E0198
    purification system (ESRD). E1610, E1615
    softening system (ESRD) E1625
    sterile A4712, A4714, A4319
    tanks (dialysis). A4880
Wedges, shoe. L3340-L3420
Wet mount Q0111
Wheel attachment, rigid pickup walker. E0155
Wheelchair E0950-E1298, K0001-K0108
    accessories. E0192, E0950-E1030, E1065-E1069,
    . . . . E2211-E2226, E2300-E2399
    amputee. E1170-E1200
    back, fully reclining, manual E1226
    battery A4631
    component or accessory, not otherwise specified. K0108
    cushions. E2601-E2619
    motorized. E1210-E1213
    narrowing device. E0969
    power add-on E0983-E0984
    shock absorber E1015-E1018
    specially sized E1220, E1230
    stump support system K0551
    tire E0996, E0999, E1000
    transfer board or device E0705
    tray K0107

Wheelchair—*continued*

   van, non-emergency. A0130

   youth E1091

WHFO with inflatable air chamber L3807

WHO, wrist extension. L3914

Whirlpool equipment. E1300-E1310

Wig. A9282

Wipes A4245, A4247

Wound cleanser. A6260

Wound cover

   alginate dressing A6196-A6198

   collagen dressing. A6020-A6024

   foam dressing. A6209-A6214

   hydrocolloid dressing. A6234-A6239

   hydrogel dressing A6242-A6247

   non-contact wound warming cover, and accessory. E0231, E0232

   specialty absorptive dressing A6251-A6256

Wound filler

   alginate dressing. A6199

   collagen based A6010

   foam dressing. A6215

   hydrocolloid dressing A6240, A6241

   hydrogel dressing A6248

   not elsewhere classified. A6261, A6262

Wound pouch A6154

Wrist

   disarticulation prosthesis. L6050, L6055

   hand/finger orthosis (WHFO). E1805, E1825, L3800-L3954

XYZ

Xenon Xe 133, ... Q3004

Xylocaine HCL, ... J2000

X-ray equipment, portable, ... Q0092, R0070, R0075

Zidovudine, ... J3485

Ziprasidone mesylate, ... J3486

Zoledronic acid, ... J3487